Nursing and Society

Nursing and Society

Editors

Elena Fernández-Martínez
Lisa Alves Gomes
Cristina Liébana-Presa

MDPI • Basel • Beijing • Wuhan • Barcelona • Belgrade • Manchester • Tokyo • Cluj • Tianjin

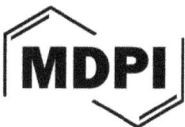

MDPI

Editors

Elena Fernández-Martínez
Nursing and Physiotherapy
Universidad de León
León
Spain

Lisa Alves Gomes
Nursing
University of Minho
Braga
Portugal

Cristina Liébana-Presa
Nursing and Physiotherapy.
Campus de Ponferrada
Universidad de Leon
Ponferrada (Leon)
Spain

Editorial Office
MDPI
St. Alban-Anlage 66
4052 Basel, Switzerland

This is a reprint of articles from the Special Issue published online in the open access journal *International Journal of Environmental Research and Public Health* (ISSN 1660-4601) (available at: www.mdpi.com/journal/ijerph/special_issues/nursing_society).

For citation purposes, cite each article independently as indicated on the article page online and as indicated below:

LastName, A.A.; LastName, B.B.; LastName, C.C. Article Title. *Journal Name* **Year**, *Volume Number*, Page Range.

ISBN 978-3-0365-1724-7 (Hbk)
ISBN 978-3-0365-1723-0 (PDF)

Contents

About the Editors

Elena Fernández-Martínez

Elena Fernandez-Martínez has a university degree in Nursing from the Universidad de León (Spain), a Bachelor of Psychology from the Universidad Nacional de Educacion a Distancia (UNED-Spain) and a PhD from the Universidad de León. Associate Professor of the Department of Nursing and Physiotherapy of the Universidad de León (Spain).

Lisa Alves Gomes

Lisa Alves Gomes born in Boston Massachusetts, has a Nursing degree, a Master degree in Educational Sciences, a Specialist Degree in Nursing Rehabilitation and a PhD in Nursing Sciences from the Catholic University of Portugal, Institute of Health Sciences Porto. Researcher at Health Sciences Research Unit: Nursing (UICISA: E) of the Nursing School of Coimbra. Adjunct Professor at the Nursing School, University of Minho Braga, Portugal.

Cristina Liébana-Presa

Cristina Liébana-Presa has a university degree in Nursing from the Universidad de León (Spain), a Bachelor of Social and Cultural Anthropology from the Universidad Nacional de Educacion a Distancia (UNED-Spain) and a PhD from the Universidad de Córdoba. Associate Professor of the Department of Nursing and Physiotherapy of the Universidad de León (Spain).

Preface to "Nursing and Society"

Papers in this book from the Special Issue of the International Journal of Environmental Research and Public Health will explore the contribution of nurses to society. The year 2020 is considered by the World Health Organization as the International Year of the Nurse and Midwife. This book serves as an incentive to support the visibility of the contribution of nurses to society, emphasizing the crucial role of nurses in achieving greater attention to community health and the social and environmental determinants that intervene in the health of the population. Nurses are the heart of health teams. They play an essential role in developing new community care models, health promotion, disease prevention, and treatment.

Elena Fernández-Martínez, Lisa Alves Gomes, Cristina Liébana-Presa
Editors

International Journal of
Environmental Research and Public Health

MDPI

Article

Heart Disease, Now What? Improving Quality of Life through Education

Lisa Gomes [1], Cristina Liébana-Presa [2,*], Beatriz Araújo [3], Fátima Marques [4] and Elena Fernández-Martínez [5]

1   Nursing School, Minho University, 4710-057 Braga, Portugal; lgomes@ese.uminho.pt
2   SALBIS Research Group, Faculty of Health Sciences, Campus of Ponferrada, Universidad de León, 24401 Ponferrada, Spain
3   Institute of Health Sciences, Universidade Católica Portuguesa, 4169-005 Porto, Portugal; baraujo@porto.ucp.pt
4   Intensive Care Coronary Unit, Centro Hospitalar De Trás-Os-Montes E Alto Douro, E.P.E., 5000-508 Vila Real, Portugal; fatimaecmarques@sapo.pt
5   SALBIS Research Group, Faculty of Health Sciences, Universidad de León, 24071 León, Spain; elena.fernandez@unileon.es
*   Correspondence: cliep@unileon.es

Citation: Gomes, L.; Liébana-Presa, C.; Araújo, B.; Marques, F.; Fernández-Martínez, E. Heart Disease, Now What? Improving Quality of Life through Education. *Int. J. Environ. Res. Public Health* 2021, 18, 3077. https://doi.org/10.3390/ijerph18063077

Academic Editor: Paul B. Tchounwou

Received: 5 February 2021
Accepted: 15 March 2021
Published: 17 March 2021

Abstract: Introduction: The management of chronic illness assumes a level of demand for permanent care and reaches a priority dimension in the health context. Given the importance of nursing care to post-acute coronary syndrome patients, the objective of this study is to evaluate the impact of an educational intervention program on quality of life in patients after acute coronary syndrome. Method: Quasi-experimental study with two groups: an experimental group exposed to the educational intervention program and the control group without exposure to the educational intervention program. Results: The results showed statistically significant differences between both groups ($p < 0.001$). Although only valid for the specific group of subjects studied, the educational intervention program enabled significant gains in quality of life. Conclusions: According to the findings of the study, a systematized and structured educational program, integrated into the care organization and based on transition processes, is effective in developing self-care skills and improves the quality of life in patients after acute coronary syndrome.

Keywords: coronary disease; cardiac rehabilitation; health education; quality of life; self-care

1. Introduction

Cardiovascular diseases (CVD) are the main cause of death [1,2] decade after decade and self-care is not at the top of the pyramid of best practices for chronic disease management.

Changes in the population's health/disease patterns pressure worldwide health care systems' sustainability. These changes include an aging population, an increasing number of individuals with CVD risk factors, and the prevalence of multimorbidity [3]. The burden of heart disease in Europe indicates that we are presently far from achieving the expected success [4]. Health care systems believe that people who seek and need health care will obey the recommendations proposed by professionals.

Patients with heart disease have needs in various dimensions of their lives that require continuous health care, which the current systems have difficulties in satisfying. In the health–disease transition, rehabilitation depends largely on health literacy, adherence to rehabilitation programs, and the patient's active participation in the management of their therapeutic regime [5]. Skills and ability development, behavior, and lifestyle changing is a challenge given the complex treatment regimes.

In the specific case of acute coronary syndrome (ACS), disease control requires a rigorous and long-lasting therapeutic plan. There is a need for patient and family involvement and compliance with the set of proposed recommendations [6]. Non-compliance with therapeutic adherence reaches such proportions that it can be considered a new cardiovascular risk factor [7].

Therefore, it is essential to develop strategies that promote greater adherence to the prescribed treatment. These educational programs can represent an important strategy in the fight against heart disease because they enable the development of self-care skills necessary for patients to reach their potential and quality of life (QoL) [8].

However, cardiac patients have difficulties in identifying and managing signs and symptoms related to heart disease, in adhering to therapy, in performing daily life activities, and even in interpersonal management [9]. For these reasons, self-care education is fundamental because it is about influencing behavior change by increasing knowledge, changing attitudes, and developing skills. Education goals include cardiac patients' participation in decision making for lifelong continuing care, awareness-raising, and functional performance [10].

The educational process is gradual, systematized, and personalized. In clinical practice, nurses find it difficult to implement these educational programs due to the high cost of hospitalizations and scientific advances in treatment that have shortened the length of hospital stays for patients with heart disease. This implies that in the rehabilitation plan the educational process begins on the first day of hospitalization [11].

Cardiac rehabilitation programs (CRP) have a strong educational component. Recognized in recent decades as an intervention with a cost-effective impact, CRP assume an integral part of the multidimensional treatment. They improve prognosis, reduce the number of readmissions and health expenses, as well as increase QoL [12]. However, in Portugal, as in other countries, the rate of admission to cardiac rehabilitation programs is very low [13]. The uncertainty about what will happen after discharge and how the patient can adapt to their new health condition justifies a care practice that facilitates the process of making informed decisions. Given that not everyone has access to CRP, the need for implementing educational interventions during hospitalization becomes even more important to improve patient outcomes.

Aware of the importance of nursing care for the post-ACS patient, the objective of this research is to design, implement, and evaluate the impact of an educational intervention program during the hospitalization period on the development of self-care skills and QoL. This article also adds data to the study previously published by Gomes and Reis (2019), and contributes to a better understanding of the importance of nurse-led educational intervention [14].

2. Materials and Methods

2.1. Study Design and Setting and Procedure

The authors conducted quasi-experimental research, with the establishment of two groups—an experimental group, and a control group. The control group received standardized nursing care, and the experimental group, in addition to the standardized nursing care, had access to the educational intervention program. The 67 participants were adult/elderly patients diagnosed with ACS, hospitalized at an intensive care coronary unit (ICCU) in the northern region of Portugal, who spoke and understood Portuguese, had preserved cognitive and verbal ability, and agreed to participate in the study [14].

However, we encountered the impossibility of randomizing the groups due to the organization of the ICCU and the cardiology unit. If randomization were the choice, the participants of the control group would attend the educational intervention program since the ICCU is an open space and the cardiology unit does not have single rooms. To solve this problem, we opted for the consecutive series method, which consisted of testing the educational intervention in a non-parallel way [15]. Throughout 2016, during two-week periods, patients were included in the intervention group and, the following week new patients were included in the control group and so on, until reaching the required number of participants for our study. Despite the non-randomization, this method allows the same probability of the patient being included in one of the groups [16]. Table 1 shows the distribution of the groups by weeks/months.

Table 1. Distribution of participants by the experimental and control groups.

Week	March	April	May	June	July
1st Week	Experimental	Control	Experimental	Control	Experimental
2nd Week	Experimental	Control	Experimental	Control	Experimental
3rd Week	Control	Experimental	Control	Experimental	Control
4th Week	Control	Experimental	Control	Experimental	Control

Each phase of the program has specific objectives, as well as different strategies for action. Table 2 summarizes these phases. The four sessions provided moments for intrinsic motivation, learning, and reflection. Nurse–patient interviews conducted during hospitalization and one month after discharge was the strategy adopted for data collection. Due to the geographical dispersion of the hospital's affluence area, authors opted to contact patients by telephone.

Table 2. Sessions developed during the educational intervention program for patients with acute coronary syndrome.

Sessions	Education Strategies	Objective
1st session (1st day of hospitalization)	Video/nurse and patient session	Develop patient's awareness of their chronic disease Describe heart function and disease
2nd session	Group session	Improve adherence to treatment
3rd session (Hospital discharge day)	Patient and family session	Signs and symptoms management Medication management Promote lifestyle changes
4th session (1 month after hospital discharge)	Telephone follow-up	Develop healthy eating habits Practice physical activity and exercise Express and understand psychological aspects

The ethics committee and administration council of the institution and the medical director of the ICCU approved the study protocol. This study did not entail any cost to the participant or institution. It did not involve therapeutic actions; invasive, radiological procedures; or the collection of biological products. Each patient filled out a declaration of informed consent.

2.2. Educational Intervention Program

To obtain significant learning for the development of self-care skills, the program had a structured and systematic approach with four sessions [14,17] and involved three educational areas. At the end of the sessions, the patient should be able to: (i) know the risks of heart disease (cognitive area); (ii) know how to control the signs and symptoms of heart disease and know how to perform their most instrumental self-care (psychomotor area); (iii) understand that changing their behaviors increases their QoL (affective area). Figure 1 illustrates the educational intervention program framework and the outcome indicators.

Given that hospitalization is increasingly shorter and that there is a need to repeat information for processing, the authors used the theoretical model of social learning of Bandura [18]. Based on the statement of Bandura's theory of self-efficacy, that expectations of self-efficacy are dependent on contexts and situations of achievement, patients are encouraged to imagine success, anticipate potential outcomes, and so respond confidently with more adaptive strategies to overcome barriers. The patients need to trust their abilities to achieve the proposed goals. The more confident and motivated the patient, the greater the success and opportunity to enhance a new health behavior.

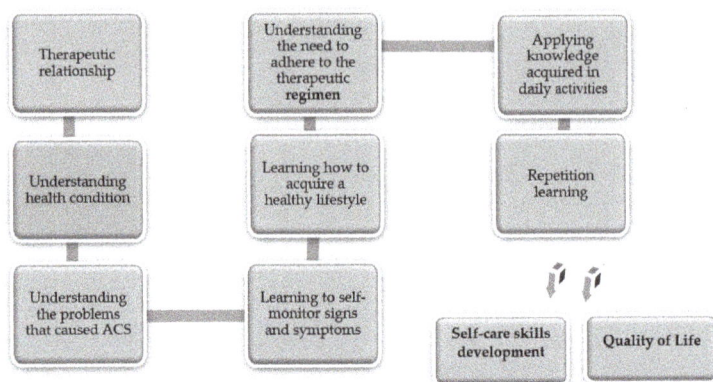

Figure 1. Educational intervention program framework and outcome indicators.

The educational intervention program had the following pedagogical strategies: (i) interviews with the nurse rehabilitation specialist; (ii) an educational video; (iii) checklist/pamphlet; (iv) telephone follow-up interview. The first session began in the ICCU, 12 to 24 h after hospitalization and depending on the hemodynamic stability of the patient. The nurse rehabilitation specialist conducted an interview with didactic resources; the authors opted for the visualization of a video with the following themes and contents:

- How does the heart function?
- What is coronary heart disease?
- Diagnosis of coronary disease;
- Therapeutic management;
- Modifiable risk factors;
- Healthy lifestyle.

The second session was a group session and held the following day, aimed at identifying the patient's knowledge regarding the contents exposed in the video, and clarifying doubts and misassumptions. The authors used this strategy since the patients' beliefs about the disease and the personal experience also result from the social experience. Loring and Holman explain that social persuasion can improve the perception of self-efficacy [19]. During the third session held on the day of hospital discharge, the nurse used a checklist with the contents of the video. The checklist had the following purpose: (i) organize and systematize the information so that the nurse can identify difficulties, and (ii) serve as a leaflet for patient guidance. The fourth and last session occurred one month after discharge, with the aim of monitoring the patient and reinforcing information.

2.3. Instruments Used to Collect Data

For data collection, authors used a sociodemographic and clinical context questionnaire, the therapeutic self-care scale and the MacNew heart disease health-related QoL questionnaire.

Doran et al. [20] developed the therapeutic self-care scale (TSCS) with the objective of assessing the capacity for self-care in acute care contexts. This scale assesses the person's ability to perform four categories of self-care activities: taking medication as prescribed by the doctor; identifying and managing symptoms; performing activities of daily living; and managing changes in health status. The maximum score is 60 points and corresponds to a high level of performance in therapeutic self-care. The original version of the instrument by Doran et al. was translated, validated, and adapted for the Portuguese population by Cardoso, Queirós, Fontes Ribeiro, and Amaral [21].

The MacNew heart disease questionnaire is a self-administered modification of the original quality of life after myocardial infarction (QLMI) instrument [22]. It assesses the feelings of patients who have suffered an acute myocardial infarction and are attending a CRP. Höfer et al. [23] states that the MacNew QLMI scale is a specific QoL assessment instrument, but it is used also in other cardiac pathologies, such as angina. To calculate the scores of the questionnaires, the authors used the average of all items and for the total QoL. For presentation and interpretation of results, the variable QoL has the following intervals: 1 to 3, 3 to 5, and 5 to 7. Patients with averages in the range 1 to 3 have worse QoL, patients with averages between 3 and 5 are considered to have moderate QoL, and high QoL is assumed for patients with an average between 5 and 7 points. Leal et al. [24] validated the MacNew QoL version for the Portuguese population.

2.4. Data Analysis

For data treatment, the authors used descriptive and inferential statistical techniques and used the Statistical Package for Social Science (SPSS) software, version 23 for statistical analysis. The statistical techniques applied were frequency (absolute and relative), measures of central tendency (arithmetic mean and median), measures of dispersion or variability (minimum value, maximum value, and standard deviation), and tests (Chi-square test, Fisher's exact test, Mann–Whitney U test, Wilcoxon test, Spearman's correlation coefficient significance test, and the Shapiro–Wilk test as a normality test). For all tests, the value of 0.05 was set as the limit of significance, that is, the null hypothesis was rejected when the probability of type I error (probability of rejection of the null hypothesis when it was true) was lower than the set value, when $p < 0.05$, that is, $p < 5\%$.

3. Results

The results obtained for sociodemographic characteristics are set out in Table 3. In both groups, the majority of the patients were male, with the percentages being 90.6% in the experimental group and 71.4% in the control group. The ages of the patients in the experimental group extended between 40 and 80 years, with an average age of 57.72 ± 10.55 years. In this group, 28.1% of patients were under 50 years old; the same percentage was between 50 and 60 years old and between 60 and 70 years old. Half of the patients are older than 56.50 years old and the frequency distribution departed significantly from the characteristics of a normal or Gaussian curve ($p = 0.022$). We found that most patients of both groups reported being married or cohabiting, with percentages of 81.3% and 60.0%, respectively, in the experimental group and in the control group. In the experimental group, 43.8% of the patients had primary-level education, and in the control group, this percentage was even higher at 74.3%. No participant was illiterate.

Table 3. Sociodemographic characteristics.

Variables		Experimental n = 32 (100%)		Control n = 35 (100%)		p Value
				Group		
Sex	Female	3 (9.4%)		10 (28.6%)		0.047
	Male	29 (90.6%)		25 (71.4%)		
Marital Status	Married/Cohabiting	26 (81.3%)		21 (60%)		0.036
Education Level	Primary (elementary) school	14 (43.8%)		26 (74.3%)		0.102
		M ± SD	Min–Max	M ± SD	Min–Max	0.015
Age		57.72 ± 10.55	40–80	65.09 ± 11.05	45–89	

Note: M; Mean. SD; Standard Deviation. Min–Max; Minimum–Maximum.

The results illustrated in Table 4 allow us to know the clinical characteristics of the patients. The authors found that most elements of both groups had acute myocardial infarction diagnosis, with the percentages being 90.6% and 88.6%, respectively in the experimental and control group. This was followed by unstable angina (9.4% and 11.4%). The Chi-square test revealed that the observed difference is not statistically significant ($p = 0.784$). As for risk factors, it appears that in both groups, dyslipidemia predominates,

5

with percentages of 78.1% and 71.4%, followed by arterial hypertension, with percentages of 53.1% and 54.3%, followed by smoking—37.5% and 34.3%, and diabetes mellitus—34.4% and 31.4%, respectively. It appears that the most common risk factors are present in both groups. The Chi-square test revealed that the differences observed between the two groups are not statistically significant ($p = 0.999$). Regarding the weight status, 37.5% of the patients in the experimental group were revealed to be in the pre-obesity situation, followed by 34.4% classified as Stage I obese. In the control group, 45.7% of the patients are pre-obese and 22.9% classified as Stage I obese. Through the application of the Mann–Whitney U test, to compare the body mass index, authors found that the differences observed between the two groups were not statistically significant ($p = 0.292$). Above-normal weight predominates in both groups.

Table 4. Clinical characteristics of the groups.

Variable		Experimental n = 32 (100%)	Control n = 35 (100%)	*p* Value
		Group		
Medical diagnostic	Acute myocardial infarction	29 (90.6%)	31 (88.6%)	0.784
	Unstable chest angina	3 (9.4%)	4 (11.4%)	
Risk factors	Dyslipidemia	25 (78.1%)	25 (71.4%)	0.999
	Arterial hypertension	17 (53.1%)	19 (54.3%)	
	Smoking	12 (37.5%)	12 (34.3%)	
	Diabetes mellitus	11 (34.4%)	11 (31.4%)	
Weight status	Pre-obesity	12 (37.5%)	16 (45.7%)	0.292
	Stage I obesity	11 (34.4%)	8 (22.9%)	

The results also suggest improvements in the development of self-care skills and QoL in patients undergoing an educational intervention. Applying the Wilcoxon test to compare the two groups between each evaluation moment, the authors verified the existence of statistically significant differences in both cases ($p < 0.001$). The comparison of the mean and median values suggests that, between the first and in the second evaluation, the elements of the experimental group tended to improve their therapeutic self-care, while in the elements of the control group the trend was the opposite, that is, there was a deterioration in therapeutic self-care (Table 5). Authors also observed that all patients of the experimental group obtained results equal to 60 points (maximum value of the therapeutic self-care assessment scale). Consequently, the average value was 60.00 ± 0.00 points, the median had the same value, and the frequency distribution cannot be considered normal ($p = 0.000$). In the control group, the results ranged between 21 and 58 points, with an average value of 38.77 ± 7.74 points. It appears that half of the patients in this group had values equal to or greater than 39 points and the frequency distribution reveals characteristics similar to that of a normal distribution ($p = 0.883$). The application of the Mann–Whitney U test revealed the existence of significant differences between the two groups ($p < 0.001$) and a comparison of the values of the measures of central tendency reveals that the participants in the experimental group indicated better therapeutic self-care than those in the control group.

Table 5. Pre-intervention and post-intervention therapeutic self-care assessment scale results.

Questionnaire		**Pre-Intervention Group**			**Post-Intervention Group**		
		Experimental n = 32 (100%)	Control n = 35 (100%)	*p*-Value	Experimental n = 32 (100%)	Control n = 35 (100%)	*p*-Value
Therapeutic self-care	M ± SD	58.31 ± 1.20	43.54 ± 6.57	<0.001	60 ± 0.00	38.77 ± 7.74	<0.001
	Me	58	43		60	39	
	Min–Max	54–60	31–60		60–60	21–58	
	p-value *	<0.001	0.299		0.00	0.883	

Note: M; Mean. SD; Standard Deviation. Me; Median; Min–Max; Minimum-Maximum. * *p*-values for normal distribution.

The results illustrated in Table 6 regarding the MacNew questionnaire for the patients in the experimental group showed minimum values and maximum values between 3.22 and 6.26 points, with an average value of 4.74 ± 0.65 points. This means that patients on average perceived their QoL positively. Half of the elements in this group showed results equal to or greater than 4.76 points, and the frequency distribution departed significantly from the characteristics of a normal distribution (p = 0.114). In the control group, we observed results between 1.74 and 4.96 points. The average value was 3.78 ± 0.66 points, with a median of 3.74 points. The frequency distribution can be considered normal (p = 0.249).

Table 6. Quality of life assessment scale results.

Questionnaire QoL		Group		
		Experimental n = 32 (100%)	Control n = 35 (100%)	p-Value
Quality of life—global	M ± SD	4.74 ± 0.65	3.78 ± 0.66	<0.001
	Me	4.76	3.74	
	Min–Max	3.22–6.26	1.74–4.96	
	p-value *	0.114	0.249	
Quality of life—physical	M ± SD	4.34 ± 0.63	3.43 ± 0.59	<0.001
	Me	4.40	3.40	
	Min–Max	3.20–5.60	2.40–5.00	
	p-value *	0.375	0.182	
Quality of life—emotional	M ± SD	4.80 ± 0.77	3.84 ± 0.74	<0.001
	Me	4.93	3.93	
	Min–Max	3.21–6.57	1.43–5.00	
	p-value *	0.687	0.029	
Quality of life—social	M ± SD	5.29 ± 0.79	4.17 ± 0.91	<0.001
	Me	5.33	4.17	
	Min–Max	3.00–6.67	1.83–6.17	
	p-value *	0.042	0.543	

Note: M; Mean. SD; Standard Deviation. Me; Median; Min–Max; Minimum-Maximum. * p-values for normal distribution.

For the physical dimension of QoL, the authors observed, in the experimental group, results that ranged between 3.20 and 5.60 points, with an average value of 4.34 ± 0.63 points. Half of the respondents in this group had values equal to or greater than 4.40 points, and the frequency distribution can be considered normal (p = 0.375). In the control group, the authors observed values between 2.40 and 5.00 points, with an average of 3.43 ± 0.59 points. Half of the elements in this group obtained results above 3.40 points, which shows that the perception of the QoL is close to the value of 3.50 points that represents the average value of the scale. The values are lower than those of the experimental group. The frequency distribution departed significantly from a normal distribution (p = 0.182).

In the emotional dimension for the experimental group, values between 3.21 and 6.57 points were observed, with a mean value of 4.80 ± 0.77 points and a median of 4.93 points. The frequency distribution showed characteristics close to a normal curve (p = 0.687). In the control group, the observed values were between 1.43 and 5.00 points, with an average of 3.84 ± 0.74 points. Half of the individuals that constituted this group obtained results above 3.93 points and the frequency distribution departed significantly from the characteristics of a normal curve (p = 0.029).

In the social-life dimension, the authors found in the experimental group values between 3.00 and 6.67 points, with the mean value being 5.29 ± 0.79 points. Half of the elements in this group showed results greater than 5.33 points. The frequency distribution cannot be considered normal (p = 0.042). For the control group, authors found values between 1.83 and 6.17 points, with an average of 4.17 ± 0.91 points. Half of the sample elements showed values equal to or greater than 4.17 points. The frequency distribution shows characteristics close to a normal curve (p = 0.543).

Applying the Mann–Whitney U test, the authors can conclude that between both groups there is a statistically significant difference ($p < 0.001$) in global, physical, emotional, and social QoL. The comparison of the values of the measures of central tendency reveals that the elements of the experimental group showed significantly better QoL than those of the control group.

4. Discussion

As for the sociodemographic characterization, the authors found that in both groups, the patients are mostly male, with low literacy. The average age of the participants in the experimental group is 57.72, while the average age of the patients in the control group is 65.09. These results reflect the profile of coronary patients in the Portuguese population, according to governmental reports [25], in which the prevalence of coronary disease is higher in males, with low literacy and incidence between 50 and 70 years old. Regarding the level of education, the findings of this study revealed that for individuals with a low level of education, risk factors were more prevalent. These results were consistent with the findings of the study conducted by Marques da Silva et al. (2019). They studied the prevalence of cardiovascular risk factors and other comorbidities in patients with hypertension in Portuguese primary health care populations. However, despite the higher prevalence of individuals with low levels of education, it is worth highlighting the trend of a gradual increase in risk factors among individuals with higher education levels [26,27].

There was also a higher prevalence in both groups of married/cohabiting patients. In the Okwose et al. [28] study, patients reported that family members are a strong motivating factor. Having a partner or relative to support them and participate in new activity routines is important. Family can promote patients' emotional support and enable therapeutic regimen adherence.

Data suggests that the educational program promotes improvements in the cardiac patient's self-care skills and in global, physical, emotional, and social QoL. The program made patients more proactive in decision-making and assuming responsibilities for their health conditions. In the Riegel et al. [29] study, the behavior-change factors address habits, motivation, decision-making, and the challenges of persistence. However, it is important to consider that illness-related factors address specific issues that make self-care exceedingly difficult—multimorbidity, symptoms, and stressful life events.

The results of the Goodman, et al. [30] study carried out in patients with decompensated heart failure (HF), suggest that low scores in self-care skills can be related to difficulties in decision-making and lack of motivation, and not so much to learning difficulties. Therefore, in the Rice et al. [31] study, results suggest that nurse-led patient education for adults with HF improves QoL and reduces hospital admissions and readmissions—a major cause of health-care costs [32]. However, for this study the authors did not consider readmissions as an outcome. The randomized controlled trial study conducted in Iran with 60 patients that had HF also concluded that a self-management education program is an appropriate strategy for improving QoL in patients with HF [33].

Educational programs implemented during hospitalization aim to enable patients to deal more effectively with the chronic disease after hospital discharge. Improving patient's health outcomes by increasing knowledge and behaviors related to the cause of the disease, treatment, and coping strategies can prevent complications and better QoL [34]. In our opinion, this educational program can be adapted and implemented among other chronic disease patients, since teaching skills can be generalized.

The results indicate that behavioral changes and self-care skills depend on educational programs for patients to learn and practice. The educational sessions are not just for transmitting information but also should involve moments of elucidation, reflection, and discussion accompanied by didactic material such as pamphlets and audiovisual media for better understanding. For practice implications, Rice et al. [31] considered diverse pedagogical methods, such as nurse-led education strategies.

The study design should be considered as a limitation; it would have been interesting to compare two intervention groups with each other. Furthermore, it would be desirable to carry out longitudinal studies to confirm the differences between the groups in the long term after the intervention.

5. Conclusions

This study revealed a positive relationship between the development of self-care skills and the QoL of the post-ACS patient. However, the period of one month between the two assessment moments (hospitalization and one month after discharge) may not have been enough to observe permanent changes in self-care skills and QoL. In future studies, it will be necessary to evaluate the effectiveness of the educational intervention program in a longer follow-up period.

Knowledge alone does not influence self-care behaviors. It is a complex decision-making process. The patient uses values and experiences in decision-making and these experiences emerge from situational awareness, their perceptions, and the meanings given to the cardiac event. Each option and response create a set of standards.

In making complex decisions, the nurse supports and helps the post-ACS patient to recognize decision-making situations and provide strategies to facilitate effective responses.

The nurse's educational intention alone is not enough. This intentionality involves implementing educational interventions guidelines, so that patients and families are informed (knowledge development), trained (skills development), and involved in their health care. Nurses being patients' partners in decision-making can indicate the path towards adaptation, autonomy, and QoL, because these decisions will be compatible with personal life goals.

Author Contributions: Conceptualization, L.G. and B.A.; methodology, L.G., B.A., and F.M.; software, L.G., E.F.-M., and C.L.-P.; validation, L.G., E.F.-M., and C.L.-P.; formal analysis, L.G., E.F.-M., C.L.-P., and B.A.; investigation, L.G., B.A., and F.M.; resources, L.G. and F.M.; data curation, L.G., E.F.-M., C.L.-P.; writing—original draft preparation, L.G.; writing—review and editing, L.G., E.F.-M., and C.L.-P.; visualization, L.G., E.F.-M., C.L.-P., B.A., and F.M. supervision, L.G., E.F.-M., C.L.-P., B.A., and F.M.; project administration, L.G., E.F.-M., C.L.-P., B.A., and F.M. All authors have read and agreed to the published version of the manuscript.

Funding: This research received no external funding.

Institutional Review Board Statement: The study was conducted according to the guidelines of the Declaration of Helsinki, and approved by the Ethics Committee of Centro Hospitalar de Trás-os-Montes e Alto Douro, E.P.E, date of approval 27 April 2016.

Informed Consent Statement: Informed consent was obtained from all subjects involved in the study.

Conflicts of Interest: The authors declare no conflict of interest.

References

1. Benjamin, E.J.; Blaha, M.J.; Chiuve, S.E.; Cushman, M.; Das, S.R.; de Ferranti, S.D.; Floyd, J.; Fornage, M.; Gillespie, C.; Isasi, C.R.; et al. Heart disease and stroke statistics—2017 update a report from the American heart association. *Circulation* **2017**, *135*, e146–e603. [CrossRef]
2. Townsend, N.; Wilson, L.; Bhatnagar, P.; Wickramasinghe, K.; Rayner, M.; Nichols, M. Cardiovascular disease in Europe: Epidemiological update 2016. *Eur. Heart J.* **2016**, *37*, 3232–3245. [CrossRef]
3. de Almeida Simões, J.; Augusto, G.F.; Fronteira, I.; Hernández-Quevedo, C. Portugal. *Health Syst. Transit.* **2017**, *19*, 1–184.
4. Wilkins, E.; Wilson, L.; Wickramasinghe, K.; Bhatnagar, P. European Cardiovascular Disease Statistics 2017. Available online: www.ehnheart.org (accessed on 3 February 2021).
5. Oscalices, M.I.L.; Okuno, M.F.P.; Lopes, M.C.B.T.; Batista, R.E.A.; Campanharo, C.R.V. Health literacy and adherence to treatment of patients with heart failure. *Rev. Esc. Enferm. USP* **2019**, *53*, e03447. [CrossRef] [PubMed]
6. WHO. *Hearts Technical Package for Cardiovascular Disease Management in Primary Health Care: Risk Based CVD Management*; World Health Organization: Geneva, Switzerland, 2020.
7. Gale, C. Acute coronary syndrome in adults: Scope of the problem in the UK. *Br. J. Cardiol.* **2017**, *24*, 3–9. [CrossRef]

8. Ruppar, T.M.; Cooper, P.S.; Johnson, E.D.; Riegel, B. Self-care interventions for adults with heart failure: A systematic review and meta-analysis protocol. *J. Adv. Nurs.* **2018**, *75*, 676–682. [CrossRef] [PubMed]
9. Grant, J.; Graven, L.; Fuller, K. Problems experienced in the first month after discharge from a heart failure-related hospitalization. *J. Patient Cent. Res. Rev.* **2018**, *5*, 140–148. [CrossRef] [PubMed]
10. Loghmani, L.; Monfared, M.B. The effect of self-care education on knowledge and function of patients with heart failure hospitalized in Kerman city hospitals in (2017). *Electron. J. Gen. Med.* **2018**, *15*, 47. [CrossRef]
11. Jung, H.G.; Yang, Y.K. Factors influencing health behavior practice in patients with coronary artery diseases. *Health Qual. Life Outcomes* **2021**, *19*, 1–9. [CrossRef]
12. Piepoli, M.F.; Hoes, A.W.; Agewall, S.; Albus, C.; Brotons, C.; Catapano, A.L.; Cooney, M.T.; Corra, U.; Cosyns, B.; Deaton, C.; et al. 2016 European Guidelines on cardiovascular disease prevention in clinical practice. *Eur. Heart J.* **2016**, *37*, 2315–2381. [CrossRef]
13. Abreu, A.; Mendes, M.; Dores, H.; Silveira, C.; Fontes, P.; Teixeira, M.; Clara, H.S.; Morais, J. Mandatory criteria for cardiac rehabilitation programs: 2018 guidelines from the Portuguese Society of Cardiology. *Rev. Port. Cardiol.* **2018**, *37*, 363–373. [CrossRef] [PubMed]
14. Gomes, L.; Reis, G. Effectiveness of an Educational Program to Enhance Self-care Skills After Acute Coronary Syndrome: A Quasi-Experimental Study. In *Communications in Computer and Information Science*; Springer: Berlin/Heidelberg, Germany, 2019; Volume 1016, pp. 269–279.
15. Gray, J.; Grove, S.K.; Sutherland, S. *Burns and Grove's the Practice of Nursing Research: Appraisal, Synthesis, and Generation of Evidence*; Elsevier: St. Louis, MS, USA, 2017.
16. Hulley, S.B.; Cummings, S.R.; Browner, W.S.; Grady, D.G.; Newman, T.B. *Designing Clinical Research*, 4th ed.; Lip-Pincott Williams and Wilkins: Philadelphia, PA, USA, 2013.
17. Riegel, B.; Dickson, V.V.; Faulkner, K.M. The Situation-Specific Theory of Heart Failure Self-Care. *J. Cardiovasc. Nurs.* **2016**, *31*, 226–235. [CrossRef] [PubMed]
18. Bandura, A. The Explanatory and Predictive Scope of Self-Efficacy Theory. *J. Soc. Clin. Psychol.* **1986**, *4*, 359–373. [CrossRef]
19. Holman, H.; Lorig, K. Patient Self-Management: A Key to Effectiveness and Efficiency in Care of Chronic Disease. *Public Health Rep.* **2004**, *119*, 239–243. [CrossRef]
20. Doran, D.; Harrison, M.B.; Laschinger, H.; Hirdes, J.; Rukholm, E.; Sidani, S.; Hall, L.M.; Tourangeau, A.E.; Cranley, L. Relationship between nursing interventions and outcome achievement in acute care settings. *Res. Nurs. Health* **2006**, *29*, 61–70. [CrossRef] [PubMed]
21. Cardoso, A.F.; Queirós, P.; Ribeiro, C.; Amaral, A. Cultural Adaptation and Psychometric Properties of the Portuguese Version of the Therapeutic Self-Care Scale. *Int. J. Caring Sci.* **2014**, *7*, 426–436.
22. Lim, L.-Y.; Valenti, L.; Knapp, J.; Dobson, A.; Plotnikoff, R.; Higginbotham, N.; Heller, R. A self-administered quality-of-life questionnaire after acute myocardial infarction. *J. Clin. Epidemiol.* **1993**, *46*, 1249–1256. [CrossRef]
23. Höfer, S.; Lim, L.; Guyatt, G.; Oldridge, N. The MacNew Heart Disease health-related quality of life instrument: A summary. *Health Qual. Life Outcomes* **2004**, *2*, 3. [CrossRef] [PubMed]
24. Leal, A.; Paiva, C.; Höfer, S.; Amado, J.; Gomes, L.; Oldridge, N. Evaluative and Discriminative Properties of the Portuguese MacNew Heart Disease Health-related Quality of Life Questionnaire. *Qual. Life Res.* **2005**, *14*, 2335–2341. [CrossRef]
25. Ferreira, R.; Macedo, M.; Pinto, F.; Neves, R.; Andrade, C.; Santos, G. Programa Nacional Para as Doenças Cérebro-Cardiovasculares 2017. 2017. Available online: http://comum.rcaap.pt/handle/10400.26/21114 (accessed on 15 December 2020).
26. Da Silva, P.M.; Lima, M.J.; Neves, P.M.; De Macedo, M.E. Prevalência de fatores de risco cardiovascular e outras comorbilidades em doentes com hipertensão arterial assistidos nos Cuidados de Saúde Primários: Estudo Precise. *Rev. Port. Cardiol.* **2019**, *38*, 427–437. [CrossRef]
27. Zajacova, A.; Lawrence, E.M. The Relationship Between Education and Health: Reducing Disparities Through a Contextual Approach. *Annu. Rev. Public Health* **2018**, *39*, 273–289. [CrossRef] [PubMed]
28. Okwose, N.C.; O'Brien, N.; Charman, S.; Cassidy, S.; Brodie, D.; Bailey, K.; MacGowan, G.A.; Jakovljevic, D.G.; Avery, L. Overcoming barriers to engagement and adherence to a home-based physical activity intervention for patients with heart failure: A qualitative focus group study. *BMJ Open* **2020**, *10*, e036382. [CrossRef] [PubMed]
29. Riegel, B.; Dunbar, S.B.; Fitzsimons, D.; Freedland, K.E.; Lee, C.S.; Middleton, S.; Stromberg, A.; Vellone, E.; Webber, D.E.; Jaarsma, T. Self-care research: Where are we now? Where are we going? *Int. J. Nurs. Stud.* **2019**, *103402*, 103402. [CrossRef] [PubMed]
30. Goodman, H.; Firouzi, A.; Banya, W.; Lau-Walker, M.; Cowie, M.R. Illness perception, self-care behaviour and quality of life of heart failure patients: A longitudinal questionnaire survey. *Int. J. Nurs. Stud.* **2013**, *50*, 945–953. [CrossRef] [PubMed]
31. Rice, H.; Say, R.; Betihavas, V. The effect of nurse-led education on hospitalisation, readmission, quality of life and cost in adults with heart failure. A systematic review. *Patient Educ. Couns.* **2018**, *101*, 363–374. [CrossRef]
32. Weibel, L.; Massarotto, P.; Hediger, H.; Mahrer-Imhof, R. Early education and counselling of patients with acute coronary syndrome. A pilot study for a randomized controlled trial. *Eur. J. Cardiovasc. Nurs.* **2016**, *15*, 213–222. [CrossRef] [PubMed]
33. Vandenberghe, D.; Albrecht, J. The financial burden of non-communicable diseases in the European Union: A systematic review. *Eur. J. Public Health* **2020**, *30*, 833–839. [CrossRef]
34. Abbasi, A.; Ghezeljeh, T.N.; Farahani, M.A. Effect of the self-management education program on the quality of life in people with chronic heart failure: A randomized controlled trial. *Electron. Physician* **2018**, *10*, 7028–7037. [CrossRef]

International Journal of
Environmental Research and Public Health

MDPI

Article

Translation and First Pilot Validation Study of the "Undergraduate Nursing Student Academic Satisfaction Scale" Questionnaire to the Spanish Context

María Dolores Guerra-Martín [1,*], Alejandro Cano-Orihuela [2], Raúl Martos-García [3] and José Antonio Ponce-Blandón [3,*]

1   Department of Nursing, University of Seville, 41009 Seville, Spain
2   University Hospital Son Espases, 07120 Palma de Mallorca, Spain; alejandrocanoorihuela@gmail.com
3   Red Cross Nursing School, University of Seville, 41009 Seville, Spain; rmartos@cruzroja.es
*   Correspondence: guema@us.es (M.D.G.-M.); japonce@cruzroja.es (J.A.P.-B.)

Citation: Guerra-Martín, M.D.; Cano-Orihuela, A.; Martos-García, R.; Ponce-Blandón, J.A. Translation and First Pilot Validation Study of the "Undergraduate Nursing Student Academic Satisfaction Scale" Questionnaire to the Spanish Context. *Int. J. Environ. Res. Public Health* **2021**, *18*, 423. https://doi.org/10.3390/ijerph18020423

Received: 15 November 2020
Accepted: 4 January 2021
Published: 7 January 2021

Publisher's Note: MDPI stays neutral with regard to jurisdictional claims in published maps and institutional affiliations.

Abstract: Satisfaction helps nursing students to develop skills and improve their academic performance, hence the importance of assessing it by means of a reliable instrument. The objective was to translate and culturally adapt the "Undergraduate Nursing Student Academic Satisfaction Scale" (UNSASS) instrument to the Spanish context. A cross-sectional study was conducted with a representative sample of 354 fourth-year nursing students from University of Seville, Seville, Spain. The validation process was carried out in five phases as follows: direct translation, synthesis of the translations, back translation, consolidation by a panel of experts, and pilot test with nursing students. After two rounds among two expert committees, the Content Validity Index (CVI) varied from 0.85 to 1, obtaining a CVI above 0.8 with the global questionnaire. A scale composed of 48 items and 4 subscales was obtained, resulting in a Cronbach's α coefficient of 0.96. Within the subscales, this coefficient varied between 0.92 and 0.94. No statistically significant differences were found between the total satisfaction of the scale and gender and teaching unit. An inversely proportional relationship was found between the age and the "Support & Resources" scale. The "Escala de Satisfacción Académica del Estudiante de Enfermería" (ESAEE) scale was obtained, translated, and adapted to the Spanish context from the UNSASS scale, with satisfactory consistency and validity.

Keywords: personal satisfaction; students; nursing; surveys and questionnaires; validation studies

1. Introduction

The new focus of universities is to become facilitating centers for teaching, where the students are able to acquire knowledge through friendly methods and where the institutions base their efforts on promoting a healthy environment of well-being [1,2].

Critical and creative thinking is demanded from health professionals, and nursing education has evolved to adapt to these new requirements. This process has gradually taken place thanks to efficient professional competences aimed at obtaining a high level of satisfaction for the user of the educational system [3].

Students' satisfaction helps build self-confidence and is a source of support to develop skills and acquire knowledge, thus helping to improve academic performance [4,5].

The current generation of students is flooded with a great variety of stimuli, with an element that reinforces the motivation to learn in the students being important; in this sense, satisfaction is very much connected to the increase in motivation, through which they learn more and better, which is useful for their future professional practice [6]. However, satisfaction in relation to obtaining any degree is complemented by stressors such as suffering, diseases, disabilities, or death of patients [7].

The non-intellectual competences involved in academic performance can be important resources for promoting academic adjustment and satisfaction, favoring the retention and persistence processes in college. In the same way, working on the non-cognitive skills closely linked with study satisfaction could also improve performance and academic success, thereby increasing domain-specific satisfaction. In this case, for example, individual work on intrinsic motivation or group work that enhances the ability to relate to one's fellow students could improve satisfaction with one's study habits [8].

Furthermore, some studies support the finding that the environment at university can be perceived as stressful and that developing the ability to handle negative situations effectively increases perceived support from peer relationships and can create a virtuous cycle that helps students improve this competence [9]. Thus, some authors suggest the importance of developing one's own scale to measure the satisfaction of Nursing Degree students [7], carrying out experiences in which it is clear that these students complement the stressors that young people commonly have with those additional derived from the practical environment, in which day by day they find stress-generating stimuli. Moreover, there is the need that these students have to establish relationships with other health professionals, and the fact of having to play a new role for which they have not yet been fully trained.

Thus, there are various studies whose objective was to validate standardized scales targeted at evaluating nursing students' satisfaction, by dealing with either one or more of its aspects or factors, and directed towards a specific idiomatic and/or cultural context. Currently, there are validated scales that evaluate satisfaction and effectiveness in the clinical learning setting, as well as satisfaction in clinical practices [10–13]. In the case of Asadizaker et al. [4], with their "Satisfaction with First Clinical Practical Education" (SFCPE) scale, they evaluated in a more comprehensive manner this realm of nursing education, through the "Instructor performance" ($\alpha = 0.92$), "Integrated plan" ($\alpha = 0.82$)", "Feelings and perceptions" ($\alpha = 0.78$), "Learning atmosphere" ($\alpha = 0.73$), "Scheduling" ($\alpha = 0.70$), "Facilities" ($\alpha = 0,65$), and "Access to professionals" ($\alpha = 0.60$) subscales. Furthermore, given the importance that the first experience in a clinical setting, the main factor assessed by this scale, is the cornerstone of the future in professional nursing for all nursing students, the authors defend the use of this instrument, concluding that it is valid and reliable.

In the scope of the European Space of Higher Education, Lepiani et al. [14] conducted a study focused on the satisfaction of first-year nursing students when addressing Basic knowledge, the Organization of teaching, the Skills developed, the Teaching–learning process, Access and attention in the students, and the Curriculum and its structure as study factors. Satisfaction assessment scales have also been described in the university context, not only in the nursing field, which have shown to be useful and could also be applied in contexts of assessment of the satisfaction of undergraduate nursing students [15].

In contrast, among the scales of multidimensional appreciation are studies such as the one focused on determining nursing students' satisfaction [16], where a level of satisfaction in 11 factors was determined. Additionally, the study developed by Gloria and Ortiz [1] established the quality of life level and the factors related to it in such students, when applying the "Calidad de Vida y Satisfacción" (Q-LES-Q) questionnaire.

Despite the usefulness of all these instruments, a multidimensional, validated, and reliable "Undergraduate Nursing Student Academic Satisfaction Scale" (UNSASS) was found focusing on the measurement of satisfaction of nursing students with a Nursing Degree and all the integral aspects that make up the student's learning period. This scale was developed by Dennison and El-Masri [17] and validated in the Canadian context, whose function is to evaluate the level of satisfaction over four dimensions, namely "In-Class Teaching", "Clinical Teaching", "The Program", and "Support & Resources", where each scale obtained Cronbach's alpha coefficients of 0.92, 0.91, 0.91, and 0.74, respectively, and of 0.96 for the entire scale, which denoted an excellent overall internal consistency.

It is true that other instruments have been developed to evaluate the satisfaction of nursing students, in different cultural contexts, such as the work of Chen and Lo [18], validating the "Nursing Student Satisfaction Scale" (NSSS) instrument for its use in the USA context with high internal consistency ($\alpha = 0.96$), where satisfaction was evaluated in three factors, namely Curriculum and teaching, Environment, and Professional social interaction. Subsequently, Domingues et al. [19] once again validated this tool, the NSSS scale, although in this case for the Brazilian context. It was composed of three factors, namely "Curricular dimension and teaching", "Environmental dimension", and "Social/Professional interactions". Despite the recognition of the usefulness of this scale in different contexts, it clearly covers a smaller set of scenarios in its studied dimensions, excluding aspects as relevant as the support and necessary resources and the differentiation between clinical learning environments and academic environments ("in-class" learning). These aspects are however effectively addressed by the UNSASS scale, proving to be one of the most complete due to its properties of internal consistency, reliability, measurement of errors, construct validity, structural validity, and criterion validity. Furthermore, the scale follows the standardized quality assessment criteria methodology of studies on measurement properties of health status measurement instruments [20].

Thus, a translation and validation research of the aforementioned scale to the Spanish context were justified. We therefore proposed the research as this study's objective to translate and culturally adapt the multidimensional, validated, and reliable "Undergraduate Nursing Student Academic Satisfaction Scale" instrument to the Spanish context. The study also aimed to verify the level of satisfaction of fourth-year nursing students and the existing relationships between the level of satisfaction and gender, age, or the teaching units to which they belonged.

2. Materials and Methods

2.1. Design and Participants

A validation study of the "Undergraduate Nursing Student Academic Satisfaction Scale" (UNSASS) questionnaire adapted to the Spanish context was conducted, which included a non-experimental, quantitative, descriptive, and cross-sectional pilot test, between December 2018 and July 2019, where data collection took place in April 2019.

The study population were the 354 fourth-year nursing students belonging to the Virgen Macarena, Virgen del Rocío, or Virgen de Valme teaching units, from the School of Nursing, Physiotherapy and Podiatry of the University of Seville, Seville, Spain, where a stratified sampling was conducted respecting the proportion of students of the target population. The students were recruited by means of e-mail messages, and the instrument was provided online using the Google Forms tool. From the study population divided by teaching unit composed of 74 from Virgen del Rocío, 226 from Virgen Macarena, and 54 from Virgen de Valme, a final sample of 32 students (9.04%) of the entire school was obtained, of which 7 (9.46%), 19 (8.41%), and 6 (11.11%) were from each of the teaching units, respectively, numbers that fall within the 30–40 students estimated in the scientific literature [21].

In addition to asking about gender, age, and teaching unit, the instrument was applied to fourth-year students since they were immersed in the context of undergraduate nursing studies for a longer period of time and, therefore, possessed more knowledge, excluding those who did not understand Spanish and who did not attend the previous years in that school.

2.2. Translation and Cultural Adaptation Process

The instrument used for validation in the Spanish context was the "Undergraduate Nursing Student Academic Satisfaction Scale" (UNSASS) [17]. To this end, the guidelines for cultural adaptation and validation of health questionnaires by Ramada, Serra, and Declós [22] and by Romero-Martín, Gómez-Salgado, De la Fuente-Ginés, Macías-Seda, García-Díaz, and Ponce-Blandón [23] were followed, consisting of five phases, namely direct translation, synthesis, back translation, consolidation by expert committees, and pilot test of the questionnaire.

Initially, two independent and bilingual nurses with work experience and knowledge of the Spanish university system in force conducted a linguistic, cultural, and conceptual translation of the instrument [24]. Subsequently, the researchers synthesized both translated versions comparing by pairs, where the existing discrepancies between the two versions were identified and discussed, reaching consensus. The consensual version in Spanish was back-translated into English by two independent translators, who did not have access to the original version. Subsequently, pair corrections were made, and the prototype of the scale called "Escala de Satisfacción Académica del Estudiante de Enfermería (ESAEE)" was created. For logical appearance validity, two expert committees were created with a total of 13 participants—one was made up of 7 professors from diverse university settings and the other was constituted by 6 fourth-year nursing students [21]. The objective of both expert committees was to assess whether each item was understandable, with sufficient clarity in each of them.

2.3. Applicability and Feasibility

In the pilot phase, each of the participants was asked to complete the version of the ESAEE instrument translated and adapted to the Spanish context and, later on, they were given the choice to express if they found any difficulty in understanding any of the items, as well as to leave comments on them. In this sense, if at least 15% of the students had difficulties with any item, it should be reviewed; but none of the participants found any difficulty in answering the questions. We also asked them to indicate the time they needed to answer the survey, the result being slightly less than 15 min.

Likewise, it was considered that, in adaptations, it is relevant not only to show evidence of a possible linguistic equivalence between the original and the adapted instruments, but also to state that the adaptations are equivalent from a conceptual point of view [24].

When calculating the relevance or validity of the questionnaire, the "Content Validity Index" (CVI) was used, in which, for each item to be considered acceptable in the final questionnaire, its relevance had to be assessed with a value of 3 or 4 out of 4 on a Likert scale by more than 78% of the experts [25,26], that is, a CVI equal to or higher than 0.78, and that it was understandable for at least 80% of the experts [21,27].

Those items that did not meet the aforementioned requirements were reviewed and reassessed, contacts being made with the primary translators and with those in charge of the back translation, in order to verify that the changes we were going to implement faithfully reflected the original scale. With the translators' approval, a series of changes were introduced in some items; the others were kept unchanged following the translators' suggestions.

2.4. Statistical Analysis

When assessing the internal consistency or reliability of the questionnaire, its Cronbach's alpha coefficient was calculated, where a value above 0.7 was considered acceptable, which reveals a strong relationship among the questions of the test, either in each dimension or subscale or in the entire questionnaire [28]. For the construct validity, a confirmatory factor analysis (CFA) was used, and a previous verification of the suitability was checked with the Bartlett sphericity test and the Kaiser–Meyer–Olkin (KMO) coefficient. A significance of $p < 0.05$ for the Bartlett test and a value of KMO > 0.60 were considered acceptable as recommended in the literature [29]. The extraction method used to perform the CFA was the principal component analysis, and the rotation method used was the Varimax method with Kaiser normalization.

When describing the gender, age, and teaching unit variables, the subscales and items of the questionnaire, means, standard deviations and percentages were used.

The Shapiro–Wilk test and the Levene's test were used to observe normality distribution, as well as to determine whether there was homogeneity in the variances, in addition to parametric tests such as the Student's *t*-test and the ANOVA test or non-parametric ones, like Kruskal-Wallis or Mann-Whitney U. For the relationship of two continuous quantitative variables, Pearson's correlation test was performed.

In order to perform the statistical data analysis, the SPSS© statistical software, version 21.0 (IBM Corp., Armonk, NY, USA) was used.

2.5. Ethical Considerations

Prior to the translation and validation process, authorization was asked from the authors of the UNSASS questionnaire, and they gave permission to use the UNSASS scale for its adaptation and use in the present study [17].

The participants of both expert committees (professors and students) and the students who participated in the pilot test were previously informed about the purpose of the study and they provided informed voluntary written consent. Their information was registered anonymously so it would not be possible to identify participants´ answers, guaranteeing anonymity and data confidentiality at all times. The study was approved by the Research Ethics Committee from the Spanish Red Cross Nursing College, University of Seville, with reference number 10/2018. According to this report, the study meets the requirements for research with human beings and complies with current regulations in Spain and the European Union regarding research issues.

3. Results

3.1. Translation and Adaptation Phase

After the described translation process and assessment, the initial version of the instrument, after going through the expert panel, can be found as supplementary information to this article (Table S1, Supplementary Materials), with its variables (type and operational definition) summarized in Table 1.

Table 1. Variables, types, and operational definitions.

Variable	Type	Operational Definition
Age	Discreet and quantitative	Years old
Gender	Dichotomous, nominal, and qualitative	Man, Woman
Teaching Unit	Nominal and qualitative	Virgen del Rocío, Virgen de Valme, Virgen Macarena
Satisfaction (Scale total)	Quantitative	48–240
Satisfaction (In-Class Teaching subscale)	Quantitative	16–80
Satisfaction (Clinical Teaching subscale)	Quantitative	15–75
Satisfaction (Program Design and Delivery subscale)	Quantitative	12–60
Satisfaction (Support & Resources subscale)	Quantitative	5–25

3.2. Item Creation Process and Content Validity

When presenting a CVI above 0.78 or when being considered clear by at least 80% of the experts in both the first and second rounds, the reevaluated items were accepted as relevant and were included in the final version of the scale.

In the first round of item appreciation by the expert committees, seven items (3, 15, 28, 30, 31, 42, and 44) did not reach the clarity appreciation cutoff point in at least 80% of the experts, and there were also six items (4, 15, 28, 31, 44, and 45) with a CVI below 0.78. Those items were subjected to a second evaluation round with the improvements proposed by the experts and a reassessment of the translation process. In any case, in this first round of the expert panel of professors, some of the suggestions for improvement that the experts proposed for each of the items that did not meet the validity or relevance criteria were taken into account.

Unlike in the panel of professors, the panel of students did not find objections in the items when assessing their clarity and relevance.

Therefore, the items in which professors had discrepancies were reevaluated, rechecking each of the steps previously performed, again comparing the previous versions of the scale, and contacting the primary and native translators who carried out the translations, to verify that the modifications that we were going to make could be a reflection of the original scale, in order to maintain fidelity in the process, since it was not possible to move away from its essence. With the approval of the translators, some modifications were introduced in the items, and in others, they were kept the same following the suggestions of the translators.

Once the items had been modified, a second analysis was made by the panel of professors in order to verify that the changes made were the ideal ones to achieve optimal clarity and relevance of each of the items. In this second round of the validation process, all the reevaluated items obtained a CVI above 0.78 (Table 2), the reason why they were accepted as relevant and were included in the final version of the scale. They observed that, in its integrity, the scale was expressed with sufficient clarity, thereby concluding this phase of the validation process, including all items for the final version of the scale, even the reassessed items.

Table 2. Content Validity Index (CVI) of the reevaluated items after the last round with the expert committees.

No.	Item	Content Validity Index
4	Faculty members make an effort to understand difficulties I might be having with my course work	0.85
15	Faculty members create a good overall impression	0.85
28	Clinical instructors provide enough opportunities for independent practice in the lab and clinical sites	1
31	Faculty members behave professionally	0.85
44	The secretaries are caring and helpful	0.85
45	The secretaries behave professionally	1

CVI: Content Validity Index.

3.3. Results of the Pilot Study

The ESAEE scale was administered to a sample of 32 students. A total of 78.1% of participants ($n = 25$) were women. The mean age of the sample was 22.2 years (21–27), SD = 1.62). The distribution of participants among the different teaching units was 21.8% ($n = 7$), 59.3% ($n = 19$), and 18.7% ($n = 6$) for "Virgen del Rocío", "Virgen Macarena", and "Virgen de Valme" units, respectively.

Table 3 shows the descriptive of the score obtained (mean, standard deviation, and the percentage of the mean score related to the maximum value of each of the subscales and the ESAEE scale as a whole). The subscale 4 "Support & Resources" was the best valued subscale by nursing students. No comprehension or legibility problems were identified for any of the items.

Table 3. Mean, standard deviation, and percentage of the mean score in relation to the possible maximum of each of the subscales and of the entire "Escala de Satisfacción Académica del Estudiante de Enfermería" (ESAEE) scale.

Descriptive Parameter	In-Class Teaching Subscale	Clinical Teaching Subscale	Program Design and Delivery Subscale	Support & Resources Subscale	Total Satisfaction
Mean	3.54	3.92	3.63	4.19	3.75
Standard Deviation	0.22	0.19	0.27	0.08	0.30
Percentages	70.8%	78.4%	72.6%	83.8%	75.0%

Table 4 presents the mean and standard deviation for each of the items and for each of the subscales.

Table 4. Mean values and standard deviation for items, subscales, and total ESAEE scale.

	Items	Mean	SD		Items	Mean	SD
	"In-Class Teaching" subscale	3.54	0.22		**"Clinical Teaching" subscale**	3.92	0.19
1.	I can freely express my academic and other concerns to faculty members	3.81	1.03	17.	Clinical instructors are approachable and make students feel comfortable about asking questions	4.00	0.84
2.	Faculty members are easily approachable	3.69	0.82	18.	Clinical instructors provide feedback at appropriate times, and do not embarrass me in front of others (classmates, staff, patients and family members)	4.00	1.02
3.	Faculty members make every effort to assist students when asked	3.72	0.81	19.	Clinical instructors are open to discussions and difference in opinions	3.75	0.95
4.	Faculty members make an effort to understand difficulties I might be having with my course work	3.44	0.98	20.	Clinical instructors give me sufficient guidance before I perform technical skills	4.09	0.86
5.	Faculty members are usually available after class and during office hours	3.75	0.80	21.	Clinical instructors view my mistakes as part of my learning	4.00	1.05
6.	I can freely express my academic and other concerns to the administration	3.56	0.95	22.	Clinical instructors give me clear ideas of what is expected from me during a clinical rotation	3.78	1.07
7.	Faculty are fair and unbiased in their treatment of individual students	3.66	0.90	23.	Clinical instructors facilitate my ability to critically assess my client's needs	3.72	1.08
8.	Faculty members provide adequate feedback about students' progress in a course	3.34	0.90	24.	Clinical instructors assign me to patients that are appropriate for my level of competence	4.13	0.87
9.	I receive detailed feedback from faculty members on my work and written assignments	3.19	1.15	25.	Clinical instructors give me verbal and written feedback concerning my clinical experience	3.91	1.03
10.	Channels for expressing students' complaints are readily available	3.09	1.30	26.	Clinical instructors demonstrate a high level of knowledge and clinical expertise	3.97	0.86
11.	Faculty members are good role models and motivate me to do my best	3.59	0.80	27.	Clinical instructors are available when needed	3.84	0.88
12.	The administration shows concern for students as individuals	3.34	1.07	28.	Clinical instructors provide enough opportunities for independent practice in the lab and clinical sites	3.81	1.00
13.	Faculty members demonstrate a high level of knowledge in their subject area	3.69	0.78	29.	Clinical instructors encourage me to link theory to practice	3.69	0.97
14.	Faculty members take the time to listen/discuss issues that may impact my academic performance	3.44	1.05	30.	Instructions are consistent among different clinical and lab instructors	3.78	0.97
15.	Faculty members create a good overall impression	3.91	0.73	31.	Faculty members behave professionally	4.44	0.62
16.	I am generally given enough time to understand the things I have to learn	3.47	0.92				

Table 4. *Cont.*

Items	Mean	SD		Items	Mean	SD
"Program Design and Delivery" subscale	3.63	0.27		**"Support & Resources" subscale**	4.19	0.98
32. This program provides a variety of good and relevant courses	3.69	1.03	44.	The secretaries are caring and helpful	4.06	0.98
33. The program enhances my analytical skills	3.59	0.95	45.	The secretaries behave professionally	4.22	0.75
34. Most courses in this program are beneficial and contribute to my overall professional development	3.56	0.95	46.	Support at the clinical and computer labs is readily available	4.13	1.00
35. The quality of instruction I receive in my classes is good and helpful	3.72	0.81	47.	Computer and clinical labs are well equipped, adequately staffed, and are readily accessible to meet	4.25	0.67
36. I usually have a clear idea of what is expected of me in this program	3.28	0.89	48.	The facilities (class rooms, clinical and computer labs) facilitate my learning	4.31	0.69
37. The program is designed to facilitate team work among students	3.72	0.92				
38. The program enhances my problem solving or critical thinking skills	3.72	0.89				
39. There is a commitment to academic excellence in this program	3.38	1.07				
40. As a result of my courses, I feel confident about dealing with clinical nursing problems	3.09	1.23				
41. Going to class helps me better understand the material	3.88	0.90				
42. I am able to experience intellectual growth in the program	4.06	0.84				
43. Overall, the program requirements are reasonable and achievable	3.88	0.94		Total ESAEE Scale	3.75	0.30

3.4. Internal Consistency and Reliability

The four subscales that constitute the ESAEE scale obtained Cronbach's alpha coefficients of 0.94 (In-Class Teaching subscale), 0.94 (Clinical Teaching subscale), 0.92 (Program Design and Delivery subscale), and 0.92 (Support & Resources subscale). The ESAEE scale obtained the highest Cronbach's alpha coefficient, i.e., 0.96.

3.5. Internal Validity of the Scale

Regarding the confirmatory factor analysis (CFA), before the CFA, KMO = 0.93 and $p < 0.001$ was achieved in the Bartlett test. The CFA results revealed and confirmed the four original factors that accounted for 67.3% of the total variance and a factor loading above 0.4 in all the items. Table 5 presents, through the rotated component matrix, the values of the CFA model and the standardized coefficients of the model items that best fit (only factor loading values above 0.4 are expressed).

3.6. Hypothesis Contrast Analysis

The relationship of gender and teaching unit with the satisfaction of the surveyed students was analyzed, not only in each of the factors or dimensions but also in the entire scale, and no relationship was observed. However, in the case of the relationship between age and satisfaction there was no relation between them, both in the entire scale and in all the subscales, except for the "Support & Resources" subscale ($p = 0.003$; Pearson's correlation coefficient of -0.513), which indicated an inversely proportional relationship, with moderate intensity.

Table 5. Confirmatory factor analysis (CFA) for ESAEE (rotated component matrix and Cronbach's alpha coefficient).

"In-Class Teaching" Subscale (Items 1–16) (Cronbach's α = 0.94)	Factor 1	Factor 2	Factor 3	Factor 4
3. Faculty members make every effort to assist students when asked	0.729			
14. Faculty members take the time to listen/discuss issues that may impact my academic performance	0.725	0.498		
1. I can freely express my academic and other concerns to faculty members	0.718			
2. Faculty members are easily approachable	0.706			
9. I receive detailed feedback from faculty members on my work and written assignments	0.699			
16. I am generally given enough time to understand the things I have to learn	0.683			
13. Faculty members demonstrate a high level of knowledge in their subject area	0.654			0.442
4. Faculty members make an effort to understand difficulties I might be having with my course work	0.637	0.485		
11. Faculty members are good role models and motivate me to do my best	0.633			
7. Faculty are fair and unbiased in their treatment of individual students	0.632			
8. Faculty members provide adequate feedback about students' progress in a course	0.624	0.464		
15. Faculty members create a good overall impression	0.617			0.421
12. The administration shows concern for students as individuals	0.604	0.520		
6. I can freely express my academic and other concerns to the administration	0.596			
5. Faculty members are usually available after class and during office hours	0.589			
10. Channels for expressing students' complaints are readily available	0.588			
"Clinical Teaching" subscale (items 17–31) (Cronbach's α = 0.94)	Factor 1	Factor 2	Factor 3	Factor 4
20. Clinical instructors give me sufficient guidance before I perform technical skills		0.881		
28. Clinical instructors provide enough opportunities for independent practice in the lab and clinical sites		0.808		
30. Instructions are consistent among different clinical and lab instructors		0.799		
23. Clinical instructors facilitate my ability to critically assess my client's needs		0.785		
25. Clinical instructors give me verbal and written feedback concerning my clinical experience		0.784		
18. Clinical instructors provide feedback at appropriate times, and do not embarrass me in front of others (classmates, staff, patients and family members)		0.781		
24. Clinical instructors assign me to patients that are appropriate for my level of competence		0.775		
27. Clinical instructors are available when needed		0.735		
19. Clinical instructors are open to discussions and difference in opinions		0.728		
22. Clinical instructors give me clear ideas of what is expected from me during a clinical rotation		0.718		
29. Clinical instructors encourage me to link theory to practice		0.713		
26. Clinical instructors demonstrate a high level of knowledge and clinical expertise		0.676		
21. Clinical instructors view my mistakes as part of my learning		0.637		
17. Clinical instructors are approachable and make students feel comfortable about asking questions	0.430	0.543		
31. Faculty members behave professionally		0.450		

Table 5. *Cont.*

	Factor 1	Factor 2	Factor 3	Factor 4
"In-Class Teaching" Subscale (Items 1–16) (Cronbach's α = 0.94)	Factor 1	Factor 2	Factor 3	Factor 4
"Program Design and Delivery" subscale (items 32–43) (Cronbach's α = 0.92)			Factor 3	
34. Most courses in this program are beneficial and contribute to my overall professional development			0.868	
32. This program provides a variety of good and relevant courses			0.787	
40. As a result of my courses, I feel confident about dealing with clinical nursing problems			0.705	
36. I usually have a clear idea of what is expected of me in this program			0.701	
39. There is a commitment to academic excellence in this program			0.675	
41. Going to class helps me better understand the material			0.677	
38. The program enhances my problem solving or critical thinking skills		0.406	0.650	
35. The quality of instruction I receive in my classes is good and helpful			0.632	
33. The program enhances my analytical skills		0.538	0.613	
42. I am able to experience intellectual growth in the program	0.553		0.671	
37. The program is designed to facilitate team work among students			0.588	
43. Overall, the program requirements are reasonable and achievable	0.471		0.553	
"Support & Resources" subscale (items 44–48) (Cronbach's α = 0.92)	Factor 1	Factor 2	Factor 3	Factor 4
46. Support at the clinical and computer labs is readily available				0.875
47. Computer and clinical labs are well equipped, adequately staffed, and are readily accessible to meet				0.760
48. The facilities (class rooms, clinical and computer labs) facilitate my learning				0.746
45. The secretaries behave professionally			0.406	0.648
44. The secretaries are caring and helpful				0.598
Eigen Value	43.835	11.732	8.675	3.070
% of variability	43.835	55.567	64.242	67.312
% of cumulative variability	43.835	55.567	64.242	67.312

Only factor loading values above 0.4 are expressed.

4. Discussion

The final version of the ESAEE scale is composed of 48 items divided into 4 subscales (In-Class Teaching, Clinical Teaching, Program Design and Delivery, and Support & Resources), identically to the original UNSASS scale [17]. All the items, as Dennison and El-Masri [17] did in their development of the UNSASS scale, were evaluated both in terms of clarity and of relevance, this last characteristic by means of the CVI. Similarly, in order to maintain fidelity with the original in the adaptation of the instrument, the same Likert-type scale scoring was followed, and no strata were proposed for the classification of satisfaction.

By means of the expert committees (professors and students), it was verified that the ESAEE scale presents logical appearance validity. The reliability of the UNSASS scale was assessed using Cronbach's alpha, and showed excellent reliability for the entire scale and for the subscales, with the ESAEE scale presenting reliability levels even higher than the original. However, it is necessary to highlight that the calculation of Cronbach's alpha was not performed from the perspective of a scale made up of 5-point ordinal variables, as suggested by some in the literature [30,31] but rather as nominal polycotomic variables. However, in any case, this same literature suggests that with this type of analysis the Cronbach's alpha would probably have been even higher.

With respect to the "Satisfaction with First Clinical Practical Education" (SFCPE) questionnaire developed by Asadizaker et al. [4] to assess satisfaction in the nursing students with their first clinical setting, it consists of seven factors, and there are similarities when analyzing the nursing student's satisfaction between the two scales, although the ESAEE scale is more compact for having fewer factors, four specifically.

In the first subscale of ESAEE, mostly devoted to theoretical teaching in classrooms, there is no correlation with the SFCPE scale, since the latter is more focused on the clinical scope. However, the second subscale, "Clinical Teaching", is in fact widely adopted and, at the same time, subdivided into several factors that can relate between the subscales. In this sense, the SFCPE adopts factors like "Feelings and perceptions" (Factor 3) (related to items 18, 19, and 29 from ESAEE), "Clinical atmosphere" (Factor 4) (related to items 21, 23, and 25 from ESAEE), "Instructor performance" (Factor 1) (related to items 22, 24, 26, 30, and 31 from ESAEE), or "Access to professionals" (Factor 7) (related to items 17, 20, and 27 from ESAEE). The third subscale in ESAEE, "Program Design and Delivery", is related to the SFCPE scale in the following factors: 2. "Integrated plan" and 5. "Scheduling". Finally, the "Support & Resources" subscale from ESAEE is related to Factor 6. "Facilities" of the SFCPE scale.

In relation to gender, no statistically significant difference was found between satisfaction and this variable. This coincides with the study by Salamonson et al. [32], in which no relationship was found between satisfaction and the age of the nursing students, coinciding with the results obtained in the ESAEE scale, with the exception of the "Support & Resources" subscale, where the relationship with satisfaction was in fact statistically significant. Studies such as the ones by Milton-Wildey et al. [33] and Domingues et al. [19] set forth that younger students present greater satisfaction levels than older students, which is in agreement with the results obtained in the "Support & Resources" subscale from ESAEE.

In the ESAEE scale, total satisfaction was high (75%). Regarding the decreasing order of the students' satisfaction levels with the different subscales, we found that the "Support & Resources" subscale (83.8%) was the best valued, followed by "Clinical Teaching" (78.4%), "Program Design and Delivery" (72.6%), and, in fourth and last place, "In-Class Teaching" (70.8%).

The "In-Class Teaching" subscale from ESAEE obtained a higher result than that obtained in the "Cuestionario de Satisfacción del Estudiante" by Jiménez et al. [34], where the "Desempeño del profesor" factor (related to the "In-Class Teaching" subscale from ESAEE), was in second place, but with a percentage of 64%. The results obtained in our study (mean of 3.54) are in agreement with those obtained by Domingues et al. [19] with a mean of 3.57 for the "Curricular dimension and teaching" factor.

The results obtained for the "Clinical Teaching" subscale (78.4%) from ESAEE were consistent with those obtained in the study by Espeland and Indrehus [10], where 70% of the students were satisfied with the "Clinical practice".

The "Program Design and Delivery" from ESAEE is related in the study by Lepiani et al. [18] with the "Organization of teaching" factor, which obtained a mean score of 3.81 in the students' satisfaction levels, similarly to our study (3.63). In the study by Domingues et al. [19], this subscale is related to the "Curricular dimension and teaching" factor, which obtained a mean score of 3.57, also similar to the result obtained in the "Program Design and Delivery" subscale.

The results of the "Support & Resources" subscale from ESAEE, with items related to the infrastructures and to the administration and services staff, are in agreement with those obtained in the study by Pecina [3], where the areas best evaluated were "IT services" and "Infrastructures". In the study by Lepiani et al. [14], the "Facilities" factor was the worst evaluated (mean of 2.87); however, this result does not coincide with the higher satisfaction level obtained in subscale 4 (mean of 4.19).

A very high reliability was obtained in the ESAEE scale (α: 0.96), coinciding with the values obtained in the studies by Asadizaker et al. [4] and Baykal et al. [14]. In addition, Domingues et al. [19] and Dennison and El-Masri [17] reached Cronbach's α coefficients of 0.92, 0.97, 0.93, and 0.96, respectively; however, lower results, though reliable, were obtained in Pecina [3] and in Salamonson et al. [29], namely 0.83 and 0.80, respectively.

As a limitation of this research, we can mention having conducted an exploratory study of the ESAEE questionnaire, without accompanying it with a reliability test (test and re-test), in addition to only selecting students from the last year of the nursing program. This would have allowed us to calculate the interclass correlation coefficients, which would have given much more consistency to the study. Thus, as an improvement proposal, we shall conduct a reliability test, by having the participants complete the ESAEE questionnaire a second time 15 days after its first application, in addition to expanding the selection to students from the third year, who also have clinical practices as well as theoretical classes. Another limitation to highlight is the absence of an external evidence of validity, given that, due to the scarcity of specific scales available of this type, it would also be very difficult to identify a "gold standard". As it is a first pilot validation study of the scale and, therefore, a line of research in which the authors continue to investigate, the inclusion of a comparison with an external evidence of validity could be suggested for the future.

5. Conclusions

Obtaining the satisfaction level of undergraduate nursing students represents an opportunity to know the aspects that can be improved, in order to implement measures leading to better quality in the studies, from the point of view not only of the curricula, but also of their transposition to theoretical classes, care practices, and the organization of the Nursing School. The aforementioned will improve how the students cope with their entry in the near future into the nursing profession and, with that, into the professional health care provided to people. This research could also be useful for a future review of the aforementioned aspects, either by the Nursing Schools or by the universities.

The Escala de Satisfacción Académica del Estudiante de Enfermería (ESAEE) scale was developed through a 5-phase validation process, adapted to the Spanish context. It consists of 48 items encompassed in four appreciation dimensions (In-Class Teaching, Clinical Teaching, Program Design and Delivery, and Support & Resources), with a Content Validity Index and a Cronbach's α sufficiently high and similar to the original version of the validated questionnaire (UNSASS), which signifies sufficiently high internal consistency and validity of the content of the questionnaire for its validation. Only one moderate negative correlation was observed between the "Support & Resources" subscale and age.

For the future, we intend to conduct a multicenter research study with Nursing Schools from other universities, with a larger sample of nursing students and from different years, in addition to conducting not only a quantitative but also a qualitative approach, since in the world of perceptions and feelings, as in the case of the study of satisfaction, it is necessary to know more in depth what those students feel.

Supplementary Materials: The following are available online at https://www.mdpi.com/1660-460 1/18/2/423/s1, Table S1: "Escala de Satisfacción Académica del Estudiante de Enfermería" (ESAEE scale) after translation, expert committee modifications, and piloting.

Author Contributions: Conceptualization, M.D.G.-M. and A.C.-O.; methodology, M.D.G.-M., A.C.-O., and J.A.P.-B.; software, M.D.G.-M., A.C.-O., and R.M.-G.; validation, formal analysis, and data curation, M.D.G.-M. and A.C.-O.; writing—original draft preparation, M.D.G.-M. and A.C.-O.; writing—review and editing, R.M.-G and J.A.P.-B.; visualization, A.C.-O. and R.M.-G.; supervision, M.D.G.-M. and J.A.P.-B. All authors have read and agreed to the published version of the manuscript.

Funding: This research received no external funding.

Institutional Review Board Statement: The study was conducted according to the guidelines of the Declaration of Helsinki, and approved by the Research Ethics Committee from the Spanish Red Cross Nursing College, University of Seville, with reference number 10/2018.

Informed Consent Statement: Informed consent was obtained from all subjects involved in the study.

Conflicts of Interest: The authors declare no conflict of interest.

References

1. Gloria-Barraza, C.; Ortiz-Moreira, L. Factores relacionados a la calidad de vida y satisfacción en estudiantes de enfermería. *Cienc. Enfermería* **2012**, *18*, 111–119. [CrossRef]
2. Reig, A.; Cabrero, J.; Ferrer, R.I.; Richart, M. *La Calidad de Vida y el Estado de Salud de los Estudiantes Universitarios*; Universidad de Alicante: Alicante, Spain, 2001.
3. Pecina-Leyva, R. Satisfacción académica del estudiante de enfermería en una Universidad Pública en México. Available online: https://www.ctes.org.mx/index.php/ctes/article/view/639 (accessed on 6 January 2021).
4. Asadizaker, M.; Saeedi, A.S.; Abedi, H.; Saki, A. Development of a psychometric scale to measure student nurse satisfaction with their first practical clinical education. *Acta Med. Mediterr.* **2015**, *31*, 1337–1344.
5. Levett-Jones, T.; McCoy, M.; Lapkin, S.; Noble, D.; Hoffman, K.; Dempsey, J.; Arthur, C.; Roche, J. The development and psychometric testing of the satisfaction with simulation experience scale. *Nurse Educ. Today* **2011**, *31*, 705–710. [CrossRef]
6. Negrao, R.C.; Amado, J.C.; Carneiro, M.F.; Mazzo, A. Satisfacción de los estudiantes con las experiencias clínicas simuladas: Validación de escala de evaluación. *Rev. Lat.-Am. Enferm.* **2014**, *22*, 709–715. [CrossRef]
7. López-Medina, I.M.; Sánchez-Criado, V. Percepción del estrés en estudiantes de enfermería en las prácticas clínicas. *Enfermería Clínica* **2005**, *15*, 307–313. [CrossRef]
8. Magnano, P.; Lodi, E.; Boerchi, D. The role of non-intellective competences and performance in college satisfaction. *Interchange* **2020**, *51*, 253–276. [CrossRef]
9. Hartley, M.T. Examining the relationships between resilience, mental health, and academic persistence in undergraduate college students. *J. Am. Coll. Health* **2011**, *59*, 596–604. [CrossRef] [PubMed]
10. Espeland, V.; Indrehuz, O. Evaluation of students' satisfaction with nursing education in Norway. *J. Adv. Nur.* **2003**, *42*, 226–236. [CrossRef] [PubMed]
11. D'Souza, M.S.; Nalry, S.; Parahoo, K.; Venkatesaperumal, R. Perception of and satisfaction with the clinical learning environment among nursing students. *Nurse Educ. Today* **2015**, *35*, 833–840. [CrossRef]
12. Antohe, I.; Riklikiene, O.; Tichelaar, E.; Saarikoski, M. Clinical education and training of student nurses in four moderately new European Union countries: Assessment of students' satisfaction with the learning environment. *Nurse Educ. Pract.* **2016**, *17*, 139–144. [CrossRef]
13. Admi, H.; Moshe-Eilon, Y.; Sharon, D.; Mann, M. Nursing students' stress and satisfaction in clinical practice along different stages: A cross-sectional study. *Nurse Educ. Today* **2018**, *68*, 86–92. [CrossRef] [PubMed]
14. Lepiani, I.L.; Dueñas, M.; Meadialdea, M.J.; Bocchino, A. Satisfacción de estudiantes de enfermería con el proceso formativo adaptado al Espacio Europeo de Educación Superior. *Enfermería Docente* **2013**, *101*, 22–28.
15. Lodi, E.; Boerchi, D.; Magnano, P.; Patrizi, P. College satisfaction scale (CSS): Evaluation of contextual satisfaction in relation to college student life satisfaction and academic performance. *BPA Appl. Psychol. Bull.* **2017**, *65*, 51–64.
16. Baykal, U.; Sokmen, S.; Korkmaz, S.; Akgun, E. Determining student satisfaction in a nursing college. *Nurse Educ. Today* **2005**, *25*, 255–262. [CrossRef] [PubMed]

17. Dennison, S.; El-Masri, M.M. Development and psychometric assessment of the undergraduate nursing student academic satisfaction scale (UNSASS). *J. Nurs. Meas.* **2012**, *20*, 75–89. [CrossRef] [PubMed]
18. Chen, H.C.; Lo, H.S. Development and psychometric testing of the nursing student satisfaction scale for the associate nursing programs. *J. Nurs. Educ. Pract.* **2012**, *2*, 25–37. [CrossRef]
19. Domingues, C.; Devos, E.L.; Tomaschewski, J.G.; Silva, R.; Pinho, D. Predictive and associated factors with nursing students' satisfaction. *Acta Paul. Enferm.* **2015**, *28*, 566–572. [CrossRef]
20. Mokkink, L.B.; Terwee, C.B.; Patrick, D.L.; Alonso, J.; Stratford, P.W.; Knol, D.L.; Bouter, L.M.; de Vet, H.C.W. The COSMIN checklist for assessing the methodological quality of studies on measurement properties of health status measurement instruments: An international Delphi study. *Qual. Life Res.* **2010**, *19*, 539–549. [CrossRef]
21. Souza, V.D.; Rojjanasrirat, W. Translation, adaptation and validation of instruments or scales for use in cross-cultural health care research: A clear and user-friendly guideline. *J. Eval. Clin. Pract.* **2011**, *17*, 268–274. [CrossRef]
22. Ramada, J.M.; Serra, C.; Declós, G.L. Adaptación cultural y validación de cuestionarios de salud: Revisión y recomendaciones metodológicas. *Salud Publica Mex.* **2013**, *55*, 57–66. [CrossRef]
23. Romero-Martín, M.; Gómez-Salgado, J.; De la Fuente-Ginés, M.; Macías-Seda, J.; García-Díaz, A.; Ponce-Blandón, J.A. Assessment of reliability and validity of the Spanish version of the nursing students' perception of instructor caring (S-NSPIC). *PLoS ONE* **2019**, *14*, e0212803. [CrossRef] [PubMed]
24. Carretero-Dios, H.; Pérez, C. Normas para el desarrollo y revisión de estudios instrumentales: Consideraciones sobre la selección de tests en la investigación psicológica. *Int. J. Clin. Health Psychol.* **2007**, *7*, 863–882.
25. Polit, D.; Tatano-Beck, C. The content validity index: Are you sure you know what's being reported? Critique and recommendations. *Res. Nurs. Health* **2006**, *29*, 489–497. [CrossRef] [PubMed]
26. Lozano, L.M.; Turbani, J.V. Psicometría; Meneses, J., Ed.; Editorial UOC: Barcelona, Spain, 2013; pp. 141–197.
27. Merino-Soto, C. Percepción de la claridad de los ítems: Comparación del juicio de estudiantes y jueces-expertos. *Rev. Latinoam. Cienc. Soc. Niñez Juv.* **2016**, *14*, 1469–1477. [CrossRef]
28. Bójorquez-Molina, J.; López-Aranda, L.; Hernández-Flores, M.E.; Jiménez-López, E. Utilización del alfa de Cronbach para validar la confiabilidad de un instrumento de medición de satisfacción del estudiante en el uso de Software Minitab. In Proceedings of the Innovation in Engineering, Technology and Education for Competitiveness and Prosperity, 11th Latin American and Caribbean Conference for Engineering and Technology, Cancún, México, 14–16 August 2013.
29. McCoach, D.B.; Gable, R.K.; Madura, J.P. Evidence based on the internal structure of the instrument: Factor analysis. In *Instrument Development in the Affective Domain*; Springer: New York, NY, USA, 2013. [CrossRef]
30. Elossua, P.; Zumbo, B.D. Coeficientes de fiabilidad para escalas de respuesta categórica ordenada. *Psicothema* **2008**, *20*, 896–901.
31. Zumbo, B.D.; Gadermann, A.M.; Zeisser, C. Ordinal versions of coefficients alpha and theta for Likert rating scales. *J. Mod. Appl. Stat. Methods* **2007**, *6*, 21–29. [CrossRef]
32. Salamonson, Y.; Metcalfe, L.; Alexandrou, E.; Cotton, A.; McNally, S.; Murphy, J.; Frost, S. Measuring final-year nursing students' satisfaction with the vivaassessment. *Nurse Educ. Pract.* **2015**, *16*, 1–6. [CrossRef]
33. Milton-Wildey, K.; Kenny, P.; Parmenter, G.; Hall, J. Educational preparation for clinical nursing: The satisfaction of students and new graduates from two Australian universities. *Nurse Educ. Today* **2014**, *34*, 648–654. [CrossRef]
34. Jiménez-González, A.; Terriquez-Carrillo, B.; Robles-Cepeda, F.J. Evaluación de la satisfacción académica de los estudiantes de la Universidad Autónoma de Nayarit. *Rev. Fuentes* **2011**, *3*, 46–56.

International Journal of
Environmental Research and Public Health

MDPI

Article

Study of the Strengths and Weaknesses of Nursing Work Environments in Primary Care in Spain

Vicente Gea-Caballero [1,2], José Ramón Martínez-Riera [3,*], Pedro García-Martínez [1,2,*], Jorge Casaña-Mohedo [4], Isabel Antón-Solanas [5,6], María Virtudes Verdeguer-Gómez [7], Iván Santolaya-Arnedo [8,9] and Raúl Juárez-Vela [8,9]

[1] Nursing School La Fe, Adscript Center of Universidad de Valencia, 46026 Valencia, Spain; gea_vic@gva.es
[2] Research Group GREIACC, Health Research Institute La Fe, Avda. Fernando Abril Martorell, 106, Pabellón Docente Torre H, Hospital La Fe, 46026 Valencia, Spain
[3] Departamento Enfermería Comunitaria, Medicina Preventiva y Salud Pública e Historia de la Ciencia, Universidad de Alicante, 03080 Alicante, Spain
[4] Health Department, Universidad Católica de Valencia, C/Quevedo 2, 46001 Valencia, Spain; jorge.casana@ucv.es
[5] Department of Physiatry and Nursing, Faculty of Health Sciences, University of Zaragoza, C/Domingo Miral s/n, 50009 Zaragoza, Spain; ianton@unizar.es
[6] Research Group Nursing Research in Primary Care in Aragón (GENIAPA) (GIIS094), Institute of Research of Aragón, Avenida San Juan Bosco, 13, 50009 Zaragoza, Spain
[7] Departament de Salut La Ribera, Atención Primaria, Ctra. Corbera, Alzira, 46600 Valencia, Spain; mariviverdeguer@gmail.com
[8] Centro de Investigación Biomédica de la Rioja, Logrono, 26006 La Rioja, Spain; isantolalla@riojasalud.es (I.S.-A.); raul.juarez@unirioja.es (R.J.-V.)
[9] Department of Nursing, University of La Rioja, Logroño, 26006 La Rioja, Spain
* Correspondence: jr.martinez@ua.es (J.R.M.-R.); garcia_pedmarb@gva.es (P.G.-M.)

Citation: Gea-Caballero, V.; Martínez-Riera, J.R.; García-Martínez, P.; Casaña-Mohedo, J.; Antón-Solanas, I.; Verdeguer-Gómez, M.V.; Santolaya-Arnedo, I.; Juárez-Vela, R. Study of the Strengths and Weaknesses of Nursing Work Environments in Primary Care in Spain. *Int. J. Environ. Res. Public Health* **2021**, *18*, 434. https://doi.org/10.3390/ijerph18020434

Received: 24 November 2020
Accepted: 1 January 2021
Published: 7 January 2021

Publisher's Note: MDPI stays neutral with regard to jurisdictional claims in published maps and institutional affiliations.

Abstract: Background: Nursing work environments are defined as the characteristics of the workplace that promote or hinder the provision of professional care by nurses. Positive work environments lead to better health outcomes. Our study aims to identify the strengths and weaknesses of primary health care settings in Spain. Methods: Cross-sectional study carried out from 2018 to 2019. We used the Practice Environment Scale of the Nursing Work Index and the TOP10 Questionnaire of Assessment of Environments in Primary Health Care for data collection. The associations between sociodemographic and professional variables were analyzed. Results: In total, 702 primary care nurses participated in the study. Responses were obtained from 14 out of the 17 Spanish Autonomous Communities. Nursing foundation for quality of care, management and leadership of head nurse and nurse–physician relationship were identified as strengths, whereas nurse participation in center affairs and adequate human resources to ensure quality of care were identified as weaknesses of the nursing work environment in primary health care. Older nurses and those educated to doctoral level were the most critical in the nursing work environments. Variables Age, Level of Education and Managerial Role showed a significant relation with global score in the questionnaire. Conclusion: Interventions by nurse managers in primary health care should focus on improving identified weaknesses to improve quality of care and health outcomes.

Keywords: nursing; primary care; workplace; quality of health care; nurse's role

1. Introduction

The nursing workforce plays a crucial role in health systems globally. According to the World Health Organization (WHO) [1], nurses must work to their full potential if countries are to achieve universal health coverage for the population. Nurses are a key element in the sustainability of the health service, enhancing quality of care and promoting patient safety, satisfaction and confidence [2,3]. These reasons have justified the implementation of the international campaign "Nursing Now" and the declaration of the year 2020 as the International Year of the Nurse.

In order to achieve the highest possible quality of nursing care, it is essential to analyze the elements contributing to the delivery of such care; the sum of these elements is the nursing work environment (NWE). Thus, NWE is defined as the characteristics of the workplace that promote or hinder the delivery of quality nursing care [4]. Positive NWEs are characterized by lower rates of mortality, morbidity and adverse events [5–7]; reduced administrative costs and absenteeism [8]; a lower level of burnout and increased patient satisfaction with nursing care and the health organization [9]. Improving health outcomes, the sustainability of the health system and user satisfaction are common goals for healthcare managers, which can be addressed from the perspective of NWE with positive conditions for care. The Magnet Hospital program, for example, accredits centers of excellence and quality of care based on evidence-based practice [10–12]. Magnet centers promote the development of a culture of safety and quality care, staff recognition programs, interdisciplinary communication and horizontal management that contribute positively to the work environment [13,14].

NWE studies have been extensive in hospital settings [15]. However, there is a lack of evidence about the impact of positive primary health care (PHC) NWE on patient outcomes. This may be a handicap for optimizing PHC services, where the configuration of the microenvironment should be conducive to the provision of excellent care. Previous studies [4] have pointed to a possible association between positive PHC NWE and patient outcomes, but the evidence is still scarce.

Previous studies [4,16–18] have assessed the PHC NWE in Spain, concluding that management and leadership of the head nurse, nurse–physician relationship and nursing foundation for quality of care are the most highly valued aspects by primary care nurses, whereas adequate human resources to ensure quality of care is frequently among the least valued characteristics of the workplace. A recent scoping review of the literature suggested that the reality of the PHC NWE is different from that of the hospital NWE. This is due to differences in the decision-making and organizational processes and the relationships between team members. Thus, the evidence available on the hospital NWE may not be applicable to the reality of the PHC NWE [19]. According to Lucas and Nunes [19], the work environment is the most influential factor with the greatest impact on nursing outcomes and on the perceptions of the quality of care and client safety. In order to assess and thus improve the quality of the NWE, Poghosyan et al. [20] developed a global model for optimizing the PHC NWE. In their model, they propose the integration of institutional policies, organizational innovation and research.

We argue that positive PHC NWE can increase the quality of nursing care and, subsequently, improve patient outcomes. However, in order to achieve this goal, it is necessary to analyze the strengths and weaknesses of the PHC NWE. Therefore, we aim to analyze the characteristics of NWE in PHC settings in Spain, identifying these environments' strengths and weaknesses. In addition, we aim to analyze the associations between sociodemographic and professional variables in our sample, as well as the nursing professionals' perception of their NWE.

2. Materials and Methods

2.1. Design

Cross-sectional study of the strengths and weaknesses of NWE in PHC settings in Spain.

2.2. Participants and Study Location

We recruited a non-probabilistic, multi-stage sample of qualified nurses working in PHC settings in Spain. Due to the limited resources for data collection and the geographical dispersion of PHC professionals, the maximum possible number of participants was proposed as a sampling target during the set data collection period. Inclusion criteria for participation in this study were: being qualified as a nurse, having worked in the same

PHC setting for at least 3 months and signing the consent form. Data collection was paused during vacation periods in order to limit the possibility of bias arising from staff turnover.

A total of 817 questionnaires were received, of which 115 (14.7%) were excluded. The reasons for their exclusion were: 7 (6.09%) nurses who did not work at PHC, 27 (23.48%) did not complete the questionnaires correctly and 81 (70.43%) did not meet the criteria for participation in the study.

First, the researchers disseminated the study through social networks (Twitter, Facebook) obtaining an unrestricted sample [21]. Simultaneously, direct dissemination among PHC nurses was achieved by contacting key informants via institutional e-mail (on two occasions, one month apart) to encourage and remind them to participate in the study. This was done between June 2018 and June 2019.

A data collection pack containing the consent form, a questionnaire of sociodemographic variables developed ad hoc and the Practice Environment Scale of the Nursing Work Index (PES-NWI) questionnaire was sent via email to the participants. We used Google Forms®, with a limited response via Internet Protocol (IP), to collect the data electronically. A letter of invitation to participate in the study was also attached, as well as a request to contribute to the dissemination of the study with the purpose of reaching a greater number of PHC nurses through a snowball sampling technique.

2.3. Instruments of Data Collection

An ad hoc questionnaire was designed to collect sociodemographic and professional variables including age, gender, level of education, professional specialization, work experience in PHC settings and management role and responsibilities.

There are multiple measurement tools for the study of NWE [22]. The PES-NWI is among the most widely used and has high levels of consistency and reliability (Cronbach's Alpha 0.807–0.916) [9,23,24]. We used the Spanish version of the PES-NWI, which was adapted and validated for use in Spanish PHC settings by de Pedro-Gómez et al. [25] in 2012. The Spanish PES-NWI is divided into 5 dimensions, namely, nurse participation in center affairs (nine items) (D1), nursing foundation for quality of care (10 items) (D2), management and leadership of head nurse (five items) (D3), adequate human resources to ensure quality of care (four items) (D4) and nurse–physician relationship (three items) (D5). This tool includes a total of 31 items measured on a 4-point Likert scale, with scores ranging between 4 to 124. A favorable environment receives scores of >2.6, neutral or controversial environments receive scores between 2.6 and 2.4 and an unfavorable NWE receives scores of >2.4 for each dimension. Total scores are interpreted as follows: values ≥80.6 are interpreted as positive environments for nursing work, values between 74.5 and 80.5 are identified as controversial environments and values ≤74.4 are classed as negative environments for nursing work [26]. For the present study, Cronbach's alpha for the PES-NWI was 0.937, with a reliability range between 0.836 and 0.935 for each dimension.

More recently, an abbreviated version of the PES-NWI tool was developed by Gea-Caballero et al. [26] with the aim of synthetizing and prioritizing the essential elements for improving PHC settings in the Spanish context. The TOP10 Questionnaire of Assessment of Environments in Primary Health Care (hereinafter TOP10) is divided into 3 dimensions, namely, nurse participation in center affairs (D1a), quality of care (D2a) and human resources (D3a). It comprises 10 items identified as the "essential elements of care"; if not positive, these essential elements of care can seriously affect the quality of care in any given NWE. The total score of the TOP10 questionnaire ranges between 10 and 40. The higher the score, the more favorable the NWE. Cronbach's alpha for the TOP10 questionnaire was reported at 0.816 in a previous study [26]; for the present study, Cronbach's alpha was 0.805. The TOP10 questionnaire was completed by the researchers based on the results obtained from the Spanish version of the PES-NWI tool.

The information for the analysis of the TOP10 was extracted from the PES-NWI questionnaire, since the 10 essential items are part of the 31 that make up the PES-NWI.

2.4. Statistical Analysis

We used descriptive statistics to analyze the sociodemographic and professional characteristics of our sample. Mean and standard deviation for quantitative variables and frequencies, and percentages for qualitative variables, were calculated.

We calculated the Cronbach's alpha coefficient of both the PES-NWI and TOP10 questionnaire to assess internal consistency and reliability as a whole, and for each dimension separately. Reliability was considered excellent when Cronbach Alpha was greater than 0.90; good between 0.80 and 0.89; acceptable between 0.70 and 0.79; questionable between 0.60 and 0.69; poor between 0.50 and 0.59 and unacceptable below 0.50 [27].

We carried out a normality test using Shapiro–Wilk and Kolmogorov–Smirnov tests as appropriate for the quantitative variables. Four variables were found to have a non-normal distribution, namely, dimensions D1, D3, D4 and D5, and were analyzed using non-parametric methods. For the bivariate analyses of variables with a normal distribution (D2 and TOP10), we used a *t*-test for independent samples for dichotomous variables and ANOVA for polytomous variables. If significant differences in the ANOVA were found, the Bonferroni test was applied to determine which pairs of categories presented significant differences between them.

The SPSS v23 statistical package was used for the statistical analysis, and a significance level of $p = 0.05$ was adopted.

2.5. Ethical Considerations

We safeguarded our participants' confidentiality and anonymity according to Spanish/European data protection regulations (Organic Law 3/2018). The participants were informed about the methods and aims of the study and gave their consent to take part in this investigation. This study was approved by the Research Ethics Committee of the Valencian Community (Xàtiva/Ontinyent, Valencia, Spain). The participants did not receive any compensation for completing the questionnaires.

3. Results

The final sample consisted of 702 qualified PHC nurses. The participants were mainly women (71.9%), aged 40 years or older (61.1%) and with more than 10 years of work experience (52.4%). Most of our participants were educated to degree level (64.3%), 5.4% were nurse specialists and 11.8% were nurse managers or coordinators. Responses were obtained from 14 out of the 17 Spanish Autonomous Communities, with a greater representation from the Valencian Community and the Canary Islands (76.3%).

The results of the PES-NWI are shown in Table 1. The NWE in Spanish PHC settings was positive with a total average score of 82.4. Three dimensions were identified as strengths, namely, nursing foundation for quality of care (D2), management and leadership of head nurse (D3) and nurse–physician relationship (D5), and one dimension was identified as a weakness in the PHC settings studied: adequate human resources to ensure quality of care (D4). Nurse participation in center affairs (D1) was considered as neutral or controversial. Specifically, 17 items were identified as strengths, and only 9 were classed as weaknesses of the PHC settings (items 6, 7, 9, 12, 16, 25–28). The reliability of the PSE-NWI in our sample was confirmed with a Cronbach's alpha 0.937 and a range between 0.836 and 0.935 for each of its dimensions.

The average score from the TOP10 questionnaire was 29.7. Two of its dimensions were identified as strengths: participation in center affairs (D1a) and quality of care (D2a), and one was identified as a weakness: human resources (D3a). The reliability of the TOP10 tool in our sample was confirmed with a Cronbach's alpha 0.805.

Table 1. Total scores by dimensions and items from the PES-NWI.

	Score Mean (SD)		
	Strengths	Neutral	Weaknesses
Dimension 1: Nurse participation in the center affairs		2.50 (0.7)	
1 *: Staff nurses are formally involved in the internal management of the center (boards, decision-making bodies)		2.47 (0.9)	
2: Nurses at the center have opportunities to participate in decisions affecting the various policies developed by the center		2.47 (0.9)	
3: Many opportunities exist for the professional development of nurses		2.41 (0.9)	
4: Management listens and responds to the concerns of its nurses		2.55 (0.9)	
5: The Director of Nursing is accessible and easily "visible"	2.90 (1.0)		
6: A professional career can be developed or there are opportunities for promotion in the clinical career			2.27 (1.0)
7: Managers consult with nurses about problems and ways of doing things on a day-to-day basis			2.34 (1.0)
8: Staff nurses have opportunities to participate in the center's committees, such as the committee on research, ethics, infections	2.87 (0.9)		
9: Nursing managers are at the same level of power and authority as other managers in the center			2.34 (1.0)
Dimension 2: Nursing foundation for quality of care	2.72 (0.6)		
10: Nursing diagnostics are used	2.88 (1.0)		
11 *: There is an active quality assurance and improvement programme		2.59 (0.9)	
12: There is a programme for welcoming and mentoring new nurses	2.68 (0.9)		
13: Nursing care is based on a nursing model rather than a biomedical model	3.14 (0.9)		
14 *: Assigning patients to each nurse promotes continuity of care	2.63 (0.9)		
15 *: There is a common, well-defined nursing philosophy that permeates the environment in which patients are cared for		2.44 (0.9)	
16: There is a written and updated plan of care for each patient	2.58 (0.9)		
17: Center managers are concerned that nurses provide high-quality care	2.97 (0.9)		
18 *: A program of continuing education is developed for nurses	2.97 (0.9)		
19 *: The nurses in the center have adequate clinical competence	3.03 (0.8)		2.25 (1.1)
Dimension 3: Management and leadership of head nurse	2.93 (0.9)		
20 *: The coordinator/supervisor is a good manager and leader	2.88 (1.0)		
21: The supervisor/coordinator supports the staff in their decisions, even if the conflict is with medical staff	2.94 (1.0)		
22: The supervisor/coordinator uses mistakes as opportunities for learning and improvement, not as criticism	2.87 (1.0)		
23: The supervisor/coordinator is sympathetic and advises and supports the nurses	3.07 (1.0)		
24: Work well done is recognised and praised	2.90 (1.0)		

31

Table 1. *Cont.*

	Score Mean (SD)		
	Strengths	Neutral	Weaknesses
Dimension 4: Adequate human resources to ensure quality of care			2.33 (0.8)
25 *: There are enough employees to do the job properly			2.28 (1.0)
26 *: There are sufficient numbers of registered nurses to provide quality care			2.35 (1.0)
27: Support services (wardens, administrative staff, etc.) are adequate and make it easier to spend more time with patients			2.38 (0.9)
28: There is sufficient time and opportunity to discuss care issues with the other nurses			2.32 (0.9)
Dimension 5: Nurse–physician relationship	2.87 (0.7)		
29: A lot of teamwork is done between doctors and nurses	2.63 (0.9)		
30: There are good working relationships between doctors and nurses	3.10 (0.7)		
31 *: Practice between nurses and doctors is based on appropriate collaboration	2.87 (0.8)		
TOP10 questionnaire	Strengths	Neutral	Weaknesses
Dimension 1a: Participation in center affairs	2.73 (0.7)		
Dimension 2a: Quality of care	2.92 (0.7)		
Dimension 3a: Human resources			2.31 (1.0)
Overall result			
PES-NWI total	82.43 (17.4)		
TOP10 total	29.68 (6.2)		

SD: standard deviation; strength: score > 2.6; neutral or controversial: score between 2.4–2.6; weakness: score < 2.4; positive environment: PES-NWI score > 80.6; controversial environment: PES-NWI score 74.4–80.6; negative environment: PES-NWI score < 74.4; * TOP10 items.

32

The bivariate analysis of the results from PES-NWI and the sociodemographic and professional variables are shown in Table 2. Age was statistically significant for the PES-NWI and 3 out of its 5 dimensions (D2, D3 and D5). The participants' level of education was statistically significant for the overall PES-NWI and 4 of its dimensions (D1, D2, D3 and D5), and management role was found to be statistically significant for the PES-NWI and 4 of its dimensions (D1, D2, D3 and D4). We did not find a statistically significant correlation between PES-NWI and the rest of the sociodemographic and professional variables.

Table 2. Bivariate analysis of the results from PES-NWI and the sociodemographic and professional variables.

					Scoring M(SD)		
		Global			Dimensions		
			D1	D2	D3	D4	D5
Age (years)	p [a]	0.016 *	0.123	0.047 *	0.041 *	0.467	0.000 *
Less than or equal to 30		84.98 (15.9)	2.63 (0.6)	2.74 (0.6)	3.00 (0.8)	2.44 (0.7)	3.04 (0.7)
31–40		84.99 (17.7)	2.55 (0.6)	2.83 (0.7)	3.06 (0.9)	2.31 (0.8)	3.06 (0.7)
41–50		81.56 (17.3)	2.48 (0.7)	2.70 (0.6)	2.92 (0.9)	2.29 (0.8)	2.82 (0.7)
>50		80.22 (17.6)	2.46 (0.7)	2.65 (0.6)	2.82 (0.9)	2.33 (0.8)	2.71 (0.7)
Managerial role	p [b]	<0.000 *	<0.000 *	<0.000 *	<0.000 *	<0.000 *	0.296
Yes		94.65 (14.4)	3.01 (0.6)	3.06 (0.5)	3.52 (0.6)	2.63 (0.8)	2.96 (0.7)
No		80.55 (17.3)	2.44 (0.6)	2.67 (0.6)	283 (0.9)	2.28 (0.8)	2.86 (0.7)
Level of education	p [a]	<0.000 *	0.026 *	<0.000 *	0.011 *	0.518	0.017 *
Diploma		84.73 (17.4)	2.56 (0.7)	2.82 (0.6)	3.02 (0.9)	2.36 (0.8)	2.95 (0.8)
Degree		81.21 (16.1)	2.52 (0.6)	2.67 (0.6)	2.89 (0.9)	2.28 (0.7)	2.76 (0.7)
Specialisation		80.91 (16.1)	2.53 (0.6)	2.58 (0.6)	2.93 (0.8)	2.39 (0.7)	2.73 (0.7)
Master		80.49 (17.7)	2.45 (0.6)	2.66 (0.6)	2.81 (0.9)	2.30 (0.8)	2.83 (0.7)
PhD		71.13 (16.5)	2.16 (0.7)	2.53 (0.6)	2.53 (0.8)	2.09 (0.7)	2.63 (0.7)

M: mean; SD: standard deviation; D1: participation of nursing staff; D2: nursing foundation in quality of care; D3: capacity, leadership and support of nursing staff by managers; D4: the size of staff and adequacy of human resources; D5: relationships between nursing and medical professionals; * significant values $p < 0.05$; p [a]: ANOVA; p [b]: Student's t-test.

We investigated gender inequalities in our sample (Table 3). Our results show that most of the nurses were aged ≤50 years ($p = 0.031$). The representation of women at higher education levels (masters or doctorate) is proportionally lower than that of men ($p = 0.024$) but, paradoxically, women achieve a higher percentage of specialist training ($p = 0.048$).

Table 3. Distribution and comparison of socio-demographic and occupational data by gender.

		Gender	
		Man (%)	Woman (%)
Age (years)	$p = 0.031$ *		
less than or equal to 30		22.7	77.3
31–40		28.6	71.4
41–50		22.3	77.7
>50		34.0	66.0
Level of education	$p = 0.024$ *		
Diploma		29.6	70.4
Degree		21.8	78.2
Specialisation		16.5	83.5
Master		29.3	70.7
PhD		46.7	53.3
Specialist training	$p = 0.048$ *		
Yes		15.8	84.2
No		20.7	79.3
Working experience (years)	$p = 0.206$		
<2		22.0	78.0
2–4		21.6	78.4
5–10		31.2	68.8
>10		29.3	70.7
Managerial role	$p = 0.204$		
Yes		21.7	28.4
No		78.3	71.6

p: chi square test; * $p < 0.05$

4. Discussion

The main objective of this study was to identify strengths and weaknesses in the PHC work environment in Spain. Our results suggest that positive NWEs in PHC in Spain are characterized by nursing foundations for quality care (D2), management and leadership of the head nurse (D3) and the nurse–physician relationship (D5). This is consistent with previous studies in our context [16,17]. Nurse participation in center affairs (D1) was identified as neutral or controversial in our study as opposed to a previous study by Gea-Caballero et al. [16], where it was identified as a strength. Overall, our results differ from those obtained by de Pedro-Gómez et al. [28], who classified the NWE in PHC settings in the Balearic Islands as controversial (80.4 points).

This study fits well with the improvement model proposed by Poghosyan et al. [20]. Political decision-making and organizational innovation in PHC settings are key to improve identified weaknesses. Furthermore, research in healthcare settings is essential to not only increase knowledge of, and improve, both processes and procedures, but also to create an organizational culture that promotes the integration of the best available evidence [18], thus improving patient outcomes and increasing service user satisfaction.

Given the difficulty in finding other studies in the PHC setting, and due to their conceptual proximity, we compared our results with those reported in studies about magnet hospitals (as described in the introduction). Our results show that dimensions D2, D3 and D5 are associated with a positive NWE. This is in agreement with the results from previous studies carried out in "non-magnet hospitals". These are encouraging findings, but they are still far from those obtained in "magnet hospitals", where every single dimension of the PES-NWI was identified in historical studies as a strength [29,30]. This is an encouraging finding as it demonstrates that the transformation of weak or controversial dimensions into strengths is possible, as evidenced by the results obtained in magnet and excellent work environments.

In Spanish hospitals, the same three dimensions, namely, D2, D3 and D5, were shown to be neutral or controversial for the NWE [31]. This diversity in the results suggests that the quality of the NWE in the hospital context depends on external as well as internal characteristics of the healthcare service. Therefore, interventions to improve the NWE in the PHC context should be individualized and based on the results obtained from each separate healthcare institution (microenvironment). The same reflection is applicable to PHC work environments. However, a study by de Pedro et al. [28] identified D2 and D3 only as strengths in hospitals with 300–500 beds. Paradoxically, in international studies about the characteristics of the NWE, we find a greater diversity of scenarios; some identify all the dimensions of the PES-NWI as strengths [32,33], others show management and leadership of the head nurse and nurse–physician relationship as strengths (D3 and D5) [34], and some identify management and leadership of the head nurse as the only strength (D3) [35].

In the PHC NWE in Spain, the size of the workforce or human resources (D4) is identified as a clear weakness, coinciding with national studies in both PHC [16,17,28] and hospital [28,31,36] work environments. These results coincide with those portrayed in international studies about NWE in the hospital setting [34,35]. The comparative studies between "magnet and non-magnet hospitals" reported similar results in historical studies, with human resources (D4) being identified as a weakness in "non-magnet hospitals"; it was not identified as a weakness in "magnet hospitals", but it was the worst valued dimension [29,30]. This same situation was also observed in international studies, both European [32] and Asian [33], with human resources usually being the worst valued dimension. The problem with human resources is particularly serious in Spain, where the nurse–patient ratio is 567 per 100,000 inhabitants, well below the European average (811/100,000) and far from the more industrialized countries, such as Finland, Denmark or Belgium (1500/100,000) [37]. Despite the efforts made in recent years to increase the nursing workforce, and the commitment to nurses as health agents, it is still a limitation that compromises patient safety and quality of care. Furthermore, the nurse–physician ratio in Spain is severely unbalanced. According to the Organisation for Economic Co-operation and Development (OCED) [38], the number of physicians per inhabitant in Spain is above average (7th place and above countries such as Italy, Australia, France and Finland), but the number of nurses is well below the average worldwide (23rd place out of 26 countries). Finland and Germany triple the number of nurses in Spain, and Norway quadruples it. It should not be forgotten that there is a direct correlation between the ratio of nurses and patient mortality, as well as other unwanted events and health outcomes [5–9].

These facts, framed in a global SARS-COV-2 pandemic, reveal and exacerbate existing problems within the healthcare service. For example, the COVID-19 pandemic has added undue pressure to the health services in Spain, thus highlighting the lack of qualified nurses. As suggested by Seccia Ruggero [39], the replenishment of material resources can be achieved relatively easily, but reinforcement with qualified nurses is difficult to achieve and cannot be done over a short period of time. An adequate nursing provision could contribute to improved outcomes in health crises, such as at the peak of the COVID pandemic, which has led the WHO in April 2020 to call for more investment in nurses [40]. Key stakeholders and those responsible for decision making on healthcare service planning should consider the need to increase the Spanish nursing workforce and draw a plan accordingly in the years to come.

The results from the TOP10 scale [26] were fully consistent with the PES-NWI results, identifying participation of nurses in the affairs of the center (D1a) and the nursing foundations for quality of care (D2a) as strengths, and human resources (D3a) as a weakness. We argue that TOP10 is a simpler way of identifying the strengths and weaknesses associated with the NWE, making it easier and simpler for nurse managers to identify weakness or areas for improvement within their PHC work environments. In addition, the results from the TOP10 scale are valid and reliable as supported by a recent study by Martínez-Riera et al. [41], where a group of community care experts considered that 9 out of the 10 items of the TOP10 scale were essential elements to the PHC NWE.

The comparative study of the sociodemographic and professional variables and the perception of the PHC NWE shows significant differences associated with age, level of education and the level of management in which the professionals were involved. Older nurses (50+) were the most critical with their work environments. In addition, significant differences were found for dimensions D2, D3 and D5 separately. The age-related differences found in Spanish studies should be assessed with caution due to the average age difference between nurses employed in public and private services, with greater representation in privately managed centers of the age range under 40 years [16].

Nurses educated to doctoral level identified the Spanish PHC NWE as a negative environment for nursing care and also pointed to the dimensions of nursing participation in center affairs (D1), nursing foundations for quality of care (D2) and human resources (D4) as weaknesses. Interestingly, the dimension nursing foundations for quality of care (D2) was identified as a weakness by doctoral nurses and as a strength by the rest of the nursing professionals. The same was observed in a previous study [17] in the Community of Madrid. This may suggest a lower level of job satisfaction among the most the nursing professionals with a highest level of education [33], or perhaps it may reflect a greater capacity for critical thinking. This situation is paradoxical. PHC nurses look after an ageing population with highly complex and chronic conditions. Thus, it would seem reasonable to integrate nurses with high levels of training and those in advanced practice roles in PHC settings [42]. The International Council of Nurses [43] defines advanced nurse practitioners as professionals who have acquired the theoretical knowledge, complex decision-making skills and clinical competencies for extended practice in the country and context for which they are accredited. Advanced training, such as a master's or doctoral degree, is recommended for an advanced nursing practice qualification [44]. Our results show that highly qualified nurses (doctoral level) value their work environment the least, reflecting the fact that the work environment may not be adapted to the academic level of these professionals. We argue that it is necessary to ensure that highly qualified nurses and those in advanced practice roles [45] are able to work to their full potential within PHC settings in Spain, and recommend that aspects such as the nurses' level of training and expertise, and not simply their seniority and years of experience, are taken into account when designing nursing career pathways. Advanced practice nursing.

The nurses in a management role identified nursing participation in the affairs of the center (D1), nursing foundations in the quality of care (D2), management and leadership of the head nurse (D3) and human resources (D4) as strengths, with their score being higher than that of their staff nurse colleagues. This was also the case in previous studies carried out in Spain [16,17]. Interestingly, the human resources dimension (D4), which was recognized as a weakness in our study, as well as in previous studies [16], was not identified as such by the nurse managers, who considered it to be a strength. We believe that this phenomenon should be analyzed further through in-depth qualitative interviews with nurse managers, as well as other key stakeholders, in order to fully understand the root cause of this problem. Namely, it is possible that there are specific factors which are affecting the participants' assessment of the impact of the nursing workforce on the NWE. This may include the level of participation of the highest trained professionals and the quality of the relationship between the nurse managers and the rest of the staff.

Finally, from a gender perspective, no significant differences were observed when comparing the NWE with the gender of the participants in our study.

Limitations

We wish to highlight a number of limitations. First, our cross-sectional design does not allow us to infer causality in the relationships between variables. Second, although our sample is larger than that of previous PHC NWE studies, we cannot guarantee the representativeness of the entire nursing population in Spain as some of the Spanish territories are either not represented or under-represented. Third, although precautions were taken to control for duplicate responses, it is possible that some scaped our scrutiny. For these reasons, we recommend that further studies analyzing the NWE in PHC settings with more powerful samples are carried out in order to confirm these data.

5. Conclusions

The NWE in PHC settings in Spain is positive and comparatively better than the NWE in hospital settings. We identified the following strengths: (1) nursing foundation for the delivery of care, (2) management and leadership of the head nurse and (3) nurse–physician relationship, and the following weakness: (1) participation of nurses in the affairs of the center and (2) human resources. We argue that there is room for improvement of the NWE in PHC settings in Spain, and that efforts should be directed towards the neutral and negative aspects identified. Two groups of nurses were particularly critical of their NWE, namely, older nurses and those educated to doctoral level. Nurse managers did not identify human resources as a weakness, contrary to the results from previous national and international investigations. We found no evidence of gender influence on the results obtained.

Author Contributions: Conceptualization, V.G.-C., R.J.-V. and J.R.M.-R.; methodology, V.G.-C., R.J.-V., M.V.V.-G., I.A.-S. and P.G.-M.; software, R.J.-V., J.C.-M., I.S.-A. and P.G.-M.; validation, V.G.-C. and J.R.M.-R.; formal analysis, P.G.-M., J.C, I.S.-A. and R.J.-V.; investigation, V.G.-C., R.J.-V., M.V.V.-G., I.A.-S., M.V.V.-G., J.C.-M. and M.V.V.-G.; resources, J.C.-M., I.S.-A. and M.V.V.-G.; data curation, P.G.-M., J.C.-M., I.A.-S., I.S.-A. and R.J.-V.; writing—original draft preparation, V.G.-C., J.R.M.-R., J.C.-M., M.V.V.-G., I.A.-S., I.S.-A. and P.G.-M.; writing—review and editing, V.G.-C., R.J.-V. and P.G.-M.; visualization, J.R.M.-R. and M.V.V.-G.; supervision, R.J.-V., J.R.M.-R. and M.V.V.-G.; project administration, V.G.-C. and J.R.M.-R. All authors have read and agreed to the published version of the manuscript.

Funding: This research received no external funding.

Int. J. Environ. Res. Public Health **2021**, *18*, 434

Institutional Review Board Statement: The study was conducted according to the guidelines of the Declaration of Helsinki, and approved by the Ethics Committee of Health Department of Xàtiva/Ontinyent (26-2-13), and others Ethics Committes: Health Department of Elx-Crevillent (21-3-14), Health Department of Elx Hospital General (6-11-13), Health Department of Torrevieja (21-3-14), and Health Services of Canary Islands (19-6-17).

Informed Consent Statement: Informed consent was obtained from all subjects involved in the study.

Data Availability Statement: Not applicable.

Conflicts of Interest: The authors declare no conflict of interest.

References

1. All-Party Parliamentary Group on Global Health (APPG). *Triple Impact: How Developing Nursing Will Improve Health, Promote Gender Equality and Support Economic Growth*; APPG: London, UK, 2016. Available online: https://www.who.int/hrh/com-heeg/triple-impact-appg/en/ (accessed on 3 February 2020).
2. Jurado, I. Actitudes, uso y propuestas sobre el sistema sanitario español. *Encuentros Multidiscip.* **2012**, *14*, 37–47. Available online: http://dialnet.unirioja.es/servlet/oaiart?codigo=3980519 (accessed on 10 October 2019).
3. Bayle, M.S. La contrarreforma sanitaria. *Pap. Relac. Ecosociales Cambio Glob.* **2013**, *123*, 63–72. Available online: https://www.fuhem.es/papeles_articulo/la-contrarreforma-sanitaria/ (accessed on 15 October 2019).
4. Gea-Caballero, V.; Castro-Sánchez, E.; Júarez-Vela, R.; Díaz-Herrera, M.Á.; de Miguel-Montoya, I.; Martínez-Riera, J.R. Elementos esenciales de los entornos profesionales enfermeros en Atención Primaria y su influencia en la calidad del cuidado. *Enferm. Clín.* **2018**, *28*, 27–35. [CrossRef]
5. Trinkoff, A.M.; Johantgen, M.; Storr, C.L.; Han, K.; Liang, Y.; Gurses, A.P.; Hopkinson, S. A comparison of working conditions among nurses in magnet® and non-magnet® hospitals. *J. Nurs. Admin.* **2010**, *40*, 309–315. [CrossRef] [PubMed]
6. Jarrín, O.; Flynn, L.; Lake, E.T.; Aiken, L.H. Home health agency work environments and hospitalizations. *Med. Care* **2014**, *52*, 877. [CrossRef]
7. Aiken, L.H.; Sloane, D.M.; Bruyneel, L.; Van den Heede, K.; Griffiths, P.; Busse, R.; McHugh, M.D. Nurse staffing and education and hospital mortality in nine European countries: A retrospective observational study. *Lancet* **2014**, *383*, 1824–1830. [CrossRef]
8. Liu, C.F.; Sharp, N.D.; Sales, A.E.; Lowy, E.; Maciejewski, M.L.; Needleman, J.; Li, Y.F. Line authority for nurse staffing and costs for acute inpatient care. *INQUIRY J. Health Care* **2009**, *46*, 339–351. [CrossRef]
9. Lake, E.T. Development of the practice environment scale of the Nursing Work Index. *Res. Nurs. Health* **2002**, *25*, 176–188. [CrossRef]
10. Bashaw, E.S. Fusing Magnet® and just culture. *Am. Nurse Today* **2011**, *6*, 42–45. Available online: https://www.myamericannurse.com/fusing-magnet-and-just-culture/ (accessed on 20 January 2020).
11. Bashaw, E.S.; Rosenstein, A.H.; Lounsbury, K. Culture trifecta: Building the infrastructure for Magnet® and just culture. *Am. Nurse Today* **2012**, *7*, 38–41. Available online: https://www.myamericannurse.com/culture-trifecta-building-the-infrastructure-for-magnet-and-just-culture/ (accessed on 25 January 2020).
12. Drenkard, K. Magnet momentum: Creating a culture of safety. *Nurse Lead.* **2011**, *9*, 28–46. [CrossRef]
13. Petit dit Dariel, O.; Regnaux, J.P. Do Magnet®-accredited hospitals show improvements in nurse and patient outcomes compared to non-Magnet hospitals: A systematic review. *JBI Database Syst. Rev.* **2015**, *13*, 168–219. [CrossRef]
14. Anderson, V.L.; Johnston, A.N.; Massey, D.; Bamford-Wade, A. Impact of MAGNET hospital designation on nursing culture: An integrative review. *Contemp. Nurse* **2018**, *54*, 483–510. [CrossRef] [PubMed]
15. Lake, E.T.; Sanders, J.; Duan, R.; Riman, K.A.; Schoenauer, K.M.; Chen, Y. A meta-analysis of the associations between the nurse work environment in hospitals and 4 sets of outcomes. *Med. Care* **2019**, *57*, 353–361. [CrossRef]
16. Gea-Caballero, V.; Díaz-Herrera, M.A.; Juárez-Vela, R.; Ferrer-Ferrándiz, E.; Tenías-Burillo, J.M.; Martínez-Riera, J.R. Perception of the professional nursing care in primary care in the Valencian Community, in departments with public and private management. *An. Sist. Sanit. Navar.* **2018**, *42*, 159–168. [CrossRef]
17. Parro-Moreno, A.; Serrano, P.; Ferrer, C.; Serrano, L.; de la Puerta, M.L.; Barberá, A.; de Pedro, J. Influence of socio-demographic, labour and professional factors on nursing perception concerning practice environment in Primary Health Care. *Aten. Prim.* **2013**, *45*, 476–485. [CrossRef] [PubMed]
18. De Pedro-Gómez, J.; Morales-Asencio, J.M.; Sesé Abad, A.; Bennasar Veny, M.; Artigues Vives, G.; Perelló Campaner, C. Nursing practice settings and competence to incorporate evidence into decisions: Analysis of the situation in the Balearic Islands (Spain). *Gac. Sanit.* **2011**, *25*, 191. [CrossRef] [PubMed]
19. Lucas, P.; Nunes, E. Nursing practice environment in Primary Health Care: A scoping review. *Rev. Bras. Enferm.* **2020**, *73*, e20190479. [CrossRef] [PubMed]
20. Poghosyan, L.; Boyd, D.R.; Clarke, S.P. Optimizing full scope of practice for nurse practitioners in primary care: A proposed conceptual model. *Nurs. Outlook* **2016**, *64*, 146–155. [CrossRef]
21. Van Selm, M.; Jankowski, N.W. Conducting online surveys. *Qual. Quant.* **2006**, *40*, 435–456. [CrossRef]
22. Norman, R.M.; Sjetne, I.S. Measuring nurses' perception of work environment: A scoping review of questionnaires. *BMC Nurs.* **2017**, *16*, 66. [CrossRef] [PubMed]

23. Gajewski, B.J.; Boyle, D.K.; Miller, P.A.; Oberhelman, F.; Dunton, N. A multilevel confirmatory factor analysis of the Practice Environment Scale: A case study. *Nurs. Res.* **2010**, *59*, 147–153. [CrossRef] [PubMed]
24. Alzate, L.C.C.; Bayer, G.L.A.; Allison Squires, B.S.N. Validation of a Spanish version of the Practice Environment Scale of the Nursing Work Index in the Colombian context. *Hisp. Health Care Int.* **2014**, *12*, 34. [CrossRef]
25. De Pedro-Gómez, J.; Morales-Asencio, J.M.; Sesé-Abad, A.; Bennasar-Veny, M.; Pericas-Beltran, J.; Miguélez-Chamorro, A. Psychometric testing of the Spanish version of the practice environment scale of the nursing work index in a primary healthcare context. *J. Adv. Nurs.* **2012**, *68*, 212–221. [CrossRef] [PubMed]
26. Gea-Caballero, V.; Juárez-Vela, R.; Díaz-Herrera, M.Á.; Mármol-López, M.I.; Blazquez, R.A.; Martínez-Riera, J.R. Development of a short questionnaire based on the Practice Environment Scale-Nursing Work Index in primary health care. *PeerJ* **2019**, *7*, e7369. [CrossRef]
27. George, D.; Mallery, P. *SPSS/PC + Step by Step: A Simple Guide and Reference*; Wadsworth Publishing Company: Belmont, CA, USA, 1994.
28. De Pedro-Gómez, J.; Morales-Asencio, J.M.; Sesé Abad, A.; Bennasar Veny, M.; Artigues Vives, G.; Perelló Campaner, C. Entorno de práctica de los profesionales de enfermería y competencia para la incorporación de la evidencia a las decisiones: Situación en las Islas Baleares. *Gac. Sanit.* **2011**, *25*, 191–197. Available online: http://scielo.isciii.es/scielo.php?script=sci_arttext&pid=S0213-91112011000300004&lng=es (accessed on 15 October 2019). [CrossRef]
29. Kramer, M. Magnet hospital nurses describe control over nursing practice. *West. J. Nurs. Res.* **2003**, *25*, 434–452. [CrossRef]
30. Kramer, M.; Schmalenberg, C. Essentials of a magnetic work environment part 1. *Nursing* **2004**, *34*, 50–54. [CrossRef]
31. Fuentelsaz-Gallego, C.; Moreno-Casbas, T.; López-Zorraquino, D.; Gómez-García, T.; González-María, E. Percepción del entorno laboral de las enfermeras españolas en los hospitales del Sistema Nacional de Salud. Proyecto RN4CAST-España. *Enferm. Clín.* **2012**, *22*, 261–268. [CrossRef]
32. Mainz, H.; Baernholdt, M.; Ramlau-Hansen, C.H.; Brink, O. Comparison of nurse practice environments in Denmark and the USA. *Int. Nurs. Rev.* **2015**, *62*, 479–488. [CrossRef]
33. Wang, Y.; Dong, W.; Mauk, K.; Li, P.; Wan, J.; Yang, G.; Hao, M. Nurses' practice environment and their job satisfaction: A study on nurses caring for older adults in shanghai. *PLoS ONE* **2015**, *10*, e0138035. [CrossRef] [PubMed]
34. Topçu, I.; Türkmen, E.; Badır, A.; Göktepe, N.; Miral, M.; Albayrak, S.; Özcan, D. Relationship between nurses' practice environments and nursing outcomes in Turkey. *Int. Nurs. Rev.* **2016**, *63*, 242–249. [CrossRef]
35. Tei-Tominaga, M.; Sato, F. Effect of nurses' work environment on patient satisfaction: A cross-sectional study of four hospitals in Japan. *Jpn. J. Nurs. Sci.* **2016**, *13*, 105–113. [CrossRef] [PubMed]
36. Escobar-Aguilar, G.; Gómez-García, T.; Ignacio-García, E.; Rodríguez-Escobar, J.; Moreno-Casbas, T.; Fuentelsaz-Gallego, C.; Contreras-Moreira, M. Entorno laboral y seguridad del paciente: Comparación de datos entre los estudios SENECA y RN4CAST. *Enferm. Clín.* **2013**, *23*, 103–113. [CrossRef] [PubMed]
37. Consejo General de Enfermería. Informe Sobre Recursos Humanos Sanitarios en España y la Unión Europea 2014. Análisis Comparativo de la Situación de Médicos y Enfermeras. Available online: https://www.consejogeneralenfermeria.org/sala-de-prensa/doc-interes/send/19-documentos-de-interes/567-informe-sobre-recursos-humanos-sanitarios-en-espana-y-la-union-europea-2015 (accessed on 23 November 2020).
38. Organisation for Economic Co-operation and Development. 2020. Available online: https://stats.oecd.org/Index.aspx?DataSetCode=HEALTH_REAC (accessed on 28 September 2020).
39. Seccia, R. The Nurse Rostering Problem in COVID-19 emergency scenario. In *Technical Report*; Sapienza University of Rome: Rome, Italy, 2020; Available online: http://www.optimization-online.org/DB_FILE/2020/03/7712.pdf (accessed on 23 November 2020).
40. World Health Organization. La OMS y Sus Asociados Hacen un Llamamiento Urgente para que se Invierta en el Personal de Enfermería. Available online: https://www.who.int/es/news-room/detail/07-04-2020-who-and-partners-call-for-urgent-investment-in-nurses (accessed on 28 September 2020).
41. Martínez-Riera, J.R.; Juárez-Vela, R.; Díaz-Herrera, M.Á.; Montejano-Lozoya, R.; Doménech-Briz, V.; Benavent-Cervera, J.V.; Cabellos-García, A.C.; Melo, P.; Nguyen, T.H.; Gea-Caballero, V. Qualitative Analysis by Experts of the Essential Elements of the Nursing Practice Environments Proposed by the TOP10 Questionnaire of Assessment of Environments in Primary Health Care. *Int. J. Environ. Res. Public Health* **2020**, *17*, 7520. [CrossRef] [PubMed]
42. Naylor, M.D.; Kurtzman, E.T. The role of nurse practitioners in reinventing primary care. *Health Aff.* **2010**, *29*, 893–899. [CrossRef]
43. International Council of Nurses. Nurse Practitioner/Advanced Practice Network: Definitions and Characteristics of the Role. Available online: https://international.aanp.org/Practice/APNRoles (accessed on 25 April 2020).
44. Gysin, S.; Sottas, B.; Odermatt, M.; Essig, S. Advanced practice nurses' and general practitioners' first experiences with introducing the advanced practice nurse role to Swiss PHC: A qualitative study. *BMC Fam. Pract.* **2019**, *20*, 1–11. [CrossRef] [PubMed]
45. Swan, M.; Ferguson, S.; Chang, A.; Larson, E.; Smaldone, A. Quality of PHC by advanced practice nurses: A systematic review. *Int. J. Qual. Health Care* **2015**, *27*, 396–404. [CrossRef]

International Journal of
Environmental Research and Public Health

MDPI

Article

Friendship and Consumption Networks in Adolescents and Their Relationship to Stress and Cannabis Use Intention

María Cristina Martínez-Fernández [1], Cristina Liébana-Presa [1,*], Elena Fernández-Martínez [2], Lisa Gomes [3] and Isaías García-Rodríguez [4]

1   SALBIS Research Group, Faculty of Health Sciences, Campus de Ponferrada, Universidad de León, 24401 Ponferrada, Spain; mmartf@unileon.es
2   SALBIS Research Group, Faculty of Health Sciences, Universidad de León, 24071 León, Spain; elena.fernandez@unileon.es
3   Nursing School, Minho University, 4704-553 Braga, Portugal; lgomes@ese.uminho.pt
4   SECOMUCI Research Groups, Department of Electric, Systems and Automatics Engineering, Universidad de León, 24071 León, Spain; isaias.garcia@unileon.es
*   Correspondence: cliep@unileon.es

Abstract: Background: Cannabis is an illegal psychoactive substance that's use is widespread among adolescents. During adolescence, many changes can cause stress. In this phase, the group of friends becomes increasingly important, being a situation of vulnerability for the beginning of cannabis use, either as an escape mechanism or due to peer's influence. Therefore, the purpose of this study is to describe and analyze the structure of the consumption and friendship network, the intention to use cannabis, and the stress in a secondary school class. Methods: An online platform with validated self-reported questionnaires were used for data collection. Results: The sample consisted of adolescents (*n* = 20) aged 14–16 from a third-year class of compulsory secondary education in Ponferrada (León, Spain). Significant differences were obtained concerning consumption intention and the different network metrics in both the friendship and consumption networks. Subsequently, the representation of these networks was carried out. Conclusions: Social Network Analysis is a very useful tool that provides a picture of the context in which adolescents are located. In the consumption network, there are central actors who have not yet consumed cannabis; this is a crucial moment to implement prevention strategies.

Keywords: cannabis; adolescents; stress; social network analysis; network; friendship

check for updates

Citation: Martínez-Fernández, M.C.; Liébana-Presa, C.; Fernández-Martínez, E.; Gomes, L.; García-Rodríguez, I. Friendship and Consumption Networks in Adolescents and Their Relationship to Stress and Cannabis Use Intention. *Int. J. Environ. Res. Public Health* **2021**, *18*, 3335. https://doi.org/10.3390/ijerph18073335

Academic Editor: Paul B. Tchounwou

Received: 26 February 2021
Accepted: 21 March 2021
Published: 24 March 2021

Publisher's Note: MDPI stays neutral with regard to jurisdictional claims in published maps and institutional affiliations.

1. Introduction

According to the World Health Organization (WHO), cannabis is the most widely consumed drug among young people in 2018; approximately 4.7% of young people aged 15 to 16 years had consumed it at least once [1]. In Spain, the most recent data indicate that cannabis is the illegal psychoactive substance with the highest prevalence of use, with an average age of onset of 14.8 years; in fact, 398,600 students aged 14 to 18 years had consumed cannabis during 2016 [2]. Substance use is related to multiple risk factors, including school failure and problematic behaviors [3]. Additionally, substance use can lead to physical, psychological and social disorders that demand the design of effective prevention policies [4]. Substance use and abuse is, therefore, one of the main risk factors for health, where adolescent users are more likely to manifest social and personal issues, lower psychological adjustment and emotional competence [5].

Adolescence is a period of change. A key characteristic of youth is that it is a relevant phase in the consolidation, gain or loss of previously acquired habits and lifestyles, which has an impact on the future health status of individuals [6]. Emotional and behavioral adjustment problems have been seen as mediators between cannabis use and psychosis risk [7]. Early initiated cannabis use results as a significant marker of mental health and behavioral risk [8]. Therefore, well-being in adolescents plays a key role in preventing substance use [7]. Moreover, burnout experienced by adolescents in high school can have an influence on cannabis use, being relevant to the consideration of academic stress in the prevention of cannabis use, since its use causes a loss of academic expectations and motivation [9].

As previously mentioned, cannabis use may appear as an escape mechanism from stress [10]; in fact, those adolescents who do not use cannabis cope with stress in a more flexible way [11]. There are cognitive schemes based on beliefs of grandiosity and insufficient self-control that are significantly associated with drug use [12]. The theory of planned behavior provides an explanation for cannabis use and describes the relationship between cognitive characteristics of individuals and the development and maintenance of behavioral patterns [13]. Developmental theories indicate that the transition to adolescence is decided by an increase in the frequency of peer interactions, the adoption of more sophisticated interpersonal behaviors, new social roles and experiences, adolescents' motivation to develop a stable sense of identity, and young people's reliance on peer feedback (and their perceived status by peers) [14].

In this context, the concept of Social Network Analysis (SNA) emerged, is proving an impact on the health. Peers are fundamental in the social organization of adolescents, as they are present in the academic environment and activities. Likewise, during adolescents' development, they increasingly acquire more autonomy and independence from their family environment [15,16]. SNA has been widely applied in public health, social support, social capital, influences on health behaviors, and the social structure of information dissemination [17]. Many studies have been carried out using the SNA in adolescents, indicating how the position in the peer group and popularity have an influence on relevant aspects, such as leisure activities and eating behaviors that spread in the friendship network, influencing overweight [18] and even sleeping habits, where the most popular adolescents sleep less than the rest of the individuals in the network [19].

SNA is a theoretical and methodological paradigm that makes possible to evaluate the relational context empirically and to capture contexts of social interaction, which determine the behavior of the actors that are part of that context [17]. Thus, one of the key components in adolescent well-being are social networks. The literature has found that having friends or being connected to friendship networks that exhibit risky behaviors (smoking or drinking alcohol) implies an increased risk of engaging in these behaviors, both initially and over time [20]. SNA can be helpful in better understanding the mechanisms underlying the connection between friendships and risk behaviors [20]. Adolescent contacts are important for the establishment of adolescent health, as well as for the acquisition and maintenance of risk behaviors [21,22].

Peer influence is defined as a phenomenon characterized by the presence of both selection and socialization. By understanding why adolescents fit in with their peers, it is possible to develop preventive measures that alternatively address the psychological motivations that lead to conformity at present [14]. However, peer influence from adolescence to adulthood has been found to be later much less clear [23].

Following the exposed problem, this study has the following question: what is the relationship between the structural characteristics of friendship and cannabis use networks, an individual's intention to use cannabis and young adolescents' stress? The SNA can become a useful tool that will allow us to know the behavioral pattern of the network in order to plan concrete and effective interventions on the identified risk behaviors (cannabis use intention and stress), in short, to promote healthy and sustainable networks. Therefore, the aim of this study is to describe the structure of the consumption and friendship network, the intention to use cannabis and the stress of young adolescents in a secondary school class, and, furthermore, to analyze the relationships between network structural variables, consumption intention and stress and to represent these relationships in order to identify peer leaders and plan interventions that promote health (less stress and less consumption).

2. Materials and Methods

A cross-sectional, descriptive and correlational study was conducted. A nonproba-bilistic convenience sample was selected. The sample is composed of all students enrolled in a 3rd-year class in a Compulsory Secondary Education (E.S.O.) center in the city of Ponferrada (León, Spain) during the 2019/2020 academic year. The criteria for selecting this class are twofold: (i) the age of the students is at the age of initiation of cannabis use and (ii) previous academic courses that ensure the coexistence of students. The selected class has 20 students.

2.1. Variables and Measuring Instruments

Stress: Stress was measured using the Student Stress Inventory–Stress Manifestations (SSI–SM) [24] validated in Spanish for adolescents [25]. This questionnaire consists of 22 items, with a five-point Likert-type scale (not at all, rarely, sometimes, often and totally). These items are distributed in three factors: emotional ($\alpha = 0.79$), physiological ($\alpha = 0.62$) and behavioral ($\alpha = 0.66$).

Cannabis use: To measure cannabis use, the Spanish Survey on Drug Use in Secondary Education (ESTUDES) [2] is used. This questionnaire is composed of different items, according to the substances, from which we selected those referring to the block of cannabis use. The section is made up of 10 items related to the time that cannabis has been used, the first time it was used and how it is used.

Cannabis Use Intention: The validated Cannabis Use: Intention Questionnaire (CUIQ) was used for the youth population [26]. This questionnaire comprises 12 items. Each one of the items is evaluated by means of a Likert-type scale from 1 to 5 points.

Networks: To determine the classroom consumption and friendship network, a limited census of actors is used that is matched to the list of classroom peers. Students are asked to nominate only those actors/peers in their class with whom they would go out to consume. With the data collected, a sociocentric matrix is obtained. In the same way, to obtain the classroom friendship network, students were asked to nominate from the census of actors those classmates with whom they share their free time. A 4-point Likert-type scale was used, where 0 means "I never share my free time," and 4 means "We are always together."

2.2. Procedure

Data were collected by online questionnaire. Authorization was obtained by the corresponding Compulsory Secondary Education center, and the teacher of the class involved was contacted to make them aware of the procedure. Data collection took place on different days in February 2020. The online questionnaire was carried out in different web programming languages, PHP (Zend, Minneapolis, MN, USA) and MySQL (Oracle, Santa Clara, CA, USA) for its dynamization, together with a front-end based on HTML5 (World Wide Web Consortium (W3C), Cambridge, MA, USA), CSS (World Wide Web Consortium (W3C), Cambridge, MA, USA), JavaScript (Oracle, Santa Clara, CA, USA) (and jQuery (The OpenJS Foundation, San Francisco, CA, USA)), complying with different standards and measures that facilitate its visualization on different devices (responsive design).

2.3. Data Analysis

Qualitative variables are shown as frequencies and percentages. Quantitative variables were expressed as mean and standard deviation. After verifying that the quantitative variables did not follow a normal distribution, using the Kolmogorov–Smirnov test with Lilliefors correction, nonparametric correlations were performed, and Spearman's rho coefficients were obtained. Statistical analyses were carried out using Statistical Package for the Social Sciences software (SPSS v. 26.0) (IBM, Armonk, NY, USA).

For network analysis, the data obtained were transferred to Excel and processed using the UCINET V 6.0 program and NetDraw [27]. Centrality measures (see Table 1) were calculated for the participants.

Table 1. Definitions of the Social Network Analysis (SNA) centrality metrics.

Concept	Definition
InDegree Centrality	Number of people who ask the actor for advice [28].
Betweenness centrality	Extent to which an actor serves as a potential "go-between" for other pairs of actors in the network by occupying an intermediary position on the shortest paths connecting other actors [28].
Closeness centrality	Measures how close an actor is to the other actors in the network [29].
Eigenvector Centrality	Measure of actor centrality that takes into account the centrality of the actors to whom the focal actor is connected. Thus, an actor whose three friends have many connections will have higher Eigenvector centrality than an actor whose three friends have few connections [28].

2.4. Ethical Considerations

The anonymity and confidentiality of the study subjects were considered at all times. Being underage minors, prior authorization was received from their parents or legal guardians for participation in the study, as well as the informed consent of the participants. The data obtained from the research will be treated in accordance with both the Constitutional Law 3/2018, of December 5, on the Protection of Personal Data and Guarantee of Digital Rights and the General Data Protection Regulation of the European Union EU 2016/679 (GDPR). In addition, permission was requested from the educational center and the competent body for education in the region (Consejería de Educación de la Junta de Castilla y León). The study was approved by the ethics committee (ETICA-ULE-035-2019) of the University of León (Spain), which ensures compliance with ethical and legal aspects.

3. Results

The sample consisted of a total of 20 adolescents, of which 10% were female ($n = 2$), and 90% male ($n = 18$), with an age measurement of 14.45 $\pm$ 0.61 (min = 14; max = 16).

First, regarding the results of cannabis use, the data obtained place the prevalence of cannabis use at 10% ($n = 2$). Of these, one individual's last cannabis use was 40 days ago, while the other shows a more habitual use, being the last use 3 days ago. The age of onset of use was 13 years old. One of the two consumers used cannabis mixed with tobacco. When asked that, if cannabis consumption were legal would they consume it, 20% of the students said that they would consume it, while 15% of the sample had already tried it (including consumers). Finally, it is worth noting that one student consumed cannabis alone quite often, while the other indicated that he had never consumed cannabis alone. Regarding the cannabis use intention, the total values are 1.35 $\pm$ 1.13; however, we find a high maximum, that result in the equivalence table indicates that it is above the 90th percentile. This means that 90% of young people of the same age have a lower intention to consume than this one.

Secondly, the descriptive results obtained for the variable stress and are set out in Table 2. Stress obtained total values of 37.65 $\pm$ 18.45.

Table 2. Descriptive statistics of stress.

Questionnaire		n	Min–Max	M $\pm$ SD	Me
SSI–SM	Emotional	20	0–40	18.85 $\pm$ 9.99	18
	Physiological	20	0–17	9.15 $\pm$ 4.46	9
	Behavioral	20	0–25	9.65 $\pm$ 5.93	8.5
	Total	20	0–77	37.65 $\pm$ 18.45	37.5

Note: SSI–SM; Student Stress Inventory–Stress Manifestations. Min–Max; Minimum–Maximum. M; Mean. SD; Standard Deviation. Me; Median.

Thirdly, Table 3 shows the values of the structure of the consumption and friendship networks, the actors who may be in more central positions in the networks and with greater degree of influence. The following parameters are described: indegree, outdegree, degree of proximity (out/in closeness), betweenness, and influence through the eigenvector. It is found that networks are similar in terms of values and density, which may suggest that adolescents select their friends as the peers with whom they would go out to consume.

Table 3. Descriptive indicators of centrality in consumption and friendship networks.

SNA Centrality Metrics		Min–Max.	M ± SD
Consumption Network	Indegree	0–0.42	0.22 ± 0.18
	Outdegree	0–0.89	0.22 ± 0.25
	Out closeness	0.25–0.83	0.43 ± 0.18
	In closeness	0.25–0.41	0.37 ± 0.03
	Betweenness	0–11.41	1.84 ± 3.20
	Eigenvector	0–54.26	28.38 ± 14.30
Friendship Network	Indegree	0–0.30	0.20 ± 0.20
	Outdegree	0–0.63	0.20 ± 0.10
	Out closeness	0.25–0.83	0.54 ± 0.21
	In closeness	0.25–0.51	0.45 ± 0.06
	Betweenness	0–6.39	1.46 ± 1.83
	Eigenvector	0–53.87	28.43 ± 14.21

Note: Min–Max; Minimum–Maximum. M; Mean. SD; Standard Deviation.

Figure 1 illustrates the distribution of normalized betweenness in the friendship network, showing that a large number of individuals have a very low intermediation capacity. In fact, 30% of the individuals have no intermediation capacities at all.

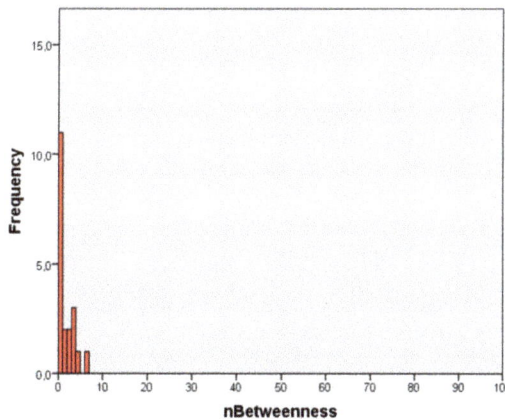

Figure 1. Normalized Betweenness (nBetweenness) centrality distribution.

A correlational analysis between the different variables, stress, cannabis use intention and friendship and consumption networks is shown in Table 4.

43

Table 4. Correlations between centrality metrics of friendship and consumption networks, stress and cannabis use intention.

			SSI–SM				
			Emotional	Physiological	Behavioral	Total	CUIQ
Consumption Network	Indegree	Rho	−0.354	−0.150	0.191	−0.088	−0.034
	Outdegree	Rho	−0.024	0.191	0.376	0.192	0.525 *
	Out closeness	Rho	−0.015	0.174	0.346	0.182	0.500 *
	In closeness	Rho	−0.272	−0.181	0.084	−0.121	−0.249
	Betweenness	Rho	0.048	0.265	0.421	0.278	0.549 *
	Eigenvector	Rho	−0.302	0.014	0.394	0.007	0.285
Friendship Network	Indegree	Rho	−0.328	0.021	0.125	-0.50	0.265
	Outdegree	Rho	0.138	0.446 *	0.530 *	0.401	0.596 **
	Out closeness	Rho	0.181	0.414	0.541 *	0.399	0.531 *
	In closeness	Rho	−0.511 **	-0.188	0.074	−0.270	0.016
	Betweenness	Rho	0.153	0.417	0.496 *	0.375	0.598 **
	Eigenvector	Rho	−0.295	0.194	0.297	0.063	0.337
SSI–SM. Total		Rho	0.825 **	0.925 **	0.799 **		
CUIQ		Rho	0.510 *	0.687 **	0.479 *	0.622 **	

Note. CUIQ; Cannabis Use: Intention Questionnaire. SSI–SM; Student Stress Inventory–Stress Manifestations. Rho: Spearman's correlation. * Correlation is significant at the 0.05 level. ** Correlation is significant at the 0.01 level.

No significant correlations were found for cannabis use with these data, given the small sample size of the consumers. Behavioral manifestations of stress involve behaviors, such as acting defensively, neglecting friendships or showing negative attitudes in different interpersonal relationships. In this regard, it is noteworthy that a statistically significant correlation was found between the behavioral manifestations of stress dimension and the metrics of out closeness ($r = 0.541$), outdegree ($r = 0.530$) and the degree of betweenness ($r = 0.496$). In addition, statistically significant correlations were found in this network for in closeness ($r = −0.511$), emotional manifestations and physical manifestations and outdegree ($r = 0.446$). The cannabis use intention appears statistically significantly correlated with different network metrics: for the friendship network, outdegree ($r = 0.596$), out closeness ($r = 0.531$) and betweenness ($r = 0.598$), while, in the consumption network, outdegree ($r = 0.252$), out closeness ($r = 0.500$) and betweenness ($r = 0.549$). On the other hand, it shows a statistically significant correlation with total stress ($r = 0.622$) and its different manifestations: emotional ($r = 0.510$), physiological ($r = 0.687$) and behavioral ($r = 0.0479$).

Figure 2 represents the classroom friendship network, where males are represented with a blue color and females with a pink color. Cannabis users are identified as square-shaped nodes and nonusers as circles. The size of the nodes varies according to their total stress. The intensity of the relationships is measured through the strength of the ties (0–4), where a greater strength indicates that these students are united by a bond of friendship by spending a large part of their free time together. The size of the nodes varies as a function of the total stress scores. Thus, we find how individuals who are consumers are close and could be considered friends. These nodes, although they have relationships with those actors who are more central, establish ties of greater intensity with actors who are on the periphery. However, it stands out how the girl who uses cannabis establishes ties of friendship with the central actors, being, in addition, one of the individuals with higher levels of stress. In general, we found a dense network, where relationships of varying intensity were high. We found an isolated node and a node on the periphery that only maintains a relationship with two individuals from the others in the class, being also one of the individuals with the highest level of general stress.

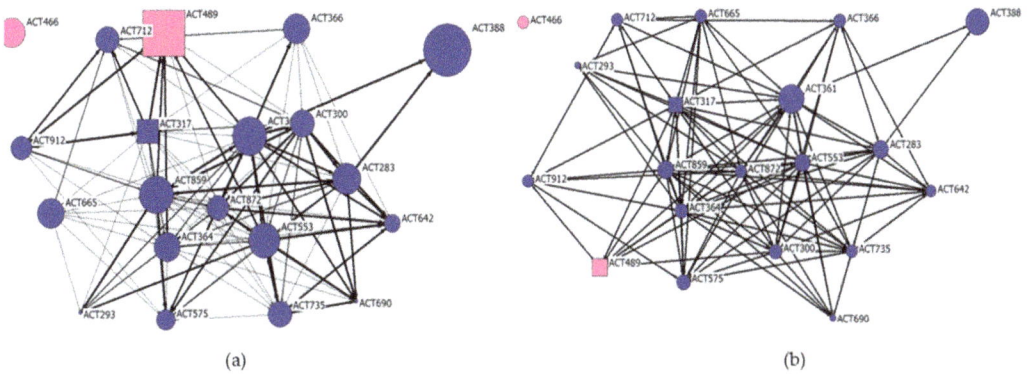

Color. Pink: Female / Blue: Male. Shape. Square: Cannabis user / Circle: Non-Cannabis user
Node size: according to behavioral manifestations. Bond density: according to friendship intensity (0- 4)

Figure 2. Friendship network structure and the study variables; (**a**) total of Student Stress Inventory–Stress Manifestations, (**b**) bbehavioral of Student Stress Inventory–Stress Manifestations.

Figure 3 shows the classroom consumption network from which students were asked to select, out of all their classmates, those individuals with whom they would consume. As in the previous case, the size of the nodes varies as a function of the total stress scores or the behavioral manifestations of stress. The structure is similar to the friendship network, since the central actors are maintained, in this case, the central actor being a cannabis user. Consequently, it may be an indication that the friendship network influences cannabis consumption, being that this consumption is accepted by those nodes with whom they share more time.

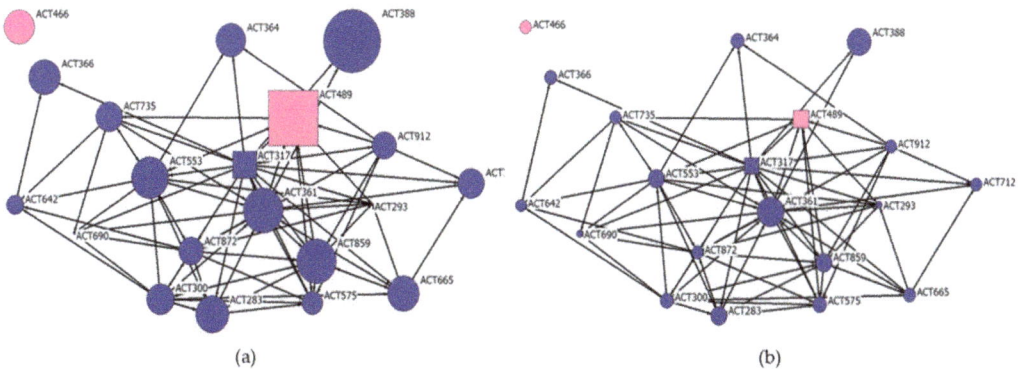

Color: Pink: Female / Blue: Male. Shape: Square: Cannabis user / Circle: Non-Cannabis user
Node size: According to behavioral manifestations.

Figure 3. Consumption network structure and the study variables; (**a**) total of Student Stress Inventory–Stress Manifestations, (**b**) behavioral of Student Stress Inventory–Stress Manifestations.

Figure 4 shows the two networks, but, in this case, the size of the node varies depending on the cannabis use intention. Although most of the subjects obtained scores according to the mean, we found nodes of greater size, whose scores were indicative of an intention higher than normal. These actors are found both in the periphery and in the center of the network and are individuals in whom action must be taken through different intervention strategies when they are in a situation of risk at the beginning of cannabis use.

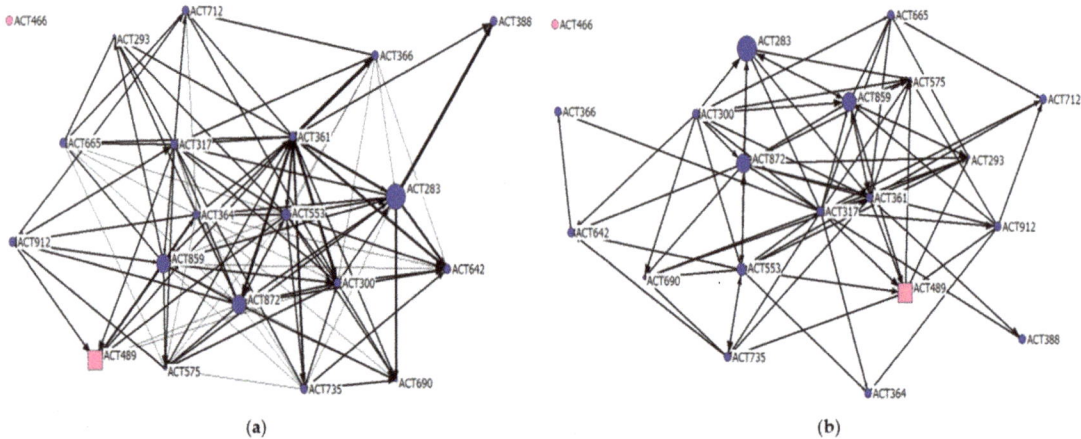

(a)   (b)

Color: Pink: Female / Blue: Male. Shape: Square: Cannabis user / Circle: Non-Cannabis user
Node size: According to cannabis use intention

Figure 4. Cannabis use intention (a) consumption network; (b) friendship network.

4. Discussion

The aim of this article is to describe the consumption and friendship network of adolescents and to relate it to stress in its different manifestations and the cannabis use intention. Subsequently, the representation of the friendship and consumption network is carried out for those variables in which significant results have been obtained: the intention to use cannabis, total stress and behavioral manifestations of stress, which are related to acting defensively, neglecting friendships, talking more about peers and teachers, picking on others, etc.

SNA allows us to locate those individuals with positions of influence within the network. Although multiple factors influence cannabis use, the literature indicates that family stressors have a direct impact on the progression to problematic cannabis use, as well as their consequent indirect effects through the school experience of young people [30]. Furthermore, cannabis use causes difficulties in school performance, creating a lack of motivation and interest that feeds back by increasing cannabis use [9]. In adolescence, there is a change in the relationship system of young people, from focusing on the family to associating with peers; in this sense, the SNA helps to explain personal attachment to the community from a local level in the structure of the friendship network and supports the peer influence theory [31]. Previous experiences have employed the SNA in school settings with adolescents to identify those who are considered leaders among their peers and train them to deliver e-cigarette prevention programs to the rest of the class [32]. In this case, through SNA, we have identified the most central actors, two individuals who are in central positions in the consumption network, who may be in positions of risk of initiation, problematic consumption or ability to transmit these behaviors to the rest of their peers, and through whom to carry out prevention strategies and interventions customized for each setting.

In addition, it is necessary to consider the emotional and behavioral adjustment problems that mediate the relationship between cannabis use and risk of psychosis [7], as this study points out, highlighting the importance of prevention by focusing on the mediating role of emotional and behavioral problems to train young people in socioemotional competencies in school contexts [7]. The literature highlights the importance of prevention and addressing adolescents before actual cannabis use takes place; as [33] says, adolescents who think more positively about being under the influence of marijuana, those with greater approval from their social environment, and those with less confidence in their ability to abstain from using have a greater intention to initiate marijuana use [33]. In addition, adolescents will have a more favorable attitude toward drug use if their contacts with environments and inciting companies and the contacts with drugs maintained by friends are greater [34]. Thus, SNA can be used as an intervention strategy to promote behavioral changes, since networks influence the health of their members by generating a context with its own behavior and norms where members can influence each other through persuasion, information exchange or support [35]. In this sense, the correlation found in this study between the betweenness centrality metric and the intention to use cannabis could be a potential danger, regarding the spreading of this unhealthy habit, as the individuals with higher betweenness values play an important role in the dissemination of behavior through the networks. This is especially relevant if one takes into account that 30% of the individuals have no intermediation capacities in the network.

This study presents advances in the area of cannabis use, since it is the first study to analyze the friendship and consumption network, stress and cannabis use intention. However, it has some limitations that should be considered: This is a small sample, which is not representative of the population, and the results should be interpreted with caution. In addition, there is a possibility that some participants did not declare their consumption, as can be seen in the classroom consumption network with very central actors not consuming, where it can be seen that those who have consumed are very central, but not all of them. In addition, in future studies, it would be useful to carry out longitudinal designs that can indicate how these variables behave over time and be able to carry out causal explanations, as well as designs where health education interventions are proposed to these population groups.

5. Conclusions

SNA is a useful tool that provides a picture of the context where adolescents are located. It allows identifying those that are more isolated, which is considered a disadvantage, and the most popular, who can be chosen as role models by their peers. After knowing the consumption network of the class, we find central actors who that have not initiated cannabis consumption. This indicates a crucial moment to carry out prevention strategies adapted to each school context. These strategies should be implemented at earlier ages, since we found several cannabis-consuming students who may have been influenced by their peers.

Author Contributions: Conceptualization, M.C.M.-F., C.L.-P. and I.G.-R.; methodology, M.C.M.-F., C.L.-P. and I.G.-R.; software, M.C.M.-F., C.L.-P. and I.G.-R.; validation, M.C.M.-F., C.L.-P. and I.G.-R.; formal analysis, M.C.M.-F., C.L.-P., E.F.-M., L.G. and I.G.-R.; investigation, M.C.M.-F., C.L.-P., E.F.-M., L.G. and I.G.-R.; resources, M.C.M.-F., C.L.-P., E.F.-M., L.G. and I.G.-R. data curation, M.C.M.-F., C.L.-P. and I.G.-R.; writing—original draft preparation, M.C.M.-F., C.L.-P. and I.G.-R.; writing—review and editing, E.F.-M. and L.G.; visualization, M.C.M.-F., C.L.-P. and I.G.-R.; supervision, C.L.-P. and I.G.-R. All authors have read and agreed to the published version of the manuscript.

Funding: This research received no external funding.

Institutional Review Board Statement: The study was conducted according to the guidelines of the Declaration of Helsinki and approved by Ethics Committee of University de Leon (ETICA-ULE-035-2019).

Informed Consent Statement: Informed consent was obtained from all subjects involved in the study.

Data Availability Statement: Not Applicable.

Acknowledgments: We thank Benítez-Andrades J.A. for his contribution and help in the management of data collection and Marqués-Sánchez P. for her willingness, help and vision throughout the process.

Conflicts of Interest: The authors declare no conflict of interest.

References

1. World Health Organization. Adolescent Mental Health. Available online: https://www.who.int/es/news-room/fact-sheets/detail/adolescent-mental-health (accessed on 8 January 2021).
2. Observatorio Español de las Drogas y las Adicciones. ESTUDES 2018/19. Encuesta sobre el Uso de Drogas en Enseñanzas Secundarias en España (1994–2018). Available online: http://www.pnsd.mscbs.gob.es/profesionales/sistemasInformacion/sistemaInformacion/pdf/ESTUDES_2018-19_Informe.pdf. (accessed on 3 January 2021).
3. Espada, J.P.; Griffin, K.W.; Botvin, G.J.; Méndez, X. Adolescencia: Consumo de Alcohol y Otras Drogas. *Papeles Del Psicólogo* **2003**, *23*, 9–17.
4. Palacio, A.B.; Santana, J.D.M.; Monroy, M.F.; Sánchez, I.G.; Meneses, G.D. Modelo Explicativo Del Comportamiento De Los Jóvenes Ante El Botellón Y El Cannabis Desde La Perspectiva Del Marketing Social. *Rev. Española Investig. Mark ESIC* **2012**, *16*, 87–111. [CrossRef]
5. Extremera, N.; Fernández-Berrocal, P. The Subjective Happiness Scale: Translation and Preliminary Psychometric Evaluation of a Spanish Version. *Soc. Indic. Res.* **2014**, *119*, 473–481. [CrossRef]
6. Fernández Villa, T.; Alguacil Ojeda, J.; Ayán Pérez, C.; Bueno Cavanillas, A.; Cancela Carral, J.M.; Capelo Álvarez, R.; Delgado Rodríguez, M.; Jiménez Mejías, E.; Jiménez Moleón, J.J.; Llorca Díaz, J.; et al. UNIHCOS Project: Dynamic cohort of Spanish college students to the study of drug and other addictions. *Rev. Esp. Salud. Publica.* **2013**, *87*, 575–585. Available online: http://www.ncbi.nlm.nih.gov/pubmed/24549356 (accessed on 9 January 2021). [CrossRef]
7. Fonseca-Pedrero, E.; Lucas-Molina, B.; Pérez-Albéniz, A.; Inchausti, F.; Ortuño-Sierra, J. Experiencias Psicóticas Atenuadas y Consumo de Cannabis En Adolescentes de La Población General. *Adicciones* **2019**, *32*, 41. [CrossRef]
8. Hawke, L.D.; Wilkins, L.; Henderson, J. Early cannabis initiation: Substance use and mental health profiles of service-seeking youth. *J. Adolesc.* **2020**, *83*, 112–121. [CrossRef] [PubMed]
9. Walburg, V.; Dany, M.; Aurélie, M. Burnout among High-School Students and Cannabis Use, Consumption Frequencies, Abuse and Dependence. *Child Youth Care Forum* **2015**, *44*, 33–42. [CrossRef]
10. Low, N.C.P.; Dugas, E.; O'Loughlin, E.; Rodriguez, D.; Contreras, G.; Chaiton, M.; O'Loughlin, J. Common stressful life events and difficulties are associated with mental health symptoms and substance use in young adolescents. *BMC Psychiatry* **2012**, *12*, 116. [CrossRef] [PubMed]
11. Kruczek, A. Mood and Coping Flexibility in a Group of Adolescents Using Marijuana. *Alcohol. Drug Addict. Alkohol. Narkom.* **2017**, *30*, 85–102. [CrossRef]
12. Calvete, E.; Estévez, A. Consumo de Drogas En Adolescentes: El Papel Del Estrés, La Impulsividad y Los Esquemas Relacionados Con La Falta de Límites. *Adicciones* **2019**, *21*, 49–56. [CrossRef]
13. Ajzen, I. The Theory of Planned Behavior. *Organ. Behav. Hum.* **1991**, *50*, 179–211. [CrossRef]
14. Brechwald, W.A.; Prinstein, M.J. Beyond Homophily: A Decade of Advances in Understanding Peer Influence Processes. *J. Res. Adolesc.* **2011**, *21*, 166–179. [CrossRef]
15. Moody, J. Peer Influence Groups: Identifying Dense Clusters in Large Networks. *Soc. Netw.* **2001**, *23*, 261–283. [CrossRef]
16. Osgood, D.W.; Feinberg, M.E.; Wallace, L.N.; Moody, J. Friendship Group Position and Substance Use. *Addict. Behav.* **2014**, *39*, 923–933. [CrossRef]
17. Luke, D.A.; Stamatakis, K.A. Systems Science Methods in Public Health: Dynamics, Networks, and Agents. *Annu. Rev. Public Health* **2012**, *33*, 357–376. [CrossRef] [PubMed]
18. De La Haye, K.; Garry, P.M.; Carlene, W. Obesity-Related Behaviors in Adolescent Friendship Networks. *Soc. Netw.* **2010**, *32*, 161–167. [CrossRef]
19. Li, X.; Kawachi, I.; Buxton, O.M.; Haneuse, S.; Onnela, J.P. Social Network Analysis of Group Position, Popularity, and Sleep Behaviors among U.S. Adolescents. *Soc. Sci. Med.* **2019**, *232*, 417–426. [CrossRef] [PubMed]
20. Jeon, K.C.; Goodson, P. US Adolescents' Friendship Networks and Health Risk Behaviors: A Systematic Review of Studies Using Social Network Analysis and Add Health Data. *PeerJ* **2015**, *3*, e1052. [CrossRef] [PubMed]
21. De la Haye, K.; Green, H.D., Jr.; Kennedy, D.P.; Pollard, M.S.; Tucker, J.S. Selection and Influence Mechanisms Associated with Marijuana Initiation and Use in Adolescent Friendship Networks. *J. Res. Adolesc.* **2013**, *23*, 474–486. [CrossRef] [PubMed]
22. Tucker, J.S.; de la Haye, K.; Kennedy, D.P.; Green, H.J., Jr.; Pollard, M.S. Peer Influence on Marijuana Use in Different Types of Friendships. *J. Adolesc. Health* **2014**, *54*, 67–73. [CrossRef] [PubMed]
23. Pollard, M.S.; Tuckera, J.S.; Greena, H.D.; de la Hayeb, K.; Espelagec, D.L. Adolescent Peer Networks and the Moderating Role of Depressive Symptoms on Developmental Trajectories of Cannabis Use. *Addict. Behav.* **2018**, *76*, 34–40. [CrossRef] [PubMed]
24. Fimian, M.J.; Philip, A.; Fastenau, J.H.; Tashner, A.; Cross, H. The Measure of Classroom Stress and Burnout among Gifted and Talented Students. *Psychol. Sch.* **1989**, *26*, 2, 139–153. [CrossRef]
25. Escobar, M.; Blanca, M.J.; Fernández-Baena, F.J.; Trianes, M.V. Adaptación Española de La Escala de Manifestaciones de Estrés Del Student Stress Inventory (SSI-SM). *Psicothema* **2011**, *23*, 475–485.

26. Lloret, D.; Morell-Gomis, R.; Laguia, A.; Moriano, J.A. Design and Validation of a Cannabis Use Intention Questionnaire (CUIQ) for Adolescents. *Adicciones* **2018**, *30*, 54–65. [CrossRef]
27. Borgatti, S.P.; Everett, M.G.; Freeman, L.C. *Ucinet 6 for Windows: Software for Social Network Analysis*; Analytic Technologies: Harvard, MA, USA, 2002.
28. Kilduff, M.; Tsai, W. *Social Networks and Organizations*; Sage: Thousand Oaks, CA, USA, 2003.
29. Borgatti, S.P.; Everett, M.G. Network Analysis of 2-Mode Data. *Soc. Netw.* **1997**, *19*, 243–269. [CrossRef]
30. Butters, J.E. Family stressors and adolescent cannabis use: A pathway to problem use. *J. Adolesc.* **2002**, *25*, 645–654. [CrossRef]
31. Chang, C.Y.; Wu, C.I. The friend influence in network neighbourhood context on adolescents' community attachment. *Int. J. Adolesc. Youth* **2020**, *25*, 536–550. [CrossRef]
32. Chu, K.H.; Sidani, J.; Matheny, S.; Rothenberger, S.D.; Miller, E.; Valente, T.; Robertson, L. Implementation of a cluster randomized controlled trial: Identifying student peer leaders to lead E-cigarette interventions. *Addict. Behav.* **2021**, *114*, 106726. [CrossRef]
33. Malmberg, M.; Overbeek, G.; Vermulst, A.A.; Monshouwer, K.; Vollebergh, W.A.M.; Engels, R.C.M.E. The theory of planned behavior: Precursors of marijuana use in early adolescence? *Drug Alcohol. Depend.* **2012**, *123*, 22–28. [CrossRef] [PubMed]
34. Jiménez, M.V.M.; Díaz, F.J.R.; Ruiz, C.S. Factores relacionados con las actitudes juveniles hacia el consumo de alcohol y otras sustancias psicoactivas. *Psicothema* **2006**, *18*, 52–58.
35. Knox, J.; Schneider, J.; Greene, E.; Nicholson, J.; Hasin, D.; Sandfort, T. Using social network analysis to examine alcohol use among adults: A systematic review. *PLoS ONE* **2019**, *14*, e0221360. [CrossRef] [PubMed]

International Journal of
*Environmental Research
and Public Health*

MDPI

Article

Living with the Memories—Parents' Experiences of Their Newborn Child Undergoing Heart Surgery Abroad: A Qualitative Study

Ólöf Kristjánsdóttir [1,*], Annica Sjöström-Strand [2] and Gudrún Kristjánsdóttir [1]

1   Faculty of Nursing, University of Iceland, Eirberg, Eiriksgata 34, 101 Reykjavík, Iceland; gkrist@hi.is
2   Department of Health Sciences, Faculty of Medicine, Lund University, Box 157, 22100 Lund, Sweden; annica.sjostrom-strand@med.lu.se
*   Correspondence: olofk@hi.is

Received: 22 October 2020; Accepted: 24 November 2020; Published: 28 November 2020

check for
updates

Abstract: Parents of children with a congenital heart defect needing complex heart surgery are at high risk of developing health problems. One can assume that parents whose child undergoes heart surgery abroad will undoubtably face added and unique stressors and health vulnerabilities. The aim of this qualitative study was to explore the transition experiences of parents of children who underwent a complex heart surgery abroad as newborns 1–5 years ago. The qualitative content analysis methodology by Graneheim and Lundman was used. A purposive sample of twelve parents, whose child had undergone a heart surgery abroad, participated in face-to-face, semi-structured interviews. Interviews were transcribed and analyzed using inductive qualitative content analysis. The overarching theme of "living with the memories" emerged from parents' experiences, emphasizing the long-lasting impact this stressful event had on their lives. These experiences were characterized by four main categories: (1) being in an unknown situation; (2) feeling connected; (3) wishing to be accepted; and (4) finding closure. The findings show that the transition of having a newborn child undergo heart surgery abroad superimposed on the expected parenthood. That parents need to feel connected and included as legitimate clients was highlighted in their stories of experienced vulnerabilities. The results highlight the need for interdisciplinary teams to support these vulnerable families, particularly with follow-up care.

Keywords: child; parent; congenital heart disease; heart surgery; qualitative research; content analysis; cross-border care; transitions

1. Background

Having a child with a critical congenital heart defect (CCHD) is recognized as an extremely distressing experience for parents [1], inevitably leading to vast supportive care needs that begin at the child's congenital heart defect (CHD) diagnosis and continue through surgery and childhood [2,3]. CHDs are the most common congenital abnormality among infants, with the global yearly prevalence estimated at about 1% [4]. Of these, 25% are predicted to have CCHD, which is a life-threatening condition requiring urgent heart surgery and intensive care at birth, followed by life-long medical follow-ups and often further surgery [5]. It is estimated that up to 30% of parents of children with CCHD develop post-traumatic stress disorder and 25–50% develop depression or anxiety [6]. This is problematic because a parent's ability to care for their child diminishes if their own needs are not met [2,7]. Unfortunately, these parents continue to be at a higher risk of developing mental health problems due to a lack of social support, information, and mental support [2,3].

Transitions in hospital environments (e.g., from the pediatric intensive care unit (PICU) to a clinical ward) are known as challenging experiences for parents of critically ill children [8], including those with CCHD [9,10]. Under these circumstances, insecurity, fear, stress, and anxiety are reported to be experienced by parents due to, for example, the unfamiliarity and uncertainty of the new environments. Subsequently, these may result in various changes, impacting parental and child health and well-being [8–10].

Due to the highly specialized hospital treatments complex pediatric heart surgeries require, this medical service is not always available "at home". In these instances, children may be referred overseas, where they receive state-funded cross-border care [11,12]. These unprecedented circumstances inevitably introduce heightened stress, and unique challenges to already vulnerable families. Currently, our understanding of state-funded cross-border care for children with CCHD and their families is limited. Given this dearth of knowledge, using a qualitative approach to the parental transition experience, is seen as a prerequisite for understanding the supportive care needs of these families. State-funded cross-border, or the transfer of patients between two health care systems where funding agreements are in place, is different from medical tourism, which implies patients traveling abroad to receive "out-of-pocket and third-party payments medical treatments" [13]. Both cross-border care and medical tourism involve the movement of patients and families between countries, cultures, and health care systems. This inevitably creates added stress, challenges, and burden. Even so, the contexts are very different, for example, the severity and acuity of newborn's CCHD needing cross-border care is inevitably different from medical tourism.

Scarce literature exists regarding child medical tourism [14,15]. Only three studies were found looking at parents' experiences [16–18], all focusing on older children (not newborns) receiving cancer or blood-related treatments in the United States. Two include Spanish-speaking parents from low-income countries [16,17] and one English-speaking parents from a high-income country [18]. Overall, these studies showed that transitions into new cultural environments create stress and extra burdens on families [16–18].

According to Meleis's transitions theory [19], transition is the movement from one life condition to another and involves an adaption to change. Transitions can be triggered by events that require geographical changes (e.g., relocation), where sudden and rapid adjustments to different environments are needed. This inadvertently increases individuals' stress and depletes and disrupts their usual sources of support. Therefore, creating an imbalance which can affect individual's vulnerability risk, health, and wellbeing [19]. The transitions experienced by parents of newborn children with CCHD needing heart surgery abroad, surely create an imbalance. Understanding these experiences is thus an important first step in developing quality health care for these families. Therefore, the aim of this study was to elucidate and describe parents' transition experiences of having a newborn suffering from a heart defect and having to undergo heart surgery abroad.

2. Methods

2.1. Design and Sample

A qualitative exploratory design, based on Graneheim and Lundman's content analysis methodology, was chosen to describe parents' experiences of their child undergoing heart surgery abroad [20,21]. This approach is well suited to capture a deeper understanding of a topic and to obtain a sense of individuals' experiences from their own perspective. Here, the meaning of an experience is described in terms of what and how it is experienced, and surfaces from the actual text using manifest (categories) and latent (themes) content analysis. This type of analysis is preferable when populations or topics have limited research because it helps create new knowledge that can be woven into a new or existing theory [20,21]. To ensure quality, the consolidated criteria for reporting qualitative research (COREQ) guidelines were followed in preparing this manuscript, and are provided in Supplementary Table S1.

A purposive sampling method was used to select the participants based on whether parents identified as having a child (0–18 years old) with CHD who underwent heart surgery at a university hospital in the southern part of Sweden between 2014 to 2019. Participants were included if they were over 18 years, able to speak and understand Icelandic, and if no more than 5 years had passed since their child underwent heart surgery in Sweden.

2.2. Setting and Recruitment of Participants

Participants were initially recruited from a patient database at the largest hospital in Reykjavik, Iceland. After participating in a survey, parents were asked if the researchers could contact them again in the future for an interview study. Those who provided consent were contacted by the first author (Ó.K.) via email, during which they were informed about the current study's goal and invited to participate. In total, 25 parents were invited to participate, and of these, 11 declined to participate. The final study sample consisted of 12 parents because two parents dropped out due to unforeseen events conflicting with the study.

Table 1 shows the sociodemographic and specific characteristics of the parents with regards to the travel and their child. Of the 12 participants, 7 were mothers and 5 fathers. Of these, three traveled abroad more than once, two had a child that underwent more than one surgery, one had a child that experienced severe complications and disability after surgery, and one parent had a child that died. All children were newborns when they traveled abroad for the first time for surgery. The time from child's heart surgery abroad and parents interview ranged from 1-to-5 years.

Table 1. Family demographics and background (*n* = 12).

Parent Information	*n* (%)
Role	
Mother	7 (58)
Father	5 (42)
Age [a]	
20–29 years	5 (45)
30–39 years	5 (45)
40–49 years	1 (10)
Marital status [a]	
Married/common law	7 (63)
Living separately	3 (27)
Divorced	1 (10)
Education	
Highschool diploma or vocational education	5 (42)
Tertiary (collage/university)	5 (42)
Advanced college/university	2 (16)
Total monthly family income [a]	
≤789,000 ISK	4 (37)
790,000–1.29 million ISK	5 (45)
≥1.3 million ISK	2 (18)
Other children at the time (no)	8 (67)
Both parents traveled abroad (yes)	12 (100)
Relatives traveled abroad with parents (yes)	8 (67)
Length of stay abroad [a]	
≤14 days	4 (36)
15–21 days	5 (46)
>22 days	2 (18)
Multiple travels abroad (no)	9 (75)
Time from travel abroad to study [a]	
1–2 years	5 (45)
3–5 years	6 (55)

Table 1. *Cont.*

Child Information	*n* (%)
Gender (boy)	10 (83)
Age of child at first travel abroad	
1–10 days old	7 (58)
11–30 days old	3 (25)
>31 days old	2 (17)
Delivery type (vaginal)	7 (58)
Time of diagnosis (postnatal)	9 (75)
Diagnosed heart defect (ICD-10) [b]	
Congenital malformations of great arteries (Q25)	6 (50)
Congenital malformations of pulmonary and tricuspid valves (Q22)	2 (17)
Congenital malformations of cardiac septa (Q21)	3 (25)
Discordant ventriculoarterial connection (Q20.3)	1 (8)

[a] Demographic data missing for one participant. [b] Category based on the International Classification of Diseases, Tenth Revision.

2.3. Data Collection

Data were collected between November 2019 and February 2020 via 12 individual face-to-face semi-structured interviews. The interview guide used was developed by the authors, informed by their previous work [22], confirmed in the authors group, and pilot tested both with one mother and during the first three interviews, which resulted in minor revisions. Each interview started with the broad question: "Can you please describe how you experienced having to travel to Sweden for your infant's heart surgery?" Probing questions were asked to encourage participants to describe their experience as much as possible (e.g., "Could you please explain what you mean by that?"). Selected interview questions are listed in Table 2.

Table 2. Selected interview questions.

- Could you tell me what it was like learning that your child needed heart surgery abroad?
- Could you please tell me what it was like while you were waiting to travel abroad for your child in surgery?
- Could you please tell me what it was like traveling abroad for your child surgery abroad?
- Could you tell me what it was like while you were waiting for your child in surgery?
- Could you tell me how you experienced the hospital stay abroad?
- Could you tell me how you experienced the support provided by the health care staff?
- Could you tell me what it was like being away from your family (e.g., other children)?
- Could you tell me about the things that made this experience stressful for you?
- Could you tell me about what helped you during stressful time periods?
- Could you tell me your experiences with the discharge process?
- Could you tell me how this experience has affected your health? Relationships?
- Could you tell me your experience of flying with your child back home?
- Could you tell me how it was like coming back home after the surgery?
- Could you please describe your life after you were discharged from the hospital abroad and back home?

Before the interviews started, a written informed consent form was provided and signed by the participants, and the interviewer explained her role in the research. No prior personal relationship existed between any of the researchers and the participants. All authors are female, registered pediatric nurses, with clinical experience and a research background (Masters and Doctorate degrees).

All of the interviews were carried out by the first author (Ó.K.) and took place in accordance with the parents' wishes. That is to say, 11 were conducted in a separate interview room at a university in Iceland, and one was conducted in a private room at the participant's workplace. The interviews lasted between 45 and 136 min, during which time only the interviewer and interviewee were present in the room. At the end of the interview, parents were thanked for their time and willingness to share their stories. Parents did not receive any financial reward for participating in the study.

2.4. Data Analysis

The data were analyzed using Graneheim and Lundman's [20,21] content analysis approach. The codebook was developed from the initial analysis of the data (a posterior) using an inductive method. All interviews were audio recorded, transcribed verbatim by a professional transcriber, checked for accuracy, and translated from Icelandic to English to make them available to all of the authors. The data analysis process started with the three authors reading and rereading the transcribed text individually to familiarize themselves with the material. Next, the three authors created meaning units from the text that comprised of several words or sentences that helped answer the research question. The meaning units were then condensed and labeled with codes that were understood in relation to the context (i.e., an open coding process). Initial codes were created by the three authors, who also referred to the literature when creating the final coding list. These codes facilitated the identification of concepts. Next, the authors used a categorization process to identify categories and subcategories, followed by the identification of a theme. The authors used a process of reflection and discussion to agree on the codes, categories, and themes. This resulted in the creation of a coding tree; provided as a Supplementary Table S2. This process was well documented throughout.

2.5. Ethical Considerations

Each potential participant was provided with verbal and written information stating that: (a) participation was voluntary; (b) withdrawal from the study could be made at any time without reason; and (c) all data were confidential. Each participant was provided with a written informed consent form. All parents were informed that a registered psychologist would be available to them following the interview. Permission for the study was obtained from the National Bioethics Committee of Iceland (no. 18/204) and the Icelandic Data Protection Authority.

3. Results

The overarching theme of "living with the memories" emerged from parents' closeness with their experiences, and its lasting presence in their lives. Although up to five years had passed since parents had traveled abroad for their child's heart surgery, their memories and emotions were still vivid. In all instances, parents became emotional at some point during their interview. Table 3 illustrates the overarching theme, and the four categories and eight subcategories from which this theme emerged.

Table 3. Overarching theme, main categories, and subcategories.

Overarching Theme: Living with the Memories	
Categories	**Subcategories**
1. Being in an unknown situation	a. Disrupted life b. Life on hold
2. Feeling connected	a. Supportive environment b. Handling the experience
3. Wishing being accepted	a. Parenting roles and needs b. Feeling overlooked: Culture and system
4. Finding closure	a. Surviving b. Showing compassion

3.1. Being in an Unknown Situation

Parents memories of their child's CHD diagnosis and heart surgery abroad revealed the superimposition of unanticipated and unwanted transitions on an expected transition of parenting a healthy and normal newborn. One father described this unexpected transition of the news vividly: *"just a complete shock to hear this just like that ... [you thought] your child was going for a 15-minute routine test [at the hospital], but comes home 16 days later somehow ... this is like [being on] a rollercoaster, you have no control. You just have to sit."* (Father 5). In these unknown situations, parents' lives were disrupted and somehow placed on hold.

3.1.1. Disrupted Life

All parents were shocked upon receiving the news of their child's CHD diagnosis and stunned when told that their child needed to travel overseas for complex heart surgery. Parents previous envision and expectations of a normal parenthood were superimposed by previously unknown reality, or as one mother described, *"it was surreal when he [doctor] said: He must go to Sweden. We just stared at him: What are you talking about? ... Go to Sweden? He was just born."* (Mother 7). In this situation, parents' lives changed instantaneously and often without any warning, leaving them feeling powerless. The chain of unanticipated changes and disruption was described as overwhelming and leaving parents at a loss for what to do, *"there was this overwhelming overflow of anxiety of all the tasks that lay ahead. You just asked yourself: What am I supposed to do now."* (Father 2).

In such strange and unknown situations, parents' habitats were constantly changing, which forced them to adjust to new environments, with new rules and regulations. Hospital rules, such as only allowing one parent to stay overnight at the cardiac ward, having to share a room with other families, were felt to restrict parents' ability to share habitats freely. Access to healthy food was also described as problematic, and sometimes it seemed that parents lived in a suitcase and sleep was a luxury: *"We got a room to stay in ... Of course, she [the mother] just wanted to be next to him ... I checked on them several times during the night. So, I did not sleep much, but it was still good to get a room and a shower, and we were there with the suitcases."* (Father 5). Within these changing circumstances parents had to learn how to care for their child and themselves, in addition to maintaining a healthy relationship with their support systems in Iceland and Sweden. Creating an equilibrium within these situations was difficult.

Following the surgery and throughout childhood, the child's illness continued to create disruptions in parents' lives. This was exemplified by parents' descriptions of their child's continuous follow-up medical appointments, long-term therapies, and multiple surgeries abroad. The daily stress was evident in parents' interviews, described by one mother as feeling like *"a balloon about to burst"* (Mother 3) following the aftermath, but today, three years post-surgery, her daughter goes *"weekly to physiotherapy and occupational therapy, then there are regular team meetings at the kindergarten ... and then she naturally has regular follow-ups with her cardiologist and an orthopedic surgeon, an ophthalmologist, and the neurologist."* (Mother 3).

3.1.2. Life on Hold

Amidst this turmoil of changes, parents simultaneously experienced the feeling that their lives were on hold. This feeling was mostly described as waiting for event to happen or milestones to be hit. The events and milestones identified as important, varied by parents.

However, all parents talked about the day of the surgery as particularly hard. The anxiety and uncertainty before were followed by either joy and thankfulness when the outcome was positive, but grief, sadness, and anger when it was negative. The stress of waiting was perhaps most palpable in parents' stories as 'phone-call': *"we just wandered around and kill time. And then he [surgeon] phoned when the surgery was over ... Everybody jumped up when the phone rang and just Oh My God!"* (Mother 12).

Following the surgery, parents then began waiting for the child's recovery. In this regard, the PICU discharge was a significant milestone for parents. Although this time-point created anxiety, parents also understood how significant this milestone was for the child and the family as a whole. As described by one mother, *"it was a big step for him to get there [cardiac ward], it was just amazing, just for all the three of us to be together."* (Mother 7).

Parents with other children at home expressed the stress of being separated from them. Some parents had never been away from their children before, and for the smaller children, explaining their absence was hard. Waiting to return home and reunite with their children, but not knowing at what date, was very distressing for the whole family: *"What was hardest was not knowing when we would go back home ... every night she [the daughter at home] asked: Mama when are you coming home?"* (Mother 1).

This feeling of waiting continued for parents. Parents described anxiety as they waited for the child to hit developmental milestones and their worries as they waited for child's next follow-up appointment with the cardiologist: *"But before the follow-up appointments, I become nervous. I always got a headache afterwards, sort of like de-stressing."* (Mother 7). This waiting placed a strain on parents and put their lives on hold.

3.2. Feeling Connected

As parents moved through their unexpected and unwanted transitions of their child's illness, supportive environment that provided comfort, familiarity, and connection, appeared in parents' interviews as a situational condition that facilitated a healthy transition. In particular, the importance of feeling connected—to the child, the siblings, the spouse, the grandparents, the health professionals, and other families of peers—was evident.

3.2.1. Supportive Environment

As parents prepared for the travel to Sweden, they asked questions and sought support from various sources. The pediatric cardiologist was described by all parents as their key person within the health care system that provided them support, being referred to as the *"rock"* (Father 4) and *"the main man"* (Father 5). Following parents return home, the cardiologist continued to be that key person and almost the only professional support.

Spark, a nonprofit CHD parent organization, was mentioned by all parents as instrumental in preparing and supporting them throughout the journey. Their peer-to-peer program, parental Facebook groups, website, and staff was described as immaculate for seeking knowledge and information, as well as being a safe space in which parents were understood and able to envision the future. One father described Spark as a *"rescue squad"* (Father 10); a metaphor exemplified in mother's rumination of her struggles leading up to the travel on of how to explain the situation, and say goodbye to her other daughters: *"we disagreed [she and her husband] ... so I sought advice from other mothers [via Spark's website] about how to best explain this to my daughters ... I didn't want to lie to them about where we were going."* (Mother 3).

Parents always sheltered themselves by seeking closeness and support from the grandparents, who traveled abroad with the parents, except if they needed to care for the siblings at home. Both parents traveled with their child to Sweden in all instances, but siblings always stayed at home. But a supportive spouse was likely the most important source of support for all parents: *"We [he and his wife] were just going to solve this together and just hope for the best."* (Father 2).

As parents transitioned between countries, hospitals, and wards, it was important for them to build a safe and comforting habitat for the family. Here, the Ronald McDonald House was described as having the welcoming "home away from home" environment they needed. Furthermore, Icelandic countrymen in Sweden (i.e., grandparents, other families, and health professionals) were instrumental in creating familiarity and security: *"And our moms were also there with us. They often prepared food for us which was home-like and very helpful ... as was having other three Icelandic families staying at the same time, also with children undergoing heart surgery."* (Mother 11).

All parents felt that their child received quality health care both by health professionals in Sweden and Iceland, and were remembered for their competence and skills: *"The staff ... was wonderful ... I experienced so much professionalism and security while I was there and if I'd need to do this again, I'd insist on it being in Lund."* (Mother 9). However, in seeking support for themselves, Icelandic health professionals working at the hospital in Sweden were frequently described as a significant source of support and help. Parents portrayed them as selfless and voluntary; these professionals provided the parents with what seemed like a crucial yet unofficial support network. They stepped in and touched many parents' lives: "*And during that time … an Icelandic anesthesiologist, he … just stepped into a role, he had not needed to do this. I don't know how we would have coped without having him there.*" (Father 6). The Icelandic health professional provided important security in their cultural familiarity, both in the care setting or as a support during medical meetings. It was clear that parents welcomed and preferred support from Icelandic health professionals because it helped them to better understand their situation: "*Because you knew nothing [prior to transferring to a cardiac ward] … we got some brochures and stuff … but there was an Icelandic nurse working on that ward, which was very nice. And she spoke to us in Icelandic about exactly everything.*" (Mother 12).

3.2.2. Handling the Experience

Parents' ability to cope following the news of their child's CHD diagnosis and surgery abroad varied. Some parents seemed more resilient and quickly found their new normal. The unknown situation and challenges were seen as an assignment and personal qualities a facilitator: "*I was incredibly strong … I was so convinced that this would work out well.*" (Mother 1). Furthermore, parents took charge and became engaged in their healing. They created "*photo album*" (Father 2) of the journey, intentionally accepted help offered to them by the community, "*My boss said: Just go and as see a psychologist, just pick one you like … So we [him and his wife] went together to see a psychologist.*" (Father 10), as well as seeking out and asking for the help they felt they needed, "*I asked if it would not be a good idea if I talked to a psychologist or something …*" (Mother 1).

Parents' ability to face their fears, however varied. They struggled with the unexpected path their life had taken. Parents were worried about their child's future and how their own future would be influenced by the illness, as illustrated by one father: "*If all goes wrong … then you'll naturally go to a dark place … even if you decide not to hang yourself, you're going to live with it, then life is still useless, so you're just such a passenger.*" (Father 10).

Knowledge and skills helped parents face the fear and handle their experiences. The act of knowing symbolized a need for control and hope. Parents' need for knowledge varied, however. Some sought a deeper understanding of their situation, while others felt that too much information created fear and anxiety. Parents described how their own education enabled them to seek and gain resources. However, a lack of knowledge (e.g., of the Swedish language) created vulnerability and a feeling of disconnect. One father explained this when he said: "*Some of the Swedish nurses, just didn't want to speak English … they just avoided talking [to us].*" (Father 4). Further, knowledge and information were often described in opposition. For example, information was provided or not received, or was helpful or paradoxical. When information contradicted parents' hopes for a normal future for their child, it was described as threatening, even when signs of their child's permanent disability were evident.

Talking about their experiences was a coping mechanism used by all parents. However, their readiness to share this experience varied, and some needed a long time before they were ready, "*Yes, at that time there were no tears … I really do not remember much from this time. And it was not until after a year had passed [since the heart surgery abroad] that I could talk about it.*" (Mother 11). Memories also emerged, that parents did not want to talk about. One father described how he wanted to forget some memories: "*[There are] unspeakable things I've … forgotten and blocked out, this is somehow such a tribulation.*" (Father 6).

After returning home, some parents sought help from professionals to handle their experiences and help them to recover. No parent, however shared memories of faith or religion in their coping. Furthermore, with the exception of walking, physical or spiritual activities were seldom mentioned by parents as a way of coping, although one father found it helpful: "*I started to meditate … sometimes I did yoga … I started to run long distance.*" (Father 10).

3.3. Wishing Being Accepted

Parents situational conditions could also inhibit a healthy transitional experience. In the interviews, not being seen as a legitimate client, emerged as an important inhibitor. Overall parents did not feel accepted, neither by the Icelandic or Swedish health care systems. They expressed a need to be accepted as a legitimate client, meaning both as a parent—with continuous and multiple parenting roles, and as a client—with complex health care needs. When overlooked, parents' vulnerabilities emerged, and their risk of developing traumatic experiences seemed to increase.

3.3.1. Parenting Roles and Needs

Parents felt it was important for them to fulfill their parenting roles of presence and caretaking as best they could throughout the child's traveling and hospitalization. If overlooked by health professionals, parents described feeling distressed and dismissed: "*I found it very difficult that someone [at the PICU] could just drive me away from my child ... that all of a sudden [somebody could] just [say]: You can't be with your daughter, now you just have to leave.*" (Mother 3).

At the same time, the extremely stressful situations, and environments that parents found themselves in made parenting a challenge. Understanding how best to care for their child was not only difficult but also frightening: "*We just sat with him [in the PICU], which was extremely strange and surrealist to be sitting there and he was attached to 300 lines and all kinds of drugs and everything is beeping, and you do not know what is actually happening. That was a strange life experience. And you are like, should I be here or not? You just do not know how to behave.*" (Mother 1).

Parenting also involved creating relationships with health professionals. Here transparency and honesty about the child's condition was a fundamental component of trust building. When parents were not included in the decision making concerning their child, as described by one father regarding his son's critical condition, they felt as if their parental rights were being violated: "*You'd never keep such information [CHD condition severity] from a patient, you'd tell him exactly what the situation was. And I think it should be exactly the same for parents.*" (Father 6).

Furthermore, the disruption of the illness put a strain on spousal relationships. Parents described disagreements in their understanding of the illness and its ramifications. It seemed that if an underlying relationship problem existed previously, it was magnified by this stressful situation. In some cases, it triggered the disintegration of the family: "*I got sick [in Sweden] ... and my ex's reaction was so upsetting, that like, I got this kind of confirmation that we couldn't be married anymore.*" (Mother 1). Of the 12 parents interviewed, four separated following their arrival back home.

As parents transitioned between health care systems, they often felt their needs were overlooked by health professionals both in Iceland and Sweden. The needs parents were overlooked varied, but mothers more than fathers talked about their psychological issues during and following their child's hospitalization. Parents described how they felt alone in dealing with their health problems and their need for support: "*There is nobody thinking about the parents ... I realized that there was no mental support provided abroad. And not here at home either.*" (Mother 8).

Parents' vulnerabilities were expressed in their memories of distress. All mothers were recovering from childbirth when they traveled the first time with their infant to Sweden. Nevertheless, mother's postpartum problems such as "*lactation mastitis*" (Mother 1), "*lactation suppression*" (Father 6), "*post-partum depression*" (Mother 3), and "*postpartum pain*" (Mother 12) were always secondary. Mothers described how they experienced physical pain and became sick following childbirth. Memories of this physical suffering were frequently associated with the traveling: "*I remember this extreme pain; I was walking down some long [airport] terminals.*" (Mother 1). This left first-time mothers feeling particularly vulnerable. Overall, parents were sleep deprived and tired during the child's hospitalization period. However, the fatigue and emotional aftershock usually appeared after they arrived back home, following which, some mothers described they developed psychological problems: "*When she was eight months old, then I began experiencing traumatic stress and anxiety ... It had been escalating since she came home."* (Mother 3). For some, these health problems were only short-term, whereas in others they became long-term health issues.

3.3.2. Feeling Overlooked: Culture and System

On their arrival in Sweden, parents had to adjust to a foreign environment, language, costumes, and regulations. In this situation, parents inevitably experienced cultural barriers. However, the parents' ability to speak or understand English or Swedish was not assessed before they traveled to Sweden. These abilities were simply assumed.

Language barriers were the most common issues raised by parents. While most parents were able to communicate in English or Swedish, some were not. Those that were unable to speak English did not seek help from a translator. Indeed, the mere idea of a translator seemed awkward and even shameful; rather, parents described how they did their best or relied on other family members to help them: *"I'm very poor in English . . . but my mom and her boyfriend . . . helped me understand."* (Mother 12).

Most parents felt welcomed during their stay in Sweden, although some mentioned cultural insensitivities from health professionals. In a few cases, parents noted that health professionals' proficiency in English was lacking. This was surprising to parents and in retrospect they regretted not asking for better service.

Parents talked about how they felt that unrealistic expectations and responsibilities were being placed on them. Sometimes parents felt as if they were being taken for granted, even treated as employees: *"We were just in a part-time job, actually we were providing intensive care by watching over her the whole night."* (Mother 3). Parents described how health professionals expected them to cope, under what they felt were unrealistic and extreme circumstances for them, that left them traumatized. These traumatic events were mostly related to their child's suffering during medical procedures: *"My only memory is when a line was being removed, this was a long line, all the way into the heart. I just remember how much he screamed."* (Mother 11).

When in Iceland, parents did not receive any follow-up support and there was no interdisciplinary team assigned to help the families. Parents were mostly left to navigate the systems and bureaucracy on their own to find help and support. They expressed surprise at the scarcity of resources available to them and described a gap in the system: *"Perhaps the biggest problem with the process is what happened afterwards. Because he died . . . We just came home and there was nobody that contacted us . . . We had to seek everything ourselves like psychological help and all that."* (Father 6). Some parents were so concerned with these systemic flaws that they sought ways to help repair the system. These parents advocated for a multidisciplinary health care team to assist the whole family.

3.4. Finding Closure

The time span of parent's situational transitions varied, but *"[getting] off the rollercoaster"* (Father 5) and finding closure was desired by all parents. Parents did not always describe a specific endpoint, but when they did it seemed fluid and sometimes attached to 'ritual(s)'. The process of finding closure was expressed in surviving and compassion, with personal growth indicating a healthy transition.

3.4.1. Surviving

All parents interviewed were survivors, they had been through tremendous challenges, stress, and even trauma, and were able to share this. The meaning parents placed on survival varied, however. For some, the stressful life event itself was their focus: *"It is a huge undertaking to go abroad. When I think back to this time, I just get shivers down my spine and if I had to do this again, I would have a nervous breakdown."* (Mother 9). This was also exemplified in one father's recollection of this time: *"we as parents, so often think back to this time with a sense of horror, it was a really dreadful time."* (Father 4). In other cases, parents described this stressful experience as something they needed to endure in order to survive: *"I just wanted this to be over. Just to get through this and have it over with."* (Mother 7).

Parents also described survival as a process of moving on and finding a new normal. This was illustrated by for example in growing their families or ending a spousal relationship. However, this process was perhaps most clearly illustrated by one father: *"Then you go off the rollercoaster and you just know: Wow! . . . but then you just keep going, just forward, and finally you start picking up the threads of a healthy life."* (Father 5). In addition, recovering was also found in parents interviews as an indicator of closure: *"This is such a huge shock . . . recovering could've been much harder for us . . . but I think we're just lucky."* (Mother 7).

Parents who struggled the most were grieving some type of loss. To be able to move on, they had to reevaluate their experience and even reshape their memories. This was illustrated by one mother, whose daughter developed long term complications, in her statement that, *"my existence now is trying to make peace with my life . . . you know her difficult life. The life she will lead . . . trying to find meaning . . . "* (Mother 3).

3.4.2. Showing Compassion

Parents expressed their compassion for parents in the same situation as them, especially those who were more vulnerable. They questioned whether the current system was tailored for these specific groups and had concerns: *"[It] is absolutely necessary to ask people before they travel abroad [about English skills], because individuals with intellectual disabilities are having children for example, or parents who didn't even finish elementary school and or aren't good in languages. Then it is necessary . . . to have someone to translate for them."* (Mother 9).

Following their experiences of traveling abroad, some parents joined peer-to-peer groups to support other parents and others even started lobbying within the Icelandic hospital system, for health care reforms: *"we have criticized the process, asked for changes . . . we are told a new protocol is in place . . . I just hope that if something like this happens again [child dies abroad], it goes better for those people."* (Father 6).

Empathy-based survival guilt towards the suffering of other parents was also expressed by many parents. This empathy was directed towards other parents who either lost their child or had a much sicker child: *"After the funeral . . . the guilt I felt towards my sister- and brother-in-law. We'd just got through this and it went so well and then . . . their son just dies."* (Mother 9).

4. Discussion

This study elicited parents' experiences of their child's CHD diagnosis, heart surgery abroad, and journey beyond. The overarching theme, living with the memories, highlighted the superimposition of this stressful live event on the expected transition to parenthood, where parents' vivid memories still impacted their lives up to five years later. The most concerning finding was parents' negative memories of the transition back home and their descriptions of roadblocks to recovery that followed.

According to Meleis's transitions theory [19], the constructs that define transitions are its nature (e.g., critical event), conditions (i.e., facilitators and inhibitors), and patterns of response (e.g., indicators of a healthy transition). Furthermore, all transitions are believed to build on universal commonalities, where disconnectedness is seen as the most pervasive one [19].

A parental transition triggered by child's CCHD and need for heart surgery abroad has not been previously documented. However, other types of parental transitions focusing on child medical tourism [16–18] and hospitalizations of critically ill children [8–10] have been studied. Concurrently, our findings support the diverse and universal nature of transition experiences [19], although all parents experienced situational transitions, its nature—complexity, suddenness, degree of stress, and social support required —was particularly different. Thus, the uniqueness of our findings relates to the transitional conditions experienced by our parents.

Our findings showed both facilitators and inhibitors in parents' environmental conditions. Connectivity represented itself both as a facilitator (e.g., in networks of health professionals and peer-groups) and an inhibitor (e.g., separation from child's siblings). Separation or feeling separated is associated with personal, familial, socio-cultural, and geographical factors. However, separation from family and home life is hard on individuals in hospital settings and can lead to vulnerability, loneliness, and dependency [23].

The distance between home and hospital created a feeling of disconnection in parents in our study. Concurrently, others have shown that separation caused by geographical distance can negatively impact family relationships during child's hospitalization. Specifically, parents' likelihood of relationship difficulties with other family members tend to grow as the distance between hospital and home increases [24]. In our study, several parents described relationship tensions during their stay in Sweden, with some attributing this tension to the distance from home. Further, the separation from the child's siblings at home was also hard on parents, and aligns with the findings of others [16]. Parents used modern technology (e.g., Facebook, Skype, Facetime) to connect with the left-behind siblings. This seemed however disjointed to their feeling of disconnectedness due to the physical distance. Another contributing factor may be siblings age, as all were relatively young, which might have made the utilization of technology perplexing.

In hospital settings, separation from home triggers a need for comfort and support that can be found through cultural connection. This includes seeking familiarity in terms of language and food, in addition to developing a sense of belonging in terms of social support networks [23]. Consistent with a meta-analysis and systematic reviews of parental coping with their child's CHD [3], our participants used various coping strategies from surgery to childhood. However, their means of becoming culturally connected while abroad—particularly in the security, safety, and trust they placed in countrymen—is unique to our findings. Here, child's grandparents and the health professionals working at the hospital abroad were of significance in creating this cultural connection.

Similar to that in other studies [3,25], grandparents were a significant source of support to parents in our study. Grandparents were a cornerstone in their habitat building, either caring for the child's siblings at home or traveling with them abroad, thus creating familiarity through food and language. In hospital settings, such comfort can counterbalance negative emotions associated with being away from home and home life [23]. Importantly, the findings showed that the support provided by countrymen working as health professionals at the hospital abroad, created unique networks and relationships essential to the parents. These professionals provided parents with services ranging from direct medical care to assistance with practical matters, all seemingly done voluntarily. The shared culture and language appear to have created a feeling of safety, understanding, and familiarity, and a sense of belonging. Cultural competence in health care involves streamlining care and facilitating communication [26]. This could be done by matching patients and providers based on their cultural similarities [27,28]. Our results suggest that cultural competence in health care can be achieved by providing families traveling abroad with access to the medical care of health professionals who are fellow countrymen.

A key element facilitating healthy parental transitions from the PICU to a clinical ward is effective communication and information flow [8]. Furthermore, clarity in patient-provider communication is needed for facilitating and managing transitions, also imperative to securing quality care [29]. Our findings show that parents' experienced communication challenges with health professionals while abroad, which amplified the imbalance of social capitals inherent in the client-providers encounters. The clearest communicational challenges reported related to language and other cultural barriers. Similar findings are reported in child medical tourism [16,17]. Although no participant asked for medical translator, they sought assistance from their fellow countrymen (i.e., family and health professionals) when needed.

Language discrepancies between clients and health clinicians contribute to communication errors, especially if both speak a second language [30,31]. Furthermore, within these language-discrepant medical communication settings, individuals' distress and vulnerabilities are likely to increase [30,32]. This is problematic and implies that assessing and anticipating families' need for support prior to traveling (e.g., a medical translator) is necessary, as has been suggested by others [14]. It is therefore surprising that our participants and apparent health professionals did not anticipate this, even though both parties had to communicate in a second language (i.e., English).

The transitions experienced by our parents following their child's CHD diagnosis and cardiac surgery were extremely stressful. In a brief period, parents transitioned from expecting to go home with a healthy baby to having a critically ill newborn needing cardiac surgery abroad. Some even had to make this journey abroad three times. Parents' descriptions of their aftershock, unmet needs, and short- and long-term health problems following their arrival back home, concur with the pediatric cardiac literature [6]. Similar findings are however not reported in the child medical tourism literature [16–18].

Personal growth and empowerment are a positive outcome of transitions [19], described by few parents in our study. This growth was best exemplified in the compassion and empathy parents showed toward their peers in similar situations, and in parents' efforts to reform the current health care system. Concurrently, in a qualitative study, looking at parents mostly from low-income countries, majority of parents experienced personal growth (e.g., greater compassion for others) as a result of coming to the United States to seek medical treatment for their child [16]. In addition, a quantitative study [33] reported nearly 40% of parents experienced posttraumatic growth after their child's admission to PICU. The different contexts and samples used in these studies compared to ours, may explain the inconsistency of experienced personal growth by our parents. Even so, all parents in our study described a path to recovery as they tried to fit the transition into their life story in a meaningful way.

Our findings suggest an urgent need for follow-up care and support for this population, but currently, no such support is provided by health professionals in either Iceland or Sweden. A significant feature of transitional care is comprehensive and continued follow-up care for patients and families [19]. This is in line with pediatric cardiology guidelines [34] which recommend that a multidisciplinary health team supports children with CHD and their parents throughout their whole journey, including with follow-up care. Systematic reviews examining parents after their child's PICU admission [35] and meta-analyses examining adult ICU survivors and their relatives [36] have indicated that follow-up appointments can improve mental health for these groups. These findings stress the urgency of offering the same follow-up service for families of children with CHD, particularly for at-risk groups such as those traveling abroad.

eHealth is considered a promising aid to lower psychiatric morbidity in families of children with CHD [34,37] and is particularly relevant for the population of the current study. This mode of health care creates opportunities for interactive communication between all stakeholders, allowing health care teams at home and abroad to collaborate more easily with parents as they transition between systems. Furthermore, via website apps, psychological follow-up care could, for example, permit parents to make virtual revisits to the hospital abroad.

This study has both limitations and strengths for consideration. Of the seven mothers and five fathers who participated, only eight children with CHD were represented. The range of possible experiences might thus have been restricted because both parents could participate. However, parent couples' experience of a stressful event often varies greatly [38]. A written request was sent to 25 parents via e-mail. Fifteen parents replied to the e-mail, but only 12 parents participated in the study. It is unclear whether the 13 parents who did not participate are in some way demographically different from those who did. The nearly equal number of mothers and fathers, and the wide range of sociodemographic characteristics in the participant sample, however, strengthened the study findings. Additionally, the primary categories reappeared in all of the interviews, thus creating a saturation that strengthened the results. The study findings may not be generalized to other populations, but may be transferable to other parents of children with CHD traveling abroad for cardiac surgery. The sample size was relatively small. However, the fact that similar sample sizes have been used in other studies [39,40] and the emphasis on richness rather than sample size in content analysis [41] provides strength to our findings. The trustworthiness of the study findings lies in the methods used and the experience of the three authors. All authors are registered nurses with pediatric clinical experience. The second author (A.S.S.) has extensive experience with pediatric acritical care cardiology and working with parents of children with CCHD. Although all authors are experienced researchers, the second author also has extensive experience in qualitative content analysis methods.

5. Conclusions

The lived experiences of parents when their child underwent complex heart surgery abroad are filled with difficult memories and emotions. Parents' readiness and need for support was heightened after arriving home from abroad. However, these needs were not met by either of the health care systems involved. Culturally competent care for the families must be designed and implemented, starting with an assessment of language skills prior to the travel. Assigning families to multidisciplinary health care teams and providing them with follow-up support are necessary. Here, the use of eHealth interventions to improve interactive communication between all stakeholders is promising.

Supplementary Materials: The following are available online at http://www.mdpi.com/1660-4601/17/23/8840/s1, Table S1: COREQ checklist, Table S2: Coding tree.

Author Contributions: Conceptualization, Ó.K., G.K. and A.S.-S.; methodology, Ó.K., G.K. and A.S.S.; validation, Ó.K., G.K. and A.S.-S.; formal analysis, Ó.K., G.K. and A.S.-S.; investigation, Ó.K.; resources, G.K.; data curation, G.K.; writing—original draft preparation, Ó.K.; writing—review and editing, Ó.K., G.K. and A.S.-S.; visualization, Ó.K.; supervision, G.K. and A.S.-S.; project administration, Ó.K.; funding acquisition, Ó.K. and G.K. All authors have read and agreed to the published version of the manuscript.

Funding: This research was funded by the Landspítali Háskólasjúkrahús (A-2020-016), Félag Íslenskra Hjúkrunarfræðinga (B-2020-2004), and Forskningsrådet om Hälsa, Arbetsliv och Välfärd (2018-01399).

Acknowledgments: The researchers are most grateful to the parents who shared their experiences, and all those who supported this project.

Conflicts of Interest: The authors declare no conflict of interest.

References

1. McMahon, E.; Chang, Y.-S. From surviving to thriving—Parental experiences of hospitalised infants with congenital heart disease undergoing cardiac surgery: A qualitative synthesis. *J. Pediatr. Nurs.* **2020**, *51*, 32–41. [CrossRef] [PubMed]
2. Biber, S.; Andonian, C.; Beckmann, J.; Ewert, P.; Freilinger, S.; Nagdyman, N.; Kaemmerer, H.; Oberhoffer, R.; Pieper, L.; Neidenbach, R.C. Current research status on the psychological situation of parents of children with congenital heart disease. *Cardiovasc. Diagn.* **2019**, *9*, S369–S376. [CrossRef] [PubMed]
3. Lumsden, M.R.; Smith, D.M.; Wittkowski, A. Coping in parents of children with congenital heart disease: A systematic review and meta-synthesis. *J. Child. Fam. Stud.* **2019**, *28*, 1736–1753. [CrossRef]
4. Liu, Y.; Chen, S.; Zühlke, L.; Black, G.C.; Choy, M.-K.; Li, N.; Keavney, B.D. Global birth prevalence of congenital heart defects 1970–2017: Updated systematic review and meta-analysis of 260 studies. *Int. J. Epidemiol.* **2019**, *48*, 455–463. [CrossRef] [PubMed]
5. Bakker, M.K.; Bergman, J.E.; Krikov, S.; Amar, E.; Cocchi, G.; Cragan, J.; De Walle, H.E.; Gatt, M.; Groisman, B.; Liu, S. Prenatal diagnosis and prevalence of critical congenital heart defects: An international retrospective cohort study. *BMJ Open* **2019**, *9*, e028139. [CrossRef] [PubMed]
6. Woolf-King, S.E.; Anger, A.; Arnold, E.A.; Weiss, S.J.; Teitel, D. Mental health among parents of children with critical congenital heart defects: A systematic review. *J. Am. Heart Assoc.* **2017**, *6*, e004862. [CrossRef]
7. Bruce, E.; Lilja, C.; Sundin, K. Mothers' lived experiences of support when living with young children with congenital heart defects. *J. Spec. Pediatr. Nurs.* **2014**, *19*, 54–67. [CrossRef]
8. Suleman, Z.; Evans, C.; Manning, J.C. Parents' and carers' experiences of transition and aftercare following a child's discharge from a paediatric intensive care unit to an in-patient ward setting: A qualitative systematic review. *Intensive Crit. Care Nurs.* **2019**, *51*, 35–44. [CrossRef]
9. Obas, K.A.; Leal, J.M.; Zegray, M.; Rennick, J.E. Parental perceptions of transition from intensive care following a child's cardiac surgery. *Nurs. Crit. Care* **2016**, *21*, e1–e9. [CrossRef]
10. Gaskin, K.L. Patterns of transition experience for parents going home from hospital with their infant after first stage surgery for complex congenital heart disease. *J. Pediatr. Nurs.* **2018**, *41*, e23–e32. [CrossRef] [PubMed]

11. Neistinn. Hjartagáttin, Meðfæddur Hjartagalli. Available online: http://neistinn.is/hjartagattin/ (accessed on 30 January 2020).

12. Gunnarsdóttir, B. Greining alvarlegra meðfæddra hjartagalla á Íslandi 2014–2017. Bachelor's Thesis, University of Iceland, Reykjavik, Iceland, 14 May 2018.

13. World Health Organization. *Cross-Border Health Care in the European Union: Mapping and Analysing Practices and Policies*; World Health Organization. Regional Office for Europe: Geneva, Switzerland, 2011.

14. Hamlyn-Williams, C.; Lakhanpaul, M.; Manikam, L. Child medical tourism: A new phenomenon. In *Handbook on Medical Tourism and Patient Mobility*; Lunt, N., Horsfall, D., Hanefeld, J., Eds.; Edward Elgar: Cheltenham, UK, 2015; pp. 360–369. [CrossRef]

15. Lorraine Culley, N.H.; Baldwin, K.; Lakhanpaul, M. Children travelling for treatment: What we don't know. *Arch. Dis. Child.* **2013**, *98*, 442–444. [CrossRef]

16. Margolis, R.; Ludi, E.; Pao, M.; Wiener, L. International adaptation: Psychosocial and parenting experiences of caregivers who travel to the United States to obtain acute medical care for their seriously ill child. *Soc. Work Health Care* **2013**, *52*, 669–683. [CrossRef] [PubMed]

17. Crom, D.B. The experience of South American mothers who have a child being treated for malignancy in the United States. *J. Pediatric Oncol. Nurs.* **1995**, *12*, 104–112. [CrossRef]

18. Cockle, S.G.; Ogden, J. The 'radiation vacation': Parents' experiences of travelling to have their children's brain tumours treated with proton beam therapy. *Health Psychol. Open* **2016**, *3*, 2055102916649767. [CrossRef] [PubMed]

19. Meleis, A.I. *Transitions Theory: Middle Range and Situation Specific Theories in Nursing Research and Practice*; Springer Publishing Company: New York, NY, USA, 2010.

20. Graneheim, U.H.; Lundman, B. Qualitative content analysis in nursing research: Concepts, procedures and measures to achieve trustworthiness. *Nurse Educ. Today* **2004**, *24*, 105–112. [CrossRef] [PubMed]

21. Graneheim, U.H.; Lindgren, B.M.; Lundman, B. Methodological challenges in qualitative content analysis: A discussion paper. *Nurse Educ. Today* **2017**, *56*, 29–34. [CrossRef] [PubMed]

22. Terp, K.; Sjostrom-Strand, A. Parents' experiences and the effect on the family two years after their child was admitted to a PICU—An interview study. *Intensive Crit. Care Nurs.* **2017**, *43*, 143–148. [CrossRef] [PubMed]

23. Wensley, C.; Botti, M.; McKillop, A.; Merry, A.F. A framework of comfort for practice: An integrative review identifying the multiple influences on patients' experience of comfort in healthcare settings. *Int. J. Qual. Health Care* **2017**, *29*, 151–162. [CrossRef]

24. Yantzi, N.; Rosenberg, M.W.; Burke, S.O.; Harrison, M.B. The impacts of distance to hospital on families with a child with a chronic condition. *Soc. Sci. Med.* **2001**, *52*, 1777–1791. [CrossRef]

25. Rempel, G.R.; Ravindran, V.; Rogers, L.G.; Magill-Evans, J. Parenting under pressure: A grounded theory of parenting young children with life-threatening congenital heart disease. *J. Adv. Nurs.* **2013**, *69*, 619–630. [CrossRef]

26. White, J.; Plompen, T.; Tao, L.; Micallef, E.; Haines, T. What is needed in culturally competent healthcare systems? A qualitative exploration of culturally diverse patients and professional interpreters in an Australian healthcare setting. *BMC Public Health* **2019**, *19*, 1096. [CrossRef] [PubMed]

27. Hsueh, L.; Hirsh, A.T.; Maupomé, G.; Stewart, J.C. Patient–provider language concordance and health outcomes: A systematic review, evidence map, and research agenda. *Med. Care Res. Rev.* **2019**. [CrossRef] [PubMed]

28. Flores, G. The impact of medical interpreter services on the quality of health care: A systematic review. *Med. Care Res. Rev.* **2005**, *62*, 255–299. [CrossRef] [PubMed]

29. Meleis, A. Facilitating and Managing Transitions: An Imperative for Quality Care. *Investig. En Enfermería: Imagen Y Desarro.* **2018**, *21*. [CrossRef]

30. de Moissac, D.; Bowen, S. Impact of language barriers on quality of care and patient safety for official language minority francophones in Canada. *J. Patient Exp.* **2019**, *6*, 24–32. [CrossRef]

31. Gudykunst, W.B. *Theorizing about Intercultural Communication*; Sage: Thousand Oaks, CA, USA, 2005.

32. Bowen, S. *Language Barriers in Access to Health Care*; Health Canada: Ottawa, ON, Canada, 2001.

33. Rodríguez-Rey, R.; Palacios, A.; Alonso-Tapia, J.; Pérez, E.; Álvarez, E.; Coca, A.; Mencía, S.; Marcos, A.M.; Mayordomo-Colunga, J.; Fernández, F.; et al. Posttraumatic growth in pediatric intensive care personnel: Dependence on resilience and coping strategies. *Psychol. Trauma Theory Res. Pract. Policy* **2017**, *9*, 407–415. [CrossRef]

34. Utens, E.; Callus, E.; Levert, E.M.; Groote, K.; Casey, F. Multidisciplinary family-centred psychosocial care for patients with CHD: Consensus recommendations from the AEPC psychosocial working group. *Cardiol. Young* **2018**, *28*, 192–198. [CrossRef]

35. Baker, S.C.; Gledhill, J.A. Systematic review of interventions to reduce psychiatric morbidity in parents and children after PICU admissions. *Pediatr. Crit. Care Med.* **2017**, *18*, 343–348. [CrossRef]

36. Rosa, R.G.; Ferreira, G.E.; Viola, T.W.; Robinson, C.C.; Kochhann, R.; Berto, P.P.; Biason, L.; Cardoso, P.R.; Falavigna, M.; Teixeira, C. Effects of post-ICU follow-up on subject outcomes: A systematic review and meta-analysis. *J. Crit. Care* **2019**, *52*, 115–125. [CrossRef]

37. Williams, T.S.; McDonald, K.P.; Roberts, S.D.; Chau, V.; Seed, M.; Miller, S.P.; Sananes, R. From Diagnoses to Ongoing Journey: Parent Experiences Following Congenital Heart Disease Diagnoses. *J. Pediatr. Psychol.* **2019**, *44*, 924–936. [CrossRef]

38. Feinberg, M.E.; Jones, D.E.; McDaniel, B.T.; Liu, S.; Almeida, D. Chapter II: New fathers' and mothers' daily stressors and resources influence parent adjustment and family relationships. *Monogr. Soc. Res. Child. Dev.* **2019**, *84*, 18–34. [PubMed]

39. Sjostrom-Strand, A.; Terp, K. Parents' experiences of having a baby with a congenital heart defect and the child's heart surgery. *Compr. Child. Adolesc. Nurs.* **2017**, *42*, 10–23. [CrossRef] [PubMed]

40. David Vainberg, L.; Vardi, A.; Jacoby, R. The experiences of parents of children undergoing surgery for congenital heart defects: A holistic model of care. *Front. Psychol.* **2019**, *10*, 2666. [CrossRef] [PubMed]

41. Bengtsson, M. How to plan and perform a qualitative study using content analysis. *Nurs. Open* **2016**, *2*, 8–14. [CrossRef]

Publisher's Note: MDPI stays neutral with regard to jurisdictional claims in published maps and institutional affiliations.

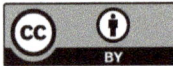

International Journal of
Environmental Research and Public Health

MDPI

Article

Physical Activity, Resilience, Sense of Coherence and Coping in People with Multiple Sclerosis in the Situation Derived from COVID-19

María Mercedes Reguera-García [1], Cristina Liébana-Presa [1,*], Lorena Álvarez-Barrio [2], Lisa Alves Gomes [3] and Elena Fernández-Martínez [1]

1 SALBIS Research Group, Faculty of Health Sciences, Campus of Ponferrada, University of León, 24401 Ponferrada, Spain; mercedes.reguera@unileon.es (M.M.R.-G.); elena.fernandez@unileon.es (E.F.-M.)
2 Department of Nursing and Physiotherapy, Faculty of Health Sciences, Campus of Ponferrada, University of León, 24401 Ponferrada, Spain; lalvb@unileon.es
3 Nursing School, Minho University, 4710-057 Braga, Portugal; lgomes@ese.uminho.pt
* Correspondence: cliep@unileon.es

Received: 2 October 2020; Accepted: 4 November 2020; Published: 6 November 2020

check for updates

Abstract: The confinement forced by COVID-19 can have repercussions on the health of people diagnosed with multiple sclerosis. The objective of this study is to analyze the relationships between physical activity, a sense of coherence, resilience and coping among people diagnosed with Multiple Sclerosis during the health emergency situation. To achieve this goal, this transversal descriptive study included 84 patients that belonged to multiple sclerosis associations during the period of confinement. Participants filled out the Physical Activity (IPAQ-SF), Sense of Coherence (SOC-13), Resilience Scale (ER-14) and coping (COPE-28) questionnaires. The results showed that the average age was 46.9 and that 67.9% had Relapsing Remittent Multiple Sclerosis diagnosed on average 13.9 years ago. They had a high degree (33.3%) and moderate degree (34.5%) of physical activity, high levels of resilience, while the level of a sense of coherence was average and the most commonly used strategies for coping were active confrontation and religion. Physical activity was not related to the rest of the studied variables, but there were correlations between the other variables. The people with multiple sclerosis who belong to patient associations have remained physically active during the obligatory confinement period and have elevated degrees of resilience and an average sense of coherence, as well as using suitable coping strategies, which is why the social-health resource of belonging to a patient association could be boosting these variables that are beneficial to their health.

Keywords: multiple sclerosis; COVID-19; physical activity; resilience; sense of coherence; coping

1. Introduction

The world is currently going through a pandemic due to a new strain of coronavirus, the severe acute respiratory syndrome (SARS-CoV-2). There are many aspects that remain unknown about this illness. At the moment there are no treatment strategies, nor is there a vaccine [1], and many countries have adopted social distancing and/or quarantining to break the chain of transmission of the COVID-19 illness. In Spain, a state of alarm was declared in order manage the health crisis situation brought about by COVID-19 in March 2020, the Royal Decree 463/2020 of 14 March [2], in response to the growing number of cases of coronavirus in Spain; it imposed a national quarantine as a health measure. On 21 June 2020, the country entered the dubbed "new normality", introducing health measures such as the use of facemasks and social distancing. Current research [3] referring to the psychological impact of quarantine suggests that it is necessary to take into account the stress factors resulting from the situation (duration, fear of infection, frustration, fear, boredom, anger, insufficient information, lack of basic supplies, financial losses and stigma) in order to ensure that the experience of quarantining be as tolerable as possible for the population [3,4].

It is not known how duration might affect the different collectives of people who already suffer from prior illnesses such as multiple sclerosis (MS). MS is chronic and autoimmune, affecting the central nervous system [5] and with an unstable clinical course with a wide range of cognitive and neurological effects [6]. It affects women more than men (3:1) [7] and is usually diagnosed between 20 and 40 years of age. Certain characteristics of MS, such as its unknown origin, its unpredictable course, its multiple symptoms and the current nonexistence of a definitive cure, affect the adherence to the treatment as well as the quality of life [8]. MS patients suffer functional deterioration, fatigue, psychological anxiety and limitations in their social relationships, all of which leads to a lesser quality of life for these people at both the physical and psychological level [9,10], giving rise to them experiencing a low self-efficacy due to the limitations of the illness itself [8]. Furthermore, this population of MS sufferers is more sensitive to suffering cognitive dysfunctions and mental health problems, especially depression followed by anxiety, since this affects them at a larger scale than the general population (more than 20% of the population) [11,12]. Those people who suffered problems of mental health before the quarantine and social distancing may be more vulnerable to adverse psychological effects [1]. Recent research indicates that exposure risks are the cause of COVID-19 infection in the MS population. Younger people with a lower socioeconomic status will have a higher risk of exposure and are potential targets for educational intervention and medical support to limit exposure. Delays in therapies and the interruption of MS care have also been observed [13].

There is a lack of previous research that includes the consequences deriving from the COVID-19 virus pandemic at the physical and psychological level in people suffering from MS. This is why research into physical activity, resilience, coping and a sense of coherence has been selected, as these are the variables related to well-being and the promotion of health.

In people with MS, the degree of physical activity is usually reduced, making them less physically active than the general population [14]. It is related to the degree of general incapacity and the limitation for walking in people with MS [15]. In these patients, vigorous activities are reduced, leading to the predominance of light activities and the fact that they spend quite a lot of time being inactive during the day [16]. The reduced participation, the limitation of movement and the degree of incapacity factors mean that the physical activity of the MS population is less than that of the general population, and consequently they do not obtain the benefits that come from carrying out physical exercise, leading to a greater propensity for their suffering certain illnesses, especially cardiovascular ones [17]. It is necessary to promote physical activity and include it in intervention programs, since a greater degree of physical activity is related to personal factors such as sociodemographics, the level of education, their work situation, mechanisms for self-regulation and the perception of barriers, especially those related to physical activity [16].

Resilience is characterized by the ability to achieve, retain or recover a degree of physical or emotional health after adversity [17]. In people with MS, disability is associated with success in adapting and recuperation. Greater levels of resilience are associated with a reduction in fatigue (20% less), greater participation and exercise, greater social and financial support, a healthier diet and better psychological health [17]. People with MS have reported that higher levels of resilience are associated with healthy behaviors and a more successful adaptation to changes in the life of the patients that result from their illness [18]. This variable has been studied in different populations [19], but rarely in patients with MS.

The sense of coherence is understood as a way of perceiving the world that allows stressful factors to be faced [20]. MS is a chronic illness with an unpredictable evolution [21], which includes suffering physical limitations and psychosocial difficulties that affect the quality of life of these people, threatening their sense of cohesion [8,22]. A greater sense of cohesion gives rise to better mental health and a lower negative effect, as well as warding off depression [8,23].

People with MS use different coping strategies in the different stages of the illness. In the first stages, emotional and avoidance-type strategies prédominate; meanwhile, in the intermediate stages of the illness, the use of more active coping strategies predominate [24]. On certain occasions, the use of emotional-type strategies are related to a better psychological adaptation and those of avoidance are related to the prevention of a depressive reaction through the rejection of negative thoughts about the future progression of the illness when they are used in the first stages following the diagnosis of the illness [23]. Psychological interventions centered on one's resources to cope more effectively with the MS are necessary to bring a positive adaptation to the adverse situation [25].

Based on the aforementioned points, the following study has been carried out to obtain greater knowledge on the influence of this pandemic on the health/illness of people with MS. The objective will be to discover and analyze the relationships between physical activity, a sense of coherence, resilience and coping in people diagnosed with MS during the emergency health situation brought about by COVID-19.

2. Materials and Methods

A cross-sectional, descriptive and correlational study was conducted.

2.1. Participants

The population is made up of 1236 people with MS belonging to multiple sclerosis associations in Castilla y León (Spain) (See Table 1). Through a nonprobabilistic convenience sampling, 84 participants were selected.

Table 1. Multiple sclerosis associations of the Castilla y León region (Spain).

PROVINCE	Associations name	WEB
Leon	SIL association for multiple sclerosis. Ponferrada ASILDEM.	https://aedem.org/quick-show/151-vacio/215-asociacie-em-de-fuentes-nuevas-le
	Leon multiple sclerosis association ALDEM.	https://esclerosismultipleleon.org/
Valladolid	Valladolid multiple sclerosis association AVEM.	https://www.emvalladolid.es/
Burgos	Association of relatives and sufferers of multiple sclerosis AFAEM.	https://www.esclerosismultipleburgos.org/contacto/
	Burgos multiple sclerosis association ASBEM.	http://www.asbemiranda.org/
	Ribera de Duero multiple sclerosis association AREM.	https://aedem.org/noticias-asociaciones/noticias-ribera-de-duero/76-asociaciibera-de-duero-de-esclerosis-mple-actividades-del-a003
Salamanca	Salamanca multiple sclerosis association ASDEM.	www.asdem.org/
Segovia	Segovia multiple sclerosis association ASGEM.	www.segoviaesclerosis.org/
Zamora	Zamora multiple sclerosis association AZDEM.	www.azdemzamora.es
Palencia	Palencia multiple sclerosis association APEM.	https://esclerosismultiple.com/entidades/asociacion-palentina-de-esclerosis-multiple-apem/
Avila	Avila multiple sclerosis association ADEMA.	www.ademavila.com/
Soria	Soria multiple sclerosis association ASOEM.	https://aedem.org/ini/1888-informe-bernat-soria

2.2. Instruments Used to Collect Data

The short-format of the (IPAQ-SF) international questionnaire, validated in Spanish [26], is used with young adults and middle-aged people (15–69). It consists of four generic items to obtain information on physical activity related to health. It provides separate results for the three types of activity: vigorous intensive activities, activities of moderate intensity and walking. Obtaining the final result requires the totaling of the duration (in minutes) and frequency (in days) of these three types of activity, from which the physical activity is categorized in three levels: low, moderate and high. The "sitting time" is also registered. This is time dedicated to carrying out a sedentary activity [27].

The Resilience Scale, (ER-14), has 14 items to evaluate the degree of individual resilience [19]. The version was validated into Spanish by Sánchez–Teruel and Robles–Bello [28]. The ER-14 measures two factors: on the one hand, personal competence (11 items), and on the other hand, the acceptance of oneself and of life (three items). This scale presents a suitable internal consistency ($\alpha = 0.79$) and validity of the calculated criterion with other measurements of general resilience (CD-RISC) ($r = 0.87$; $p < 0.01$). According to the scores: 98–82: very high resilience; 81–64: high resilience; 63–49: normal; 48–31: low; and between 30–14: very low. The reliability indices are suitable, demonstrating that it is a good instrument for measuring this variable [28].

The questionnaire on the Sense of Coherence (SOC 13) [20] is the Spanish-adapted version [29]. This scale consists of 13 items that are scored using a Likert-type scale of seven points. It contains three scales corresponding to the three dimensions of the construct: compression ($\alpha = 0.630$), direction ($\alpha = 0.596$) and significance ($\alpha = 0.594$), and a total score ($\alpha = 0.799$).

The questionnaire on coping COPE-28 [30] is the Spanish version (COPE-28) [31]. It is composed of 28 items scored using a Likert-type scale that goes from 0 (absolutely nothing) to 3 (a lot). These items are grouped together in pairs, producing 14 modes of coping: active coping ($\alpha = 0.452$), instrumental support ($\alpha = 0.630$), acceptance ($\alpha = 0.516$), self-distraction ($\alpha = 0.482$), venting ($\alpha = 0.302$), planning ($\alpha = 0.585$), religion ($\alpha = 0.880$), denial ($\alpha = 0.458$), self-blaming ($\alpha = 0.617$), substance use, emotional support, positive reframing ($\alpha = 0.602$), humor ($\alpha = 0.835$) and behavioral disengagement ($\alpha = 0.654$).

2.3. Procedure

The data for the study was gathered online by means of Google Forms (https://forms.gle/yu1gfoSX8h6L1HnV9). Prior to sending the questionnaire, all of the MS associations of Castilla y León (Spain) were contacted by telephone and e-mail. The members diagnosed with MS were requested to participate in the questionnaire using e-mail or WhatsApp. The gathering of the data took place between 28 March and 3 June 2020, during the period of confinement, due to the state of alarm imposed by the Spanish government for the management of the health crisis situation.

2.4. Data Analysis

The analysis of the data was descriptive, analytical and correlational. It was checked that the adjustment did not comply with the normal distribution of the data by means of the Kolmogorov–Smirnov test with the Lilliefors significance correction. For this reason, nonparametric tests were carried out (U of Mann–Whitney) for the comparisons of averages between the groups. Nonparametric correlations were carried out in order to evaluate the associations between the quantitative variables, and the Spearman rho coefficients were obtained. A value of $p < 0.05$ was considered statistically significant.

The database and the statistical analyses cited were carried out using the SPSS 26.0 (Statistical Package for the Social Sciences) computer program (IBM, New York, NY, USA).

2.5. Ethical Considerations

The people participating in the study were considered anonymous and the data confidential. Prior informed consent was requested for their collaboration. The data are collected and handled respecting all of their rights and guarantees in accordance with those established in the UE2016/679 Regulation and in the Constitutional Law 3/2018 of 5 December on the Protection of Personal Data and digital rights guarantees. The study was approved by the ethics committee (ETICA-ULE-016-2020) of the University of León (Spain), which guarantees that the questions are both ethical and legal.

3. Results

The sociodemographic characteristics of the participants are set out in Table 2. 84 people diagnosed with MS in the Spanish Autonomous Community of Castilla y León participated in the study. The results of the average and the standard deviation in terms of age were 46.9 ± 9.7 years old (M±SD). In relation to the clinical characteristics of the illness, the greatest part of the sample, 67.9%, was diagnosed with Relapsing Remittent Multiple Sclerosis (EMRR), followed by 25% diagnosed with its Secondary Progressive Multiple Sclerosis (EMPS). The descriptive values for the years of diagnosis of the MS were 13.9 ± 8.3 (average 15 years old, maximum 35 and minimum 1).

Table 2. Sample description.

		Total 84 (100%)
Gender	Man	34 (40.5%)
	Women	50 (59.5%)
City	Aranda de Duero	1 (1.2%)
	Ávila	4 (4.8%)
	Burgos	17 (20.2%)
	Miranda de Ebro	4 (4.8%)
	Palencia	13 (15.5%)
	Ponferrada	15 (17.9%)
	Segovia	4 (4.8%)
	Soria	6 (7.1%)
	Valladolid	20 (23.8%)
Type of multiple sclerosis	Primary Progressive	5 (6.0%)
	Progressive Recurrent	1 (1.2%)
	Secondary Progressive	21 (25.0%)
	Relapsing Remittent	57 (67.9%)
Number of people you live with	0	8 (9.5%)
	1	29 (34.5%)
	2	28 (33.3%)
	3	15 (17.9%)
	4	4 (4.8%)
Living with children under 14 years of age	0	63 (75.0%)
	1	13 (15.5%)
	2	7 (8.3%)
	3	1 (1.2%)
Have you had COVID-19?	Yes	0 (0%)
	No	68 (81.0%)
	Maybe	16 (19.0%)

Table 2. *Cont.*

		Total 84 (100%)
	Yes	0 (0%)
Do you have COVID-19?	No	77 (91.7%)
	Maybe	7 (8.3%)
	Yes	0 (0%)
Have you lived or do you live with people with COVID-19?	No	71 (84.5%)
	Maybe	12 (14.3%)

The results obtained for the physical activity variable are set out in Table 3. The U Mann–Whitney test has been carried out, and no differences have been found between men and women. As regards the scores for the questions on physical activity, 28 participants (33.3%) have scored high, 18 (21.4%) low and 29 (34.5%) have achieved a moderate degree of physical activity.

Table 3. Descriptive statistics of physical activity in minutes per week.

	Questionnaires	*n*	Minimum	Maximum	M ± SD	Me *	IR *
	Vigorous activity (V)	66	0	7200	1042.42 ± 1568.32	340	1480
	Moderate activity (M)	65	0	3600	870.77 ± 1005.62	540	1200
IPAQ *	Walk (W)	74	0	4258	956.0 ± 1158.65	495	1328.25
	TOTAL physical activity	75	0	10,890	2614.7 ± 2472.40	1986	3186
	Sitting time	61	15	1380	430.08 ± 282.59	360	270

Note: * minutes/week. M; Mean. SD; Standard Deviation. Me; Median. IR; Interquartile Ranges.

The descriptive statistics of the resilience, sense of coherence and coping variables are set out in Table 4. No differences have been found in the sex of the participants for the scores of these variables. In the case of resilience, 30 (35.7%) participants were perceived as having a very high resilience, 37 (44%) were evaluated as having high levels, 14 (16.7%) scored within what is considered normal, and 2 (2.4%) and 1 (1.2%) obtained low values or very low values, respectively.

Table 5 details the correlations between the variables of the study. The results indicate that physical activity does not correlate significantly with any of the other studied variables; however, although in some cases they are weak, correlations are observed between resilience, sense of coherence and coping. Thus, the highest levels of personal competence (CP), acceptance of oneself and of life (De) for resilience are related to the highest scores of compression (CO), direction (Dir) and significance (Sig) for the sense of coherence. As regards coping, the strategies for active coping (A), acceptance (Ac) and positive reframing (Pr) are positively related to the total and to the two dimensions of resilience of personal competence (CP) and acceptance of oneself and of life (AV), as well as to the factor of significance (Sig) of the sense of coherence variable. The strategies of denial (D), self-blaming (Sb) and behavioral disengagement (Bd) show negative correlations with resilience and the sense of coherence which have been evaluated in the study. Substance use as a strategy (Su) correlates negatively with resilience, in particular with the dimension of accepting oneself and life (De).

Table 4. Descriptive statistics of resilience, sense of coherence and coping.

	Questionnaires	*n*	Items	Minimum	Maximum	M ± SD
ER-14	Personal competence	84	11	14	77	59.71 ± 11.26
	Acceptance of oneself and life	84	3	4	21	15.19 ± 3.90
	Total	84	24	18	97	74.90 ± 14.39
SOC-13	Compression	84	5	11	32	22.50 ± 5.13
	Direction	84	4	7	27	18.26 ± 4.79
	Signification	84	4	7	28	20.42 ± 4.31
	Total	84	13	29	82	61.18 ± 12.25
COPE-28	Active coping	84	2	0	6	4.37 ± 1.27
	Instrumental support	84	2	0	6	3.48 ± 1.52
	Acceptance	84	2	1	6	3.65 ± 1.59
	Self-distraction	84	2	0	6	2.80 ± 1.42
	Venting	84	2	0	6	1.20 ± 1.66
	Planning	84	2	0	6	3.54 ± 1.73
	Religion	84	2	0	6	4.55 ± 1.38
	Denial	84	2	0	6	0.90 ± 1.40
	Self-blaming	84	2	0	6	2.57 ± 2.16
	Substance use	84	2	0	6	3.52 ± 1.72
	Emotional support	84	2	0	6	1.63 ± 1.66
	Positive reframing	84	2	0	6	0.83 ± 1.19
	Humor	84	2	0	6	2.23 ± 1.52
	Behavioral disengagement	84	2	0	6	0.26 ± 0.97

Note: ER-14: Resilience Scale. SOC-13: Sense of Coherence. COPE-28: Coping. SD: standard deviation. M: mean.

Table 5. Spearman's rho correlations of physical activity, resilience, sense of coherence and coping.

Questionnaires		W	M	V	T	CP	DE	T	CO	Dir	Sig	T
		IPAQ				ER-14			SOC-13			
IPAQ	W	1.000										
	M	0.406 **	1.000									
	V	0.074	0.447 **	1.000								
	T	0.601 **	0.815 **	0.656 **	1.000							
ER-14	CP	−0.003	0.055	0.112	0.113	1.000						
	De	−0.073	−0.014	0.066	0.006	0.724 **	1.000					
	T	−0.011	0.039	0.106	0.092	0.980 **	0.834 **	1.000				
SOC-13	Co	−0.001	−0.026	−0.088	−0.046	0.433 **	0.498 **	0.467 **	1.000			
	Dir	−0.103	−0.041	−0.011	−0.068	0.366 **	0.382 **	0.384 **	0.745 **	1.000		
	Sig	0.059	−0.062	0.112	0.009	0.426 **	0.390 **	0.445 **	0.517 **	0.500 **	1.000	
	T	−0.020	−0.036	−0.015	−0.043	0.467 **	0.489 **	0.496 **	0.891 **	0.877 **	0.772 **	1.000
COPE-28	A	0.041	0.038	−0.096	0.051	0.405 **	0.351 **	0.433 **	0.097	0.035	0.266 *	0.148
	I	−0.138	−0.183	0.061	−0.175	−0.018	−0.062	−0.030	−0.144	−0.130	−0.021	−0.129
	Ac	−0.104	0.094	−0.094	−0.015	0.587 **	0.564 **	0.620 **	0.359 **	0.223 *	0.373 **	0.376 **
	Sd	0.023	0.015	−0.001	0.062	0.127	−0.016	0.109	−0.105	−0.232 *	−0.310 **	−0.248 *
	V	−0.125	−0.229	−0.004	−0.111	0.023	−0.049	0.030	−0.234 *	−0.187	−0.124	−0.215 *
	P	−0.101	0.002	0.056	0.098	0.215 *	0.186	0.228 *	0.045	−0.015	0.131	0.070
	R	−0.014	0.011	0.020	−0.030	−0.038	−0.077	−0.044	−0.078	0.071	−0.007	−0.039
	D	0.058	0.063	0.043	0.009	−0.190	−0.248 *	−0.213	−0.332 **	−0.314 **	−0.312 **	−0.390 **
	Sb	−0.162	−0.072	0.003	−0.069	−0.115	−0.290 **	−0.155	−0.348 **	−0.317 **	−0.395 **	−0.428 **
	Su	−0.177	−0.113	0.175	−0.040	−0.088	−0.219 *	−0.127	−0.104	−0.113	−0.077	−0.124
	E	0.010	−0.018	0.117	0.052	−0.005	−0.042	−0.011	−0.087	−0.018	0.143	0.005
	Pr	0.064	0.070	0.236	0.197	0.518 **	0.352 **	0.517 **	0.136	0.095	0.278 *	0.166
	H	0.094	0.019	0.142	0.044	0.129	0.047	0.115	−0.051	−0.078	0.062	−0.021
	Bd	−0.133	0.014	0.061	−0.013	−0.394 **	−0.286 **	−0.392 **	−0.251 *	−0.220 *	−0.355 **	−0.323 **

Note: *: $p < 0.05$, **: $p < 0.01$, T: total, W: Walk, M: Moderate activity, V: Vigorous activity, CP: competence personal, De: Acceptance of oneself and of life, Co: Compression, Dir: Direction, Sig: Signification, A: active coping, I: instrumental support, Ac: acceptance, Sd: self-distraction, V: venting, P: planning, R: religion, D: denial, Sb: Self-blaming, Su: substance use, E: emotional support, Pr: Positive reframing, H: humor, Bd: behavioral disengagement.

4. Discussion

The results revealed that the clinical and personal characteristics of the participants in the present study were similar to other studies conducted on patients with multiple sclerosis during the COVID-19 pandemic [1,13,32].

If we compare the time spent sitting down per week collected with the IPAQ of our sample with the study carried out by Moti et al. [33], which analyzed people with MS in America, we find that our population has a slightly higher value. Furthermore, our data show elevated levels of physical activity. These data seem to indicate a high participation in the activities proposed by the different associations and that they are concerned about their physical condition during this period of confinement. On the other hand, Hubbard et al. [34] observed that people with slight MS tended to do less physical activity in comparison with healthy people.

The results showed that people with multiple sclerosis who participate in associations presented high levels of resilience [19] overall and in the domains of personal competence and acceptance of oneself and of life. These values of adaptation to adverse situations are important for the well-being of people, as the studied sample went through 11 weeks of quarantine and time is considered as a predictive factor for acute stress disorder [3]. Furthermore, the effect of interventions that focus on promoting resilience and other personal resources are necessary to effectively cope with multiple sclerosis [25]. If the present study is compared to the work of Plowman et al. [17] in people with MS, the total resilience factors are very similar. On the contrary, the total resilience values and the I factor (personal competence) obtained in our sample are higher than those reached in the study carried out by Sánchez–Teruel et al. [28] in young healthy people. The case of populations with painful chronic pathologies such as fibromyalgia [35] highlights that our results are much higher (almost double) for this variable. It will be interesting to analyze the role of the associations in the promotion of the health of patients diagnosed with MS.

According to the data on the sense of coherence, those with multiple sclerosis who frequently attended associations in the Autonomous Community of Castilla y León had a total sense of coherence of 61.19 ± 12.252 during the confinement period. If we compare our data with the study of the sense of coherence in health personnel during the COVID-19 pandemic, we observe that our sample obtained higher mean values although they did not present symptoms of COVID [36]. Nonetheless, lower values than those of the present study are observed in populations with MS [37,38]. Conversely, persons with late effects of polio have obtained higher values, which could be due to their perception of the disability being less acute and to the fact that, upon having a later start, they have developed the capacity to understand, manage and be motivated when faced with stressful events and problems that come up during their lives [39]. If we compare our data with people without neurological problems and with a cardiac pathology, we observe that cardiac patients obtain worse values since they tend to be associated with other pathologies such as depression [40]. However, if we compare our sample with people older than 65–75, 76–80 and over 80, we see that all of the older people have higher scores in total (74 ± 3.44) and for decompression (27 ± 0.49), direction (23 ± 0.83) and significance (23 ± 1.09) [40].

The coping of the people with multiple sclerosis who participated in associations showed diverse levels according to the strategies used in comparison with people with multiple sclerosis who coped with the prognosis of their illness [29]; we observe that our population presented higher levels in terms of instrumental support 3.48 ± 1.52, substance use 3.52 ± 1.72, self-blaming 2.57 ± 2.16 and religion 4.55 ± 1.38. This leads us to think that they have less functional strategies when facing the COVID-19 situation due to their low self-esteem, perceived high levels of stress or psychological unease, as observed in French people facing serious illness or trauma [12]. In addition, people with MS can show increased discomfort due to having psychological problems due to alterations of cognitive dysfunctions, information processing, and immediate and episodic memory typical of MS [41]. Furthermore, the high values in religious coping lead us to think that they indicate a lower satisfaction with the decision that was taken to resolve the existence of stress [42]. Comparing our results on coping with values for healthy people, we find that emotional support, humor and positive revaluation present lower values in our study [43]. These data are logical because people with MS offer to undertake maladaptive coping strategies [12].

Finally, the results of this study indicate that the level of physical activity of a person with MS, which is measured in terms of the mastery of activity (vigorous, moderate), the total and the time spent sitting down, is not related to resilience, coping or sense of coherence in the social confinement situation that derives from the COVID-19 virus. However, we have found theoretical studies which support that psychological aspects can be influenced by physical activity [9,44].

Regarding the relationships between resilience and sense of coherence, this study observed that there was a positive relationship between them. This means that the most resilient people present greater levels of a sense of coherence and vice versa. This could benefit patients with MS, since there is evidence that supports a relationship between positive dimension factors (resilience and/or optimism) and subjective emotional well-being [45]. Recent research on the impact of COVID-19 on German public health supports our data, proposing to improve the sense of coherence to improve resilience to stressors [46]. According to the results of the relationships between coping and resilience, we observe that if a patient has a higher score in the strategies of active coping, acceptance, emotional support and planning, he or she will present greater levels of resilience and will have a greater capacity for adapting to adverse situations; that is, strategies for positive coping or task orientation are related to a better mental health [47,48]. In the same way, coping strategies such as denial, self-blame, substance abuse, venting and behavioral disconnection are negatively related to resilience, since they are strategies that maintain stress, as has been observed by other researchers [43,49]. Concerning the relationships between sense of coherence and coping, they depend on the strategies, as not everybody behaves in the same way. However, we can highlight the negative relationship between both venting and behavioral disengagement and the dimension of compression of the sense of coherence. According to recent studies, the behavior of our sample is the same as in Bedouin women older than 61 with little education and few possibilities for finding a job [50]. In both populations, one can observe that when there is a sensation of there being no control over the results or of being at the mercy of luck, it is probable that they will have a sensation of impotence and use passive or evasive strategies such as behavioral disconnection or the strategy of venting, which consists in verbally expressing the negative parts of a stressful situation. For all of the points mentioned above in relation to the COVID-19 scenario, researchers such as Ornell et al. support three main factors for developing mental health strategies: (1) multidisciplinary teams; (2) regular and precise clear communications about the outbreak situation; and (3) psychological counseling services through electronic applications for the community in general and especially for vulnerable people [4].

This study presents limitations, such as the method of sampling and the selection of the participants, which may exclude MS patients who do not belong to associations; furthermore, other variables such as the level of education, degree of incapacity and the medication used could have been included. Furthermore, it would be desirable to carry out longitudinal studies during similar adverse situations in people with multiple sclerosis, which might include variables such as resilience, sense of cohesion and coping strategies, as well as other more specific physical capacities altered by the illness, such as balance, walking or strength.

5. Conclusions

The majority of the participants in associations in Castilla y León (Spain) suffer from a type of Relapsing Remittent Multiple Sclerosis, followed by Secondary Progressive Multiple Sclerosis. In spite of the confinement/quarantine, the greatest part obtains high and moderate scores in physical activity. Although no relationship has been found between physical activity and the psychological variables, there is evidence of the influence of the latter on the well-being of the patients. It can be observed as those people who achieve high values in resilience, as well as in sense of coherence. Furthermore, the use of coping strategies in the sample confirms that active coping, acceptance, positive reframing, denial, self-blaming, behavioral disengagement and venting are negatively related to resilience and the sense of coherence.

This research may be useful in describing the degree of coping, sense of coherence, physical activity and coping strategies of people with multiple sclerosis in the confinement/quarantine situation deriving from the COVID-19 virus in Spain. Likewise, to detect possible problems and be able to establish psychological and or physical interventions for the associations of those affected with MS, this research might be repeated again in the future in order to promote health in similar situations.

Author Contributions: Conceptualization, M.M.R.-G., E.F.-M., C.L.-P. and L.Á.-B.; data curation, M.M.R.-G., L.Á.-B., C.L.-P. and E.F.-M.; formal analysis, E.F.-M., C.L.-P., M.M.R.-G. and L.Á.-B.; investigation, M.M.R.-G., L.Á.-B., E.F.-M. and C.L.-P.; methodology, E.F.-M., C.L.-P., L.Á.-B. and M.M.R.-G.; Project administration E.F.-M., C.L.-P., M.M.R.-G., L.Á.-B. and L.A.G.; resources, M.M.R.-G., E.F.-M., C.L.-P., L.Á.-B. and L.A.G.; software C.L.-P., E.F.-M., M.M.R.-G. and L.Á.-B.; supervision, M.M.R.-G., C.L.-P., E.F.-M., L.Á.-B. and L.A.G.; validation, E.F.-M., C.L.-P., M.M.R.-G., L.Á.-B. and L.A.G.; visualization, C.L.-P., E.F.-M., M.M.R.-G., L.Á.-B. and L.A.G.; writing—original draft, M.M.R.-G., L.Á.-B., C.L.-P. and E.F.-M.; writing—review and editing, E.F.-M., C.L.-P., M.M.R.-G., L.Á.-B. and L.A.G. All authors have read and agreed to the published version of the manuscript.

Funding: This research received no external funding.

Conflicts of Interest: The authors declare no conflict of interest.

References

1. Seyed, M.; Sahraian, M.A.; Rezaeimanesh, N.; Naser, A. Psychiatric Advice During COVID-19 Pandemic for Patients with Multiple Sclerosis. *Iran. J. Psychiatry Behav. Sci.* **2020**, *14*, e103243. [CrossRef]
2. *Real Decreto 463/2020, de 14 de marzo, por el que se declara el estado de alarma para la gestión de la situación de crisis sanitaria ocasionada por el COVID-19; Documento BOE-A-2020-3692*; BOE: Beijing, China, 2020; Volume 67, pp. 25390–25400. Available online: https://www.boe.es/diario_boe/txt.php?id=BOE-A-2020-3692 (accessed on 31 July 2020).
3. Brooks, S.K.; Webster, R.K.; Smith, L.E.; Woodland, L.; Wessely, S.; Greenberg, N.; Rubin, G.J. The psychological impact of quarantine and how to reduce it: Rapid review of the evidence. *Lancet (Lond., Engl.)* **2020**, *395*, 912–920. [CrossRef]
4. Ornell, F.; Schuch, J.B.; Sordi, A.O.; Kessler, F.H.P. "Pandemic fear" and COVID-19: Mental health burden and strategies. *Braz. J. Psychiatry* **2020**, *42*, 232–235. [CrossRef] [PubMed]
5. Oh, J.; Vidal-Jordana, A.; Montalban, X. Multiple sclerosis. *Curr. Opin. Neurol.* **2018**, *31*, 752–759. [CrossRef] [PubMed]
6. McNulty, K. Coping with multiple sclerosis: Considerations and interventions. In *Coping with Chronic Illness and Disability: Theoretical, Empirical, and Clinical Aspects*; Springer US: New York, NY, USA, 2007; pp. 289–311, ISBN 9780387486680.
7. Sellner, J.; Kraus, J.; Awad, A.; Milo, R.; Hemmer, B.; Stüve, O. The increasing incidence and prevalence of female multiple sclerosis—A critical analysis of potential environmental factors. *Autoimmun. Rev.* **2011**, *10*, 495–502. [CrossRef] [PubMed]
8. Calandri, E.; Graziano, F.; Borghi, M.; Bonino, S. Depression, Positive and Negative Affect, Optimism and Health-Related Quality of Life in Recently Diagnosed Multiple Sclerosis Patients: The Role of Identity, Sense of Coherence, and Self-efficacy. *J. Happiness Stud.* **2018**, *19*, 277–295. [CrossRef]
9. Sá, M.J. Psychological aspects of multiple sclerosis. *Clin. Neurol. Neurosurg.* **2008**, *110*, 868–877. [CrossRef]
10. McCabe, M.P.; McKern, S. Quality of life and multiple sclerosis: Comparison between people with multiple sclerosis and people from the general population. *J. Clin. Psychol. Med. Settings* **2002**, *9*, 287–295. [CrossRef]
11. Marrie, R.A.; Fisk, J.D.; Yu, B.N.; Leung, S.; Elliott, L.; Caetano, P.; Warren, S.; Evans, C.; Wolfson, C.; Sveson, L.W. Mental comorbidity and multiple sclerosis: Validating administrative data to support population-based surveillance. *BMC Neurol.* **2013**, *13*, 1–8. [CrossRef]
12. Haji Akhoundi, F.; Sahraian, M.A.; Naser Moghadasi, A. Neuropsychiatric and cognitive effects of the COVID-19 outbreak on multiple sclerosis patients. *Mult. Scler. Relat. Disord.* **2020**, *41*, 102164. [CrossRef]

13. Moss, B.P.; Mahajan, K.R.; Bermel, R.A.; Hellisz, K.; Hua, L.H.; Hudec, T.; Husak, S.; McGinley, M.P.; Ontaneda, D.; Wang, Z.; et al. Multiple sclerosis management during the COVID-19 pandemic. *Mult. Scler. J.* **2020**, *26*, 1163–1171. [CrossRef] [PubMed]

14. Motl, R.W.; McAuley, E.; Snook, E.M. Physical activity and multiple sclerosis: A meta-analysis. *Mult. Scler. J.* **2005**, *11*, 459–463. [CrossRef] [PubMed]

15. Streber, R.; Peters, S.; Pfeifer, K. Systematic Review of Correlates and Determinants of Physical Activity in Persons with Multiple Sclerosis. *Arch. Phys. Med. Rehabil.* **2016**, *97*, 633–645.e29. [CrossRef]

16. Krüger, T.; Behrens, J.R.; Grobelny, A.; Otte, K.; Mansow-Model, S.; Kayser, B.; Bellmann-Strobl, J.; Brandt, A.U.; Paul, F.; Schmitz-Hübsch, T. Subjective and objective assessment of physical activity in multiple sclerosis and their relation to health-related quality of life. *BMC Neurol.* **2017**, *17*, 10. [CrossRef] [PubMed]

17. Ploughman, M.; Downer, M.B.; Pretty, R.W.; Wallack, E.M.; Amirkhanian, S.; Kirkland, M.C.; Fisk, J.D.; Mayo, N.; Sadovnick, A.D.; Beaulieu, S.; et al. The impact of resilience on healthy aging with multiple sclerosis. *Qual. Life Res.* **2020**, *29*, 2769–2779. [CrossRef]

18. Silverman, A.M.; Verrall, A.M.; Alschuler, K.N.; Smith, A.E.; Ehde, D.M. Bouncing back again, and again: A qualitative study of resilience in people with multiple sclerosis. *Disabil. Rehabil.* **2017**, *39*, 14–22. [CrossRef]

19. Wagnild, G. A review of the resilience Scale. *J. Nurs. Meas.* **2009**, *17*, 105–113. [CrossRef] [PubMed]

20. Antonovsky, A. The structure and properties of the sense of coherence scale. *Soc. Sci. Med.* **1993**, *36*, 725–733. [CrossRef]

21. Compston, A.; Coles, A. Multiple sclerosis. *Lancet (Lond., Engl.)* **2008**, *372*, 1502–1517. [CrossRef]

22. Štern, B.; Zaletel-Kragelj, L.; Hojs Fabjan, T. Impact of sense of coherence on quality of life in patients with multiple sclerosis. Wien. *Klin. Wochenschr.* **2020**, 1–9. [CrossRef]

23. Calandri, E.; Graziano, F.; Borghi, M.; Bonino, S. Coping strategies and adjustment to multiple sclerosis among recently diagnosed patients: The mediating role of sense of coherence. *Clin. Rehabil.* **2017**, *31*, 1386–1395. [CrossRef]

24. Keramat Kar, M.; Whitehead, L.; Smith, C.M. Characteristics and correlates of coping with multiple sclerosis: A systematic review. *Disabil. Rehabil.* **2019**, *41*, 250–264. [CrossRef] [PubMed]

25. Black, R.; Dorstyn, D. A biopsychosocial model of resilience for multiple sclerosis. *J. Health Psychol.* **2015**, *20*, 1434–1444. [CrossRef]

26. Ruiz-Casado, A.; Alejo, L.B.; Santos-Lozano, A.; Soria, A.; Ortega, M.J.; Pagola, I.; Fiuza-Luces, C.; Palomo, I.; Garatachea, N.; Cebolla, H.; et al. Validity of the Physical Activity Questionnaires IPAQ-SF and GPAQ for Cancer Survivors: Insights from a Spanish Cohort. *Int. J. Sports Med.* **2016**, *37*, 979–985. [CrossRef]

27. Lee, P.H.; Macfarlane, D.J.; Lam, T.H.; Stewart, S.M. Validity of the international physical activity questionnaire short form (IPAQ-SF): A systematic review. *Int. J. Behav. Nutr. Phys. Act.* **2011**, *8*, 115. [CrossRef]

28. Sánchez-Teruel, D.; Robles-Bello, M.A. Escala de resiliencia 14 ítems (RS-14): Propiedades psicométricas de la versión en español. *Rev. Iberoam. Diagn. Eval. Aval. Psicol.* **2015**, *2*, 103–113.

29. Virués-Ortega, J.; Martínez-Martín, P.; Del Barrio, J.L.; Lozano, L.M.; De Pedro, J.; Almazán, J.; Avellanal, F.; Boix, R.; Cerrato, E.; Medrano, M.J.; et al. Validación transcultural de la Escala de Sentido de Coherencia de Antonovsky (OLQ-13) en ancianos mayores de 70 años. *Med. Clin. (Barc)* **2007**, *128*, 486–492. [CrossRef] [PubMed]

30. Carver, C.S. You want to measure coping but your protocol's too long: Consider the brief COPE. *Int. J. Behav. Med.* **1997**, *4*, 92–100. [CrossRef]

31. Mate, A.I.; Andreu, J.M.; Peña, M.E. Propiedades psicométricas de la versión española del "inventario breve de afrontamiento" (COPE-28) en una muestra de adolescentes. *Behav. Psychol.* **2016**, *24*, 305–318.

32. Louapre, C.; Collongues, N.; Stankoff, B.; Giannesini, C.; Papeix, C.; Bensa, C.; Deschamps, R.; Créange, A.; Wahab, A.; Pelletier, J.; et al. Clinical Characteristics and Outcomes in Patients with Coronavirus Disease 2019 and Multiple Sclerosis. *JAMA Neurol.* **2020**, *77*, 1079–1088. [CrossRef]

33. Motl, R.W.; Sasaki, J.E.; Cederberg, K.L.; Jeng, B. Validity of Sitting Time Scores from the International Physical Activity Questionnaire-Short Form in Multiple Sclerosis. *Rehabil. Psychol.* **2019**, *64*, 463–468. [CrossRef]

34. Hubbard, E.A.; Motl, R.W.; Manns, P.J. The descriptive epidemiology of daily sitting time as a sedentary behavior in multiple sclerosis. *Disabil. Health J.* **2015**, *8*, 594–601. [CrossRef]

35. Cejudo, J.; García-Castillo, F.-J.; Luna, P.; Rodrigo-Ruiz, D.; Feltrero, R.; Moreno-Gómez, A. Using a Mindfulness-Based Intervention to Promote Subjective Well-Being, Trait Emotional Intelligence, Mental Health, and Resilience in Women with Fibromyalgia. *Front. Psychol.* **2019**, *10*, 2541. [CrossRef]

36. Gómez-Salgado, J.; Domínguez-Salas, S.; Romero-Martín, M.; Ortega-Moreno, M.; García-Iglesias, J.J.; Ruiz-Frutos, C. Sense of coherence and psychological distress among healthcare workers during the COVID-19 pandemic in Spain. *Sustainability* **2020**, *12*, 6855. [CrossRef]

37. Stern, B.; Socan, G.; Rener-Sitar, K.; Kukec, A.; Zaletel-Kragelj, L. Validation of the Slovenian version of short sense of coherence questionnaire (SOC-13) in multiple sclerosis patients. *Zdr. Varst.* **2019**, *58*, 31–39. [CrossRef]

38. Broersma, F.; Oeseburg, B.; Dijkstra, J.; Wynia, K. The impact of self-perceived limitations, stigma and sense of coherence on quality of life in multiple sclerosis patients: Results of a cross-sectional study. *Clin. Rehabil.* **2018**, *32*, 536–545. [CrossRef]

39. Nolvi, M.; Brogårdh, C.; Jacobsson, L.; Lexell, J. Sense of Coherence in persons with late effects of polio. *NeuroRehabilitation* **2018**, *42*, 103–111. [CrossRef] [PubMed]

40. Spadoti Dantas, R.A.; Silva, F.S.E.; Ciol, M.A. Psychometric properties of the Brazilian Portuguese versions of the 29- and 13-item scales of the Antonovsky's Sense of Coherence (SOC-29 and SOC-13) evaluated in Brazilian cardiac patients. *J. Clin. Nurs.* **2014**, *23*, 156–165. [CrossRef] [PubMed]

41. L'Encéphale—Présentation—EM Consulte. Available online: https://www.em-consulte.com/article/83225/alertePM (accessed on 24 July 2020).

42. Major, B.; Richards, C.; Cooper, M.L.; Cozzarelli, C.; Zubek, J. Personal resilience, cognitive appraisals, and coping: An integrative model of adjustment to abortion. *J. Pers. Soc. Psychol.* **1998**, *74*, 735–752. [CrossRef]

43. Madrid Álvarez, M.B.; Carretero Hernández, G.; González Quesada, A.; González Martín, J.M. Measurement of the Psychological Impact of Psoriasis on Patients Receiving Systemic Treatment. *Actas Dermo-Sifiliogr.* **2018**, *109*, 733–740. [CrossRef]

44. Learmonth, Y.C.; Motl, R.W. Physical activity and exercise training in multiple sclerosis: A review and content analysis of qualitative research identifying perceived determinants and consequences. *Disabil. Rehabil.* **2016**, *38*, 1227–1242. [CrossRef] [PubMed]

45. Eriksson, M.; Lindström, B. Antonovsky's sense of coherence scale and the relation with health: A systematic review. *J. Epidemiol. Commun. Health* **2006**, *60*, 376–381. [CrossRef]

46. Schäfer, S.K.; Sopp, M.R.; Schanz, C.G.; Staginnus, M.; Göritz, A.S.; Michael, T. Impact of COVID-19 on Public Mental Health and the Buffering Effect of a Sense of Coherence. *Psychother. Psychosom.* **2020**, *89*, 1–7. [CrossRef]

47. Thompson, G.; McBride, R.B.; Hosford, C.C.; Halaas, G. Resilience among Medical Students: The Role of Coping Style and Social Support. *Teach. Learn. Med.* **2016**, *28*, 174–182. [CrossRef]

48. Lee, S.; Kim, S.; Young Choi, J. Coping and resilience of adolescents with congenital heart disease. *J. Cardiovasc. Nurs.* **2014**, *29*, 340–346. [CrossRef]

49. Ogińska-Bulik, N.; Kobylarczyk, M. Relation between resiliency and post-traumatic growth in a group of paramedics: The mediating role of coping strategies. *Int. J. Occup. Med. Environ. Health* **2015**, *28*, 707–719. [CrossRef]

50. Braun-Lewensohn, O.; Abu-Kaf, S.; Al-Said, K.; Huss, E. Analysis of the Differential Relationship between the Perception of One's Life and Coping Resources among Three Generations of Bedouin Women. *Int. J. Environ. Res. Public Health* **2019**, *16*, 804. [CrossRef]

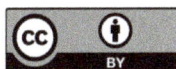

International Journal of
Environmental Research and Public Health

MDPI

Article

Daylight Saving Time and Spontaneous Deliveries: A Case–Control Study in Italy

Rosaria Cappadona [1,2,3], Sara Puzzarini [2], Vanessa Farinelli [2], Piergiorgio Iannone [1],
Alfredo De Giorgi [4], Emanuele Di Simone [5], Roberto Manfredini [1,3,4,*], Rosita Verteramo [2],
Pantaleo Greco [1,2], María Aurora Rodríguez Borrego [3,6], Fabio Fabbian [1,3,4,*]
and Pablo Jesús López Soto [3,6]

[1]   Department of Medical Sciences, University of Ferrara, 44121 Ferrara, Italy;
      rosaria.cappadona@unife.it (R.C.); pg.iannone88@gmail.com (P.I.); pantaleo.greco@unife.it (P.G.)
[2]   Obstetrics & Gynecology Unit, Department of Reproduction and Growth,
      Azienda Ospedaliero-Universitaria "S. Anna", 44124 Ferrara, Italy; s.puzzarini@ospfe.it (S.P.);
      vanessa.farinelli@edu.unife.it (V.F.); r.verteramo@ospfe.it (R.V.)
[3]   Department of Nursing, Instituto Maimónides de Investigación Biomédica de Córdoba (IMIBIC),
      14071 Córdoba, Spain; en1robom@uco.es (M.A.R.B.); n82losop@uco.es (P.J.L.S.)
[4]   Clinica Medica Unit, Department of Medicine, Azienda Ospedaliero-Universitaria "S. Anna",
      44124 Ferrara, Italy; degiorgialfredo@libero.it
[5]   Department of Biomedicine and Prevention, University of Rome Tor Vergata, I-00133 Rome, Italy;
      emanuele.disimone@uniroma1.it
[6]   Department of Nursing Pharmacology and Physiotherapy, University of Córdoba, 14071 Córdoba, Spain
*   Correspondence: roberto.manfredini@unife.it (R.M.); f.fabbian@ospfe.it (F.F.); Tel.: +39-0532-237166 (R.M.);
      +39-0532-236071 (F.F.)

Received: 1 September 2020; Accepted: 25 October 2020; Published: 3 November 2020

check for
updates

Abstract: (1) Background: Although the current literature shows that daylight saving time (DST) may play a role in human health and behavior, this topic has been poorly investigated with reference to Obstetrics. The aim of this case–control study was to evaluate whether DST may influence the number of spontaneous deliveries. (2) Methods: A low-risk pregnancy cohort with spontaneous onset of labor ($n = 7415$) was analyzed from a single Italian region for the period 2016–2018. Primary outcome was the number of spontaneous deliveries. Secondary outcomes were: gestational age at delivery, type and time of delivery, use of analgesia, birth weight, and 5-min Apgar at delivery. We compared the outcomes in the two weeks after DST (cases) to the two weeks before DST (controls). (3) Results: Data showed no significant difference between the number of deliveries occurring before and after DST (Chi-square = 0.546, $p = 0.46$). Vaginal deliveries at any gestational age showed no statistical difference between the two groups (Chi-square = 0.120, $p = 0.73$). There were no significant differences in the secondary outcomes, as well. (4) Conclusions: DST has neither a significant impact on the number of deliveries nor on the obstetric variables investigated by this study.

Keywords: daylight saving time (DST); desynchronization; circadian rhythm; chronobiology; nursing; spontaneous delivery; midwifery; obstetrics

1. Introduction

The mechanism that starts the spontaneous onset of labor still remains an unanswered question in the current literature [1]. In the obstetric field, scientific research is rich in studies, conducted both in vitro and in vivo, explaining the action of hormones in the onset and maintenance of labor during birth by correlating it with the circadian cycle [2]. Cortisol is the main stress hormone responsible for the normal adaptation of the neonate to extrauterine life. Placental corticotrophin releasing hormone

(CRH) is active from the early weeks of pregnancy and determines its duration, the time of onset of labor, and the timing of delivery; moreover, its plasma levels increase rapidly near the beginning of spontaneous labor. Data suggest that CRH may have a pivotal role in activating the mechanism of delivery [3–5]. In addition, type of delivery, e.g., vaginal or caesarean, may determine a different stress response. Recently, a study compared the activity of 11beta-hydroxysteroid dehydrogenase type 2 (11β-HSD 2) in the placenta and the umbilical cord blood cortisol level between caesarean sections, with or without uterine contraction, and vaginal delivery groups [6]. No statistically significant differences in the activity of 11β-HSD 2 were found in placentas delivered via caesarean sections compared to vaginal deliveries, while umbilical cord blood cortisol in the elective caesarean sections group was significantly lower compared to the vaginal deliveries and intrapartum caesarean sections [6]. Sleep disturbances and alterations in the circadian rhythm can lead to an increase in the levels of stress hormones and the activation of a pro-inflammatory condition can trigger and enhance the activity of prostaglandins and oxytocin, by promoting uterine contractions, the dynamic phenomena of labor, and consequently, the onset of labor [4–7]. These alternations can also be induced by shift work; in fact, women who experience an alteration of their circadian rhythm due to work are significantly more exposed to a reduction in birth rate and a lower birth weight of their newborns [8]. The purpose of the so-called "Summer time" was to capitalize on natural daylight: by turning the clock one hour forward as the days get longer in Spring, sunset is delayed by this same hour, until the clock is set back again in Autumn. After a first phase of Daylight Saving Time (DST) policy, where single countries decided their own standards, not regulated, harmonization attempts began in the 1970s to facilitate the effective operation of the internal market, and this practice is applied in over 60 countries worldwide [9]. Since light–dark alternation influences the synchronization of circadian rhythms of most human systems, DST may cause a chrono-disruption by significantly altering circadian rhythm and negatively influencing sleep quality [10]. A growing amount of evidence showed that DST transition may have negative effects on health [11–16]. Thus, based on these premises, an international consensus statement suggested that DST cannot be encouraged and therefore, should be discontinued [17].

As for female reproduction, disruptions of circadian rhythms, e.g., shift work, jet lag, and DST, have been associated with poorer fertility and early pregnancy outcomes [18]. However, very few data are available on the effect of DST on the onset of spontaneous labor. Only one recent published study showed no significant association between DST circadian rhythm and the number of spontaneous deliveries [19]. Based on this hypothesis, we evaluated whether DST might affect the number of spontaneous deliveries in a single Italian region.

2. Materials and Methods

A cohort of 7415 deliveries from low risk pregnancies with spontaneous onset of labor was enrolled in this case–control study. We used the Certificate of Childbirth Assistance (CedAP) data collection from one single Italian region, Emilia-Romagna, in the period 2016–2018. We identified the exact dates of DST during each year analyzed (Figure 1). Age and gestational age were evaluated. We defined the 2 weeks after DST as the exposure period and the 2 weeks before DST as the control period.

Exclusion criteria are shown in Table 1.

The primary outcome was defined as the number of deliveries, in particular the number of non-operative vaginal deliveries.

The rationale underlying the choice of the latter outcome was to exclude, as far as possible, the conditioning acted out by the health workers and the healthcare organizational system that weighs on the birth path, in order to bring out the influences that the endocrine and central nervous systems have on childbirth.

Secondary outcomes were:

- Gestational age delivery, defining preterm before 37 weeks, at term between 37 and 41 weeks, and post term beyond 41 weeks;
- Type of delivery: vaginal delivery, cesarean section, or operative delivery;

- Time of delivery: time when the birth occurred, combining three moments of the day—morning (08:00–15:59), afternoon (16:00–23:59), or night (00:00–07:59);
- Birth weight, divided into three distinct classes: less than 2500 g, between 2500 and 4000 g, and more than 4000 g;
- Five-minute Apgar at birth;
- Use of analgesia in labor.

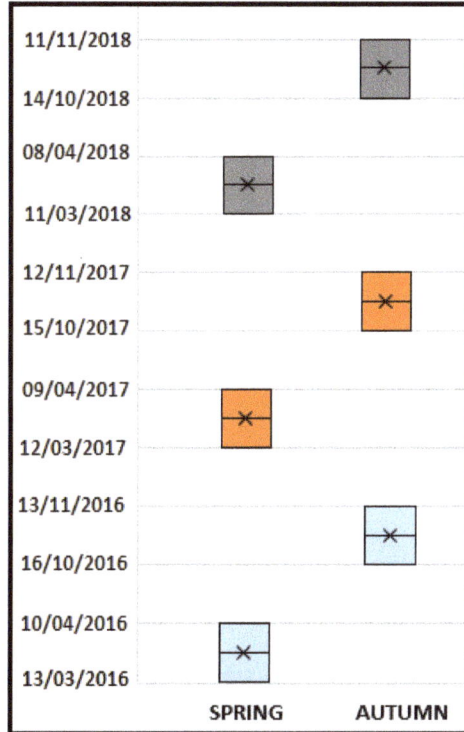

Figure 1. The two weeks belonging to the control period and the exposure period identified by daylight saving time (DST) during each year analyzed (2016–2018) are reported (grey is related with 2016, orange with 2017 and light blue with 2018).

Table 1. The table shows the exclusion criteria applied on the sample.

Exclusion Criteria
Not low risk pregnancy
Not cephalic presentation
Induction of labor
Multiple pregnancy
Fetal growth defects
Medically Assisted Procreation (MAP) pregnancies
Fetal anomalies
Stillbirth
Elective Cesarean section

We also analyzed local data relating to individual provinces. In particular, the number of at term deliveries that occurred in the three-year period was considered in the various Emilia-Romagna provinces, in order to verify whether there were any differences related to DST. The statistical analysis of the data was performed with the "chi-square" test.

We considered a 5% error with a confidence interval of 95%, standard deviation of 0.5, and z-score of 1.96.

The differences in the number of deliveries across the Spring and Autumn shifts were assessed for significance using the Poisson Means Test.

Annual birth rate was calculated as the ratio between the number of births during the two weeks pre and post DST, and the mean value of births obtained by the sum of births in the previous and the considered year divided by 2. The ratio was then multiplied by 10^3. This calculation was performed for any year considered in this study.

$$N\,(x)\;=\;\frac{N(x)}{\left[\,\frac{B(x-1)}{2}+\frac{B(x)}{2}\,\right]}*1000 \tag{1}$$

N = number of births during the index 2 weeks;
X = year considered;
x−1 = previous year;
B = total births in the Emilia-Romagna region of Italy.

In addition, we calculated the age and gestational age of participants. A logistic regression analysis was carried out, where the period including the two weeks pre and post DST was the dependent variable and the other parameters investigated in this study the independent ones. A 2-sided p-value < 0.05 was considered statistically significant. IBM Statistical Package for Social Science (SPSS 13.0 for Windows, SPSS Inc., Chicago, IL, USA) was used.

3. Results

The mean age of the 7415 women was 31.4 ± 5 years, and mean gestational age was 39.3 ± 1.4 weeks. Italian patients totaled 4801 (64.7%), whilst 35.3% were classified as non-Italian. The mean age of the women who delivered during the two weeks before DST were older than those who delivered during the two weeks post DST (31.6 ± 5.4 vs. 31.3 ± 5.3 years, $p = 0.033$); on the contrary, gestational age was not different in the two groups (39.3 ± 1.4 vs. 39.3 ± 1.4 weeks, $p = $ ns). As regarding time of delivery, 2708 births occurred in the morning (36.5%), 2022 (27.3%) in the afternoon, and 2685 (36.2%) at night. Birth rate during the Spring and Autumn shifts in the three different years of the study are shown in Table 2.

Table 2. Birth rates in the years 2016, 2017, and 2018 are shown.

Year of Study	Spring Shift		Autumn Shift	
	Control Period	Exposure Period	Control Period	Exposure Period
2016	18.39	17.42	20.89	21.21
2017	17.52	14.04	19.03	19.00
2018	16.27	17.99	17.03	17.12

Data are expressed as $* 10^3$.

3.1. Primary Outcome

Our results showed a difference in the number of deliveries between the exposed and the control groups, although it did not reach statistical significance (Table 3).

No statistical difference has been observed in the analysis of the number of deliveries ($p = 0.46$), including mode of delivery (vaginal delivery, cesarean section, or operative delivery) and gestational age (term, preterm, post term). The same result was obtained analyzing the number of spontaneous deliveries ($p = 0.73$).

The differences in the number of deliveries and number of spontaneous deliveries across the Spring and Autumn shifts assessed by the Poisson Means Test were not significant ($p = 0.37$, $p = 0.92$, $p = 0.6$, and $p = 0.65$ respectively).

Table 3. Summarized data of results of primary outcome.

Primary Outcome	Spring Shift		Autumn Shift		CHI-SQUARE	p-Value ($\alpha = 5\%$)
	Control Period	Exposure Period	Control Period	Exposure Period		
Number of deliveries	1781	1727	1950	1957	0.546	0.46
Number of spontaneous deliveries	1588	1536	1744	1716	0.120	0.73

3.2. Secondary Outcome

There were no significant differences in the secondary outcomes analyzed, between what was detected during the exposure period and what was found in the control period (Table 4).

Table 4. Summarized data of results of secondary outcomes.

Secondary Outcome	Spring Shift		Autumn Shift		CHI-SQUARE	p-Value ($\alpha = 5\%$)
	Control Period	Exposure Period	Control Period	Exposure Period		
Delivery at term	1700	1652	1860	1849	0.227	0.63
Vaginal delivery at term	1516	1468	1663	1623	0.024	0.89
Post-term delivery	22	14	18	26	2.474	0.12
Preterm delivery	52	55	65	74	0.082	0.78
Type of delivery						
Cesarean Section	103	83	104	119	3.099	0.08
Operative delivery	90	108	102	122	0.0003	0.99
Time of delivery						
Morning (5:01 a.m. to 1:00 p.m.)	605	605	667	674	0.017	0.89
Afternoon (1:01 p.m. to 9:00 p.m.)	526	506	600	585	0.025	0.87
night (9:01 p.m. to 5:00 a.m.)	650	615	681	696	0.980	0.32
Birth weight						
Less than 2500 g	30	28	43	43	0.001	0.97
Between 2500 and 4000 g	1625	1579	1771	1785	0.564	0.45
More than 4000 g	126	120	136	129	0.0005	0.98
5-min Apgar at birth						
Apgar 7 at 5 min	11	6	10	12	0.760	0.38
Apgar 8 at 5 min	22	29	28	36	0.015	0.90
Apgar 9 at 5 min	242	245	270	254	0.339	0.56
Apgar 10 at 5 min	1502	1441	1632	1643	0.899	0.34
Use of analgesia in labor	313	299	355	357	0.217	0.64

Women's age was independently associated with delivery during the two weeks post DST (OR 1.010, 95% Confidence intervals 1.002–1.019, $p = 0.021$). All the other investigated parameters were not associated with the period of the DST. Therefore, every year of increasing age of the delivering woman increased the risk of event occurrence during the two weeks after DST of 1.0% (Table 5).

Finally, we assessed the percentages of type and time of delivery during the Spring and Autumn shifts, but we could not find any difference (data not shown).

Table 5. Logistic regression analysis considering the period including the two weeks pre and post DST as the dependent variable and the other parameters investigated the independent ones.

Variables	Odds Ratios	95% Confidence Intervals	*p*
Maternal age	1.010	1.002–1.019	0.021
Gestational age	1.005	0.970–1.041	0.801
Type of delivery	0.917	0.780–1.079	0.295
Time of delivery	1.044	0.930–1.172	0.466
Birth weight	1.000	1.000–1.000	0.639
5-min Apgar at birth	1.025	0.947–1.109	0.545
Use of analgesia in labor	1.023	0.900–1.163	0.726

4. Discussion

The present study found no statistically significant differences in the number of deliveries that occurred during the two weeks following DST compared to those occurring prior to the DST shifts. The same result was obtained for each secondary outcome analyzed. These data confirm the findings by Laszlo et al. [19] also for the latitudes and climatic conditions of the Emilia-Romagna region of Italy, despite the difference in daily average hours of sunlight (approximately 180 and 50 monthly sun-hours in March and October, respectively, in Sweden, vs. 190 and 100 in March and October, respectively, in Italy). The Swedish study, in fact, showed that the number of daily and weekly deliveries in the case and control group was similar, and statistically significant (IR 1.005, 95% CI 0.990–1.019), underlining the validity of the result only for latitudes, exposure to light, and climatic conditions to which the people included in the sample are subjected. Although the characteristics just stated for Sweden and the Emilia-Romagna region are extremely different, in both studies, it is confirmed that the transition from standard time to summer time and vice versa does not impact on the number of deliveries.

These results confirm data from Roizen et al. [20] regarding the role of oxytocin in the onset and completion of childbirth and its rhythmicity. Hormone secretion, in fact, has its own circadian rhythm, not influenced by the alternation of dark and light and, therefore, not affected by the change of time. This may explain why the number of deliveries in the two weeks following the transition from standard time to summer time, and vice versa, is almost superimposable to that found in the two weeks preceding it.

The analysis of type of delivery was based on the hypothesis of a possible influence of DST on the secretion of melatonin [21–24], through the indirect evaluation of the outcome of contractile activity. In this case, we could expect to observe a greater number of operative deliveries and cesarean sections in the weeks following DST shifts, caused by dynamic or mechanical dystocia induced by anomaly or stop of contractions. This difference was more marked in the Spring period as the transition from winter time to summer time leads to the loss of one hour of darkness, with a consequent increase in light exposure and reduction in serum melatonin levels and, presumably, also in valid contractions. However, our data do not allow confirmation of this hypothesis; both the statistical analysis performed on the number of cesarean sections (*p* = 0.08) and that relating to the operative deliveries (*p* = 0.99) do not allow us to exclude that what has been detected is not attributable to simple chance.

Another relevant finding in the secondary outcome analysis was the confirmation of previous data collected in Texas, USA, by Mancuso et al. [25]. In our sample also, relating to the Emilia-Romagna region, the transition from standard time to summer time does not significantly affect the time of delivery, regardless of the gestational period and the way it occurs.

Neonatal birth weight was also investigated as a secondary outcome, to test the hypothesis of a short-term, acute effect of rhythm disruption. This is because the available data in the literature refer to studies performed on shift worker women [8], and shift work represents a chronic, long-term condition of rhythm desynchronizing effect. According to this hypothesis, the expected result could be, therefore, an increase in newborns with a low birth weight (<2500 g) in the weeks following the time change. However, the data obtained allow us to affirm that the transition from solar time to summer time and vice versa does not have a statistically significant effect on the increase in the incidence of newborns born with a low birth weight (<2500 g) ($p = 0.97$). It is possible to extend the same statement to the other investigated weight classes (2500–4000 g: p-value = 0.45; >4000 g: $p = 0.98$). Thus, we can conclude that DST shift does not have a statistically significant impact on newborn birth weight.

The rationale for the analysis of the use of epidural analgesia in periods of exposure and control was to assess whether the desynchronization induced by DST that shifts the transition could play a role in the perception of pain. In this case also, the results obtained do not allow us to exclude that the differences found are attributable to chance ($p = 0.64$).

We took into consideration age and gestational age of this low risk population and we found that the mean age of women who delivered during the two weeks before DST was older than those who delivered during the two weeks post DST and that women's age was independently associated with delivery during the two weeks post DST. We do not think that these findings could be of any relevant clinical significance due to the very small difference in age between the two groups. Moreover, these results could be related to the selection criteria aiming at evaluating only very low risk pregnancies.

We are aware of several limitations: (i) retrospective observational study; (ii) lack of perinatal complications—however, we selected only very low risk pregnancies; (iii) three years represent a short period of observation; (iv) unfortunately, we did not apply the methods used by László et al. [19] due to the different statistical package used for analysis—in fact, we used SPSS instead of SAS. Finally, (v) possible differences by race and ethnicity, since 35% of patients were not Italian. However, according to the last report of the Ministry for Health (year 2017) [26], in Italy, 21% of the births were related to mothers of non-Italian citizenship. This phenomenon is more widespread in the areas of the country with a greater foreign presence, i.e., in the Center–North, where more than 25% of births are from non-Italian mothers; in particular, in Emilia-Romagna and Lombardy, approximately 31% of births refer to foreign mothers. The most represented geographical areas of origin are Africa (27.7%), European Union (24.4%), Asia (18.1%), and South America (7.5%) [26].

However, the present study has also several strengths: (i) the large sample size, (ii) the quality of the data, and (iii) the rigorous methodology. The sample analyzed is representative of women characterized by a very low risk pregnancy, and the Emilia-Romagna region is characterized by one the best regional health systems in Italy. The choice of performing the study in a specific Italian region allowed us to obtain a reliable, good, complete, uniform, and coded source of data. The Childbirth Assistance Certificate is unique for the entire regional territory, and its compilation is mandatory following each birth in the region, independent of the structure in which it takes place.

5. Conclusions

This study shows no differences in the number of deliveries in the weeks following the change of time compared to those that precede it, neither during the Spring nor in the Autumn. This finding provides further confirmation to previous data obtained at quite different conditions of latitude, climate, and light exposure. It is possible that the multihormonal etiology of labor may explain this phenomenon. It would be interesting to extend the study to different latitudes and ethnicities, in order to verify whether our findings could be generalized or not.

Author Contributions: Conceptualization: R.C., R.V., P.G., R.M. and F.F.; methodology: R.C., S.P., V.F., A.D.G., E.D.S. and R.V.; data curation: S.P., V.F., A.D.G., P.I. and R.V.; formal analysis: S.P., V.F., P.I., A.D.G., E.D.S. and R.V.; writing—original draft preparation: R.C., S.P., V.F. and R.V.; writing—review and editing, S.P., P.I., E.D.S., P.G., R.M., M.A.R.B., F.F. and P.J.L.S.; supervision: P.G., R.M., M.A.R.B., F.F. and P.J.L.S.; project administration: R.C., S.P., E.D.S., and R.V.; funding acquisition: P.G. and R.M. All authors have read and agreed to the published version of the manuscript.

Funding: This study is supported by a scientific grant by the University of Ferrara (Fondo Incentivazione Ricerca-FIR- 2020, Roberto Manfredini).

Acknowledgments: We thank the Emilia-Romagna region, Direzione Generale 'Cura della persona, salute e welfare', for valuable and precious collaboration.

Conflicts of Interest: The authors declare no conflict of interest.

References

1. Wilcox, A.J. *Fertility and Pregnancy: An Epidemiologic Perspective*, 1st ed.; Oxford University Press: Oxford, UK, 2010.
2. Lincoln, D.W.; Porter, D.G. Timing of the photoperiod and the hour of birth in rats. *Nature* **1976**, *260*, 780–781. [CrossRef] [PubMed]
3. McLean, M.; Bisits, A.; Davies, J.; Woods, R.; Lowry, P.; Smith, R. A placental clock controlling the length of human pregnancy. *Nat. Med.* **1995**, *1*, 460–463. [CrossRef] [PubMed]
4. Spiegel, K.; Leproult, R.; Van Cauter, E. Impact of sleep debt on metabolic and endocrine function. *Lancet* **1999**, *354*, 1435–1439. [CrossRef]
5. Laugsand, L.E.; Vatten, L.J.; Bjørngaard, J.H.; Hveem, K.; Janszky, I. Insomnia and High-Sensitivity C-Reactive Protein. *Psychosom. Med.* **2012**, *74*, 543–553. [CrossRef] [PubMed]
6. Słabuszewska-Jóźwiak, A.; Włodarczyk, M.; Kilian, K.; Rogulski, Z.; Ciebiera, M.; Szymańska-Majchrzak, J.; Zaręba, K.; Szymański, J.K.; Raczkiewicz, D.; Włodarczyk, M.; et al. Does the Caesarean Section Impact on 11β HSD2 and Fetal Cortisol? *Int. J. Environ. Res. Public Health* **2020**, *17*, 5566. [CrossRef] [PubMed]
7. Hernández-Díaz, S.; Boeke, C.E.; Romans, A.T.; Young, B.; Margulis, A.V.; Mc Elrath, T.F.; Ecker, J.L.; Bateman, B.T. Triggers of spontaneous preterm delivery—Why today? *Paediatr. Perinat. Epidemiol.* **2014**, *28*, 79–87. [CrossRef]
8. Lin, Y.-C.; Chen, M.-H.; Hsieh, C.-J.; Chen, P.-C. Effect of rotating shift work on childbearing and birth weight: A study of women working in a semiconductor manufacturing factory. *World J. Pediatr.* **2011**, *7*, 129–135. [CrossRef]
9. EU Summer-Time Arrangements under Directive 2000/84/EC: Ex-Post Impact Assessment. Available online: https://www.europarl.europa.eu/thinktank/en/document.html?reference=EPRS_STU%282017%29611006 (accessed on 8 August 2020).
10. Manfredini, R.; Fabbian, F.; Cappadona, R.; Modesti, P.A. Daylight saving time, circadian rhythms, and cardiovascular health. *Intern. Emerg. Med.* **2018**, *13*, 641–646. [CrossRef]
11. Zhang, H.; Dahlén, T.; Khan, A.A.; Edgren, G.; Rzhetsky, A. Measurable health effects associated with the daylight saving time shift. *PLoS Comput. Biol.* **2020**, *16*, e1007927. [CrossRef]
12. Manfredini, R.; Fabbian, F.; Cappadona, R.; De Giorgi, A.; Bravi, F.; Carradori, T.; Flacco, M.E.; Manzoli, L. Daylight Saving Time and Acute Myocardial Infarction: A Meta-Analysis. *J. Clin. Med.* **2019**, *8*, 404. [CrossRef]
13. Manfredini, R.; Fabbian, F.; De Giorgi, A.; Cappadona, R.; Capodaglio, G.; Fedeli, U. Daylight saving time transitions and circulatory deaths: Data from the Veneto region of Italy. *Intern. Emerg. Med.* **2019**, *14*, 1185–1187. [CrossRef] [PubMed]
14. Chudow, J.J.; Dreyfus, I.; Zaremski, L.; Mazori, A.Y.; Fisher, J.D.; Di Biase, L.; Romero, J.; Ferrick, K.J.; Krumerman, A. Changes in atrial fibrillation admissions following daylight saving time transitions. *Sleep Med.* **2020**, *69*, 155–158. [CrossRef] [PubMed]
15. Malow, B.A.; Veatch, O.J.; Bagai, K. Are Daylight Saving Time Changes Bad for the Brain? *JAMA Neurol.* **2019**, *77*. [CrossRef]
16. Heboyan, V.; Stevens, S.; McCall, W.V. Effects of seasonality and daylight savings time on emergency department visits for mental health disorders. *Am. J. Emerg. Med.* **2019**, *37*, 1476–1481. [CrossRef]
17. E Cruz, M.M.; Miyazawa, M.; Manfredini, R.; Cardinali, D.; Madrid, J.A.; Reiter, R.; Araujo, J.F.; Agostinho, R.; Acuna-Castroviejo, D. Impact of Daylight Saving Time on circadian timing system. An expert statement. *Eur. J. Intern. Med.* **2019**, *60*, 1–3. [CrossRef] [PubMed]
18. Mills, J.; Kuohung, W. Impact of circadian rhythms on female reproduction and infertility treatment success. *Curr. Opin. Endocrinol. Diabetes Obes.* **2019**, *26*, 317–321. [CrossRef]
19. László, K.D.; Cnattingius, S.; Janszky, I. Transition into and out of daylight saving time and spontaneous delivery: A population-based study. *BMJ Open* **2016**, *6*, e010925. [CrossRef]

Int. J. Environ. Res. Public Health **2020**, *17*, 8091

20. Roizen, J.D.; Luedke, C.E.; Herzog, E.D.; Muglia, L.J. Oxytocin in the Circadian Timing of Birth. *PLoS ONE* **2007**, *2*, e922. [CrossRef]

21. Olcese, J. Circadian aspects of mammalian parturition: A review. *Mol. Cell. Endocrinol.* **2012**, *349*, 62–67. [CrossRef]

22. Sharkey, J.; Olcese, J. Transcriptional Inhibition of Oxytocin Receptor Expression in Human Myometrial Cells by Melatonin Involves Protein Kinase C Signaling. *J. Clin. Endocrinol. Metab.* **2007**, *92*, 4015–4019. [CrossRef]

23. Sharkey, J.T.; Puttaramu, R.; Word, R.A.; Olcese, J. Melatonin Synergizes With Oxytocin to Enhance Contractility of Human Myometrial Smooth Muscle Cells. *Obstet. Gynecol. Surv.* **2009**, *64*, 526–527. [CrossRef]

24. Olcese, J.; Beesley, S. Clinical significance of melatonin receptors in the human myometrium. *Fertil. Steril.* **2014**, *102*, 329–335. [CrossRef] [PubMed]

25. Mancuso, P.J.; Alexander, J.M.; McIntire, D.D.; Davis, E.; Burke, G.; Leveno, K.J. Timing of Birth After Spontaneous Onset of Labor. *Obstet. Gynecol.* **2004**, *103*, 653–656. [CrossRef] [PubMed]

26. Ministero della Salute. Certificato di Assistenza al Parto (CeDAP), Analisi Dell'evento Nascita—Anno 2017. Available online: http://www.salute.gov.it/portale/documentazione/p6_2_2_1.jsp?lingua=italiano&id=2931 (accessed on 28 September 2020).

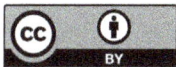

International Journal of
Environmental Research and Public Health

MDPI

Article

Implementing a Care Pathway for Complex Chronic Patients from a Nursing Perspective: A Qualitative Study

Rosario Fernández-Peña [1,2,3,*], Carmen Ortego-Maté [1,2], Francisco José Amo-Setién [1,2], Tamara Silió-García [1,2], Antoni Casasempere-Satorres [4] and Carmen Sarabia-Cobo [1,2]

1   Faculty of Nursing, University of Cantabria, 39008 Santander, Spain; carmen.ortego@unican.es (C.O.-M.); franciscojose.amo@unican.es (F.J.A.-S.); tamara.silio@unican.es (T.S.-G.); carmen.sarabia@unican.es (C.S.-C.)
2   IDIVAL Nursing Research Group, 39011 Santander, Spain
3   SALBIS Research Group, University of León, 24400 León, Spain
4   CualSoft-Qualitative Research Consulting Services, 03803 Alcoy, Spain; antoni@cualsoft.com
*   Correspondence: roser.fernandez@unican.es

Abstract: A care pathway constitutes a complex care strategy for decision-making and the organization of processes in the care of complex chronic patients, avoiding the fragmentation of care. Health professionals play a decisive role in the implementation, development, and evaluation of care pathways. This study sought to explore nurses' opinions on the care pathway for complex chronic patients three years after its implementation. The study participants were thirteen nurses with different roles who were involved in the care pathway. Thematic content analysis of the semi-structured interviews resulted in four major themes: (a) the strengths of the route; (b) the impact of the route on caregivers; (c) the weaknesses of the route; and (d) the future of the route. Overall, the pathway was positively valued for the benefits it provides to patients, the caregiver, and the administration of professional health care. Participants voiced their concerns regarding: communication and coordination difficulties among professionals across the different levels of care, the need for improved teamwork and consensus among professionals at the same center, and human and material resources. The ongoing evaluation and monitoring of facilitators and barriers is necessary throughout the implementation process, to ensure continuity and quality of care in the health system.

Keywords: care pathway; integrated health care; long-term care; quality of health care; Spain; qualitative research

Citation: Fernández-Peña, R.; Ortego-Maté, C.; Amo-Setién, F.J.; Silió-García, T.; Casasempere-Satorres, A.; Sarabia-Cobo, C. Implementing a Care Pathway for Complex Chronic Patients from a Nursing Perspective: A Qualitative Study. *Int. J. Environ. Res. Public Health* **2021**, *18*, 6324. https://doi.org/10.3390/ijerph18126324

Academic Editor: Paul B. Tchounwou

Received: 6 May 2021
Accepted: 1 June 2021
Published: 11 June 2021

Publisher's Note: MDPI stays neutral with regard to jurisdictional claims in published maps and institutional affiliations.

1. Introduction

Currently, our society is facing demographic, political, social, and economic changes that highlight the need to have health services that guarantee that the population's health needs are met, especially concerning chronic processes. Progressive population ageing, together with the increasing prevalence of chronic diseases, are the main challenges faced by health systems across Europe [1].

Integrated care is ideally suited to respond to care needs in this context via proactive and well-coordinated patient-centered multidisciplinary care, using new technologies to support patient self-management and to improve the collaboration between caregivers [1]. This transformation requires a multi-level strategy with the simultaneous and synergistic implementation of various interventions within the same territory and population [2].

Following global trends, in recent years, mortality and disability in Spain are related to NCDs (Non-Communicable Diseases), which, in 2016, according to the WHO (World Health Organization), represented up to 91% of total deaths [3]. This reality has led to a redirection in the organizational approach of the health system as well as the design of specific policies for the care of these diseases [4].

The European Pathway Association defines the care pathway as a complex intervention for the mutual decision-making and organization of care processes for a well-defined group of patients during a well-defined period, although a variety of terms have been used interchangeably in the international literature without a clear differentiation, such as critical pathway, clinical pathway, integrated care pathway, or care map [5,6]. Different studies have highlighted the strengths of implementing the care pathway, revealing an overall positive impact on the organization, coordination, and monitoring of care processes, the involvement of professionals and the improvement of process indicators [7–13]. Health professionals play a decisive role in the implementation, development, and evaluation of chronic care strategies [14,15]. Specifically, nurses carry out an important task, both as coordinators for patient care and as care liaisons between health levels, supported by their own experience in the care path and managing patients with complex chronic needs [16–18].

Adopting the Chronic Care Model as a framework for the reorientation of the health care system [15,19], chronicity management models in Spain have been developed via plans or strategies at a national and regional level in different waves from 2006 to 2015. Most of these plans are based on population models focused on the analysis of the needs of people with chronic diseases, according to the risk stratification based on the Kaiser Permanente Pyramid [20] and the model of the British Kings Fund [21]. The Strategy for Addressing Chronicity of the Spanish National Health System [22] contemplates management by integrated care processes and the definition of care pathways for the different chronic health conditions that are included in most plans or strategies for the care of chronicity across different regions in Spain [21,23].

The autonomous community of Cantabria, located in the north of Spain, has a population of 584,308 inhabitants in 2020, with an aging rate of 22.5% (population aged 65 and over, compared to the total population) [24,25].

Currently, in the community of Cantabria, there are 5802 patients identified as pluripathological. Following the guidelines of the Chronicity Care Plan in Cantabria [26], in 2016, the "Chronic Patient Care Pathway" project was created, which was aimed at all chronic patients, seeking to address different organizational models for providing care to people with different chronic diseases. In the framework of this broader project, the Pluripathological or Complex Chronic Patient Care Pathway was implemented, designed for adult patients with two or more chronic pathologies and a high level of complexity. Its objectives were to modify the natural course of their diseases, delaying their progression and improving their health by maintaining patients in their usual environment. Three nursing roles are involved in the care of the complex chronic patient included in the pathway. Firstly, the hospital liaison nurse is present in the four community hospitals with the main role of ensuring continuity of care and coordination between the different levels of care. Secondly, due to their position of leadership among other health professionals, nurse managers are essential to strengthen the quality, coordination, and integration of care [27]. Lastly, community primary care nurses are considered well-positioned regarding the nursing care of patients included in the care pathways as well as for their insights regarding the evaluation of the care pathways [28].

Although the assessment of the chronic care strategy in Cantabria has been carried out in recent years from a quantitative approach, the assessment of the Complex Chronic Patient Care Pathway has not been studied from a qualitative approach, or, more concretely, from the point of view of nursing professionals.

The aim of this study was to explore nurses' opinions on the care pathway for complex chronic patients in Cantabria, three years after its implementation, and on the different nursing roles involved in the complex chronic care pathway, specifically, the primary care nurse, the hospital liaison nurse and the nurse managers.

2. Materials and Methods

2.1. Design

A qualitative phenomenological descriptive design was conducted using semi- structured interviews. The analysis of the phenomena as they emerge from the point of view of nursing professionals' experience is necessary for a deeper understanding of their meaning [29,30]. This study adhered to the Consolidated Criteria for Reporting on Qualitative Research (COREQ) guidelines developed to evaluate qualitative research reports [31].

2.2. Research Team

The research team was formed by PhD university teachers with a background in Nursing, Psychology (CO and CS), and Anthropology (RF). In addition, a sociologist, expert in qualitive data analysis and with a PhD in Education, participated in this research. All researchers had experience in research in health sciences and none were involved in professional activity associated with the participants.

This study was part of a larger project primarily aimed at studying the impact of nursing care in the complex chronic patient on dependency, perceived satisfaction, and caregiver burden in Cantabria and the Balearic Islands. The design of this mixed methods study included participants who were patients in the Complex Chronic Patient Care Pathway, together with their caregivers [32,33]. During the fieldwork phase and after the collection of the initial quantitative and qualitative data, the research team was involved in two work sessions, in which they raised and discussed the need to include the nursing professionals involved in the complex chronic patient pathway as participants in the project. In these sessions, the research team reflected on the beliefs and motivations for this study, considering that the inclusion of this type of participants would enable the possibility of gathering a broader and more profound view of nursing care in the care pathway for complex chronic patients.

2.3. Participants

The inclusion criteria consisted of nurses working in the Cantabrian Health Service as nurse practitioners with care and management experience in handling patients labeled as complex chronic patients and included in the route, and who occupied managerial positions in the implementation of the pathway. The exclusion criterion was nurses without professional experience in the care of these patients.

In total, 13 nursing professionals participated in this qualitative study, with different nursing roles: two nurse managers, four hospital liaison nurses and seven primary care nurses, none of whom withdrew from the study. Four primary care nurses were not included in the study because they lacked experience in the management of patients included in the complex chronic patient pathway.

Sample selection was performed using purposive sampling. Key informants from the Cantabrian Health Service who held management positions were contacted to participate in the study in this professional role. These participants provided us with access to primary care nurses. For the selection of the primary care nurses, the segmentation criteria included nurses belonging to the four health areas of the public health service. The snowball technique was used to access new primary care nurses working in the different health areas of the community. Finally, we contacted the four liaison nurses of the Cantabrian Health Service working in the public hospitals of the community. Participants were contacted by telephone at their workplaces inviting them to participate in the study and informing them of the study aims and procedures.

2.4. Ethical Considerations

This project was approved by the Clinical Research Ethics Committee of University of Cantabria (Internal Code 2017.049) and was authorized for its implementation in the Cantabrian Health Service. Prior to the study, the research aims and procedures were once again informed verbally and, in writing, and informed consent was obtained from each participant. The data were treated anonymously and confidentially, conforming to the Spanish legislation and the principles of the Declaration of Helsinki.

2.5. Data Collection

The semi-structured interviews were conducted following a script and field notes were gathered to record observations related to the data collection phase. Table 1 presents the topics and questions that were asked to the participants to obtain information based on their specific nursing role.

Table 1. Semi-structured interview guide.

Topic	Questions
Professional background	Tell us about your experience and professional role regarding the complex chronic patient
Impact of the pathway	What is your opinion on the impact of the care pathway in the patients and their caregivers?
Strengths and weaknesses	Tell us about the strengths and weakness in the functioning of the pathway
Improvement strategies	Could you identify relevant strategies for improving the care pathway?
Future of the pathway	How do you rate the future of the pathway for the complex chronic patient?

Data collection was carried out during the year 2019. The face-to-face interviews were conducted by two members of the research team (RF and CS) with experience in qualitative research and with the sole presence of the participant. The interviews were mostly conducted at the hospitals and primary care centers where the nursing professionals worked, and, in four cases, they were held on university premises. The interviews were conducted and analyzed in Spanish, lasted an average of 25 min, and were audio recorded and fully transcribed by two researchers from the research team. Finally, the interview extracts shown in this article were translated into English by expert translators. All information in the transcripts regarding the participants' names and locations that could facilitate their identification was anonymized. Personal data were kept in a separate register accessible only to the project's principal investigators and those involved in data collection (CO, CS, and RF). The interviews were stored and managed in MAXQDA software (VERBI Software—Consult—Sozialforschung GmbH, Berlin, Germany), and were only accessible to researchers involved in coding and analysis.

The field work was completed when data saturation was reached, meaning that the information provided in the interviews was already collected in the agreed upon analysis categories or in the emerging categories and did not provide new concepts for analysis [34].

2.6. Data Analysis

Once transcribed, the interviews were exported to qualitative software analysis MAXQDA 2020. An inductive thematic content analysis was carried out [35,36] by four researchers from the group with the aim of enabling the emergence of categories and subcategories. Although the thematic structure served to initially organize the findings, the emergence of ideas from the data was what shaped the study themes via the appropriate analytical categories. For the analysis of the qualitative content, several analytical cycles were carried out [37–39]. First, an initial substantive coding was developed close to the data, which was complemented by in-vivo coding to track metaphors in the participants' discourse or significant terms. Subsequently, a process of categorization and recoding was performed which integrated the indicators into different categories or topics while reviewing and refining the coding system. The analysis was performed during the main data collection phase; however, it was considered mandatory to return to the field to perform more interviews to verify whether the categories raised were properly saturated. The analysis of the new data showed that no further relevant categories emerged from the data.

COREQ guidelines were followed [31], and different techniques were used to establish the trustworthiness of the data by reviewing issues concerning data credibility, transferability, dependability, and confirmability [40]. Researcher triangulation was achieved via team meetings that took place during the data collection and analysis phases, and participant triangulation was ensured by including different nursing professional roles involved in the phenomenon under study. Additionally, during the data collection, participant validation was ensured by asking the nursing professional to confirm the data obtained. A thick description of the phenomenon under study was included, and the rationale for the study was described in the framework of the wider research project. In addition, regular quality checks were made to avoid researcher bias. Furthermore, the research team adopted a reflective attitude, together with systematic attention to the context of the construction of knowledge.

3. Results

This section describes the characteristics of participants and presents the main thematic findings of our study.

In total, 13 nursing professionals (12 women, 1 man) participated in this qualitative study with a mean age of 45.9 years (range 37–54 years), and with a mean of 20.5 years professional experience as a nurse (range 12–29 years) (see Table 2). At the time of the study, all participants were working in different positions within the chronic patient care strategy of the Cantabrian Health Service: the four hospital liaison nurses in the community, primary care nurses from the different health areas, and two nurse managers.

Table 2. Profile of informants.

Informant	Sex	Age	Occupation	Professional Experience (Years)
Inf. 1	F	46	Primary Care Nurse	26
Inf. 2	F	37	Hospital liaison nurse	16
Inf. 3	F	40	Hospital liaison nurse	17
Inf. 4	M	49	Nurse manager	12
Inf. 5	F	48	Hospital liaison nurse	26
Inf. 6	F	54	Primary Care Nurse	21
Inf. 7	F	40	Nurse manager	20
Inf. 8	F	48	Primary Care Nurse	20
Inf. 9	F	46	Hospital liaison nurse	22
Inf. 10	F	45	Primary Care Nurse	17
Inf 11	F	48	Primary Care Nurse	29
Inf. 12	F	49	Primary Care Nurse	20
Inf. 13	F	47	Primary Care Nurse	21

M: Male, F: Female.

Thematic content analysis of the interviews resulted in four major themes: (a) the strengths of the route; (b) the impact of the route on caregivers; (c) the weaknesses of the route; and (d) the future of the route. The main categories and subcategories are presented in Table 3.

Table 3. Distribution of the main categories and subcategories.

	Categories
Strengths of the route	Benefits for the patient and family Benefits in the development of professional health care
Impact of the route on caregivers	It expedites the procedures and facilitates the patient's transit through the health system More accessible relationship with professionals and improved care
Weaknesses of the route	Insufficient coordination between primary care and hospital nursing professionals Need for improvement in teamwork and consensus among professionals in the same center Need for improvement of human and material resources
Future of the route	Positive future of the route Need for improvement strategies

3.1. Strengths of the Route

An emerging idea in this category that was highly valued by nursing professionals was related to the benefits of the route for patients and their families. Among the objectives that were positively evaluated as strengths, the professionals highlighted that the care pathway avoids or reduces hospital admissions, the number of visits to the hospital emergency department, as well as the number of days spent in hospital. As a result, patients spend more time in their usual social and family environment, leading to a substantial improvement in their quality of life. In addition, it favors a more individualized health care, suited to the patients' needs, and prevents them from becoming unstable.

The route increases the quality of life of patients within their pathological process (...) We are able to manage all resources better. We avoid unnecessary admissions, and therefore, at the hospital level there will be fewer admissions, which means less nosocomial diseases derived from the admissions. The greatest beneficiary is the patient, after that I think it is the family, and society. Regarding admissions, I believe there is good management, of course, it is more efficient to keep patients who are at home always well cared for, to avoid unnecessary admissions. (Informant 10)

The route is a tool that makes it possible to organize the path of these chronic patients throughout their disease process. We try to establish a connection between primary and specialized care, because what we want is for these patients to remain in their environment as long as possible, because that is what will give them stability. (Informant 7)

Secondly, participants stressed that the route is a strategy that significantly improves the professional care provided to patients and also adds satisfaction in their work as professionals. Once patients are labeled as being pluripathological, this helps alert nurses to the need to provide health care adapted to the patients' needs. Thus, patients are kept more stable, by providing care that is individualized and appropriate for their needs, without having to enter the usual care path. Moreover, the route facilitates the continuity of health care between primary care and the hospital.

Well, a care pathway, a guide, that serves us to refer patients and not to lose them in this maelstrom that we can call the health system. To have them under control in primary care and that when they get out of control of primary care, which we understand is where the patients are, and they have to go to hospital, well, they must do so without losing continuity of care and without disassociating themselves from primary care. (Informant 1)

The pluripathological label is a very important sign of alarm that puts us nurses with patients at risk, something that previously you could ignore […]. Whereas now, you continue to take care of them and follow their progress. (Informant 8)

3.2. Impact of the Route on Caregivers

The emerging ideas in relation to caregivers are related to aspects of the route that translate into improved care performance. Firstly, the route speeds up the procedures and facilitates the patient's transit between the different institutions of the health system, which avoids overloading the caregiver and represents a benefit in the care provided.

Yes, I think it is very beneficial for the caregiver or family because when they go to the hospital they don't have to wait so long and then they're discharged because they're already on their way to where they're going: to the residence or home or they get help... or they go to the social worker. They connect them in another way, without the relative or caregiver being concerned about what they have to do, or where they have to go. (Informant 13)

Secondly, the route makes it easier for caregivers to have a more accessible and closer relationship with health professionals and social workers at both the primary care and hospital levels. Likewise, this closeness makes caregivers feel more supported, with care adapted to their availability, feeling more confident with the care they provide to the patient and assume a more active role in care:

> *For the caregivers, I think they perceive important support. In the end, what they see is that they truly have an avenue of help, a resource that is close to primary care.* (Informant 7)

> *There is a very important part which is also the relevance given to the caregiver in this program. Of course, the improvement in the quality of life is evident. (...) the support that they have, the security that it gives them to have you as a reference. For example, in the hospital, they know that they can call you directly [...], it gives the caregivers security and saves them a lot of paperwork.* (Informant 5)

3.3. Weaknesses of the Route

On this subject, the informants underlined the lack of relationship and coordination between primary care and hospital nursing professionals, as a weakness in the process of implementing the care pathway. The elements involved in this lack of relationship refer to an already traditional separation between these two levels of care, difficulties in making contact between the reference nurses in primary care and the liaison nurse in the same health area as well as the lack of common spaces for contact between nurses of both care levels.

> *To me, it seems essential for a connection to exist between hospital and primary care nurses. A true connection, not only in times of instability to avoid an admission, and not just between primary care physicians and specialized internists.* (Informant 7)

Another point that stood out was the idea of insufficient joint work and consensus on the criteria and decision-making regarding complex chronic patients included in the route between professionals of the same center, especially in primary care centers, in addition to individual differences in terms of their involvement in the route as professionals. Specifically, referring to the control and power of decision that medical professionals have in the process, both in the labelling of patients and in the access to patient information during hospital visits:

> *All patient information reaches the doctors so when a patient has been discharged, my doctor has to let me know that he has been discharged, otherwise I don't know.* (Informant 1)

Thirdly, the participants highlighted a weakness concerning implementation of the route, specifically, some aspects related to human and material resources that make it difficult for the operation of the route to achieve its objectives. Thus, the high turnover of health personnel, both across centers and between levels of care, due to changes in their employment situation, interferes with continuity in knowledge and in managing the route as professionals in the same centers. Moreover, communication difficulties were emphasized between hospital and primary care professionals, as the systems used in these different centers were often different.

> *The computer applications should make it easier: if I, as a nurse, have a patient who is admitted and discharged, I should receive a discharge notice and a continuity of care report.* (Informant 7)

3.4. Future of the Route

The need for a change of model in the approach to chronicity, the benefits of the route for patients and caregivers, and the conviction of their advantages as nursing professionals, makes the participants value their future in a positive way:

> *[...] it's the trend in health care right now [...].. It's a patient-centered model. These programs must succeed either way.* (Informant 5)

> *We are convinced that this is really good.* (Informant 4)

The success of the route requires the design and implementation of certain areas of improvement. The need to improve communication and coordination between primary care nurses and hospital nurses was emphasized, by using improved resources for telematic communication, increasing the provision of nurses involved in the route, especially at the hospital level, as well as by providing continuous training on the route. Likewise, the need to redirect the role of nurses in the route by giving it more prominence and leadership was highlighted.

4. Discussion

The qualitative results of our study show that, overall, nurses have a positive assessment of the care pathway for both patients and caregivers. However, three years after its implementation, nurses stress the need for strategies to further improve in certain areas.

These areas include the need for more fluid communication and coordination channels and mechanisms between primary care nurses and hospital liaison nurses, teamwork, and consensus among professionals of the same center, as well as the improvement of human and material resources involved in the route.

The collaboration between clinical professionals from two different care levels has been carried out in Cantabria in recent years through the d'Amour questionnaire [41]. According to our findings, the quantitative results obtained from the questionnaire showed a mean score of 2.51 out of 5 in the years 2016–2019, thus suggesting equally improvable aspects in this area.

In this line, the care pathway should be considered as a process that represents a path of both success and challenges for professionals and managers, as shown in previous studies [42]. Given their dynamic nature over time, these new strategies essentially require periodic review and evaluation of their impact and assessment by both patients and professionals [11], considering the significant changes that their implementation may entail in the organizational culture and the possible need for support mechanisms to ensure their implementation in practice [7].

Inter-professional collaboration is a key element in efforts to increase the effectiveness of current health services, especially in the face of complex health problems, for which there are different conceptualizations, theoretical models [43] and assessment tools [41]. Regarding the care pathway of the complex chronic patient, the inter-professional collaboration between primary care and hospital care constitutes the vertebral axis upon which the comprehensive care between the health providers is based, thus avoiding fragmentation of care [44,45].

Other studies have focused on the role of the relational network between health professionals or health organizations from a structural point of view, in health settings and for the implementation of programs [46–50]. Thus, the multilevel model proposed by Van Houdt et al. [51] highlights the need for improved communication and coordination in the implementation of a care pathway between primary and hospital care professionals. These changes include improvements at the level of inter-organizational networks through the exchange of information and development of new communication channels, shared objectives, knowledge of the roles and competencies of the different professionals, and improved relationships. Secondly, changes in the inter-organizational mechanisms are required to change the structures of the organizations before and after the implementation of the care pathway in addition to the development of facilitating strategies to favor the creation of interpersonal networks between professionals, together with the transfer of information by electronic means [50].

The design and implementation of a new approach to health service delivery represents a challenge for managers and professionals, beginning with the preliminary planning of the implementation process, by considering the contextual, organizational, and cultural characteristics of the organizations and the intricacies of the care provided [42,52].

Int. J. Environ. Res. Public Health **2021**, *18*, 6324

5. Conclusions

The care pathway of the complex chronic patient in today's healthcare reality constitutes a valuable care strategy which responds to the needs of these patients and their caregivers in complex settings, by avoiding fragmentation of care. Due to their leadership roles, nurse managers are in an ideal position to ensure the correct implementation of these care pathways. A permanent evaluation and monitoring of facilitators and barriers to the implementation process is necessary to guarantee the continuity and quality of care in the health system.

Author Contributions: Conceptualization, R.F.-P., C.S.-C., C.O.-M., F.J.A.-S. and T.S.-G.; methodology, R.F.-P., C.S.-C., C.O.-M., F.J.A.-S. and T.S.-G., software, A.C.-S., R.F.-P., C.S.-C. and C.O.-M.; validation, R.F.-P.,C.S.-C., C.O.-M. and A.C.-S.; formal analysis, A.C.-S., R.F.-P., C.S.-C. and C.O.-M.; investigation, R.F.-P., C.S.-C., C.O.-M., F.J.A.-S., A.C.-S. and T.S.-G.; resources R.F.-P., C.S.-C., C.O.-M., F.J.A.-S., A.C.-S. and T.S.-G.; data curation, A.C.-S., R.F.-P., C.S.-C. and C.O.-M.; writing—original draft preparation, R.F.-P., C.S.-C., C.O.-M., A.C.-S., F.J.A.-S. and T.S.-G.; writing—review and editing, R.F.-P., C.S.-C., C.O.-M., A.C.-S., F.J.A.-S. and T.S.-G.; project administration, C.O.-M. and C.S.-C.; funding acquisition, C.O.-M. and C.S.-C. All authors have read and agreed to the published version of the manuscript.

Funding: This work was funded by the University of Cantabria (Spain), budget implementation 28.VU08.64662. The funders had no role in study design, data collection and analysis, decision to publish, or preparation of the manuscript.

Institutional Review Board Statement: The study was conducted according to the guidelines of the Declaration of Helsinki, and approved by the Clinical Research Ethics Committee of University of Cantabria (Internal Code 2017.049).

Informed Consent Statement: Informed consent was obtained from all subjects involved in the study.

Data Availability Statement: The data presented in this study are available on request from the corresponding author. The data are not publicly available due to privacy and ethical considerations.

Acknowledgments: We thank all the nursing professionals who agreed to participate in this work for their availability, time, and contribution to this study.

Conflicts of Interest: The authors declare no conflict of interest. The funders had no role in the design of the study; in the collection, analyses, or interpretation of data; in the writing of the manuscript, or in the decision to publish the results.

References

1. Mammarella, F.; Onder, G.; Navikas, R.; Jureviciene, E. Report on Care Pathways Approaches for Multimorbid Chronic Patients. Available online: http://chrodis.eu/wp-content/uploads/2017/02/deliverable-7-02-of-joint-action-chrodis_final.pdf (accessed on 4 December 2020).
2. Nuño-Solinís, R.; Fernández-Cano, P.; Mira-Solves, J.J.; Toro-Polanco, N.; Contel, J.C.; Guilabert Mora, M.; Solas, O. Desarrollo de IEMAC, un Instrumento para la Evaluación de Modelos de Atención ante la Cronicidad. *Gac. Sanit.* **2013**, *27*, 128–134. [CrossRef]
3. World Health Organization. *Non-Communicable Diseases Progress Monitor 2020*; World Health Organization: Geneva, Switzerland, 2020.
4. Haro, J.M.; Tyrovolas, S.; Garin, N.; Diaz-Torne, C.; Carmona, L.; Sanchez-Riera, L.; Perez-Ruiz, F.; Murray, C.J.L. The burden of disease in Spain: Results from the global burden of disease study 2010. *BMC Med.* **2014**, *12*, 1–25. [CrossRef]
5. De Bleser, L.; Depreitere, R.; De Waele, K.; Vanhaecht, K.; Vlayen, J.; Sermeus, W. Defining pathways. *J. Nurs. Manag.* **2006**, *14*, 553–563. [CrossRef] [PubMed]
6. Kinsman, L.; Rotter, T.; James, E.; Snow, P.; Willis, J. What is a clinical pathway? Development of a definition to inform the debate. *BMC Med.* **2010**, *8*, 31. [CrossRef]
7. Allen, D.; Gillen, E.; Rixson, L. Systematic review of the effectiveness of integrated care pathways: What works, for whom, in which circumstances? *Int. J. Evid. Based Healthc.* **2009**, *7*, 61–74. [CrossRef] [PubMed]
8. Daghash, H.; Lim Abdullah, K.; Ismail, M.D. The effect of acute coronary syndrome care pathways on in-hospital patients: A systematic review. *J. Eval. Clin. Pract.* **2019**, *26*, 1280–1291. [CrossRef] [PubMed]
9. Watts, T. End-of-life care pathways and nursing: A literature review. *J. Nurs. Manag.* **2013**, *21*, 47–57. [CrossRef] [PubMed]
10. Brattgjerd, M.; Olsen, R.M.; Danielsen, I.J. End-of-life care and the use of an integrated care pathway. *Qual. Rep.* **2020**, *25*, 216–237.
11. Grant, P.; Chika-Ezerioha, I. Evaluating diabetes integrated care pathways. *Pract. Diabetes* **2014**, *31*, 319–322. [CrossRef]

12. Sans Corrales, M.; Gardeñes Morón, L.; Moliner Molins, C.; Campama Tutusaus, I.; Pérez García, S.; Rozas Martínez, M. Health care pathways and expert patients: Do they improve outcomes? *Int. J. Integr. Care* **2012**, *12*, 1–6. [CrossRef]
13. Seys, D.; Bruyneel, L.; Deneckere, S.; Kul, S.; Van Der Veken, L.; Van Zelm, R.; Sermeus, W.; Panella, M.; Vanhaecht, K. Better organized care via care pathways: A multicenter study. *PLoS ONE* **2017**, *12*, e0180398. [CrossRef]
14. Yen, L.; Gillespie, J.; Jeon, Y.-H.; Kljakovic, M.; Brien, J.; Jan, S.; Lehnbom, E.; Pearce-Brown, C.; Usherwood, T. Health professionals, patients and chronic illness policy: A qualitative study. *Health Expect.* **2011**, *14*, 10–20. [CrossRef] [PubMed]
15. Coleman, K.; Austin, B.T.; Brach, C.; Wagner, E.H. Evidence on the Chronic Care Model in the new millennium. *Health Aff.* **2009**, *28*, 75–85. [CrossRef]
16. Russell, G.M.; Dahrouge, S.; Hogg, W.; Geneau, R.; Muldoon, L.; Tuna, M. Managing Chronic Disease in Ontario Primary Care: The Impact of Organizationals Factors. *Ann. Fam. Med.* **2009**, *7*, 309–318. [CrossRef] [PubMed]
17. Blakeman, T.; Macdonald, W.; Bower, P.; Gately, C.; Chew-Graham, C. A qualitative study of GPs' attitudes to self-management of chronic disease. *Br. J. Gen. Pract.* **2006**, *56*, 407–414.
18. Salmond, S.W.; Echevarria, M. Healthcare Transformation and Changing Roles for Nursing. *Orthop. Nurs.* **2017**, *36*, 12–25. [CrossRef]
19. Wagner, E.H.; Austin, B.T.; Von Korff, M. Organizing care for patients with chronic illness. *Milbank Q.* **1996**, *74*, 511–544. [CrossRef] [PubMed]
20. Schilling, L.; Deas, D.; Jedlinsky, M.; Aronoff, D.; Fershtman, J.; Wali, A. Kaiser Permanente's performance improvement system, Part 2: Developing a Value Framework. *Jt. Commun. J. Qual. Patient Saf.* **2010**, *36*, 552–560. [CrossRef]
21. Minué-Lorenzo, S.; Fernández-Aguilar, C. Critical view and argumentation on chronic care programs in Primary and Community Care. *Aten. Primaria* **2017**, *50*, 114–129. [CrossRef] [PubMed]
22. Ministerio de Sanidad Servicios Sociales e Igualdad. *Estrategia para el Abordaje de la cronicidad en el Sistema Nacional de Salud*; Ministerio de Sanidad Servicios Sociales e Igualdad: Madrid, Spain, 2012.
23. García-Goñi, M.; Hernández-Quevedo, C.; Nuño-Solinís, R.; Paolucci, F. Pathways towards chronic care-focused healthcare systems: Evidence from Spain. *Health Policy* **2012**, *108*, 236–245. [CrossRef]
24. Instituto Nacional de Estadística. Available online: https://www.ine.es/en/index.htm (accessed on 27 April 2021).
25. Instituto Cántabro de Estadística. Available online: https://www.icane.es/ (accessed on 27 April 2021).
26. Consejería de Sanidad y Servicios Sociales. *Gobierno de Cantabria. Plan de Atención a la Cronicidad de Cantabria 2015–2019*; Consejería de Sanidad y Servicios Sociales: Santander, Spain, 2015.
27. Sfantou, D.F.; Laliotis, A.; Patelarou, A.E.; Sifaki- Pistolla, D.; Matalliotakis, M.; Patelarou, E. Importance of Leadership Style towards Quality of Care Measures in Healthcare Settings: A Systematic Review. *Healthcare* **2017**, *5*, 73. [CrossRef]
28. Annells, M.; Allen, J.; Nunn, R.; Lang, L.; Petrie, E.; Clark, E.; Robins, A. An evaluation of a mental health screening and referral pathway for community nursing care: Nurses' and general practitioners' perspectives. *J. Clin. Nurs.* **2011**, *20*, 214–226. [CrossRef]
29. Caelli, K. The Changing Face of Phenomenological Research: Traditional and American Phenomenology in Nursing. *Qual. Health Res.* **2000**, *10*, 366–377. [CrossRef]
30. Korstjens, I.; Moser, A. Series: Practical guidance to qualitative research. Part 2: Context, research questions and designs. *Eur. J. Gen. Pract.* **2017**, *23*, 274–279. [CrossRef]
31. Tong, A.; Sainsbury, P.; Craig, J. Consolidated criteria for reporting qualitative research (COREQ): A 32-item checklist for interviews and focus groups. *Int. J. Qual. Health Care* **2007**, *19*, 349–357. [CrossRef]
32. Sarabia-Cobo, C.; Taltavull-Aparicio, J.M.; Miguélez-Chamorro, A.; Fernández-Rodríguez, A.; Ortego-Mate, C.; Fernández-Peña, R. Experiences of caregiving and quality of healthcare among caregivers of patients with complex chronic processes: A qualitative study. *Appl. Nurs. Res.* **2020**, *56*, 151344. [CrossRef]
33. Sarabia-Cobo, C.; Taltavull, J.; Lladó-Jordan, G.; González, S.; Molina-Mula, J.; Ortego-Mate, C.; Fernández-Peña, R. Comparison between attention and experiences of chronic complex patients: A multicentric study. *Health Soc. Care Community* **2021**. [CrossRef] [PubMed]
34. Corbin, J.; Strauss, A. *Basics of Qualitative Research: Techniques and Procedures for Developing Grounded Theory*; Sage Publications: Londres, UK, 2014; Volume 1.
35. Braun, V.; Clarke, V. Using thematic analysis in psychology. *Qual. Res. Psychol.* **2006**, *3*, 77–101. [CrossRef]
36. Kuckartz, U. Thematic Qualitative Text Analysis. In *Qualitative Text Analysis*; Sage Publications: London, UK, 2014; pp. 69–88.
37. Miles, M.B.; Huberman, A.M.; Saldana, J. *Qualitative Data Analysis: A Methods Sourcebook*, 3rd ed.; Sage Publications: London, UK, 2014.
38. Saldaña, J. *Fundamentals of Qualitative Research*; Oxford University Press: New York, NY, USA, 2011.
39. Saldaña, J. *The Coding Manual for Qualitative Researchers*, 2nd ed.; Sage Publications: London, UK, 2013.
40. Shenton, A.K. Strategies for ensuring trustworthiness in qualitative research projects. *Educ. Inf.* **2004**, *22*, 63–75. [CrossRef]
41. Nuño-Solinís, R.; Zabalegui, I.B.; Arce, R.S.; Rodríguez, L.S.M.; Polanco, N.T. Development of a questionnaire to assess interprofessional collaboration between two different care levels. *Int. J. Integr. Care* **2013**, *13*, e015. [CrossRef] [PubMed]
42. Wood, S.; Gangadharan, S.; Tyrer, F.; Gumber, R.; Devapriam, J.; Hiremath, A.; Bhaumik, S. Successes and challenges in the implementation of care pathways in an intellectual disability service: Health professionals' experiences. *J. Policy Pract. Intellect. Disabil.* **2014**, *11*, 1–7. [CrossRef]

43. D'Amour, D.; Ferrada-Videla, M.; San Martin Rodriguez, L.; Beaulieu, M.-D. The conceptual basis for interprofessional collabora-tion: Core concepts and theoretical framework. *J. Interprof. Care* **2005**, *19*, 116–131. [CrossRef]

44. Satzinger, W.; Courte-Wienecke, S.; Wenng, S.; Herkert, B. Bridging the information gap between hospitals and home. *J. Nurs. Manag.* **2005**, *13*, 257–264. [CrossRef] [PubMed]

45. Lemetti, T.; Stolt, M.; Rickard, N.; Suhonen, R. Collaboration between hospital and primary care nurses: A literature review. *Int. Nurs. Rev.* **2015**, *62*, 248–266. [CrossRef] [PubMed]

46. Cunningham, F.C.; Ranmuthugala, G.; Plumb, J.; Georgiou, A.; Westbrook, J.I.; Braithwaite, J. Health professional networks as a vector for improving healthcare quality and safety: A systematic review. *BMJ Qual. Saf.* **2012**, *21*, 239–249. [CrossRef]

47. Varda, D.; Shoup, J.A.; Miller, S. A systematic review of collaboration and network research in the public affairs literature: Implications for public health practice and research. *Am. J. Public Health* **2012**, *102*, 564–571. [CrossRef]

48. Gibbons, D.E. Interorganizational network structures and diffusion of information through a health system. *Am. J. Public Health* **2007**, *97*, 1684–1692. [CrossRef] [PubMed]

49. Valente, T.W.; Palinkas, L.A.; Czaja, S.; Chu, K.-H.; Brown, C.H. Social Network Analysis for Program Implementation. *PLoS ONE* **2015**, *10*, e0131712. [CrossRef]

50. Nguyen, O.K.; Kruger, J.; Greysen, S.R.; Lyndon, A.; Goldman, L.E. Understanding how to improve collaboration between hospitals and primary care in postdischarge care transitions: A qualitative study of primary care leaders' perspectives. *J. Hosp. Med.* **2014**, *9*, 700–706. [CrossRef]

51. Van Houdt, S.; Heyrman, J.; Vanhaecht, K.; Sermeus, W.; De Lepeleire, J. Care pathways across the primary-hospital care continuum: Using the multi-level framework in explaining care coordination. *BMC Health Serv. Res.* **2013**, *13*, 296. [CrossRef] [PubMed]

52. Leonard, M.; Graham, S.; Bonacum, D. The human factor: The critical importance of effective teamwork and communication in providing safe care. *Qual. Saf. Health Care* **2004**, *13*, i85–i90. [CrossRef] [PubMed]

International Journal of
Environmental Research and Public Health

MDPI

Article

Use of Neurodynamic or Orthopedic Tension Tests for the Diagnosis of Lumbar and Lumbosacral Radiculopathies: Study of the Diagnostic Validity

Francisco Javier González Espinosa de los Monteros [1], Gloria Gonzalez-Medina [2,*], Elisa Maria Garrido Ardila [3], Juan Rodríguez Mansilla [3], José Paz Expósito [1] and Petronila Oliva Ruiz [2]

[1] Andalusian Health Service, Hospital "Puerta Universitario del Mar", Av. Ana de Viya, 21, 11009 Cádiz, Spain; mizivaurgente@hotmail.com (F.J.G.E.d.l.M.); jose.paz.sspa@juntadeandalucia.es (J.P.E.)
[2] Nursing and Physiotherapy Department, Cadiz University, Av. Ana de Viya, 52, 11009 Cadiz, Spain; petronila.oliva@uca.es
[3] Department of Medical-Surgical Therapy, Medicine Faculty, Extremadura University, 06006 Badajoz, Spain; egarridoa@unex.es (E.M.G.A.); jrodman@unex.es (J.R.M.)
* Correspondence: gloriagonzalez.medina@uca.es; Tel.: +34-670-609-656

Received: 31 July 2020; Accepted: 22 September 2020; Published: 26 September 2020

check for updates

Abstract: Background: Lumbar radiculopathy is a nerve root disorder whose correct diagnosis is essential. The objective of the present study was to analyze the reliability diagnostic validity of eight neurodynamic and/or orthopedic tension tests using magnetic resonance imaging as the Gold Standard. Methods: An epidemiological study of randomized consecutive cases which was observational, descriptive, transversal, double blinded and was conducted following the Standards for Reporting Diagnostic accuracy studies (STARD) declaration. The sample size was 864 participants. Internal and external validity (CI = 95%) and reliability, were calculated for all tests performed independently. The diagnostic validity of the combined and multiple tests in parallel was also calculated. Results: The analysis indicated that only two tests performed independently had external validity, but neither had reliability or precision. The Straight Leg Raise test and the Bragard test performed in a multiple parallel way showed high sensitivity (97,40%), high negative predictive value (PV- 96,64%) and external validity (Likelihood Ratio- 0,05). The combined test of the Slump test and the Dejerine's triad had internal and external validity. Conclusions: The Straight Leg Raise test and the Bragard test performed in a multiple parallel way and the combined test of the Slump Test and the Dejerine's triad have clinical validity to discard lumbar or lumbar-sacral radiculopathy.

Keywords: lumbar radiculopathy; neurodynamic tension tests; orthopedic tension tests; magnetic resonance

---

1. Introduction

Lumbar radiculopathy is a dysfunction of the spinal nerve root that can be accompanied by pain, weakness, sensitivity and reflex disorders in the affected anatomical area [1]. These symptoms, in particular pain, cause a negative impact on the independence of the person which is a problem in today's society [2]. This condition causes physical disability which affects the quality of life of the person and, at the same time, has an impact on the economy of the countries.

Therefore, health care professionals need valid tools to accurately and quickly diagnose this condition. This could help to minimize the possible consequences.

Diagnosis allocates a person to a group of subjects that have a disease or with reasonable certainty [3]. An incorrect diagnosis can lead to the wrong prognosis and treatment which could harm the patient [4]. In contrast, an accurate diagnosis will lead to a correct and specific treatment [5]. In clinical practice, diagnostic tests are frequently used although its validity, precision and clinical utility are unknown [3].

Lumbosacral radiculopathies' diagnosis is generally based on the clinical history of the patient and the objective examination [6]. Therefore, these patients require a comprehensive physical and neurological assessment [7] which can avoid the unreasonable use of complementary tests [8].

Neurodynamic or orthopedic tension tests are used to examine the nerve roots of the patient. They trigger pain or other sensory symptoms that reveal the root lesion [9]. In addition, they differentiate whether the origin of the pain is neural or musculoskeletal, evaluating the mechanics and physiology of the nervous system during movement [10]. They are diagnostic tests widely used in clinical practice. Therefore, determining their validity may be the necessary basis to justify the performance of high-cost tests, such as magnetic resonance imaging, which is currently the most valid procedure for the diagnosis of lumbar radiculopathies [11]. The few studies found in the literature reveal that neurodynamic or orthopedic stress tests help the differential diagnosis of lumbar nerve root compression [12]. However, there are few studies that analyze the diagnostic validity of the tests [13] performed independently or combined. Therefore, we can affirm that there is little scientific evidence on the accuracy [14] and diagnostic precision of these tests [13,15].

In this context, we developed this research, with the aim of estimating the diagnostic validity of the following orthopedic stress tests and/or neurodynamic tests (performed individually, in combination and in parallel): Straight Leg Raise Test (SLR) or Leg Elevation Test Extended [14,16], Bragard test (B) [17], Fajersztajn test (F) [18,19], Sicard test (S) [19], Passive Neck Flexion test (PNFT) [10], Kernig (K) [20], Slump Test (S) [21] and Dejerine's triad (DT) [19]. As well as the efficacy of these tests when they are carried out in combination or in parallel, magnetic resonance imaging was used as the Gold Standard and for comparing the results; an MRI scan was used as the Gold Standard and the results were compared.

2. Materials and Methods

This was an epidemiological study of randomized consecutive cases which was observational, descriptive, transversal and double blinded. The research was conducted following the STARD (Standards for Reporting Diagnostic accuracy studies) guidelines for reporting diagnostic accuracy studies [22,23]. The ClinicalTrials.gov Study Identifier of the study is NCT04485572.

2.1. Participants

The target population (Figure 1) included all the patients referred to the Radiology Department of the "Puerta del Mar University Hospital" in Cádiz (Spain) to undertake an MRI scan of the lumbar or lumbosacral spine (1887 subjects of which 1023 were excluded). The following inclusion criteria were established: clinical suspicion of lumbar or lumbosacral radiculopathy. The exclusion criteria were: ages under 18 or over 70 years old, healthy subjects or with a radiculopathy already diagnosed, subjects with diabetes, alcoholism, HIV+, herpes zoster infection, cancer, multiple sclerosis, hereditary neuropathy, lumbar surgery, persons with pacemaker or stent, known pregnancy and persons that refused to participate in the study or undergo the MRI scan.

The study was approved by the Bioethical Research Commission of the Puerta del Mar and Bahia de Cádiz District–La Janda University Hospital in Spain (Registration number 30/14). All the ethical considerations and requirements of human clinical research mentioned in the Helsinki declaration [24] and the Data Protection Law [25] were met.

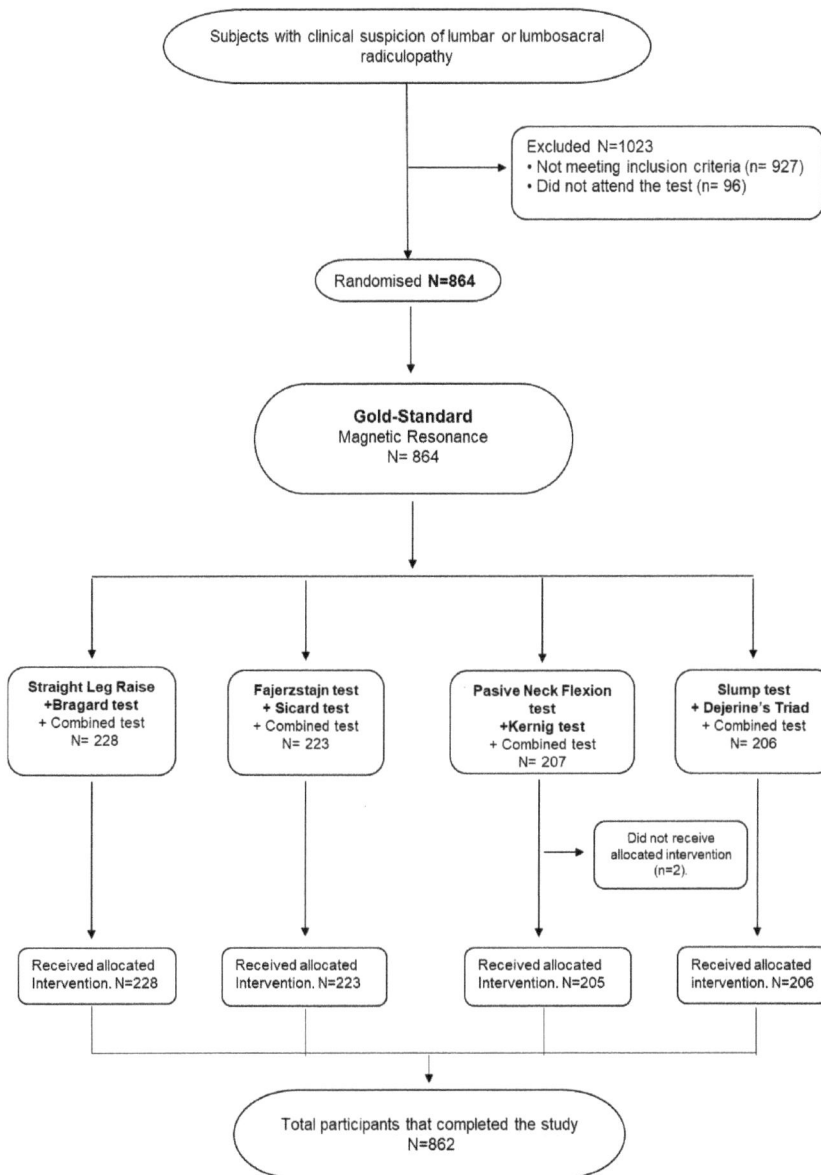

Figure 1. Target population.

2.2. Recruitment Process

Participant selection was based on the initial symptoms of lumbar or lumbosacral radiculopathy. To avoid selection bias, all the subjects referred to the Radiology Department of the "Puerta del Mar University Hospital" in Cádiz (Spain) that met the inclusion criteria were recruited consecutively and randomly.

The sample size was 864. Dividing the participants in 4 different groups was considered appropriate due to the great number of diagnostic tests that were assessed. Three diagnostic tests were performed in each group. This decision was justified and motivated by two main reasons. Firstly, neurodynamic or orthopedic tension tests trigger pain and symptoms and repeating this 12 times was not considered ethical. Secondly, systematic repetition of the tests could lead to the loss of the subjective ability of the patient to perceive changes of the symptoms.

2.3. Data Collection

Data collection was carried out in the Radiology Department of the "Puerta del Mar University Hospital" in Cádiz (Spain). This department belongs to the Diagnostic Imaging Clinical Management Unit of the hospital.

All the patients included in this study were subjected (after delivery of the information sheet and the signing of the informed consent) both to neurodynamic tests and to magnetic resonance imaging (Gold Standard), thereby avoiding bias sequence or diagnostic verification [3].

2.4. Testing Procedure

The test used as Gold Standard was MRI scan which is nowadays the test of choice to diagnose radicular pain [26]. A 1.5 Teslas Siemens MRI scan (Siemens, Erlangen, Germany) was used. The MR imaging was performed with a 4-sequence protocol performed in two planes: 1st sequence: Sagital Turbo SE-T1: TR 652, TE 14, FOV 280 mm reading, FOV phase 75%, 4 mm slice thickness, 11 slices, 4:13 min 4 h 13 min assessment time. This is the sequence of choice for morphological studies. Second sequence: Sagital Turbo SE-T2: TR 3500, TE 128, FOV 280 mm reading, FOV phase 100%, 4 mm slice thickness, 11 slices, 3:56 min assessment time. This setting is indicated to increase contrast of the spinal canal with discs and nervous structures, to visualize the connus medullaris and discs alterations and to assess spinal canal stenosis. Third sequence: Axial Turbo SE-T1: TR 438, TE 14, FOV 200 mm reading, FOV phase 5%, 4 mm slice thickness, 5 slices, 3:48 min assessment time. This sequence is used for morphological studies of the medullar canal and the vertebral foramen. Fourth sequence: Axial Turbo SE-T2: TR 3970, TE 130, FOV 1200 mm reading, FOV phase 5%, 4 mm slice thickness, 5 slices, 3:16 min assessment time. This is a sequence which is oriented towards the study of injuries and stenosis of the spinal canal.

The images of the Gold Standard were interpreted by radiologists specialized in the diagnosis of lumbar and lumbosacral magnetic resonance images. The radiologists were staff of the musculoskeletal unit of the hospital. Two of them collaborated in the study regularly and four of them collaborated discontinuously. All of them were independent to the performance of diagnostic tests (index tests) which ensure avoidance of incorporation bias. They were blind to the results of the neurodynamic and orthopaedic tests to avoid the risk of revision bias [3].

The participants of each group were assessed with two independent diagnostic tests and a third test which was the combination of both. The combined test increases the ability of the assessor to trigger symptoms and signs by stressing or easing the different neuro-musculoskeletal structures [27]. The combination of the tests was based on their similarity of the techniques and their ability to be combined. All the tests were done bilaterally, starting with the sound limb. The tests are independent and dichotomous as they are not conditional on any other test and they have a positive or negative score.

The following neurodynamic and/or orthopedic tension tests were done: The Straight Leg Raise test (SLR) [14,16], the Bragard test (B) [17] and the combined tests of both (SLR+B); the Fajersztajn test (F) [18], the Sicard test (S) [19] and the combined tests of both (F+S); the Passive Neck Flexion test (PNFT) [10], the Kernig test (K) [20] and the tests combining both (PNFT+K); the Slump test (ST) [21], the Dejerine's triad (DT) [19] and the test combining both (ST+DT). All tests were performed independently, combined and in a multiple parallel manner by a physiotherapist.

The clinical interpretation of the test was based on the changes of the patient's responses in relation to the symptoms, range of movement and resistance found. The patients were informed about the importance of their perceptions [10]. The physiotherapist that conducted the tests was independent and blind to the results of the Gold Standard. To assure the validity of the results, the data of the reference test (Gold Standard) and the neurodynamic or orthopedic tension tests (index tests) were interpreted separately.

2.5. Statistical Analysis

The statistical analysis was carried out with the IBM SPSS Statistics 22 version (IBM Corp. Released 2013. IBM SPSS Statistics for Windows, Version 22.0. IBM Corp., Armonk, NY, USA) and the EPIDAT 3.1 software version (Servizo Galego de Saúde, Spain). A descriptive analysis of the age and gender of the participants was done. Their homogeneity was verified with an analysis of the variance (ANOVA) when the validity requirements allowed it or with the Kruskal–Wallis test when they did not.

To determine internal validity, the following statistical indicators were calculated for each test: sensitivity (Sens), specificity (Spec) and the positive and negative predictive values (PV+ and PV-): 0–10% null, 10–30% very low; 30–60% low; 60–70% low moderate; 70–80% high moderate; 80–90% high; 90–100% very high.

The external validity (general utility or clinical applicability for overall population) [28–33] was estimated through the Likelihood Ratio (LR+ y LR-). The range of values and their impact on the clinical utility are: LR+: > 10 great increase, excellent test; 5–10 moderate increase, good test; 2–5: small increase, bad test; <2: minor increase, useless test. LR-: 0,5–1 minor decrease, useless test; 0,5–0.2 small decrease, bad test; 0,1–0,2 moderate decrease, good test; <0,1 great decrease, excellent test [3,34–36]. The confidence interval for all of them was 95%. The indicators of diagnostic validity were also calculated for the test performed in the multiple parallel manner.

Moreover, in order to estimate the reliability or accuracy of the diagnostic tests, the parallel method of the same test was used. This was calculated with the Kappa index (K). The range of values were: poor, <0,20; weak, between 0,21 and 0,40; moderate, between 0,41 and 0,60; good, between 0,61 and 0,80; very good, between 0,80 and 1 [3,26,27].

3. Results

Participants

The study was conducted from July 2014 until August 2016. The information related to the participants, allocated groups and tests that were performed can be seen in Table 1.

Table 1. Data collection of the participants.

Group	Starting Date	Finishing Date	Tests Performed
SLR [1]-B [2]	7 July 2014	11 November 2014	Straight Leg Raise [14] Bragard test [17]
F [3]-S [4]	13 November 2014	10 July 2015	Fajersztajn test [18] Sicard test [19]
PNFT [5]-K [6]	13 July 2015	23 March 2016	Passive Neck Flexion test [10] Kernig test [20]
ST [7]-DT [8]	28 March 2016	25 August 2016	Slump test [21] Dejerine's triad [19]

[1] SLR: Straight Leg Raise test; [2] B: Bragard test; [3] F: Fajersztajn test; [4] S: Sicard test; [5] PNFT: Passive Neck Flexion test; [6] K: Kernig test; [7] ST: Slump test; [8] DT: Dejerine's triad.

The results of the nerve root affected by group and gender are shown in Table 2.

Table 2. Nerve root affected by group and gender.

Group	Gender (%)	L1 (%)	L2 (%)	L3 (%)	L4 (%)	L5 (%)	S1 (%)	S2 (%)	S3 (%)
SLR [1]-B [2]	Male 21.05	0	0	3,07	7,01	8,77	7,89	0	0
			5,70% Right-6,57% Left-3,94% Bilateral-10,52% Lost						
	Female 18.42	0	0,43	1,31	6,14	8,33	7,89	0	0
			9,21% Right-6,57% Left-0,87% Bilateral-7,45% Lost						
F [3]-S [4]	Male 27.80	0	0	4,03	8,96	12,55	8,52	0	0
			8,07% Right-11,21% Left-13% Bilateral-1,79% Lost						
	Female 19.28	0	0,44	1,34	7,17	6,72	7,62	0	0
			Right 8,07%-Left 8,96%-Bilateral 4,03%-Lost 2,24%						
PNFT [5]-K [6]	Male 23.90	0	0	0	6.82	12.19	9.6	0	0
			7,80% Right-12,68% Left-7,31% Bilateral-0,48% Lost						
	Female 30.24	0.48	0,97	4,39	9,26	13,17	11,70	0,48	0,48
			13.65% Right-15.60% Left-9.75% Bilateral-2.43% Lost						
ST [7]-DT [8]	Male 26.21	0	0	1,94	6,31	13,59	11,65	0,48	0,48
			9,70% Right-12,13% Left-12,62% Bilateral-0% Lost						
	Female 28.64	0	0	5,82	15,53	13,59	4,85	0	0
			8,73% Right-16,01% Left-14,56% Bilateral-0,48% Lost						

[1] SLR: Straight Leg Raise test; [2] B: Bragard test; [3] F: Fajersztajn test; [4] S: Sicard test; [5] PNFT: Passive Neck Flexion test; [6] K: Kernig test; [7] ST: Slump test; [8] DT: Dejerine's triad.

Table 3 shows the results of the statistical indicators for all the diagnostic tests performed independently, combined and in a multiple parallel manner.

Table 3. Results of the validity indicators.

Test	Sens [9] (%)	Spec [10] (%)	PV+ [11] (%)	PV- [12] (%)	LR+ [13]	LR- [14]
SLR [1]	83,33	74,24	70,18	85,96	3,24	0,22
B [2]	84,38	73,48	69,83	86,61	3,18	0,21
Combined test SLR [1] + B [2]	83,38	72,73	69,23	86,49	3,09	0,21
Multiple parallel SLR [1] and B [2]	97,40	54,55	60,92	96,64	2,14	0,05
F [3]	43,12	80,70	68,12	59,74	2,23	0,70
S [4]	66,06	68,42	66,67	67,83	2,09	0,50
Combined test F [3] + S [4]	46,79	78,07	67,11	60,54	2,13	0,68
Multiple parallel F [3] and S [4]	80,69	55,21	63,27	74,94	1,80	0,35
PNFT [5]	31,53	95,74	89,74	54,22	7,41	0,72
K [6]	61,26	70,21	70,83	60,55	2,06	0,55
Combined test PNFT [5] + K [6]	64,86	68,09	70,59	62,14	2,03	0,52
Multiple parallel PNFT [5] and K [6]	73,47	67,22	72,58	68,21	2,24	0,39
ST [7]	80,17	77,78	82,30	75,27	3,61	0,25
DT [8]	19,83	96,67	88,46	48,33	5,95	0,83
Combined test ST [7] + DT [8]	93,97	77,78	84,50	90,91	4,23	0,08
Multiple parallel ST [7] and DT [8]	84,10	75,19	81,37	78,58	3,39	0,21

[1] SLR: Straight Leg Raise test; [2] B: Bragard test; [3] F: Fajersztajn test; [4] S: Sicard test; [5] PNFT: Passive Neck Flexion test; [6] K: Kernig test; [7] ST: Slump test; [8] DT: Dejerine's triad; [9] Sens: sensitivity; [10] Spec: specificity; [11] PV+: positive predictive value; [12] PV-: negative predictive value; [13] LR+: positive likelihood ratio; [14] LR-: negative likelihood ratio.

The tests assessed in this study showed no external validity (have no external applicability to this study) when they were performed independently. The SLR test and the Bragard test performed independently and in the combined test revealed internal validity. They had a high sensitivity (SLR 83,33%, B 84,38% and combined test 83,38%) and a high PV- (SLR 85,96%, B 86,61% and combined test 86,49%). However, due to the close relation to the prevalence of the condition, these results cannot be extrapolated to other populations. Therefore, the Likelihood Ratio (LR+, LR-) was calculated as this indicator is independent to the prevalence. The results obtained showed that the SLR and Bragard tests have no external validity or cannot be extrapolated to other populations, although both tests have a good reliability (0,974).

The SLR and Bragard tests performed in a multiple manner obtained high sensitivity (97,40%) and PV- (96,64%) which indicates that they have internal validity. Moreover, the results of the LR- (0,05) suggest that they have an excellent clinical utility to dismiss the condition.

No internal validity was found for the Fajersztajn and Sicard tests when they were performed individually, combined or in a multiple parallel manner. Among both tests, the Fajersztajn test had the best specificity (80,70%) and a very good accuracy or reliability (0,929).

The statistical analysis revealed that the Passive Neck Flexion test had a good internal validity as its specificity was very high (95,74%), its PV+ was high (89,74%) and the result of the LR+ was 7,41. However, the Kappa index (0,386) indicates that it has no diagnostic accuracy.

The Kernig test performed independently, combined with the passive neck flexion test and multiple in parallel, did not show internal or external validity.

The results also showed that the Slump test has internal validity with a high sensitivity (80,17%) and PV+ (82,30%). In contrast, no external validity was found for this test as the poor figures obtained in the Likelihood Ratio (LR+ 3,61. LR- 0,25) indicate. According to the Kappa index, this test has a very good reliability (0.841).

A very high specificity (96,67%) and a high PV+ (88,46%) suggest that the Dejerine's Triad has internal validity. The values of the LR+ (5,95) for this test also indicate that it has external validity but the Kappa index (0,159) does not reveal reliability or diagnostic accuracy.

The summary of the reliability of the tests calculated with the Kappa index can be seen in Table 4.

Table 4. Results of the reliability of the test.

Test	Cohen's Kappa Index
SLR [1]	0,974
B [2]	0,974
F [3]	0,929
S [4]	0,674
PNFT [5]	0,386
K [6]	0,942
S [7]	0,841
DT [8]	0,159

[1] SLR: Straight Leg Raise test; [2] B: Bragard test; [3] F: Fajersztajn test; [4] S: Sicard test; [5] PNFT: Passive Neck Flexion test; [6] K: Kernig test; [7] ST: Slump test; [8] DT: Dejerine's triad.

From all the tests analyzed in our study, the combined test of the Slump test and the Dejerine's triad is the only one that showed internal and external validity. Its sensitivity (93,97%) and PV- (90,91%) were very high, its PV+ was high (84,50%) and the value of the LR- (0.08) was excellent. All these results indicate that this combined test is effective in dismissing lumbar or lumbosacral radiculopathy. The multiple parallel test of the Slump test and the Dejerine's triad obtained high sensitivity (84,10%) and PV+ (81,37%). However, it has no external validity, which means we cannot extrapolate these results to other populations, as the results of the LR+ (3,39) and LR- (0,21) suggest.

4. Discussion

A diagnostic test has clinical utility when it shows both validity and accuracy [37,38]. The results of this study indicate that the neurodynamic or orthopedic tension tests performed independently have no clinical utility.

The only combined test that showed diagnostic validity (internal and external) was the Slump test and the Dejerine's triad. This suggests that the result could be extrapolated to other populations.

The Straight Leg Raise test and the Bragard test performed in a multiple parallel manner obtained an excellent diagnostic validity as it external and internal validity values indicate. This means that the tests can dismiss the lumbar or lumbosacral radiculopathies when its results are negative. No studies that could support these results were found in the literature.

Our study also revealed that the Straight Leg Raise test has internal validity when it is done independently. These results coincide with other studies that were conducted with high prevalence populations [39]. However, we do not coincide with other studies that have a similar design [40–42]. Regarding the safety of the test (predictive values), our results are not in accordance with the values found in other studies [43–45]. Regarding the lack of external validity of this test, we coincide with other studies that are available in the literature [41,42,46,47]. The authors of these studies also concluded that the Straight Leg Raise test has no clinical utility to confirm or dismiss the condition. Other authors also question the validity of this test [48,49]. Nevertheless, the accuracy and reliability that the test showed in our study was very high, being superior to the results shown in other studies [50–52].

As well as the Straight Leg Raise, the analysis showed that the Bragard test has internal validity but does not have external validity. We could not compare the findings related to this indicator as no studies were found in the literature to do so. The Bragard test also showed a very good reliability which was better than the results found by other authors [50].

The values obtained in the combined test of the Straight Leg Raise and the Bragard tests are similar to those obtained when the tests were performed independently. Only one study analyzing this tests was found in the research available. Nonetheless, its results were inferior to those in our study [53]. As mentioned above, the multiple parallel assessment of the Straight Leg Raise and the Bragard tests revealed excellent effectiveness to dismiss radiculopathy when the result of the test was negative. These findings were not able to be compared as no comparable studies were found published in the literature.

The Fajersztajn and Sicard tests performed independently, combined or in the multiple parallel way showed no external or internal validity. When comparing both tests, the Fajersztajn test obtained higher specificity and diagnostic reliability when it was done independently. The results related to the high specificity of this last test coincide with the results demonstrated by other authors [39,42,54–57]. However, no scientific evidence was found related to the performance of the Sicard test performed independently, combined with the Fajersztajn test or in a multiple parallel manner.

Regarding the Passive Neck Flexion test, although it has external and internal validity, its lack of diagnostic accuracy indicates that it is not clinically useful. Again, these results cannot be compared as there is no scientific evidence available in the literature. In addition, the Kernig test, the combination of the Passive Neck Flexion test and the Kernig test and their multiple parallel test showed no internal or external validity even though the Kernig test showed reliability and accuracy. This indicates that they have no clinical utility.

The analysis of the Slump test indicated that this test has internal validity which coincides with another study with a similar design to ours [58]. We are in accordance with other authors, in the high sensitivity of this test [12,44,59]. Although it showed very good reliability or accuracy, as it has no external validity, the results cannot be extrapolated to other populations. Based on these findings we consider that the Slump test has no clinical utility.

The Dejerine's triad has internal and external validity but it did not show any reliability or accuracy. These results suggest that it has no clinical utility to diagnose lumbar or lumbosacral radiculopathy. The use of this test for the diagnosis of these conditions has not been assessed in previous studies.

The multiple parallel tests of the Slump test and the Dejerine's triad have internal validity but no external validity. This indicates that they do not have clinical utility to diagnose the condition in other populations.

There are some limitations to this study. The tests were combined in pairs in order to perform the assessment. This decision was based on the fact that the neurodynamic or orthopedic tension tests trigger pain and symptoms and it was not considered ethical to over stimulate the patients. Combining all the tests among them could have shown better results to analyze which combination had the most clinical utility. Another limitation was the scarce studies related to the subject that were available in the literature. Although this made the comparison of our results difficult, it has been an opportunity to reveal gaps in the literature. We also consider that the statistical analysis could have been more complete if the reliability would have been calculated for the combined tests of all groups. For future studies, we would recommend an assessment of the accuracy of the combined test of the Slump test and the Dejerine triad as it showed to be the test with the highest diagnostic validity (internal and external).

5. Conclusions

Out of all the tests assessed in this study, only the combined test of Slump test and the Dejerine's triad and the Straight Leg Raise and Bragard test performed in the multiple parallel way had diagnostic validity (internal and external). Therefore, both tests can be considered as appropriate to diagnose lumbar or lumbosacral radiculopathy. We also recommend these tests based on their low cost and the simplicity of the technique which makes the tests very easy and quick to perform in the clinical practice. However, an MRI scan is always recommended to confirm the diagnosis.

Based on our results, the following tests have no clinical utility when performed individually: The Passive Neck Flexion test, the Dejerine's triad, the Straight Leg Raise test, the Bragard test, the Fajersztajn test, the Slump test, the Sicard test and the Kernig test.

Future research should be conducted to analyze the clinical utility of different combinations of the neurodynamic or orthopedic tension tests.

Author Contributions: Conceptualization, F.J.G.E.d.l.M., P.O.R. and J.P.E.; methodology, J.R.M.; formal analysis, J.P.E.; investigation, F.J.G.E.d.l.M.; writing—original draft preparation, G.G.-M. and J.R.M.; writing—review and editing, E.M.G.A. and G.G.-M.; visualization, F.J.G.E.d.l.M.; supervision, P.O.R. and J.P.E. All authors have read and agreed to the published version of the manuscript.

Funding: This research received no external funding.

Conflicts of Interest: The authors declare no conflict of interest.

References

1. Sánchez, S.D.; Calderón, M.M.; García Leoni, M.E.; Palazuelos, M.V. Dolores musculoesqueléticos. Radiculopatías. Afectación de partes blandas. Artritis aguda. *Medicine* **2011**, *10*, 6023–6040. [CrossRef]
2. Latka, D.; Miekisiak, G.; Jarmuzek, P.; Lachowski, M.; Kaczmarczyk, J. Treatment of lumbar disc herniation with radiculopathy. Clinical practice guidelines endorsed by The Polish Society of Spinal Surgery. *Neurol Neurochir. Pol.* **2016**, *50*, 101–108. [CrossRef] [PubMed]
3. Ochoa Sangrador, C.; González de Dios, J.; Buñuel Álvarez, J.C. Evaluación de artículos científicos sobre pruebas diagnósticas. *Evid. Pediatr.* **2007**, *3*, 24.
4. Zamora, J.; Abraira, V. Análisis de la calidad de los estudios de evaluación de pruebas diagnósticas. *Nefrología* **2008**, *28*, 42–45.
5. Murphy, D.R.; Hurwitz, E.L. A theoretical model for the development of a diagnosis based clinical decision rule for the management of patients with spinal pain. *BMC Musculoskelet. Disord.* **2007**, *8*, 60–77. [CrossRef]
6. Murphy, D.R.; Hurwitz, E.L.; Gerrard, J.K.; Clary, R. Pain patterns and descriptions in patients with radicular pain: Does the pain necessarily follow a specific dermatome? *Chiropr. Osteopat.* **2009**, *17*, 9. [CrossRef]
7. Larraguibel Salas, F. Síndrome lumbociático. *Rev. Med. Clin. Condes.* **2006**, *17*, 26–30.
8. Umaña Giraldo, H.; Henao Zuluaga, C.; Castillo Berrio, C. Semiología del dolor lumbar. *Rev. Med. Risaralda* **2010**, *16*, 43–56. [CrossRef]
9. Rodríguez-García, P.L.; Rodríguez-Pupo, L.; Rodríguez-García, D. Técnicas clínicas para el examen físico neurológico. III. Función sensitiva. *Rev. Neurol.* **2004**, *39*, 966–971. [CrossRef]
10. Butler, D.S. *Movilización del Sistema Nervioso*; Paidotribo: Barcelona, Spain, 2002; pp. 131–134.
11. Hilal, K.; Sajjad, Z.; Sayani, R.; Khan, D. Utility of Limited Protocol Magnetic Resonance Imaging Lumbar Spine for Nerve Root Compression in a Developing Country, Is It Accurate and Cost Effective? *Asian Spine J.* **2013**, *7*, 184–189. [CrossRef]
12. 7 Trainor, K.; Pinnington, M.A. Reliability and diagnostic validity of the slump knee bend neurodynamic test for upp.er/mid lumbar nerve root compression: A pilot study. *Physiotherapy* **2011**, *97*, 59–64. [CrossRef] [PubMed]

13. Davis, D.S.; Anderson, I.B.; Carson, M.G.; Elkins, C.L.; Stuckey, L.B. Upper Limb Neural Tension and Seated Slump Tests: The false positive rate among healthy young adults without cervical or lumbar symptoms. *J. Man. Manip. Ther.* **2008**, *16*, 136–141. [CrossRef]

14. Shacklock, M.; Donoso, G.; Lucha López, M. Hacia un enfoque en el diagnóstico con test neurodinámicos (tensión neural). *Rev. Fisioter.* **2007**, *29*, 288–297. [CrossRef]

15. Simpson, R.; Gemmell, H. Accuracy of spinal orthopaedic tests: A systematic review. *Chiropr. Osteopat.* **2006**, *14*, 26. [CrossRef] [PubMed]

16. Camino Willhuber GO, P.N. Straight Leg Raise Test. In *Treasure Island (FL): StatPearls Publishing*; StatPearls: Treasure Island, FL, USA, 2020.

17. Natalio Firpo, C.A. *Manual de Ortopedia y Traumatología*, 1st ed.; Carlos Natalio Firpo: Buenos Aires, Argentina, 2010; pp. 120–150.

18. Fransoo, P. *Examen Clínico del Paciente con Lumbalgia*; Paidotribo: Barcelona, Spain, 2003; pp. 100–204.

19. Ricard, F. *Tratamiento Osteopático de las Lumbalgias y Lumbociáticas por Hernias Discales*; Médica Panamericana: Madrid, Spain, 2003; pp. 7–9.

20. Ward, M.A.; Greenwood, T.M.; Kumar, D.R.; Mazza, J.J.; Yale, S.H. Josef Brudzinski and Vladimir Mikhailovich Kernig: Signs for diagnosing Meningitis. *Clin. Med. Res.* **2010**, *8*, 13–17. [CrossRef]

21. Maitland, G.D. The Slump Test: Examination and treatment. *Aust. J. Physiother.* **1985**, *31*, 215–219. [CrossRef]

22. Cohen, J.F.; Korevaar, D.A.; Altman, D.G.; Bruns, D.E.; Gatsonis, C.A.; Hooft, L.; Irwig, L.; Levine, D.; Reitsma, J.B.; De Vet, H.C.W.; et al. STARD 2015 guidelines for reporting diagnostic accuracy studies: Explanation and elaboration. *BMJ Open* **2016**, *6*, 1–17. [CrossRef]

23. Bossuyt, P.M.; Reitsma, J.B.; Bruns, D.E.; Gatsonis, C.A.; Glasziou, P.P.; Irwig, L.M. STARD 2015: An updated list of essential items for reporting diagnostic accuracy studies. *BMJ* **2015**, *351*, h5527. [CrossRef]

24. Asociación Médica Mundial. Declaración de Helsinki de la Asociación Médica Mundial. Principios éticos para las investigaciones médicas en seres humanos. *An. Sist. Sanit. Navar.* **2001**, *24*, 209–212.

25. UE. *Reglamento (UE) 2016/679 del Parlamento Europeo y del Consejo, de 27 de abril de 2016, Relativo a la Protección de las Personas Físicas en lo que Respecta al Tratamiento de datos Personales y a la Libre Circulación de estos Datos y por el que se Deroga la Directiva 95/46/CE (Reglamento General de Protección de datos)*; Diario Oficial de la Unión Europea: Madrid, Spain, 2016.

26. Comuñas, F. Dolor radicular. *Rev. Soc. Esp. Dolor* **2000**, *7* (Suppl. 2), 36–48.

27. Miller, K.J. Physical assessment of lower extremity radiculopathy and sciatica. *J. Chiropr. Med.* **2007**, *6*, 75–82. [CrossRef] [PubMed]

28. Mesa, J.C.; García, O.; Lillo, J.; Mascaró, F.; Arruga, J. Oftalmología basada en pruebas: Evaluación crítica de la literatura sobre pruebas diagnósticas. *Arch. Soc. Esp. Oftalmol.* **2008**, *83*, 639–651. [CrossRef] [PubMed]

29. Cerda, L.J.; Cifuentes, A.L. Uso de tests diagnósticos en la práctica clínica (Parte 1). Análisis de las propiedades de un test diagnóstico. *Rev. Chil. Infect.* **2010**, *27*, 205–208. [CrossRef]

30. Rupérez, F. Validez de los Elementos Diagnósticos en Endometriosis. Aplicación al Análisis de Decisión Clínica. Ph.D. Thesis, Departamento de Cirugía, Ciencias Médicas y Sociales-Universidad de Alcalá, Madrid, Spain, 2013.

31. Epidemiología General y Demografía Sanitaria, 2010–2011. Open Course Ware (16633). Epidat: Pruebas Diagnósticas. Available online: https://goo.gl/UfAwMe (accessed on 1 May 2014).

32. Ortín Ortín, E.; Sánchez Sánchez, J.A.; Menárguez Puche, J.F.; Hidalgo García, I.M. Lectura crítica de un artículo sobre diagnóstico. In *Atención Sanitaria Basada en la Evidencia: Su Aplicación a la Práctica Clínica*; Sánchez Sánchez, J.A., Ed.; Consejería de Sanidad: Murcia, Spain, 2007; pp. 233–578.

33. Hervás Angulo, A.; Lacosta Ramírez, U.; Brugarolas Brufau, C.; Díez Espino, J. Aplicabilidad en una comunidad (validez externa) de los estudios de prevención primaria de hipercolesterolemia. *Aten. Primaria* **2003**, *32*, 509–516. [CrossRef]

34. Silva Fuente-Alba, C.; Molina Villagra, M. Likelihood ratio (razón de verosimilitud): Definición y aplicación en Radiología. *Rev. Argent. Radiol.* **2017**, *81*, 204–208. [CrossRef]

35. Donis, J.H. Assessment of the validity and reliability of a diagnostic test. *Avan. Biomed.* **2012**, *1*, 73–81.

36. Camila Medina, M. Generalidades de las pruebas diagnósticas, y su utilidad en la toma de decisiones médicas. *Rev. Colomb. Psiquiat.* **2011**, *40*, 787–797. [CrossRef]

37. Ochoa Sangrador, C.; Molina Arias, M. Evaluación de la precisión de las pruebas diagnósticas (1). Variables discretas. *Evid. Pediatr.* **2017**, *13*, 1–5.

38. Cortés-Reyes, E.T.; Rubio-Romero, A.J.; Gaitán-Duarte, H. Statistical methods for evaluating diagnostic test agreement and reproducibility. *Rev. Colomb. Obstet. Ginecol.* **2009**, *61*, 247–255. [CrossRef]

39. Van der Windt, D.; Simons, E.; Riphagen, I.I.; Ammendolia, C.; Verhagen, A.P.; Laslett, M.; Deville, W.; Deyo, R.A.; Bouter, L.M.; de Vet, H.C.; et al. Physical examination for lumbar radiculopathy due to disc herniation in patients with low-back pain. *Cochrane Database Syst. Rev.* **2011**, 1–86. [CrossRef]

40. Rabin, A.; Gerszten, P.C.; Karausky, P.; Bunker, C.H.; Potter, D.M.; Welch, W.C. The sensitivity of the Seated Straight-Leg Raise Test compared with the Supine Straight-Leg Raise Test in patients presenting with Magnetic Resonance Imaging evidence of lumbar nerve root compression. *Arch. Phys. Med. Rehabil.* **2007**, *88*, 840–843. [CrossRef] [PubMed]

41. Iversen, T.; Solberg, T.K.; Romner, B.; Wilsgaard, T.; Nygaard, Ø.; Waterloo, K.; Brox, J.I.; Ingebrigtsen, T. Accuracy of physical examination for chronic lumbar radiculopathy. *BMC Musculoskelet. Disord.* **2013**, *14*, 1–9. [CrossRef] [PubMed]

42. Suri, P.; Rainville, J.; Katz, J.N.; Jouve, C.; Hartigan, C.; Limke, J.; Pena, E.; Li, L.; Swaim, B.; Hunter, D.J. The accuracy of the Physical Examination for the diagnosis of Midlumbar and Low Lumar Nerve Root Impingement. *Spine* **2011**, *36*, 63–73. [CrossRef] [PubMed]

43. Poiraudeau, S. Value of the bell test and the hyperextension test for diagnosis in sciatica associated with disc herniation: Comparison with Lasegue's sign and the crossed Lasegue's sign. *Rheumatology* **2001**, *40*, 460–466. [CrossRef] [PubMed]

44. Majlesi, J.; Togay, H.; Ünalan, H.; Toprak, S. The sensitivity and specificity of the slump and the straight leg raising tests in patients with lumbar disc herniation. *J. Clin. Rheumatol.* **2008**, *14*, 87–91. [CrossRef] [PubMed]

45. Cecin, H.A. Sinal de Cecin (Sinal "X"): Um aprimoramento no diagnóstico de compressão radicular por hérnias discais lombares. *Rev. Bras. Reumatol.* **2010**, *50*, 44–55. [CrossRef]

46. Capra, F.; Vanti, C.; Donati, R.; Tombetti, S.; O'Reilly, C.; BScPhysio(hons); Pillastrini, P. Validity of the straight-leg raise test for patients with sciatic pain with or without lumbar pain using magnetic resonance imaging results as a reference standard. *J. Manipulative Physiol. Ther.* **2011**, *34*, 231–238. [CrossRef]

47. Scaia, V.; Baxter, D.; Cook, C. The pain provocation-based Straight Leg Raise Test for diagnosis of lumbar disc herniation, lumbar radiculopathy, and/or sciatica: A systematic review of clinical utility. *J. Back Musculoskelet. Rehabil.* **2012**, *25*, 215–223. [CrossRef]

48. Ekedahl, H.; Jönsson, B.; Annertz, M. Accuracy of clinical tests in detecting disk herniation and nerve root compression in subjects with lumbar radicular symptoms. *Arch. Phys. Med. Rehabil.* **2018**, *99*, 726–735. [CrossRef]

49. Ekedahl, H.; Jönsson, B. Fingertip-to-floor test and straight leg raising test: Validity, responsiveness, and predictive value in patients with acute/subacute low back pain. *Arch. Phys. Med. Rehabil.* **2012**, *93*, 2210–2215. [CrossRef]

50. Vroomen, P.C.; De Krom, M.C.; Knottnerus, J.A. Consistency of history taking and physical examination in patients with suspected lumbar nerve root involvement. *Spine* **2000**, *25*, 91–97. [CrossRef] [PubMed]

51. Kreiner, D.S.; Hwang, S.W.; Easa, J.E.; Resnick, D.K.; Baisden, J.L.; Bess, S. An evidence-based clinical guideline for the diagnosis and treatment of lumbar disc herniation with radiculopathy. *Spine J.* **2014**, *14*, 180–191. [CrossRef] [PubMed]

52. Albert, J.; Inez Silva, L.; Liberali, M.; Yumi Kiara, P.; Marcelo Pilatti, C. Concordância entre o teste de distensão dural na posição sentada (slump test) e o teste de lasègue no diagnóstico fisioterapêutico de lombociatalgia. *FIEP Bull.* **2013**, *83*, 1–6.

53. Homayouni, K.; Jafari, S.; Yari, H. Sensitivity and specificity of Modified Bragard Test in patients with lumbosacral rediculopathy using electrodiagnosis as a reference standard. *J. Chiropr. Med.* **2018**, *17*, 36–43. [CrossRef]

54. Vroomen, P.C.; De Krom, M.C.; Knottnerus, J.A. Diagnostic value of history and physical examination in patients suspected of sciatica due to disc herniation: A systematic review. *J. Neurol.* **1999**, *246*, 899–906. [CrossRef]

55. Lurie, J.D. What diagnostic tests are useful for low back pain? *Best Pract. Res. Clin. Rheumatol.* **2005**, *19*, 557–575. [CrossRef]

56. Devillé, W.; van der Windt, D.; Dzaferagić, A.; Bezemer, P.; Bouter, L. The test of Lasègue: Systematic review of the accuracy in diagnosing herniated discs. *Spine* **2000**, *25*, 1140–1147. [CrossRef]

57. Koes, B.; Van Tulder, M.; Peul, W. Diagnosis and treatment of sciatica. *Br. Med. J.* **2007**, *334*, 1313–1317. [CrossRef]
58. M'kumbuzi, V.R.P.; Ntawukuriryayo, J.T.; Haminana, J.D.; Munyandamutsa, J.; Nzakizwanimana, E. Accuracy of straight leg raise and slump tests in detecting lumbar disc herniation: A pilot study. *Cent. Afr. J. Med.* **2012**, *58*, 5–11.
59. Urban, L.; MacNeil, B. Diagnostic Accuracy of the Slump Test for Identifying Neuropathic Pain in the Lower Limb. *J. Orthop. Sport. Phys. Ther.* **2015**, *45*, 596–603. [CrossRef]

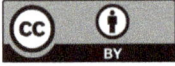

International Journal of
Environmental Research and Public Health

MDPI

Article

Spanish Validation of the "User Reported Measure of Care Coordination" Questionnaire for Older People with Complex, Chronic Conditions

Ester Risco [1], Glòria Sauch [2,*], Anna Albero [3], Nihan Acar-Denizli [4], Adelaida Zabalegui [5], Belchin Kostov [6], Paloma Amil [7], Albert Alonso [8], Ana Rios [9], Jaume Martín [10] and Núria Fabrellas [11]

[1] Intermediated Care Hospital Parc Sanitari Pere Virgili, 08035 Barcelona, Spain; erisco@perevirgili.cat
[2] Research Support Unit Catalunya Central, Fundació Institut Universitari per a la Recerca a l'Atenció Primària de Salut Jordi Gol i Gurina (IDIAPJGol), Catalan Health Institute, Catalunya Central, 08272 Sant Fruitós del Bages, Spain
[3] Emergency Department, Hospital Clínic de Barcelona, 08036 Barcelona, Spain; ALBERO@clinic.cat
[4] Department of Statistics, Faculty of Science and Letters, Mimar Sinan Fine Arts University, 34427 Istanbul, Turkey; nihan.acar@msgsu.edu.tr
[5] FEANS, Hospital Clinic de Barcelona, 08036 Barcelona, Spain; AZABALEG@clinic.cat
[6] Primary Healthcare Transversal Research Group, Institut d'Investigacions Biomèdiques August Pi i Sunyer (IDIBAPS), Primary Care Centre Les Corts, Consorci d'Atenció Primària de Salut Barcelona Esquerra (CAPSBE), 08036 Barcelona, Spain; BADRIYAN@clinic.cat
[7] Chronicity Prevention and Care Programme, Health Planning General Directorate, Ministry of Health, Government of Catalonia, 08028 Barcelona, Spain; pamil@gencat.cat
[8] Fundació Clínic per a la Recerca Biomèdica, 08036 Barcelona, Spain; AALONSO@clinic.cat
[9] Catalan Health Institute, 08007 Barcelona, Spain; a.rios@gencat.cat
[10] Research Suport Unit Barcelona, Fundació Institut Universitari per a la Recerca a l'Atenció Primària de Salut Jordi Gol i Gurina (IDIAPJGol), Catalan Health Institute Barcelona, 08025 Barcelona, Spain; jmartinr.bcn.ics@gencat.cat
[11] Department of Public Health, Mental Health and Perinatal Nursing, Universitat de Barcelona, 08907 Barcelona, Spain; nfabrellas@ub.edu
* Correspondence: gsauch.cc.ics@gencat.cat

Received: 22 June 2020; Accepted: 26 August 2020; Published: 11 September 2020

check for updates

Abstract: Introduction: Older people with complex, chronic conditions often receive insufficient or inefficient care provision, and few instruments are able to measure their perception of care provision. The "User Reported Measure of Care Coordination" instrument has been satisfactorily used to evaluate chronic care provision and integration. The aim of this study is to validate this instrument in Spanish. Methods: The questionnaire was adapted and validated in two phases: translation and cultural adaptation of the questionnaire and psychometric property measurement. Study population were chronic care conditions patients. Results: A total of 332 participants completed test re-test as part of the questionnaire validation process. The final version of the questionnaire had 6 domains: Health and Well-being (D1), Health day to day (D2), Social Services (D3), Planned Care (D4), Urgent Care (D5), and Hospital Care (D6). Cronbach's alpha for the overall questionnaire was 0.86, indicating good internal consistency. When analyzing each domain, only Planned Care (D4) and Urgent Care (D5) had Cronbach's Alphas slightly lower than 0.7, although this could be related to the low number of items in each domain. A good temporal stability was observed for the distinct subscales and items, with intraclass correlation coefficients varying from 0.412 to 0.929 ($p < 0.05$). Conclusion: The adapted version of the "User Reported Measure of Care Coordination" into Spanish proved to be a practical tool for use in our daily practice and an efficient instrument for assessment of care coordination in chronic, complex conditions in older people across services and levels of care.

Keywords: integrated care; social care; health care; older people; comorbidity; person centered care

1. Introduction

Healthcare provision to aging populations in the current economic slowdown represents a considerable challenge for major European countries, especially when readdressing policies to cover new demands related to health and social needs [1]. People with complex, chronic conditions often receive inadequate care due to poor coordination between health and social care providers [2]. This situation is even worse when dealing with people older than 65 years. Inefficient coordination is a severe limitation when trying to achieve the triple aim of optimizing health system performance: improvement of health outcomes, the patient's experience, and care cost-effectiveness [3,4].

Many integrated care initiatives responding to multiple health and social care needs have been introduced in European health systems in a variety of contexts [5,6]. Some countries, such as The Netherlands, Germany, or Austria have already worked to improve care coordination since the early 2000's [2]. The United Kingdom, with extensive experience working towards integration of care, has also developed and evaluated different potential plans to improve chronic care [7,8]. Spain has done so, with numerous actions undertaken and a variety of state-wide and regional strategies targeting different chronic conditions [9,10]. However, the impact of these strategies has hardly been evaluated, with some exceptions, such as the strategy deployed in the Basque Country [11] or the regional implementation carried out in Spain, Norway, and Greece in the context of the NEXES project (Integrated Care Services supported by Information Technologies for chronic patients with obstructive pulmonary disease, cardiac failure, and/or type II diabetes mellitus [12]).

Despite the implementation of healthcare policies and the great commitment of professionals, there are still significant weaknesses in our healthcare system as it stands: organizational and economic fragmentation between different levels of care, lack of integration between social services and healthcare, lack of coordination with family associations, and long waiting lists for diagnostic and surgical procedures.

In the region of Catalonia, Spain, the Government is already working on a new personalized model based on Person Centered Care called Interdepartmental Plan for Social and Healthcare Interaction (PIAISS) 2017–2020 [13]. This new framework contributes to the development of new strategies to improve care integration. Instruments such as the one developed by Nuño-Solinís et al. [9] have shown very good ease-of-use in daily practice, but its application is limited to the organizational level. We need new instruments to measure care coordination across all levels of care, principally when registering the perspectives of the populations [14]. Through this approach, we aim to measure the impact on the health of the population. Moreover, understanding patients' experiences is a good way to determine whether our strategies meet the expectations of populations in care coordination for chronic, complex conditions [15]. Therefore, there is a need for new validated instruments for use with Spanish-speaking population. In order to guarantee the quality of their measurements, it is essential that the instruments should be subjected to a process of validation. This process consists in adapting the instrument culturally to the setting where its psychometric characteristics are to be administered.

The "User Reported Measure of Care Coordination" questionnaire [16] is a tool developed and validated in the United Kingdom to measure the experiences of patients accessing care across organizational and professional boundaries. This tool has the potential to identify weaknesses with the goal of improving care coordination in line with the expectations of the population. The survey provides some information about how well services support patients and help users to achieve their own life goals. This instrument allows evaluation of the provision of care as well the effectiveness of future interventions for care coordination. The questionnaire consists of 46 items, divided into 7 domains: Health and well-being (D1), Health day to day (D2), Social Services (D3), Planned Care (D4), Urgent access to healthcare (D5), Hospital care (D6), and Self-information (D7). The results are expressed in a single overall numeric variable

(0–100) that is expressed as a continuous variable, in which the patients with higher scores have a more positive perception.

The aim of this study is the translation and cross-cultural adaptation of the questionnaire "User Reported Measure of Care Coordination" and the analysis of its psychometric properties.

2. Methods

2.1. Design

Adaptation and validation of the questionnaire were conducted through a descriptive cross-sectional study. This was carried out in two phases: an initial phase in which the translation and cultural adaptation of the questionnaire was performed and a second phase in which the behavior of its psychometric properties was measured. All research procedures used in this study were established in accordance with the Declaration of Helsinki; participants gave their signed informed consent, and the study was approved by the Ethics Committee at Hospital Clinic, Barcelona (HCB/2017/0731).

2.2. Translation and Cultural Adaptation of the Questionnaire

Authorization to translate the questionnaire was obtained from the copyright holders. The transcultural adaptation of the questionnaire was performed following the structured procedure described by Beaton et al. [17]. Two translations of the questionnaire from English to Spanish were done by 2 healthcare professionals working separately. A single, consolidated version of both questionnaires was then produced. This version was then back-translated into English by 2 qualified translators. Finally, both versions in English (the original version and the back-translation) were compared and found to contain no significant differences.

Content validity was performed on the pre-final version of the questionnaire by a panel of 8 expert judges, including 2 nurses and 1 physician from a primary care center, 2 social workers from social services and 1 nurse, 1 physician and 1 social worker from a tertiary hospital. Criteria for the selection of the experts were: (a) experience in evidence-based judgement and evidence-based decision-making (research, publications and experience), (b) availability and motivation to participate, and (c) impartiality. Members of the panel of experts were asked to conduct a qualitative evaluation of every item (degree of understanding, agreement with the text) and were also asked to conduct a quantitative assessment of each item following these criteria: (1) competence (items belong to theoretical established factors), (2) clarity (item is easily understood, its semantics and syntactics are suitable), (3) coherence (item is related to the factor being measured), and (4) relevance (item is essential and has to be included). Each point assessed for each item was quantified on a Likert- type scale of 3 points: (1: Agree; 2: Neither agree nor disagree; 3: Disagree). This was done in two rounds by email. In the first round, all suggestions were added to the pre-final version and the second was performed to obtain agreement among all the experts. None of the items was eliminated at this stage. Some items were adapted to our specific context, and some response categories were combined from the experts' group discussion. The self-information domain (D7) was removed from the validation process, considering that this was part of the sociodemographic data, and it could not be measured. Finally, the remaining 38 items were divided into 6 domains: Health and Well-being (D1) consisting of 6 items, Health Day to Day (D2) consisting of 14 items, Social Services (D3) consisting of 3 items, Planned Care (D4) consisting of 5 items, Urgent Care (D5) consisting of 3 items, and Hospital Care (D6) consisting of 7 items. Scored items were created by converting the individual responses to questions into scores on a scale of 0 to 100, where a score of 100 represents the best possible response, and a score of 0 represents the worst possible response. Where response options were provided that do not have any bearing on performance in terms of patient experience (such as the 'Don't know/Can't remember' option), the responses were classified as "not applicable" and no score was given. Questions without answers were not considered too. In order to compute the score for domains, a numeric value (0–100) was also established for each domain. According to this method, at least 2 questions should be answered in the Social Services (D3), Planned Care (D4), and Urgent Care (D5) domains; at least 4 questions in the Health and Well-being (D1) and Hospital Care (D6) domains; and at least 10 questions in the *Health day to day* (D2) domain. Again, higher scores mean better perception.

In order to check viability in daily practice, we conducted a pilot test administering the questionnaire to a sample of 18 patients. Patients answered the overall questionnaire and were asked to review the items, identifying words or concepts they did not understand. No relevant modifications were made.

2.3. Psychometric Properties

The characteristics of the participants were similar to those from the sample used by Crump et al. (2017) in the development and validation of the original questionnaire. To ensure a representative sample, registered nurses from across Catalonia, divided into 9 health management areas, were involved in data collection. Forty experienced registered nurses working in different primary care centers received specific training and guidelines on eligibility criteria, clinical tests, and instructions for the administration of the questionnaire. The participation of nurses was voluntary, and each nurse had to include a minimum of 5 participants. The registered nurses recruited participants during a routine visit at the health care center or at home. The participants were selected for convenience in accordance with the following inclusion and exclusion criteria. The participants should be older than 65 years old. Multimorbidity or unique condition difficult to manage according to Complex Chronic Patient (PCC) criteria or advanced chronic illness (limited prognosis, palliative orientation, advanced decisions planned) was required. Understanding oral and written Spanish was necessary. People living in long-term care institutions were excluded. All study participants signed informed consent, and the implications of participating in the study were explained through an information sheet.

A total of 40 experienced registered nurses were responsible for collecting data across Catalonia. Although all of them received specific training, some variations could appear on collecting data.

Sample size was calculated following the criteria established by Kline et al. 2010 [18], which recommend a ratio of 5–10 subjects per item.

Data analysis was performed using the R statistical software package V.3.5.0 for Windows. Descriptive statistics of the quantitative variables are presented as mean and standard deviation. Categorical variables were described according to their frequency. The descriptive analysis on the scores obtained in each domain is presented with the mean and standard deviation.

The intraclass correlation coefficient (ICC) was used to study test–retest reliability of each item between two similar assessments with an interval of 7–10 days between measurements.

The internal consistency of the questionnaire was evaluated using Cronbach's alpha, which was considered acceptable if the value was greater than 0.7. The "alpha if item deleted" index was computed to study the increase or decrease in the sample value of alpha according to the deletion of items. Correlations between the different items and domains were studied using the Spearman correlation coefficient, assuming that the various domains gather distinct information with moderate-low correlation coefficients. Correlation was considered weak when the *r* value was less than 0.3, moderate between 0.3 and 0.6, and strong when greater than 0.6. A *p* value ≤ 0.05 was considered significant.

3. Results

3.1. Patient Demographics

A total of 332 patients across Catalonia completed the study. The characteristics of these participants are shown in Table 1. The mean age of the study population was 82.1 ± 8.0 years, and 204 (56.4%) participants were women. From the overall sample, 269 (74.3%) participants lived with a family member and 13 (3.6%) with some other carer such as a friend or neighbor. The rest of the participants lived alone. Only 6 participants (1.7%) described their health status as excellent, 75 (20.7%) said it was good, 198 (54.7%) participants defined it as regular, and 83 (22.9%) described it as bad. From the overall sample, 247 (68.2%) participants did not have any help or additional assistance from a private service or institution for their daily care. The most prevalent health problems in our study sample were hypertension (79%), cardiac diseases (51.4%), diabetes (45.4%), and arthrosis or arthritis (15.7%).

Table 1. Sample characteristics (n = 362).

Variable	n (%)
Area	
0	121 (33.4%)
1	21 (5.8%)
2	38 (10.5%)
3	70 (19.3%)
4	20 (5.5%)
5	26 (7.2%)
6	26 (7.2%)
7	40 (11%)
Sex (female)	204 (56.4%)
Who they live with	
Alone	80 (22.1%)
With a family member	269 (74.3%)
Other	13 (3.6%)
Age (years), mean ± SD	82.1 ± 8.0
Person who answered the questionnaire	
The person for whom it is intended	138 (38.1%)
A friend or relative of the person for whom it is intended	86 (23.8%)
The person for whom it is intended and the friend or relative.	79 (21.8%)
The person for whom it is intended with the help of a healthcare professional	59 (16.3%)
Extra help or attention from a private service or institution	
Yes, I pay for other services with my money	76 (21%)
Yes, my family pays for extra help for my care	39 (10.8%)
No	247 (68.2%)
In general, how you describe your state of health	
Excellent	6 (1.7%)
Good	75 (20.7%)
Normal	198 (54.7%)
Poor	83 (22.9%)
Illnesses or health problems	
Hypertension	268 (74%)
Diabetes	164 (45.4%)
Heart failure or other heart problems	186 (51.4%)
Renal failure or other kidney problems	129 (35.6%)
Dementia or cognitive impairment	92 (25.4%)
Others	204 (56.4%)
Osteoarthritis	39 (10.8%)
COPD	36 (9.9%)
Osteoporosis	23 (6.4%)
Hypercholesterolemia	22 (6.1%)

The data is shown as a number and a percentage (%) unless otherwise indicated.

3.2. Descriptive Analysis

All questions were answered by the patients that participated in the study except those Conditional questions that could be skipped depending on previous answers. Table 2 shows the frequency distribution of the different questionnaire items. If we look at the non-response pattern for the items answered in the questionnaire, *Health and Well-being* (D1), *Health day to day* (D2), and *Urgent Care* (D5) had practically 99.7% of the items answered. Only in *Health Day to Day* (D2) did we find an item that had a lower score (99.7%), and item (Q8) that was 90.9%. In *Social Services* (D3), *Planned Care* (D4), and *Hospital Care* (D6) there was a lower response rate as participants skipped some questions because they were not receiving this specific care. Therefore, the answer on the perception of Social Services, Planned Care, and Hospital Care cannot be described from the population point of view.

Table 2. Frequencies of the categories for the items.

Number of Item	N	% of Responses	1	2	3	4	5	6	7	8	9
D1. Your level of Health, Welfare, and Autonomy											
Q1 (1)	362	100	102 (28.2%)	50 (13.8%)	65 (18%)	126 (34.8%)	19 (5.2%)				
Q2 (2)	362	100	103 (28.5%)	125 (34.5%)	129 (35.6%)	5 (1.4%)					
Q3 (3)	362	100	244 (67.4%)	81 (22.4%)	34 (9.4%)	3 (0.8%)					
Q4 (4)	362	100	102 (28.2%)	168 (46.4%)	82 (22.7%)	10 (2.8%)					
Q5 (5)	362	100	138 (38.1%)	132 (36.5%)	49 (13.5%)	43 (11.9%)					
Q6 (5)	362	100	90 (24.9%)	117 (32.3%)	98 (27.1%)	57 (15.7%)					
D2. Monitoring Your Health											
Q7 (6)	362	100	158 (43.7%)	125 (34.6%)	18 (5.1%)	11 (3.1%)	29 (8%)	77 (21.3%)	10 (2.8%)		
Q8 (4)	329	90.9	206 (62.6%)	107 (32.5%)	14 (4.3%)	2 (0.6%)					
Q9 (7)	361	99.7	259 (71.7%)	78 (21.6%)	18 (5%)	6 (1.7%)					
Q10 (4)	361	99.7	238 (65.9%)	94 (26%)	27 (7.5%)	2 (0.6%)					
Q11 (8)	362	100	45 (12.4%)	261 (72.1%)	56 (15.5%)						
Q12 (9)	362	100	29 (8%)	129 (35.6%)	140 (38.7%)	64 (17.7%)					
Q13 (5)	362	100	179 (49.4%)	134 (37%)	33 (9.1%)	16 (4.4%)					
Q14 (10)	362	100	26 (7.2%)	113 (31.2%)	204 (56.4%)	19 (5.2%)					
Q15 (7)	362	100	185 (51.1%)	133 (36.7%)	30 (8.3%)	14 (3.9%)					
Q16 (4)	362	100	167 (46.1%)	155 (42.8%)	32 (8.8%)	8 (2.2%)					
Q17 (4)	362	100	186 (51.4%)	142 (39.2%)	31 (8.6%)	3 (0.8%)					
Q18 (11)	362	100	253 (69.9%)	64 (17.7%)	21 (5.8%)	9 (2.5%)	14 (3.9%)	1 (0.3%)			
Q19 (12)	361	99.7	141 (39.1%)	117 (32.4%)	42 (11.6%)	29 (8%)	32 (8.9%)				
Q20 (5)	362	100	103 (28.5%)	133 (36.7%)	85 (23.5%)	41 (11.3%)					
D3. Social Services											
Q21 (13)	362	100	118 (32.6%)	244 (67.4%)							
Q22 (14)	118	32.6	58 (49.2%)	6 (5.1%)	46 (39%)	8 (6.8%)					
Q23 (15)	118	32.6	60 (50.8%)	28 (23.7%)	21 (17.8%)	1 (0.8%)	8 (6.8%)				
D4. Treatment Plan											
Q24 (16)	362	100	93 (25.7%)	181 (50%)	88 (24.3%)						
Q25 (4)	93	25.7	48 (51.6%)	40 (43%)	4 (4.3%)	1 (1.1%)					
Q26 (4)	93	25.7	35 (37.6%)	52 (55.9%)	6 (6.5%)						
Q27 (5)	174	48.1	51 (29.3%)	67 (38.5%)	10 (5.7%)	46 (26.4%)					
Q28 (4)	360	99.4	187 (51.9%)	104 (28.9%)	36 (10%)	33 (9.2%)					

Table 2. *Cont.*

Number of Item	N	% of Responses	1	2	3	4	5	6	7	8	9
D5. Emergency Treatment											
Q29 (4)	362	100	165 (45.6%)	161 (44.5%)	31 (8.6%)	5 (1.4%)					
Q30 (5)	362	100	191 (52.8%)	119 (32.9%)	27 (7.5%)	25 (6.9%)					
Q31 (17)	362	100	238 (65.7%)	16 (4.4%)	46 (12.7%)	8 (2.2%)	0	28 (7.7%)	16 (4.5%)	6 (1.7%)	4 (1.1%)
D6. Hospital Care											
Q32 (13)	362	100	177 (48.9%)	185 (51.1%)							
Q33 (18)	177	48.9	69 (39%)	56 (31.6%)	23 (13%)	18 (10.2%)	11 (6.2%)				
Q34 (4)	177	48.9	65 (36.7%)	63 (35.6%)	34 (19.2%)	15 (8.5%)					
Q35 (4)	177	48.9	67 (37.9%)	57 (32.2%)	41 (23.2%)	12 (6.8%)					
Q36 (19)	177	48.9	34 (19.2%)	130 (73.4%)	1 (0.6%)	12 (6.8%)					
Q37 (20)	177	48.9	79 (44.6%)	65 (36.7%)	33 (18.6%)						
Q38 (18)	79	21.8	37 (46.8%)	33 (41.8%)	2 (2.5%)	2 (2.5%)	5 (6.3%)				

Some 15% of respondents took question P7 to be a multiple-choice question. [1] (1) Yes, the person who helps me lives with me; (2) Yes, the person who helps me doesn't live with me; (3) Yes, the person who lives with me helps me as much as individuals who don't live with me; (4) I don't need help; (5) I need help, but I don't receive help from anyone. [2] (1) Yes, I can do all the important tasks for myself; (2) I have some difficulty in carrying out some important tasks; (3) I'm not able to carry out tasks which are important for me; (4) I don't know/I'm not sure. [3] (1) I stay in touch as much as I want with the people around me; (2) I have some contact with people, but not enough; (3) I have very little contact and I feel I somewhat lonely; (4) I have no contact with anyone. I feel completely alone. [4] (1) Yes, totally; (2) Yes, partially; (3) Disagree; (4) Completely disagree. [5] (1) Totally disagree; (2) Partially agree; (3) Disagree; (4) I'm not sure/I disagree. [6] (1) Yes, the Primary Care Physician; (2) Yes, the Primary Care Nurse; (3) Yes, the Primary Care social worker; (4) If another healthcare professional, who?; (5) No, I do it myself; (6) No, a family member or care giver does it; (7) I don't know/I'm not sure. [7] (1) Yes, completely; (2) Yes, to some degree; (3) No; (4) I don't know/I'm not sure. [8] (1) Yes; (2) No; (3) I don't know/I'm not sure. [9] (1) Never work together; (2) They sometimes work together; (3) They always work together; (4) I don't know/I'm not sure. [10] (1) None of my needs have been assessed; (2) Some of my needs have been assessed; (3) All of my needs have been assessed; (4) I don't know/I'm not sure. [11] (1) Yes, they are totally involved; (2) Yes, they are quite involved; (3) They are not sufficiently involved; (4) No, not at all involved; (5) There is no family member or care worker involved; (6) I don't want my family or a care worker to be involved. [12] (1) Yes, they receive the help they need; (2) They get help, but not as much as they need; (3) No, they get little or no help; (4) They don't need/want help; (5) There's no family member or care worker involved. [13] (1) Yes; (2) No. [14] (1) Yes, the right frequency; (2) No, I need fewer visits; (3) No, I need more visits; (4) Not applicable. [15] (1) Yes, they last the right amount of time; (2) No, I need a little more time; (3) No, I need a lot more time; (4) No, I have longer than I need; (5) Not applicable. [16] (1) Yes; (2) No; (3) I don't know/I can't remember. [17] (1) A family member; (2) A friend or neighbor; (3) Yes, the Primary Care Nurse; (3) Yes, the Primary Care social worker; (4) Yes, another healthcare professional; (5) No, the Primary Care worker; (6) The emergency services (061); (7) Another healthcare professional (not on this list) who?; (8) Another person (not on this list); (9) I don't contact anyone. [18] (1) Yes, totally; (2) Yes, partially; (3) Disagree; (4) Totally disagree; (5) I don't know. [19] (1) Not sufficiently; (2) Sufficiently; (3) Too much; (4) They didn't provide me with any information. [20] (1) Yes; (2) No; (3) I don't know/I'm not sure.

3.3. Psychometric Properties

When calculating the scores, we left out 6 items (Q1, Q7, Q21, Q24, Q31, and Q32) because they were considered additional information questions only and could not be measured. Once these items were excluded from the analysis, the Cronbach's alpha for the overall questionnaire remained at 0.86, indicating good internal consistency. When analyzing each domain, only Planned Care (D4) and Urgent Care (D5) had Cronbach's alphas slightly lower than 0.7, although this could be related to the low number of items in each domain. Furthermore, for Planned Care (D4), the Cronbach's alpha value suggested eliminating item Q28, moving internal consistency from 0.35 to 0.58. The internal consistency of each domain and correlations across domains are presented in Table 3. The scores calculated in each domain indicated moderate correlations between Health and Well-being (D1) and Health Day to Day (D2) with the subtraction of the domains. The remaining 4 domains were clearly divided into two blocks: Social Services (D3) with Planned Care (D4), and Urgent Care (D5) with Hospital Care (D6). Social Services (D3) and Planned Care (D4) were poorly correlated with Urgent Care (D5) and with Hospital Care (D6). Table 4 represents the intraclass correlation coefficient (ICC) values for test–retest results. A good temporal stability was observed for the distinct subscales and items, with intraclass correlation coefficients varying from 0.412 to 0.929 ($p < 0.05$).

In total, 9 items were excluded when calculating the scores for different dimensions. Items Q1, Q7, Q21, Q24, Q31, and Q32 were excluded as they were not considered appropriate for a score. The aforementioned questions did not evaluate performance but rather the context or background information. Item Q38 was also excluded due to a low response rate (21.8%) as well as item Q8 since it directly depended on item 7, which was also was excluded due to a low response rate. Finally, "Cronbach's Alpha if item deleted" suggested removing item Q28, raising the score for internal consistency from 0.35 to 0.58. A total of 24 items achieved one or more positive correlations greater than 0.4 with other items in the survey.

Table 3. Intercorrelation and internal consistency.

Dimensions	Dimensions						N	Mean (SD)	Cronbach's Alfa
	D1	D2	D3	D4	D5	D6			
Your level of Health, Welfare and Autonomy (D1)	1						342	62.4 (23.3)	0.73
Monitoring Your Health (D2)	0.528 *	1					334	76.1 (16.6)	0.78
Social Services (D3)	0.312 *	0.056	1				109	59.9 (42.0)	0.83
Treatment Plan (D4)	0.454 *	0.283 *	0.360 *	1			91	74.7 (17.9)	0.58
Emergency Care (D5)	0.360 *	0.462 *	0.108	0.184	1		337	76.5 (23.8)	0.62
Hospital Care (D6)	0.347 *	0.368 *	−0.052	0.088	0.404 *	1	174	67.6 (26.3)	0.77

* Spearman correlation coefficients statistically significant at the 0.05 level. SD: Standard Deviation. Mean (SD)—TOTAL: 71.1 (16.3) Cronbach's Alfa (TOTAL) = 0.86.

Table 4. Test–retest reliability.

Item Number	N	ICC$_{2,1}$	P-Value *
Your level of Health, Welfare, and Autonomy			
Q2	332	0.823	<0.001
Q3	332	0.805	<0.001
Q4	332	0.810	<0.001
Q5	332	0.789	<0.001
Q6	332	0.733	<0.001
Monitoring Your Health			
Q9	330	0.778	<0.001
Q10	330	0.622	<0.001
Q11	332	0.698	<0.001
Q12	332	0.635	<0.001
Q13	332	0.655	<0.001
Q14	332	0.412	<0.001
Q15	332	0.751	<0.001
Q16	332	0.750	<0.001
Q17	332	0.758	<0.001
Q18	332	0.644	<0.001
Q19	331	0.741	<0.001
Q20	332	0.691	<0.001
Social Services			
Q22	97	0.910	<0.001
Q23	97	0.913	<0.001
Treatment Plan			
Q25	68	0.929	<0.001
Q26	68	0.878	<0.001
Q27	131	0.743	<0.001
Emergency Care			
Q29	332	0.763	<0.001
Q30	332	0.616	<0.001
Hospital care			
Q33	153	0.734	<0.001
Q34	153	0.821	<0.001
Q35	153	0.841	<0.001
Q36	153	0.803	<0.001
Q37	151	0.829	<0.001

ICC$_{2,1}$: Intraclass Correlation Coefficient. * A value of $p < 0.05$ indicates the temporal stability between two consecutive evaluations.

4. Discussion

In this study, we translated and validated the "User Reported Measured of Care Coordination" questionnaire into Spanish. This tool aims to capture the perceptions of older people with chronic complex conditions accessing care across organizational and professional boundaries, to identify facilitators and barriers to care coordination activities in our context.

Correlation analysis indicated, on one hand, moderate correlations between Health and Well-being (D1) and Health Day to Day (D2) with other domains and, on the other hand, Social Services (D3) moderately correlated with Planned Care (D4) and Urgent Care (D5) moderately correlated with Hospital Care (D6). However, a high non-response rate was found in 3 specific domains, Social Services (D3), Planned Care (D4) and Hospital Care (D6), as these services had not recently been used by many participants in our study. The non-use of Hospital Care (D6) may be due to the health-related circumstances of each individual but access to Social Services (D3) or Planned Care (D4), considering their specific complexity very much influenced by the characteristics of healthcare and social care systems. Poor access to social services, mostly due to economic issues and system fragmentation, could directly affect the health status of the population [18]. A high percentage of the population are not aware of the existence of care planning [6]. The care plan should be a right of the population so that they can cope better with their chronic complex conditions, and this could be ensured through a formal agreement with our patients [19]. Again, there was a high percentage of missing data when studying the temporal stability in Social Services (D3), Planned Care (D4), and Hospital Care (D6) domains, as described in the original article [16]. According to the results on internal consistency, the "alpha if item deleted" index suggested to remove Q28. Authors finally decided to modify the original scale excluding this item. This was the only difference compared with the original instrument.

This instrument is adapted to our Spanish context following current policies to improve health and social care coordination with a variety of specific strategies across the country. Only a few European countries (e.g., Denmark, Portugal, and Ireland) enjoy a system that integrates social and health care horizontally. In most countries (Austria, Belgium, Spain, Italy, United Kingdom, among others), horizontal fragmentation between the social and health sectors accompanies a vertical division of responsibilities in which three levels of administration (national, regional, and local) with different allocation of power [6,20]. Thus, it is important to develop instruments to measure and improve coordination for each specific context [19]. Access, suitability, and financial sustainability as measurement indicators related to care provision are available in most countries. The quality of care coordination in chronic, complex conditions, however, is a multidimensional phenomenon that is difficult to measure; sometimes, the available data are only numeric measurements, and these do not cover the quality of care from population's point of view. It is, therefore, almost impossible to make comparisons between countries [21].

In terms of the care coordination process, the following factors appear to be important design features. At a personal level, a holistic focus that allows service users and carers to become more functional, independent, and resilient, and to live well by managing conditions in the home environment. At a service level, it is important to encourage multiple referrals to a single-entry point where care coordination can be supported. At a community level, the role of members of the local community should be seen as integral to the caregiving process. At a functional level, effective communication between members of the multidisciplinary team is essential. At an organizational level, effective targeting of service users is required to prioritize care provision. At a system level, integrated health and social care commissioning can support longer-term strategies and provide a greater degree of stability. Therefore, a political narrative that supports person-centered care coordination provides credibility when developing new ways of working [22,23].

Although the need for care coordination is clear, we have seen there are obstacles within most health care systems [24,25]. This must be overcome and has to be considered a priority. Health care systems remain disjointed and processes vary among and between primary care sites and specialty sites [26]. Patients are often unclear about why they are being referred from primary care to a specialist, and what to do after specialist visits. Referral staff deal with many different processes and lost information, which means that care is less efficient.

Addressing patient health from a broader perspective includes addressing the social determinants that influence health outcomes and engaging patients as collaborative partners in their own wellness. Health systems are beginning to recognize this dynamic interplay between an individual's social needs, healthy lifestyles, and behaviors and their corresponding health status [24,25].

Previous strategies gave us some recommendations to improve care coordination strategies: Ensure patient—and family—centeredness by identifying family needs and goals that can be supported by a care coordinator [24]. Ensure open lines of communication with the designated care coordinator [27]. Develop a shared understanding of community services and local supports for patients and families. Support interprofessional team training on implementing and measuring care coordination initiatives [28]. Use tools and measures to assess the added value of care coordination for patients and families, including patient/family experience as an outcome measure [24,29].

Our study has some limitations. The results on internal consistency should be interpreted with caution as assessing the internal consistency required omitting conditional items or self-information items. Finally, we believe it would have been preferable to determine the correlation with another tool specifically validated for measuring population perception of care coordination. However, this was impossible, since no other tool was available in the Spanish language. Moreover, although the sample was selected from the whole of Catalonia, there was a particular health management area that could not perform data collection due to a new, recently implemented research intervention.

5. Conclusions

Successful deployment of care-coordination is a big challenge that should benefit of tools capturing the experiences of patients as they access care organizational and professional boundaries. The adapted version of the "User Reported Measure of Care Coordination" into Spanish proved to be a practical tool for use in our daily practice and an efficient instrument for the evaluation of care coordination in chronic, complex conditions in older people across services and levels of care.

Further research is required to assess the extent to which survey data offer information that providers and purchasers can use to make specific changes to improve the quality of their services.

Author Contributions: Conceptualization, E.R., A.Z., P.A., A.A. (Anna Albero), G.S., A.R., J.M. and N.F.; methodology, E.R., A.Z., N.A.-D., B.K., A.A. (Albert Alonso) and A.A. (Anna Albero); software, N.A.-D. and B.K.; validation, N.A.-D., B.A. and E.R.; formal analysis, N.A.-D., B.K. and E.R.; investigation, E.R., G.S., A.Z., A.A. (Anna Albero), J.M., A.R. and A.A. (Albert Alonso); resources, E.R., G.S., A.A. (Albert Alonso), N.F., A.A. (Anna Albero), N.A.-D., P.A. and B.K.; data curation, N.A.-D., B.K. and E.R.; writing—original draft preparation, E.R., A.Z., B.K., N.A.-D. and G.S.; writing—review and editing, E.R., A.Z., B.K., N.A.-D., A.A. (Albert Alonso), J.M., A.R., N.F., G.S. and A.A. (Anna Albero); visualization, N.A.-D., A.Z., E.R., G.S., N.F., J.M. and B.K.; supervision, E.R., A.Z., P.A., A.A. (Albert Alonso), G.S., A.Z., A.R., J.M. and N.F.; project administration, E.R., G.S., A.Z., J.M. and A.A. (Albert Alonso); funding acquisition, E.R. All authors have read and agreed to the published version of the manuscript.

Funding: This work was funded by the Agència de Qualitat i Avaluació Sanitàries de Catalunya, Departament de Salut, Generalitat de Catalunya and Fundació Infermeria i Societat del Col·legi Oficial d'Infermeres i Infermers de Catalunya.

Conflicts of Interest: The authors declare no conflict of interest.

References

1. Navarro, V. The Social Crisis of the Eurozone: The Case of Spain. *Int. J. Health Serv.* **2013**, *43*, 189–192. [CrossRef] [PubMed]
2. Nolte, E.; Knai, C.; Hofmarcher, M.; Conklin, A.I.; Erler, A.; Elissen, A.; Flamm, M.; Fullerton, B.; Sönnichsen, A.C.; Vrijhoef, H.J. Overcoming fragmentation in health care: Chronic care in Austria, Germany and the Netherlands. *Health Econ. Policy Law* **2012**, *7*, 125–146. [CrossRef]
3. Institute for Healthcare Improvement. Triple Aim: Concept Design. 2009. Available online: http://www.ihi. org/Engage/Initiatives/TripleAim/Documents/ConceptDesign.pdf (accessed on 21 November 2018).
4. The Health Foundation. *Measuring Patient Experiences*; Evidence Scan; The Health Foundation: London, UK, 2013; Available online: http://www.health.org.uk/publication/measuring-patient-experience (accessed on 12 February 2018).
5. Jansen, D.L.; Struckmann, V.; Snoeijs, S. ICARE4EU: Improving care for people with multiple chronic conditions in Europe. *Int. J. Integr. Care* **2014**, *14*. [CrossRef]
6. Billings, J.; Leichsenring, K. Methodological development of the interactive INTERLINKS Framework for Long-term Care. *Int. J. Integr. Care* **2014**, *14*, e021. [CrossRef] [PubMed]
7. Graham, C.; Killpack, C.; Raleigh, V.; Redding, D.; Thorlby, R.; Walsh, J. Options Appraisal on the Measurement of People's Experiences of Integrated Care. Available online: https://www.picker.org/wp-content/uploads/2014/10/Options-appraisal-on...-integrated-care.pdf (accessed on 21 November 2018).
8. Goodwin, N.; Dixon, A.; Anderson, G.; Wodchis, W. Providing Integrated Care for Older People with Complex Needs; The King' Fund. 2014. Available online: https://www.kingsfund.org.uk/sites/files/kf/field/field_publication_file/providing-integrated-care-for-older-people-with-complex-needs-kingsfund-jan14.pdf. (accessed on 21 November 2018).

9. Nuño-Solinis, R.; Fernández-Cano, P.; Mira, J.J.; Polanco, N.T.; Contel, J.C.; Mora, M.G.; Solas, O. Desarrollo de IEMAC, un Instrumento para la Evaluación de Modelos de Atención ante la Cronicidad. *Gaceta Sanitaria* **2013**, *27*, 128–134. [CrossRef] [PubMed]

10. Cano, I.; Dueñas-Espín, I.; Hernández, C.; De Batlle, J.; Benavent, J.; Contel, J.C.; Baltaxe, E.; Escarrabill, J.; Fernández, J.M.; Garcia-Aymerich, J.; et al. Protocol for regional implementation of community-based collaborative management of complex chronic patients. *NPJ Prim. Care Respir. Med.* **2017**, *27*, 44. [CrossRef] [PubMed]

11. Nuño-Solinis, R. Desarrollo e implementación de la Estrategia de Cronicidad del País Vasco: Lecciones aprendidas. *Gaceta Sanitaria* **2016**, *30*, 106–110. [CrossRef]

12. Hernández, C.; Alonso, A.; Garcia-Aymerich, J.; Grimsmo, A.; Vontetsianos, T.; Cuyàs, F.G.; Altes, A.G.; Vogiatzis, I.; Garåsen, H.; Pellisé, L.; et al. Integrated care services: Lessons learned from the deployment of the NEXES project. *Int. J. Integr. Care* **2015**, *15*. [CrossRef]

13. Ledesma, A.; Blay, C.; Contel, J.C.; González-Mestre, A.; Sarquella, E.; Viguera, L.l. L'Atenció Centrada en la Persona en el Model D'Atenció Integrada Social i Sanitària de Catalunya: Barcelona, Spain. 2016. Available online: https://xarxanet.org/sites/default/files/gene_atencio_centrada_en_la_persona_gener_2016.pdf (accessed on 21 November 2018).

14. Guilabert, M.; Amil, P.; González-Mestre, A.; Gil-Sánchez, E.; Vila, A.; Contel, J.C.; Ansotegui, J.C.; Solas, O.; Bacigalupe, M.T.; Fernández-Cano, P.; et al. The Measure of the Family Caregivers' Experience. *Int. J. Environ. Res. Public Health* **2018**, *15*, 2040. [CrossRef]

15. Mira, J.J.; Nuño-Solinis, R.; Guilabert, M.; Solas-Gaspar, O.; Fernández-Cano, P.; González-Mestre, M.A.; Contel, J.C.; Del Río-Cámara, M. Development and Validation of an Instrument for Assessing Patient Experience of Chronic Illness Care. *Int. J. Integr. Care* **2016**, *16*, 2197. [CrossRef]

16. Crump, H.; King, J.; Graham, C.; Thorlby, R.; Raleigh, V.; Redding, D.; Goodwin, N. Developing a User Reported Measure of Care Co-ordination. *Int. J. Integr. Care* **2017**, *17*, 125. [CrossRef] [PubMed]

17. Beaton, D.; Bombardier, C.; Guillemin, F.; Ferraz, M. *Recommendations for the Cross-Cultural Adaptation of the DASH & QuickDASH Outcome Measures*; Institute for Work & Health: Toronto, ON, CA, 2007.

18. Kline, R.B. *Principles and Practice of Structural Equation Modeling*, 3rd ed.; Guilford Press: New York, NY, USA, 2010; p. 422.

19. Barnett, K.; Mercer, S.W.; Norbury, M.; Watt, G.; Wyke, S.; Guthrie, B. Epidemiology of multimorbidity and implications for health care, research, and medical education: A cross-sectional study. *Lancet* **2012**, *380*, 37–43. [CrossRef]

20. Rijken, M.P.; Lette, M.; Baan, C.; De Bruin, S.R. Assigning a Prominent Role to "The Patient Experience" in Assessing the Quality of Integrated Care for Populations with Multiple Chronic Conditions. *Int. J. Integr. Care* **2019**, *19*, 19. [CrossRef]

21. Elwyn, G.; Thompson, R.; John, R.; Grande, S.W. Developing IntegRATE: A fast and frugal patient-reported measure of integration in health care delivery. *Int. J. Integr. Care* **2015**, *15*. [CrossRef] [PubMed]

22. Bogerd, M.; Slottje, P.; Schellevis, F.G.; Giebels, A.; Rijken, M.; Van Hout, H.P.; Reinders, M.E. From protocolized to person-centered chronic care in general practice: Study protocol of an action-based research project (COPILOT). *Prim. Health Care Res. Dev.* **2019**, *20*, e134. [CrossRef] [PubMed]

23. Berntsen, G.K.R.; Strisland, F.; Malm-Nicolaisen, K.; Smaradottir, B.F.; Fensli, R.; Røhne, M.; Hernández-Quiles, C.; Valckenaers, P. The Evidence Base for an Ideal Care Pathway for Frail Multimorbid Elderly: Combined Scoping and Systematic Intervention Review. *J. Med. Internet Res.* **2019**, *21*, e12517. [CrossRef]

24. Lloyd, H.; Wheat, H.; Horrell, J.; Sugavanam, T.; Fosh, B.; Valderas, J.M.; Close, J.; Billings, J.; Benetoli, A. Patient-Reported Measures for Person-Centered Coordinated Care: A Comparative Domain Map and Web-Based Compendium for Supporting Policy Development and Implementation. *J. Med. Internet Res.* **2018**, *20*, e54. [CrossRef]

25. Kean, T. Evaluation of care coordination among healthy community-dwelling older adults finds promising but minimal impact. *Évid. Based Nurs.* **2019**, *23*, 90. [CrossRef]

26. Vimalananda, V.G.; Fincke, B.G.; Qian, S.; Waring, M.E.; Seibert, R.G.; Meterko, M. Development and psychometric assessment of a novel survey to measure care coordination from the specialist's perspective. *Health Serv. Res.* **2019**, *54*, 689–699. [CrossRef]

27. Mph, V.R.; Seltzer, A.; Xiong, L.; Morse, L.; Lindquist, L.A. Use of Electronic Health Records by Older Adults, 85 Years and Older, and Their Caregivers. *J. Am. Geriatr. Soc.* **2020**, *68*, 1078–1082.

28. Berning, M.J.; E Silva, L.O.J.; Suarez, N.E.; Walker, L.E.; Erwin, P.; Carpenter, C.R.; Bellolio, M.F. Interventions to improve older adults' Emergency Department patient experience: A systematic review. *Am. J. Emerg. Med.* **2020**, *38*, 1257–1269. [CrossRef] [PubMed]

29. Pathak, N.; Tomolo, A.; Escoffery, C. Improving Team-Based Care Coordination Delivery and Documentation in the Health Record. *Fed. Pract.* **2018**, *35*, 32–39. [PubMed]

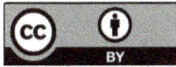

International Journal of
Environmental Research and Public Health

MDPI

Article

Sex Differences in Frail Older Adults with Foot Pain in a Spanish Population: An Observational Study

Emmanuel Navarro-Flores [1], Carlos Romero-Morales [2,*],

Ricardo Becerro de Bengoa-Vallejo [3], David Rodríguez-Sanz [3], Patricia Palomo-López [4],

Daniel López-López [5], Marta Elena Losa-Iglesias [6] and César Calvo-Lobo [3]

[1] Frailty Research Organizaded Group (FROG), Department of Nursing, Faculty of Nursing and Podiatry, University of Valencia, 46010 Valencia, Spain; emmanuel.navarro@uv.es
[2] Faculty of Sport Sciences, Universidad Europea de Madrid, 28670 Madrid, Spain
[3] Facultad de Enfermería, Fisioterapia y Podología, Universidad Complutense de Madrid, 28040 Madrid, Spain; ribebeva@ucm.es (R.B.d.B.-V.); davidrodriguezsanz@ucm.es (D.R.-S.); cescalvo@ucm.es (C.C.-L.)
[4] University Center of Plasencia, University of Extremadura, 06006 Badajoz, Spain; patibiom@unex.es
[5] Research, Health and Podiatry Group, Department of Health Sciences, Faculty of Nursing and Podiatry, Universidade da Coruña, 15403 Ferrol, Spain; daniellopez@udc.es
[6] Faculty of Health Sciences, Universidad Rey Juan Carlos, 28933 Madrid, Spain; marta.losa@urjc.es
*   Correspondence: carlos.romero@universidadeuropea.es

Received: 28 July 2020; Accepted: 19 August 2020; Published: 24 August 2020

check for updates

Abstract: Frailty is a condition that can increase the risk of falls. In addition, foot pain can influence older adults and affect their frail condition. The main objective was to measure the frailty degree in older adults in a Spanish population with foot pain from moderate to severe. Method: This is a cross-sectional descriptive study. A sample of people older than 60 years ($n = 52$), including 26 males and 26 females, were recruited, and frailty disability was measured using the 5-Frailty scale and the Edmonton Frailty scale (EFS). Results: Spearman's correlation coefficients were categorized as weak ($rs \leq 0.40$), moderate ($0.41 \leq rs \geq 0.69$), or strong ($0.70 \leq rs \geq 1.00$). There was a statistically significant correlation for the total score ($p < 0.001$) and most of the subscales of the 5-Frailty scale compared with the EFS, except for Mood ($p > 0.05$). In addition, females and males showed similar 5-Frailty and Edmonton Frail scales scores with no difference ($p > 0.05$). Conclusion: Foot pain above 5 points, i.e., from moderate to severe, does not affect the fragility more in one sex than another.

Keywords: frailty; older adults; foot deformities; foot diseases; foot pain

1. Introduction

Aging and chronical illness processes, like hyperglycemic disease, as well as muscle skeletal and heart processes can produce frailty syndrome, and as a consequence of this, be degenerative and exhibit some alterations that can affect one's mental and general health [1]. For example, aging and frailty can affect gait speed and increase fall risk due to balance alterations [2–4]. Furthermore, the presence of frailty symptoms affects the health-related quality of life (HQoL) [5] in this population group.

We can define frailty syndrome as a group of health alterations that can affect several aspects, such as the psychological, biological and social aspects, as it is a consequence of a dynamic process that reduces a person's health status [6]. Regarding foot conditions in older adult populations, foot disorders and diseases are present most frequently in the frailty population group, comprising approximately 25% [7,8].

The frequency of a frail state in people older than 65 years has been estimated between 4 and 59.1% [9].

Consultations at general practitioners related to ankle and foot conditions of osteoarticular pain origin account for more than 8% [10]. Accordingly, suffering may raise this predominance in older adults who have characteristic foot requirements that can be akin to bigger disorders [11], foot health-related quality of life (HQoL) [12], and risk of falls [13,14]

The 5-Frailty scale is a questionnaire of 5 items, which was established using an auto-administered dimension [6]. Respondents can provide affirmative or negative answers, with one punctuation to the positive response. For measuring the degree of frailty, respondents can score between zero and five points, and subjects are qualified as robust (zero point), pre-frail (one to two points), or frail (three points). The level represents their respective tiredness, resistance, ambulation, disease, and loss of weight.

Tiredness is evaluated by asking subjects if they felt tired; resistance was determined by each subject's report on their capacity to climb stairs; ambulation is represented by each subject's information on their ability to move around; illness is determined by the presence of more than five of a total of eleven pathologies, including cardiovascular diseases, diabetes, and loss of weight by a reduction of five percent during the last year [15].

The Edmonton Frailty scale (EFS) assesses nine subscales: (1) cognitive, (2) general health status, (3) independence, (4) social support, (5) pharmacologic treatment, (6) feeding, (7) mood, (8) continence, and (9) functional performance, using eleven questions. The maximum score is 17 and represents the highest degree of frailty [16]. In this case, a frailty score between zero and four does not present frailty, scores of five to six represent apparently vulnerable, scores of seven to eight represent fair frailty, scores of nine to ten represent frailty moderate, and scores of eleven or more represent severe frailty [17].

No study has yet correlated the scores of the EFS and the 5-Frailty scale. Therefore, the goal of this research was to correlate the subscales of the EFS and 5-Frailty scale in older adults and those with related foot pain.

In the literature, no references have been found regarding the frailty of older adults with foot pain related to sex, and therefore our hypothesis is that there are differences in the levels of frailty in older adults with foot pain related to sex. The objective of this study is to determine if sex can influence a greater degree of frailty.

2. Materials and Methods

The study was developed in Spain. We recruited older adult patients in a medical center, a rehabilitation service, and podiatry clinics in the Generalitat of Valencia, and all survey data were collected between September 2019 and January 2020. Researchers obtained signed informed consent from all subjects, and observational research was carried out using STROBE [18].

Considering sex distribution as the independent variable to calculate the sample size, G* Power 3.1.9.2 software (Heinrich-Heine-Universität Düsseldorf; Düsseldorf, Germany) was used after considering testing the sex differences between two independent means about sex, comparing their frailty scores. A two-tailed hypothesis, a large effect size of 0.8, an error of $\alpha = 0.05$ with a 95% confidence interval, an error $\beta = 20\%$, and a power analysis of $1 - \beta = 0.80$ were considered. Consequently, a total sample size of 52 subjects with 26 in each group was included in this study.

Prior to beginning the research, approval for conducting this study was obtained from the Ethics Committee of the University of Extremadura, 1/2020.

Informed consent was obtained from each participant after the purpose and process of the study were explained and the privacy of the participants' information was assured. The fact that their participation was entirely voluntary was also highlighted.

The inclusion criteria comprised adult patients older than 60 years who presented foot pain during the last 6 months due to toe or foot deformities, regardless of its origin or cause; higher than five points in the VAS score, excluding wounds; and able to communicate orally and provide written informed consent. VAS scores above five points, i.e., from moderate to severe, showed an intraclass correlation coefficient reliability of 0.870 [19].

130

The exclusion criteria were major neurocognitive disorder; patients who did not answer initial identification questions or who did not understand the rules of participation; and those who refused to participate in the research, i.e., no signed consent.

To recruit volunteer participants, we posted recruitment flyers in senior centers' gathering places. We also addressed groups of older adults in the center to invite them to contact us if they were willing to participate in the study. Once a potential participant expressed interest, a cognitive function evaluation was performed by a gerontological nurse practitioner (GNP) to establish the cognitive eligibility of the participant. Following evaluation by the GNP, the investigators explained the study procedures in detail to the participants.

The interview was composed of general questions of general health status, socio demographic characteristics (sex, age, BMI, height, and weight), comorbidities (e.g., anxiety, depression, diabetes, obesity, osteoarticular diseases, vascular disorders, and kidney illness) collected from medical records. Furthermore, specific items related to foot pain, such as the actual treatment or foot deformities, were assessed by a senior podiatry physician (ENF).

In this study, a total of 65 older adults expressed interest in study participation, and all met the cognitive requirements. The participants all attempted to complete the survey questionnaires. Ultimately all surveys were analyzed for the study; 14 surveys were excluded due to incomplete answers. For participants who were not able to read the questionnaires due to vision problems, the investigators read the questions aloud and marked the participants' answers on the questionnaires. Participants took about 15 min to complete the questionnaires. Participants did not get any compensation for their participation in the study.

2.1. Evaluation of Frailty

The EFS was designed to measure frailty in nine subscales: cognitive, general health status, independence, social support, pharmacologic treatment, feeding, mood, continence, and functional performance [16,20]. Total scores range from 0 to 17, and higher scores indicate more frailty, ranging from 1 = not frail; 2 = ostensibly susceptible frail; 3 = almost never; to 4 = almost always. The EFS ranged by 3 degrees. The Cronbach's α for the EFS was 0.93 [21].

First, a strong frailty mark and subjects without frailty were classified using the EFS. Subjects who scored less than five points were designated as not frail. Secondly, ostensibly susceptible frail subjects were designated as those who obtained six to eleven points. The third group included those who scored between twelve and seventeen points. The questionnaire administration required only 15 min to complete.

Participants also completed the 5-item Frailty scale [22], which has been previously validated into Spanish with an ICC = 0.82 [6,23]. This scale measured five subscales: tiredness, resistance, go around, disease, and loss of weight. Frailty scores ranged from 0 to 5, and higher scores indicate more frailty. Those participants that scored between three and five were considered frail, those that scored one or two were considered to be pre-frail, and those that obtained zero points were considered to be not frail.

The authors obtained permission from the original authors of the EFS and 5-Frailty scale to use their clinimetric tool to measure the frailty degree.

2.2. Statistical Analysis

All the variables were normally distributed, as determined by the Kolmogorov–Smirnov test ($p > 0.05$).

Regarding the results of the quantitative variables, the non-parametric data were described in terms of their median, interquartile range (IR), and minimum and maximum (range) values. Parametric data were described using means, the standard deviation (SD), and minimum and maximum (range) values.

A comparison of the quantitative data between males and females for the different questionnaire subscales of the EFS and 5-Frail scale was conducted, and significant differences were checked using an independent Student's *t*-test. Non-normal data were analyzed using Mann–Whitney U tests.

Spearman's correlation coefficients (rs) were determined between tests and qualified as low rs $\leq$ 0.40, moderate 0.41 $\leq$ rs $\geq$ 0.69, or solid 0.70 $\leq$ rs $\geq$1.00.

All analyses were considered statistically significant when the *p*-value < 0.05 with a 95% confidence interval (CI). Statistical analyses were made in SPSS (V.26.0, Chicago, IL, USA).

3. Results

3.1. Descriptive Data and Socio-Demographic Data

A normal distribution for age, height, weight, and BMI was shown ($p > 0.05$), and all items from the 5-Frailty test and the EFS showed no normal distribution ($p < 0.05$).

The size sample included 52 subjects whose mean age was 77.47 $\pm$ 10.69 years. The study subjects included 26 (50.00%) females and 26 (50.00%) males. Table 1 shows the socio-demographic characteristics. Males and females did not show statistically significant socio-demographic differences ($p > 0.05$) for age or BMI, although a higher weight and height ($p < 0.05$) were shown for males compared with females. There was no difference in the intensity of pain between sexes ($p = 0.561$).

Table 1. Descriptive and socio-demographic data of the sample.

Demographic and Descriptive Data	Total Group n = 52 Mean ± SD (Range)	Female n = 26 Mean ± SD (Range)	Male n = 26 Mean ± SD (Range)	*p* Value
Age (Years)	77.47 ± 10.69 (74.54–80.40)	79.07 ± 10.74 (75.16–82.98)	75.36 ± 10.50 (70.98–79.75)	0.224
Weight (kg)	62.47 ± 12.08 (59.16–65.78)	58.31 ± 12.44 (53.78–62.84)	67.95 ± 9.25 (64.09–71.82)	0.004
Height (m)	1.61 ± 0.08 (74.54–80.40)	1.57 ± 0.07 (1.54–1.59)	1.65 ± 0.07 (1.62–1.68)	0.000
BMI (Kg/m^2)	24.19 ± 3.96 (23.10–25.27)	23.67 ± 4.30 (22.10–25.24)	24.87 ± 3.42 (23.45–26.30)	0.286
Foot Pain	7.18 ± 3.38 (23.10–25.27)	7.28 ± 1.36 (5.00–10.00)	7.05 ± 1.43 · (5.00–10.00)	0.561

BMI: body mass index; Mean-standard deviation, range (min–max), and Student's *t*-test for independent samples were applied. In all the analyses, $p < 0.05$ (with a 95% confidence interval) was considered statistically significant.

3.2. Edmonton Frail Scale and 5-Frailty Scale Sex Distribution

As shown in Table 2, the 5-Frailty scale scores did not manifest any statistically significant difference ($p > 0.05$) for the subscales nor for the total scores between females and males with foot pain. Furthermore, the EFS scores by sex distribution are shown in Table 3, whose subscales did not show statistically significant differences ($p > 0.05$). The results of both test show that frailty in males and females with foot pain is similar.

Table 2. Comparisons of the 5-Frailty scale scores between males and females.

Frailty Scale Domains	Total Group n = 52 Mean ± SD (Range) Median (IR)	Female n =26 Mean ± SD (Range) Median (IR)	Male n = 26 Mean ± SD (Range) Median (IR)	p Value
Fatigue	0.54 ± 0.50 (0.41–0.68) 1.00 (1.00)	0.55 ± 0.35 (0.35–0.74) 1.00 (1.00)	0.54 ± 0.50 (0.31–0.77) 1.00 (1.00)	0.965
Resistance	0.47 ± 0.50 (0.33–0.60) 0.00 (1.00)	0.51 ± 0.50 (0.32–0.71) 1.00 (1.00)	0.40 ± 0.50 (0.18–0.63) 0.00 (1.00)	0.448
Ambulation	0.47 ± 0.50 (0.30–0.59) 0.00 (1.00)	0.44 ± 0.50 (0.25–0.64) 0.00 (1.00)	0.45 ± 0.50 (0.22–0.68 0.00 (1.00)	0.965
Illness	0.43 ± 0.50 (0.29–0.57) 0.00 (1.00)	0.44 ± 0.50 (0.25–0.64) 0.00 (1.00)	0.40 ± 0.50 (0.18–0.63) 0.00 (1.00)	0.782
Loss of weight	0.54 ± 0.50 (0.41–0.69) 1.00 (1.00)	0.51 ± 0.50 (0.32–0.71) 1.00 (1.00)	0.59 ± 0.50 (0.36–0.81) 1.00 (1.00)	0.604
TOTAL Frailty Scale	2.49 ± 1.50 (2.08–2.91) 3.00 (3.00)	2.51 ± 1.45 (1.96–3.07) 3.00 (2.00)	2.45 ± 1.59 (1.74–3.16) 2.50 (3.00)	0.892

CI, Confidence Interval; IR: interquartile range. Mann–Whitney U tests were used. In all the analyses, $p < 0.05$ (with a 95% confidence interval) was considered statistically significant.

Table 3. Comparisons of the Edmonton Frail Scale scores between males and females.

Edmonton Frail Scale Domains	Total Group n = 52 Mean ± SD (95%CI) Median (IR)	Female n = 26 Mean ± SD (95%CI) Median (IR)	Male n = 26 Mean ± SD (95%CI) Median (IR)	p Value
Cognition	0.78 ± 0.64 (0.60–0.96) 1.00 (1.00)	0.79 ± 0.61 (0.55–1.02) 1.00 (1.00)	0.77 ± 0.68 (0.46–1.07) 1.00 (1.00)	0.865
General health status 2A	0.66 ± 0.52 (0.49–0.84) 1.00 (1.00)	0.65 ± 0.61 (0.42–0.88) 1.00 (1.00)	0.68 ± 0.64 (0.39–0.96) 1.00 (1.00)	0.907
General health status 2B	0.82 ± 0.88 (0.57–1.97) 1.00 (1.00)	0.79 ± 0.86 (0.46–1.12) 1.00 (1.00)	0.86 ± 0.94 (0.44–1.28 1.00 (1.00)	0.845
Functional independence	0.60 ± 0.85 (0.36–0.84) 1.00 (1.00)	0.58 ± 0.82 (0.27–0.89) 0.00 (1.00)	0.53 ± 0.90 (0.23–1.03) 0.00 (1.00)	0.923
Social support	0.49 ± 0.57 (0.32–0.65) 0.00 (1.00)	0.51 ± 0.57 (0.29–0.73) 0.00 (1.00)	0.45 ± 0.59 (0.19–0.71) 0.00 (1.00)	0.648
Medication use 5A	0.60 ± 0.49 (0.46–0.74) 1.00 (1.00)	0.58 ± 0.50 (0.39–0.77) 1.00 (1.00)	0.53 ± 0.49 (0.41–0.85) 1.00 (1.00)	0.719
Medication use 5 B	0.54 ± 0.50 (0.41–0.69) 1.00 (1.00)	0.58 ± 0.50 (0.32–0.71) 1.00 (1.00)	0.50 ± 0.51 (0.27–0.72) 0.50 (1.00)	0.544
Nutrition	0.66 ± 0.47 (0.53–0.80) 1.00 (1.00)	0.65 ± 0.49 (0.47–0.83) 1.00 (1.00)	0.68 ± 0.47 (0.47–0.89) 1.00 (1.00)	0.843
Mood	0.54 ± 0.50 (0.4–0.69) 1.00 (1.00)	0.62 ± 0.49 (0.43–0.80) 1.00 (1.00)	0.45 ± 0.50 (0.22–0.68) 0.00 (1.00)	0.242
Continence	0.39 ± 0.49 (0.25–0.53) 0.00 (1.00)	0.44 ± 0.50 (0.25–0.64) 0.00 (1.00)	0.31 ± 0.47 (0.10–0.52) 0.00 (1.00)	0.351
Functional performance	1.05 ± 0.64 (0.87–1.24) 1.00 (0.00)	1.13 ± 0.58 (0.91–1.35) 1.00 (0.50	0.95 ± 0.72 (0.53–1.27) 1.00 (1.25)	0.332
Total Edmonton Frail Scale	6.969 ± 4.57 (5.67–8.24) 6.00 (7.00)	7.27 ± 4.30 (5.63–8.91) 7.00 (6.00)	6.54 ± 4.97 (4.34–8.75) 5.50 (6.50)	0.457

CI, Confidence Interval; IR: interquartile range. Mann–Whitney U tests were used. In all the analyses, $p < 0.05$ (with a 95% confidence interval) was considered statistically significant.

Table 4 shows a good correlation between items of both tests, except for the subscale nutrition ($p = 0.490$).

Table 4. Spearman's correlations between the 5-Frailty scale and Edmonton Frail Scale score domains and totals.

Edmonton Frail Scale Domains	Fatigue r (p)	Resistance r (p)	Ambulation r (p)	Illness r (p)	Loss of Weight r (p)	TOTAL Frailty Scale r (p)
Cognition	0.428 (<0.001)	0.369 (0.002)	0.513 (<0.001)	0.386 (00.001)	0.498 (<0.001)	0.773 (<0.001)
General health status 2A	0.232 (0.059)	0.174 (0.160)	0.608 (<0.001)	0.576 (<0.001)	0.623 (<0.001)	0.750 (<0.001)
General health status 2B	0.269 (0.028)	0.194 (0.116)	0.641 (<0.001)	0.562 (<0.001)	0.624 (<0.001)	0.780 (<0.001)
Functional independence	0.295 (0.015)	0.131 (0.290)	0.497 (<0.001)	0.276 (0.024)	0.383 (00.001)	0.481 (<0.001)
Social support	0.259 (0.034)	0.107 (0.390)	0.521 (<0.001)	0.334 (0.006)	0.409 (0.001)	0.510 (<0.001)
Medication use 5A	0.401 (0.401)	0.115 (0.352)	0.627 (00.401)	0.006 (<0.001)	0.417 (<0.001)	0.683 (<0.001)
Medication use 5 B	0.069 (0.579)	0.152 (0.220)	0.579 (00.579)	0.621 (<0.001)	0.379 (0.002)	0.620 (<0.001)
Nutrition	−0.097 (0.438)	−0.080 (0.518)	0.282 (0.021)	0.326 (0.007)	0.299 (0.014)	0.324 (<0.001)
Mood	0.066 (0.594)	0.075 (0.548)	0.111 (0.369)	−0.158 (0.201)	0.067 (0.590)	0.066 (0.490)
Continence	0.078 (0.529)	0.302 (0.013)	0.571 (<0.001)	0.452 (<0.001)	0.469 (<0.001)	0.575 (<0.001)
Functional performance	0.492 (<0.001)	0.434 (<00.001)	0.076 (0.542)	−0.136 (0.271)	0.149 (0.228)	0.446 (<0.001)
Total Edmonton Frail Scale	0.329 (0.006)	0.276 (0.024)	0.624 (<0.001)	0.443 (<0.001)	0.582 (<0.001)	0.842 (<0.001)

Spearman correlation coefficients (r) and *p*-values were applied. In all the analyses, *p* < 0.05 (with a 95% confidence interval) was considered statistically significant.

4. Discussion

This investigation aimed to compare the frailty degree differences between males and females with foot pain from moderate to severe using the 5-Frailty Scale and EFS. Indeed, frailty did not show statistically significant differences between the sexes. Although the total frailty score Spearman correlation was significant in Table 4, it is worthy to note that the correlation was modest, even when comparing domains, which were expected to correlate with functional independence and performance from the EFS and with resistance and ambulation from the 5-Frailty scale.

Both scales are correlated, which confers concurrent validity of each subscale to recent studies and sustains the application of the 5-Frailty score as an acceptable measurement related to frailty aspects such as ambulation, illness, or loss of weight. This aspect can be considered as an advantage with respect to other frailty scales adapted to Spanish to evaluate specific frailty aspects, like the Frailty Trait Scale (FTS) [24].

Moreover, the results from this study are different from those obtained by other researchers in functional performance related to foot pain [25,26]. Our results did not show statistically significant differences related to foot pain [5,8]. These findings are different, with similar research reported on subjects with foot pain [1], as well as with foot pain [27] as measured by employing the visual analogic scale (VAS) to determine the sex differences in healthy subjects with foot problems.

There was a statistically significant correlation in the total score and most of the subscales of the 5-Frailty scale compared with the EFS, except for Mood (*p* > 0.05).

Furthermore, prior studies have identified females who suffered from fibromyalgia and had developed foot problems as a consequence had an increased frailty degree [28].

Future studies should incorporate all other foot risk factors related with frailty syndrome. Despite the fact that the EFS has determined the frailty score [29,30].

Several limitations of this research should be taken into account. A population from different territories may be useful to ameliorate the strength of this research.

This research has only determined if foot pain can influence a greater degree of frailty by sex and we found that foot pain does not affect the frailty by sex.

Although ambulation and functional performance and risk of fall are very common in frail people [2,4], this research should also be developed for other population groups to determine the degree of frailty, for example, in widows who usually have higher frailty scores due to psychosocial aspects [29,31,32].

Furthermore, selective sampling can cause bias; for this reason, randomized sampling should be considered in future studies.

Ultimately, the correlation impact between the different foot disorders, including several genetics and acquired or traumatic alterations and chronic illness, was not studied in our research because the studied population was not suitably adjusted to develop these comparisons. The researchers therefore suggest that future research should be conducted considering different foot pathologies.

5. Conclusions

Foot pain above 5 points, i.e., from moderate to severe, does not affect the fragility more in one sex than another. Further research is needed considering different foot pathologies.

Author Contributions: Conceptualization, E.N.-F., P.P.-L., D.R.-S., R.B.d.B.-V., M.E.L.-I., C.C.-L. and D.L.-L.; methodology, E.N.-F., P.P.-L., C.R.-M., C.C.-L. and D.L.-L.; software, R.B.d.B.-V. and C.C.-L.; formal analysis, R.B.d.B.-V. and C.C.-L.; investigation, E.N.-F., P.P.-L., C.R.-M., D.R.-S. and D.L.-L.; resources, E.N.-F., P.P.-L., C.R-M., C.C.-L. and D.L.-L.; data curation, C.C.-L.; writing—original draft preparation, E.N.-F., P.P.-L., C.R.-M., C.C.-L. and D.L.-L.; writing—review and editing, E.N.-F., P.P.-L., E.N.-F., C.C.-L. and D.L.-L.; supervision, R.B.d.B.-V., M.E.L.-I., D.R.-S., C.C.-L. and D.L.-L. All authors have read and agreed to the published version of the manuscript.

Funding: This research received no external funding

Conflicts of Interest: The authors declare no conflict of interest.

References

1. López-López, D.; Becerro-de-Bengoa-Vallejo, R.; Losa-Iglesias, M.E.; Palomo-López, P.; Rodríguez-Sanz, D.; Brandariz-Pereira, J.M.; Calvo-Lobo, C. Evaluation of foot health related quality of life in individuals with foot problems by gender: A cross-sectional comparative analysis study. *BMJ Open* **2018**, *8*, e023980. [CrossRef]
2. Kamiya, K.; Hamazaki, N.; Matsue, Y.; Mezzani, A.; Corrà, U.; Matsuzawa, R.; Nozaki, K.; Tanaka, S.; Maekawa, E.; Noda, C.; et al. Gait speed has comparable prognostic capability to six-minute walk distance in older patients with cardiovascular disease. *Eur. J. Prev. Cardiol.* **2018**, *25*, 212–219. [CrossRef] [PubMed]
3. Bernhard, F.P.; Sartor, J.; Bettecken, K.; Hobert, M.A.; Arnold, C.; Weber, Y.G.; Poli, S.; Margraf, N.G.; Schlenstedt, C.; Hansen, C.; et al. Wearables for gait and balance assessment in the neurological—study design and first results of a prospective cross-sectional feasibility study with 384 inpatients. *BMC Neurol.* **2018**, *18*, 114. [CrossRef] [PubMed]
4. Thiede, R.; Toosizadeh, N.; Mills, J.L.; Zaky, M.; Mohler, J.; Najafi, B. Gait and balance assessments as early indicators of frailty in patients with known peripheral artery disease. *Clin. Biomech. (Bristol, Avon)* **2016**, *32*, 1–7. [CrossRef]
5. Navarro-Flores, E.; Pérez-Ros, P.; FM, M.-A.; Julían-Rochina, I.; Cauli, O. Neuro-psychiatric alterations in patients with diabetic foot syndrome. *CNS Neurol. Disord. Drug Targets* **2019**, *18*. [CrossRef]
6. Faller, J.W.; do Nascimento Pereira, D.; de Souza, S.; Nampo, F.K.; de Souza Orlandi, F.; Matumoto, S. Instruments for the detection of frailty syndrome in older adults: A systematic review. *PLoS ONE* **2019**, *14*, e0216166. [CrossRef]
7. Hawke, F.; Burns, J. Understanding the nature and mechanism of foot pain. *J. Foot Ankle Res.* **2009**, *2*, 1. [CrossRef]

8. Rodríguez-Sanz, D.; Tovaruela-Carrión, N.; López-López, D.; Palomo-López, P.; Romero-Morales, C.; Navarro-Flores, E.; Calvo-Lobo, C. Foot disorders in the elderly: A mini-review. *Disease-a-Month* **2018**, *64*, 64–91. [CrossRef]

9. Collard, R.M.; Boter, H.; Schoevers, R.A.; Oude Voshaar, R.C. Prevalence of frailty in community-dwelling older persons: A systematic review. *J. Am. Geriatr. Soc.* **2012**, *60*, 1487–1492. [CrossRef]

10. Menz, H.B.; Jordan, K.P.; Roddy, E.; Croft, P.R. Characteristics of primary care consultations for musculoskeletal foot and ankle problems in the UK. *Rheumatology (Oxford)* **2010**, *49*, 1391–1398. [CrossRef]

11. Benvenuti, F.; Ferrucci, L.; Guralnik, J.M.; Gangemi, S.; Baroni, A. Foot pain and disability in older persons: An epidemiologic survey. *J. Am. Geriatr. Soc.* **1995**, *43*, 479–484. [CrossRef]

12. Navarro-Flores, E.; Losa-Iglesias, M.E.; Becerro-de-Bengoa-Vallejo, R.; Lopez-Lopez, D.; Vilar-Fernandez, J.M.; Palomo-Lopez, P.; Calvo-Lobo, C. Transcultural Adaptation and Validation of the Spanish Bristol Foot Score (BFS-S). *Aging Dis.* **2018**, *9*, 861. [CrossRef]

13. Mickle, K.J.; Munro, B.J.; Lord, S.R.; Menz, H.B.; Steele, J.R. Cross-sectional analysis of foot function, functional ability, and health-related quality of life in older people with disabling foot pain. *Arthritis Care Res. (Hoboken)* **2011**, *63*, 1592–1598. [CrossRef]

14. Kaoulla, P.; Frescos, N.; Menz, H.B. A survey of foot problems in community-dwelling older Greek Australians. *J. Foot Ankle Res.* **2011**, *4*, 23. [CrossRef]

15. Aprahamian, I.; Cezar, N.O. de C.; Izbicki, R.; Lin, S.M.; Paulo, D.L.V.; Fattori, A.; Biella, M.M.; Jacob Filho, W.; Yassuda, M.S. Screening for Frailty With the FRAIL Scale: A Comparison With the Phenotype Criteria. *J. Am. Med. Dir. Assoc.* **2017**, *18*, 592–596. [CrossRef]

16. Rolfson, D.B.; Majumdar, S.R.; Tsuyuki, R.T.; Tahir, A.; Rockwood, K. Validity and reliability of the Edmonton Frail Scale. *Age Ageing* **2006**, *35*, 526–529. [CrossRef]

17. Aygör, H.E.; Fadıloğlu, Ç.; Şahin, S.; Aykar, F.Ş.; Akçiçek, F. VALIDATION OF EDMONTON FRAIL SCALE INTO ELDERLY TURKISH POPULATION. *Arch. Gerontol. Geriatr.* **2018**, *76*, 133–137. [CrossRef]

18. Vandenbroucke, J.P.; von Elm, E.; Altman, D.G.; Gøtzsche, P.C.; Mulrow, C.D.; Pocock, S.J.; Poole, C.; Schlesselman, J.J.; Egger, M. STROBE Initiative Strengthening the Reporting of Observational Studies in Epidemiology (STROBE): Explanation and elaboration. *Int. J. Surg.* **2014**, *12*, 1500–1524. [CrossRef]

19. Bijur, P.E.; Silver, W.; Gallagher, E.J. Reliability of the visual analog scale for measurement of acute pain. *Acad. Emerg. Med. Off. J. Soc. Acad. Emerg. Med.* **2001**, *8*, 1153–1157. [CrossRef]

20. Perna, S.; Francis, M.D.A.; Bologna, C.; Moncaglieri, F.; Riva, A.; Morazzoni, P.; Allegrini, P.; Isu, A.; Vigo, B.; Guerriero, F.; et al. Performance of Edmonton Frail Scale on frailty assessment: Its association with multi-dimensional geriatric conditions assessed with specific screening tools. *BMC Geriatr.* **2017**, *17*, 1–8. [CrossRef]

21. Ramírez Ramírez, J.U.; Cadena Sanabria, M.O.; Ochoa, M.E. Aplicación de la Escala de fragilidad de Edmonton en población colombiana. Comparación con los criterios de Fried. *Rev. Esp. Geriatr. Gerontol.* **2017**, *52*, 322–325. [CrossRef] [PubMed]

22. Woo, J.; Yu, R.; Wong, M.; Yeung, F.; Wong, M.; Lum, C. Frailty screening in the community using the FRAIL scale. *J. Am. Med. Dir. Assoc.* **2015**, *16*, 412–419. [CrossRef] [PubMed]

23. Rosas-Carrasco, O.; Cruz-Arenas, E.; Parra-Rodríguez, L.; García-González, A.I.; Contreras-González, L.H.; Szlejf, C. Cross-Cultural Adaptation and Validation of the FRAIL Scale to Assess Frailty in Mexican Adults. *J. Am. Med. Dir. Assoc.* **2016**, *17*, 1094–1098. [CrossRef] [PubMed]

24. Pijpers, E.; Ferreira, I.; Stehouwer, C.D.A.; Nieuwenhuijzen Kruseman, A.C. The frailty dilemma. Review of the predictive accuracy of major frailty scores. *Eur. J. Intern. Med.* **2012**, *23*, 118–123. [CrossRef] [PubMed]

25. Martinez-Amat, A.; Hita-Contreras, F.; Lomas-Vega, R.; Caballero Martinez, I.; Alvarez, P.J.; Martínez-Lopez, E. Effects of 12-week proprioception training program on postural stability, gait, and balance in older adults: A controlled clinical trial. *J. Strength Cond. Res.* **2013**, *27*, 2180–2188. [CrossRef] [PubMed]

26. Pérez-Ros, P.; Vila-Candel, R.; Martínez-Arnau, F.M. A home-based exercise program focused on proprioception to reduce falls in frail and pre-frail community-dwelling older adults. *Geriatr. Nurs. (Minneap)* **2020**. [CrossRef]

27. Navarro-Flores, E.; Losa-Iglesias, M.; Becerro-de-Bengoa-Vallejo, R.; López-López, D.; Rodríguez-Sanz, D.; Palomo-López, P.; Calvo-Lobo, C. Translation and Test–Retest of the Spanish Podiatry Health Questionnaire (PHQ-S). *Int. J. Environ. Res. Public Health* **2018**, *15*, 2205. [CrossRef]

28. Palomo-López, P.; Calvo-Lobo, C.; Becerro-de-Bengoa-Vallejo, R.; Losa-Iglesias, M.E.; Rodriguez-Sanz, D.; Sánchez-Gómez, R.; López-López, D. Quality of life related to foot health status in women with fibromyalgia: A case-control study. *Arch. Med. Sci.* **2019**, *15*, 694–699. [CrossRef]

29. Fabrício-Wehbe, S.C.C.; Cruz, I.R.; Haas, V.J.; Diniz, M.A.; Dantas, R.A.S.; Rodrigues, R.A.P. Reprodutibilidade da versão Brasileira adaptada da Edmonton Frail Scale para idosos residentes na comunidade. *Rev. Lat. Am. Enfermagem* **2013**, *21*, 1330–1336. [CrossRef]

30. Díaz de León González, E.; Gutiérrez Hermosillo, H.; Martinez Beltran, J.A.; Chavez, J.H.M.; Palacios Corona, R.; Salinas Garza, D.P.; Rodriguez Quintanilla, K.A. Validation of the FRAIL scale in Mexican elderly: Results from the Mexican Health and Aging Study. *Aging Clin. Exp. Res.* **2016**, *28*, 901–908. [CrossRef]

31. Braun, T.; Grüneberg, C.; Thiel, C. German translation, cross-cultural adaptation and diagnostic test accuracy of three frailty screening tools: PRISMA-7, FRAIL scale and Groningen Frailty Indicator. *Z. Gerontol. Geriatr.* **2018**, *51*, 282–292. [CrossRef] [PubMed]

32. Fabrício-Wehbe, S.C.C.; Schiaveto, F.V.; Vendrusculo, T.R.P.; Haas, V.J.; Dantas, R.A.S.; Rodrigues, R.A.P. Adaptación cultural y validez de la Edmonton frail scale—EFS en una muestra de ancianos Brasileños. *Rev. Lat. Am. Enfermagem* **2009**, *17*, 1043–1049. [CrossRef] [PubMed]

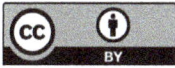

International Journal of
Environmental Research and Public Health

MDPI

Article

Individual Circadian Preference, Shift Work, and Risk of Medication Errors: A Cross-Sectional Web Survey among Italian Midwives

Rosaria Cappadona [1,2,3], Emanuele Di Simone [4,5], Alfredo De Giorgi [5], Benedetta Boari [5], Marco Di Muzio [4], Pantaleo Greco [1,2], Roberto Manfredini [1,3,5], María Aurora Rodríguez-Borrego [3,6], Fabio Fabbian [1,3,5,*] and Pablo Jesús López-Soto [3,6]

[1]   Department of Medical Sciences, University of Ferrara, 44121 Ferrara, Italy;
      rosaria.cappadona@unife.it (R.C.); pantaleo.greco@unife.it (P.G.); roberto.manfredini@unife.it (R.M.)
[2]   Obstetrics and Gynecology Unit, Azienda Ospedaliero-Universitaria S. Anna, 44121 Ferrara, Italy
[3]   Department of Nursing, Instituto Maimónides de Investigación Biomédica de Córdoba (IMIBIC),
      14071 Córdoba, Spain; en1robom@uco.es (M.A.R.-B.); n82losop@uco.es (P.J.L.-S.)
[4]   Department of Clinical and Molecular Medicine, Sapienza University of Rome, 00185 Rome, Italy;
      emanuele.disimone@uniroma1.it (E.D.S.); marco.dimuzio@uniroma1.it (M.D.M.)
[5]   Clinica Medica Unit, Azienda Ospedaliero-Universitaria S. Anna, 44121 Ferrara, Italy;
      degiorgialfredo@libero.it (A.D.G.); benedetta.boari@unife.it (B.B.)
[6]   Department of Nursing Pharmacology and Physiotherapy, University of Córdoba, 14071 Córdoba, Spain
*   Correspondence: f.fabbian@ospfe.it; Tel.: +39-0532-237071

Received: 27 July 2020; Accepted: 7 August 2020; Published: 11 August 2020

check for updates

Abstract: Background: In order to explore the possible association between chronotype and risk of medication errors and chronotype in Italian midwives, we conducted a web-based survey. The questionnaire comprised three main components: (1) demographic information, previous working experience, actual working schedule; (2) individual chronotype, either calculated by Morningness–Eveningness Questionnaire (MEQ); (3) self-perception of risk of medication error. Results: Midwives ($n = 401$) responded "yes, at least once" to the question dealing with self-perception of risk of medication error in 48.1% of cases. Cluster analysis showed that perception of risk of medication errors was associated with class of age 31–35 years, shift work schedule, working experience 6–10 years, and Intermediate-type MEQ score. Conclusions: Perception of the risk of medication errors is present in near one out of two midwives in Italy. In particular, younger midwives with lower working experience, engaged in shift work, and belonging to an Intermediate chronotype, seem to be at higher risk of potential medication error. Since early morning hours seem to represent highest risk frame for female healthcare workers, shift work is not always aligned with individual circadian preference. Assessment of chronotype could represent a method to identify healthcare personnel at higher risk of circadian disruption.

Keywords: circadian rhythm; chronotype; midwives; Morningness–Eveningness Questionnaire (MEQ); near misses; nurses; rhythms desynchronization; risk of medication errors; shift work; sleep

1. Introduction

Chronobiology is a biomedical discipline devoted to the study of biological rhythms. Biological rhythms exist at any level of living organisms and, according to their cycle length, are classified into: (a) circadian rhythms (from the Latin circa-dies, characterized by a period of ~24 h), (b) ultradian rhythms (period <24 h), and c) infradian rhythms (period >24 h) [1]. Circadian rhythms are the most commonly and widely studied biological rhythms, but they are not strictly the same in all persons, since an individual circadian preference (the so-called chronotype) closely linked to biological and psychological variables, exists. Horne & Ostberg first spoke of possible individual differences in circadian attitudes, the so-called chronotype [2]. By means of a simple a self-assessment Morningness–Eveningness Questionnaire (MEQ), they identified Morning-types (M-type, more active early in the day), Evening-types (E-type, more active later in the day), and neither type or Intermediate (I-type). As for chronotype distribution, data based on human population in the temperate region seem to show a Gaussian curve, with 10% M-type, 10% E-type, and 80% I-type [3]. Moreover, differences by sex and age exist as well, with men on average more evening-oriented than women, although these differences reduce with time [3]. In fact, young women are more morning-oriented than young men, but older women are less morning-oriented than older men [4].

Chronotype. A growing body of research indicates that evening chronotype may be associated with a series of unfavourable conditions. A review from our group analysed the available literature to evaluate the relationships between chronotype, gender, and different aspects of health, such as general health and metabolism, psychological health, and sleep and sleep-related problems (Table 1) [5,6]. As a general rule, M-types cope better with the synchrony effect than E-types and are able to adapt to unfavourable circumstances. At suboptimal times, M-types solved the analogy detection task faster, with the same accuracy and without the investment of more cognitive resources. They also showed greater alertness and wakefulness. At optimal times of day, M-types had more cognitive resources available to allocate in the case of more demanding conditions. E-types appear less able to adapt to suboptimal times, because they have to deal with social jetlag and decreased self-control [7]. In fact, a recent systematic review reported that female nurses with an evening-oriented preference suffer more problems of insomnia, sleepiness, fatigue, and anxiety [8].

Table 1. Association between chronotype and main health issues [Fabbian 2016] (Symbols: ↑ Increased; ↓ Decreased).

Main Health Issues	Chronotype	Main Findings
General and cardiovascular health	Evening-type	Unhealthy diet ↓ Physical activity ↑ Smoking Metabolic syndrome Diabetes mellitus
Psychological & psychopathological issues	Evening-type	↑ Common mental disorders ↑ Depression symptoms ↑ Anxiety symptoms Nightmares Risk-taking behaviour
	Morning-type	↑ Health-related quality of life
Sleep & sleep-related issues	Evening-type	Later bedtime and wake-up ↓ Sleep duration ↓ Sleep quality ↓ Sleep quantity ↓ Sleep efficiency

Shift work. Circadian rhythms are entrained by the light/dark alternation and a series of desynchronizing factors, such as exposure to light at night, jetlag, shift work, and daylight saving time, play a crucial role in disrupting the individual organization of circadian rhythms. Among these desynchronizing factors, shift work certainly plays crucial role, due to the wide dissemination of social request for activities warranting 24/hours/seven days a week assistance [9]. According to data from the Italian Institute of Statistics (ISTAT) survey "Working time organization: the role of atypical work schedules", shift working involves about one worker of five in Italy (20.4%). By disaggregating according to industry, social services (which includes education, health and social services, public administration) show the highest figures (26.8%), followed by manufacturing (21.9%) and trade services, including commerce, transport, and communications (21.7%). More men than women work with shifts (respectively 21.7% and 18.4%, respectively), due mainly to shift schemes which imply night work [10]. Different disorders have been associated with shift work, with stress and sleep disorders as the most frequent ones. For example, when comparing nurses and firefighters with day workers, sleep disturbances were more frequent in shift workers than day workers [11]. Moreover, different cardio-metabolic indices, including higher waist circumference, body mass index, fasting glucose, blood pressure, and cardio-metabolic risk score have been described in night workers [12], who also showed almost three times higher association with abdominal obesity independent of age and gender than day shift workers [13].

Errors. Medications errors (MEs) represent a major concern of healthcare systems worldwide, and near misses represent the most reported incidents (69.3%) [14]. According to the World Health Organization, near miss is defined as "an error that has the potential to cause an adverse event (patient harm) but fails to do so because it is intercepted" [15]. Although inadequate staffing levels, workload, and working in haste have been called the most frequent causes of increased risk for omissions and other types of error and for patient harm [16], circadian misalignment, in addition to a series of health problems in shift workers secondary to the sleep deprivation, e.g., daytime sleepiness, i.e., the difficulty maintaining wakefulness and alertness during normal waking hours [17–20], can represent a crucial favouring factor for lack of performance and any kind of errors. Attentional networks are sensitive to sleep deprivation and increased time awake, and sleep duration variability appeared to moderate the association between sleep duration with overall reaction time and alerting scores [21]. Nurses' sleep quality, immediately prior to a working 12-h shift, was shown to be more predictive of error than sleep quantity [22] and functional magnetic resonance imaging (fMRI) studies showed that task performance in nonoptimal times of the day may result in cognitive impairments leading to increased error rates and slower reaction times [23]. Moreover, sleep deprivation represents a further source of risk, not limited to the short term. In hospital shift workers, being screened positive for a sleep disorder was associated with 83% increased incidence of adverse safety outcomes in the following six months, such as motor vehicle crashes, near-miss crashes, occupational exposures, and medical errors [24].

Health professionals. Recent data from Canada, with reference to the year 2011, show that approximately 1.8 million Canadians (12% of the working population), were exposed to night shift work, and 45% were female. By occupation, professional occupations in health ranked second place (35% of workers), following occupations in protective services (37%) [25]. However, despite these numbers, and even if nurses and midwives make up almost 50% of the global healthcare shift working workforce, much of the research addressed to the shift work area used men [26]. Female nurses working in rotating night shift were found to have significantly lower mean scores in job satisfaction, sleep, and psychological well-being as compared to day shift workers [27] and even impaired sexual self-efficacy and sexual quality of life [28]. There is an extreme paucity of studies conducted on midwives, although they play an important role in medical care: a systematic review of sleep-related/fatigue-management including more than 8600 participants, 89% females, did not find studies conducted in midwives [29]. In the same year, a survey study by the American College of Nurse-Midwives Sleep and Safety Taskforce, conducted on more than 4350 certified nurse-midwives and midwives to identify sleepiness, found that midwives working shifts >12 h had higher rates of excessive daytime sleepiness compared with those who worked shifts of ≤12 h [30].

Based on these premises, the aim of this study was to evaluate the possible association between chronotype, shift work, and risk of medication errors in midwives, inviting a representative sample of these health care professionals by means of a web survey. Social media, in fact, has increased the popularity since it represents a convenient method for communicating on the Web, for recruiting participants for health research, and for conducting survey studies by questionnaires [31,32].

2. Materials and Methods

2.1. Sample

A sample of Italian midwives willing to participate in the survey were invited through the most frequently used social media, i.e., Facebook and Instagram, to complete a questionnaire. We chose this extremely smart method in order to maximize the final sample size and the willingness to fill a self-administered web survey allowed us to obtain the informed consent to take part in the survey, Thus, participation was voluntary and confidential.

Midwifes were reached through social media, and those willing to fill the questionnaire were enrolled. In this case, they were told that their personal data would not have been recorded in any way; however, we asked them to declare their job activity, and we trusted health care professionals declaring to be midwifes at the time of starting the questionnaire. We could not analyse any other data nor the reason for refusing or agreeing to participate. All cases of incomplete questionnaire were excluded from the analysis.

The survey was built on Google Forms, and sent to Italian midwifes. Data was collected starting from 14 June 2019 to 31 August 2019. The statistical power of the sample to obtain statistically significant results was determined by a freely available on-line web platform. The authors considered the appropriate sample size for an adequate study power considering a confidence level of 99% and a confidence interval of 5% on a total of about 21,000 midwives working in Italy. The analysis computed a representative sample size of 377 midwifes. The confidence interval also called margin of error is the plus-or-minus figure usually reported in opinion poll results, whilst the confidence level suggests the level of security in excluding wrong answers.

2.2. Instruments and Procedures

The questionnaire consisted of a cover page (describing the purpose of the study, as well the methods to ensure anonymity and voluntary participation), and three special sections, including several different items each. In particular, the special sections dealt with:

A. demography, actual working schedule, and working experience information;
B. the Morningness–Eveningness Questionnaire (MEQ), consisting of 19 questions about personal daily sleep-wake habits and the times of day of preference of certain activities, with assigned points from 0 to 5, giving a possible overall score ranging from 16 to 86. Five categories can be identified: definitely E-type (16–30), moderately E-type (31–41), neither type or I-type (42–58), moderately M-type (59–69), and definitely M-type (70–86). For ease of interpretation, we considered moderately E-type as E-type (16–41 points) and moderately M-type as M-type (59–86 points). Thus, we had three final subgroups: E-types, I-types, and M-types.
C. a perception of risk of medication errors survey, based on the "seven rights" (7R) rule of medication administration (right medication, right client, right dose, right time, right route, right reason, and right documentation) [33]. As for risk evaluation, we chose "near misses", i.e., accidents that do not cause the patient harm [34], since they represent the majority of medication errors [14]. The perception of risk of medication errors was evaluated on the basis of the following questions:

- Based on the 7R rule, during the last shift, how many times did you (or any of your colleagues) run the risk of making a medication error?
- Why medication error was about to occur?

2.3. Statistical Analysis

For statistical analysis, first a descriptive analysis was performed, including results derived from either MEQ calculated score and personal self-perceived chronotype. The sample was classified according to the self-perception of risk of medication errors, and subgroups by age, working schedule, years of working experience, and chronotype were then compared. Second, a logistic regression analysis was done, considering the self-perception of risk of medication errors as the dependent variable and all the other parameters as the independent ones. Third, a cluster analysis was performed, to determine the phenotype of health care professionals exposed to risk of medication errors based on demography, type of work, and chronotype. IBM Statistical Package for Social Science (SPSS 13.0 for Windows, SPSS Inc., Chicago, IL, USA) was utilized.

3. Results

3.1. Participants

The final sample included 401 Italian midwives (98.8% women), and the main characteristics are summarized in Table 2.

Table 2. Characteristics of the whole population of midwifes.

Number of Participants (*n*)	401
Female (*n* (%))	396 (98.8)
Mean age (years)	38.5 ± 10.1
age 23–30 years (*n* (%))	102 (25.5)
age 31–35 years (*n* (%))	81 (20.0)
age 36–40 years (*n* (%))	79 (19.8)
age 41–45 years (*n* (%))	37 (9.2)
age 46–50 years (*n* (%))	37 (9.2)
age 51–55 years (*n* (%))	30 (7.5)
age 56–60 years (*n* (%))	35 (8.8)
University degree (*n* (%))	32 (8)
High school degree (*n* (%))	369 (92)
Shift work schedule (*n* (%))	293 (73)
Mean working experience (years)	11.7 ± 8.9

3.2. Chronotype

As for individual chronotype (MEQ score) and age, subgroups were represented as follows: age 23–30 years: 52 ± 8.3; age 31–35 years: 56 ± 8.2; age 36–40 years: 58.2 ± 7.6; age 4–45 years: 58.7 ± 9.2; age 46–50 years: 60.5 ± 8.3; age 51–55 years: 60.4 ± 8; age 56–60 years: 58.5 ± 8.2 ($p < 0.001$).

As for individual chronotype (self-perceived), subgroups were represented as follows: M-type $n = 115$ (28.7%), I-type $n = 245$ (61%), E-type: $n = 41$ (10.2%). Mean MEQ score in groups who perceived M-type, I-type, and E-type was 64.8 ± 5.1, 54.2 ± 5.1, and 44.7 ± 7.1, respectively ($p < 0.001$).

As for individual chronotype (MEQ calculated score), subgroups were represented as follows: definite M-type: $n = 25$ (6.3%); moderately M-type: $n = 156$ (39%); I-type: $n = 202$ (50.3%); moderately E-type: $n = 16$ (4%); definite E-type: $n = 2$ (0.4%).

Figure 1 reports the distribution of groups by self-perceived and calculated chronotype. For ease of comparison, the MEQ calculated score was reported considering moderately E-type plus definite E-type as E-type and moderately M-type plus definite M-type as M-type.

3.3. Perception of Risk of Medication Errors

As for perception of risk of medication errors, subjects with response "no, never" were 208 (51.9%), and subjects with response "yes, at least once" were 193 (48.1%). The MEQ score did not show significant differences between the two groups (56.7 ± 8.4 vs. 56.5 ± 8.9, p = NS). No differences between the two groups were found for subgroups by class of age, working shift, years of working experience, and chronotype either.

Logistic regression analysis did not show any independent association with perception of risk of medication errors, whereas cluster analysis showed that perception of risk of medication errors was associated with class of age 31–35 years, shift work schedule, working experience 6–10 years, and I-type MEQ score. No perception of risk of medication errors was associated with age 46–50 years, daytime working, working experience 21–25 years, or M-type MEQ score (Figure 2).

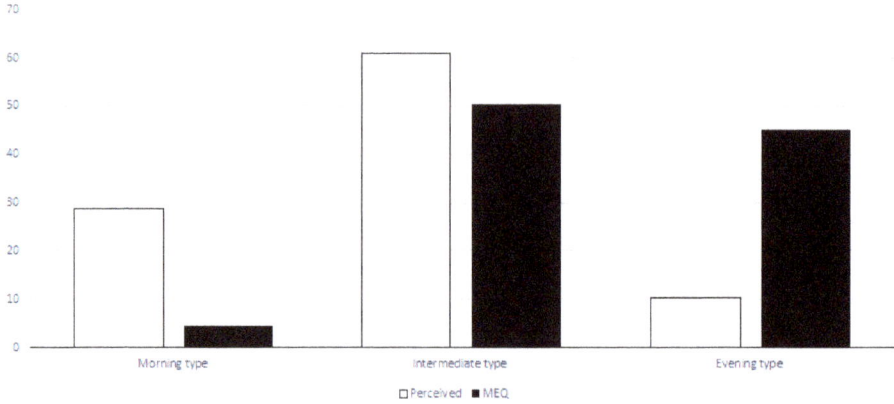

Figure 1. Self-perceived and calculated chronotype distribution of groups. For ease of comparison, the Morningness–Eveningness Questionnaire (MEQ) calculated score was reported considering moderately E-type plus definite E-type as E-type and moderately M-type plus definite M-type as M-type.

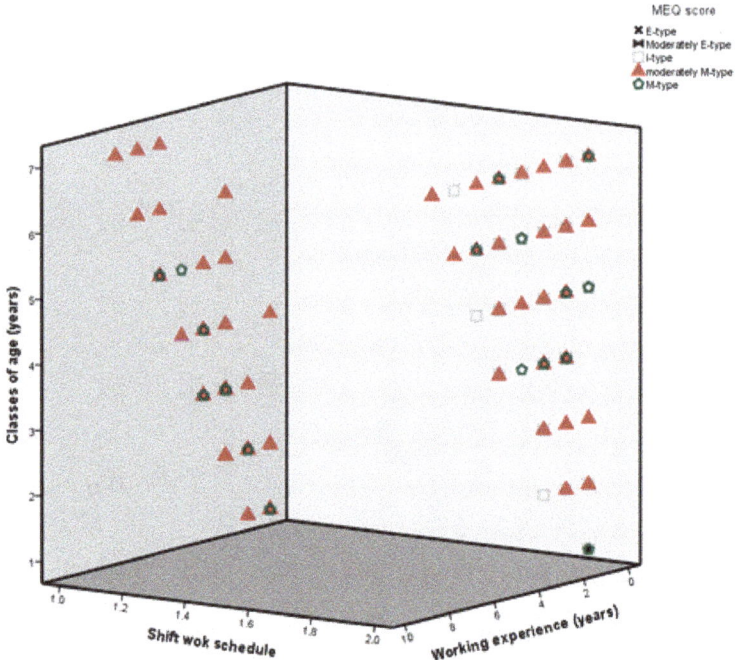

Figure 2. Cluster analysis relating age, shift work schedule, working experience, and MEQ score.

4. Discussion

The results of this study, addressed to investigate the possible relationship between chronotype and risk of medication errors in midwives, showed that the risk of medication errors was associated with younger age, shift work, relatively low working experience, and being an Intermediate chronotype. This is the first report on the association of shift work and risk medical errors in midwives. A recent multicentre Chinese study showed that sleep quality, social support, job satisfaction, occupational injuries, adverse life events, frequency of irregular meals, and employment type were statistically significant factors influencing fatigue among midwives [35]. We found that younger persons, with reduced working experiences, were more likely to report an increased risk of error. It is possible that experience may help in attenuating the decrease in performance during night shift.

Errors. Medication error incidents are more likely to be reported in the morning shift [14,36], but it is common practice that morning therapy is prearranged by the night nursing crew at the end of their shift. Rhythm desynchronization exhibits also gender-specific differences [37], and studies on the circadian and sleep-wake-dependent regulation of cognition in a forced desynchronization protocol showed that accuracy exhibited the largest sex difference in circadian modulation, with the worse performance in women in the early morning hours (at around 6 a.m.) [38]. Even risk taking, a complex form of decision-making that involves calculated assessments of potential costs and rewards, may play a role in the determination of errors. Both gender-specific and chronotype differences exist, since males report higher propensity for risk-taking, in particular E-types. However, although there is no significant difference in risk propensity or risk-taking behaviour across chronotypes in males, E-type females significantly report and take more risk than other chronotypes [39].

Chronotype. Chronotype is also strongly implicated in performance tasks, also making reference to the so-called "synchrony effects", i.e., superior performance at optimal and inferior performance at suboptimal times of day. A study aimed at evaluating the effect of individual differences in chronotype on performance task, evaluated a sample of M-type and E-type women during a driving session in morning (8 a.m.) and evening (8 p.m.). A vigilance decrement was found when E-type participants drove at their nonoptimal time of day (morning session). In contrast, driving performance in the M-type group remained stable over time on task and was not affected by time of day [40]. By contrast, studies on subjects tested for mean reaction times, error rates, and efficiency of three attentional networks (alerting, orienting, and executive control/conflict) at two time points (time 1 or baseline at 8 a.m.; time 2, after 18-h sustained wakefulness at 2 a.m.), showed that E-types participants outperformed M-types on incongruent time, i.e., deep night [21]. On one hand, negative effects of sleep impairments seem to be confirmed to affect more E-types than other chronotypes. An Australian online survey study conducted on paramedics (age 39 ± 12 years; 54% women; 85% rotating shift-workers; 57% I-types, 32% M-types, 11% E-types), showed significantly higher depression scores, anxiety, poorer sleep quality, and reduced general well-being in the E-types, compared with M-types [41]. Our study identifies Intermediate-type as the group at higher risk of error. On one hand, this result is contradictory with respect to the available literature. On the other, this result, if confirmed, is extremely interesting since Intermediate chronotype represents the most frequent circadian preference and not only in our sample. Thus, the finding that younger midwives, with relatively limited working experience, and even with chronotype extremes, are exposed to higher risk of error during their night shift, raises serious concern.

Limitations. We are aware of several limitations to this study: (a) cross-sectional design, based on data collected through a web survey, therefore the sample could be sized only by social media users only; (b) the MEQ score, even if used in the majority of studies for assessing morningness–eveningness preference, does not categorized for different ages [42]; (c) to evaluate the risk of medication error, we considered the general definition of near misses. Although it is largely the most frequent incident reported, we did not differentiate between near misses and no harm incidents [43]; (d) individual perception of the risk of medication errors is not a validated item yet; (e) logistic regression analysis did not identify independent factors; (f) we could not evaluate any gender effect, as most of the sample were women, as usually occurs for studies on nurses and midwives. However, there are also some positive aspects: (a) the web survey method warranted speed, and even in a short timeframe all different classes of age were represented; (b) we found that perception of chronotype was different from the effective profile identified by a well-validated score. This concept could help for future studies and also for practical applications since when workers (health care personnel in particular) ask for health measures, they very often make reference to personal perception.

Coping strategies. Midwifery and nursing are acknowledged as stressful occupations, and the negative impact of high stress levels often requires coping strategies. Of these, the eleven most used have been identified via interview material: drinking alcohol, smoking, using the staff social club, using social networking websites, exercising, family activities, home-based activities, outdoor activities, avoiding people, displacement, and sleep [44]. Unfortunately, it is evident that some of these coping strategies are unhealthy and extremely concerning. Moreover, due to the stress burden, absenteeism is becoming a significant global problem, and taking a "mental health day" as sickness absence is a common phenomenon, taken by more than one half of nurses and midwives, according to an online cross-sectional survey in Australia [45].

5. Conclusions

With this study, we found that younger midwives, with lower working experience, engaged in shift work and belonging to an Intermediate chronotype, seem to be at higher risk of potential medication error. At least to the best of our knowledge, this is the first web survey study addressed to the relationship between chronotype, shift work, and perceived risk of medication error in midwives. Since morning hours seem to represent highest risk frame for female healthcare workers and shift work is not always aligned with individual circadian preference, our preliminary reports could stimulate further specific research aimed to practical applications. For example, assessment of individual chronotype and sleep attitude in healthcare personnel, by means of validated questionnaires, just previously suggested in terms of prevention of metabolic diseases [46], could provide easy and inexpensive method to identify subjects at potential higher risk of circadian disruption. Again, possible countermeasures, such as time-scheduled naps during night-shifts, have been positively tested on female nurses, who showed significantly greater increments in performance between 3:00 and 7:00 a.m. on nap versus no-nap nights [47]. Last but not least, attention to shift work consequences, together with specific training programs, could help to reduce medication errors and improve patients' safety [48].

Author Contributions: Conceptualization: R.C., E.D.S., M.A.R.-B., P.J.L.-S.; Data curation: E.D.S., A.D.G., B.B.; Formal analysis: E.D.S., A.D.G., B.B., M.D.M., F.F.; Funding acquisition: P.G., M.D.M., R.M.; Investigation: R.C., E.D.S., A.D.G., B.B., M.A.R.-B., P.J.L.-S., F.F.; Methodology: R.C., E.D.S., A.D.G., P.G., M.D.M., R.M.; Project administration: R.C., E.D.S., A.D.G., B.B., F.F.; Resources: M.A.R.-B., P.G., M.D.M., R.M., P.J.L.-S.; Software: R.C., E.D.S., A.D.G., B.B., F.F.; Supervision: M.A.R.-B., P.G., M.D.M., R.M., P.J.L.-S.; Validation: R.C., E.D.S., A.D.G., B.B., M.A.R.-B., P.J.L.-S., F.F.; Visualization: R.C., A.D.G., P.G., M.D.M., R.M.; Writing—original draft: R.C., F.F.; Writing-review and editing: M.A.R.-B., P.G., M.D.M., R.M., P.J.L.-S. All authors have read and agreed to the published version of the manuscript.

Funding: This study is supported by a scientific grant by the University of Ferrara (Fondo Incentivazione Ricerca -FIR- 2020, Roberto Manfredini).

Acknowledgments: We thank Isabella Bagnaresi, Clinica Medica Unit, Department of Medical Sciences, University'of Ferrara, for precious technical support. We also thank Claudia Righini and Donato Bragatto, Biblioteca Interaziendale di Scienze della Salute, Azienda Ospedaliero-Universitaria "S.Anna", Ferrara, for helpful assistance.

Conflicts of Interest: The authors declare no conflict of interest.

References

1. Manfredini, R.; Salmi, R.; Malagoni, A.M.; Manfredini, F. Circadian rhythm effects on cardiovascular and other stress-related events. In *George Fink (Editor-in-Chief) Encyclopedia of Stress*, 2nd ed.; Academic Press: Oxford, UK, 2007; Volume 1, pp. 500–505.
2. Horne, J.A.; Ostberg, O. A self-assessment questionnaire to determine morningness-eveningness in human circadian rhythms. *Int. J. Chronobiol.* **1976**, *4*, 97–110. [PubMed]
3. Ashkenazi, I.E.; Reinberg, A.E.; Motohashi, Y. Interindividual differences in the flexibility of human temporal organization: Pertinence to jetlag and shiftwork. *Chronobiol. Int.* **1997**, *14*, 99–113. [CrossRef] [PubMed]
4. Randler, C.; Engelke, J. Gender differences in chronotype diminish with age: A meta-analysis based on morningness/chronotype questionnaires. *Chronobiol. Int.* **2019**, *36*, 888–905. [CrossRef] [PubMed]
5. Fabbian, F.; Zucchi, B.; De Giorgi, A.; Tiseo, R.; Boari, B.; Salmi, R.; Cappadona, R.; Gianesini, G.; Bassi, E.; Signiani, F.; et al. Chronotype, gender and general health. *Chronobiol. Int.* **2016**, *33*, 863–882. [CrossRef] [PubMed]
6. Ki, J.; Ryu, J.; Baek, J.; Huh, I.; Choi-Kwon, S. Association between Health Problems and Turnover Intention in Shift Work Nurses: Health Problem Clustering. *Int. J. Environ. Res. Public Health* **2020**, *17*, 4532. [CrossRef]
7. Nowack, K.; Van Der Meer, E. The synchrony effect revisited: Chronotype, time of day and cognitive performance in a semantic analogy task. *Chronobiol. Int.* **2018**, *35*, 1647–1662. [CrossRef]
8. López-Soto, P.J.; Fabbian, F.; Cappadona, R.; Zucchi, B.; Manfredini, F.; Garcia-Arcos, A.; Carmona-Torres, J.M.; Manfredini, R.; Rodriguez-Borrego, M.A. Chronotype, nursing activity, and gender: A systematic review. *J. Adv. Nurs.* **2019**, *75*, 734–748. [CrossRef]
9. Sack, R.L.; Auckley, D.; Auger, R.R.; Carskadon, M.A.; Wright, K.P., Jr.; Vitiello, M.V.; Zhdanova, I.V. Circadian rhythm sleep disorders: Part II, advanced sleep phase disorder, delayed sleep phase disorder, free-running disorder, and irregular sleep-wake rhythm. An American Academy of Sleep Medicine review. *Sleep* **2007**, *30*, 1484–1501. [CrossRef]
10. European Foundation for the Improvement of Living and Working Conditions. Available online: https://www.eurofound.europa.eu/publications/report/2009/working-time-in-the-european-union-italy (accessed on 21 March 2020).
11. Choi, S.J.; Song, P.; Suh, S.; Joo, E.Y.; Lee, S.I. Insomnia symptoms and mood disturbances in shift workers with different chronotypes and working schedules. *J. Clin. Neurol.* **2020**, *16*, 108–115. [CrossRef]
12. Ritonja, J.; Tranmer, J.; Aronson, K.J. The relationship between night work, chronotype, and cardiometabolic risk in female hospital employees. *Chronobiol. Int.* **2019**, *36*, 616–628. [CrossRef]
13. Brum, M.C.B.; Dantas Filho, F.F.; Schnorr, C.C.; Bertoletti, O.A.; Bottega, G.B.; da Costa Rodrigues, T. Night shift work, short sleep and obesity. *Diabetol. Metab. Syndr.* **2020**, *12*, 13. [CrossRef] [PubMed]
14. Aseeri, M.; Banasser, G.; Baduhduh, O.; Baksh, S.; Ghalibi, N. Evaluation of medication error incident reports at a tertiary care hospital. *Pharmacy (Basel)* **2020**, *8*, 69. [CrossRef] [PubMed]
15. World Health Organization. *World Alliance for Patient Safety: WHO Draft Guidelines for Adverse Event Reporting and Learning Systems: From Information to Action;* World Health Organization: Geneva, Switzerland, 2005.
16. Härkänen, M.; Vehviläinen-Julkunen, K.; Murrells, T.; Paananen, J.; Franklin, B.D.; Rafferty, A.M. The contribution of staffing to medication administration errors: A text mining analysis of incident report data. *J. Nurs. Scholarsh.* **2020**, *52*, 113–123. [CrossRef] [PubMed]
17. Drake, C.L.; Roehrs, T.; Richardson, G.; Walsh, J.K.; Roth, T. Shift work sleep disorder: Prevalence and consequences beyond that of symptomatic day workers. *Sleep* **2004**, *27*, 1453–1462. [CrossRef] [PubMed]
18. Rosa, D.; Terzoni, S.; Dellafiore, F.; Destrebecq, A. Systematic review of shift work and nurses' health. *Occup. Med. (Lond.)* **2019**, *69*, 237–243. [CrossRef] [PubMed]
19. Di Muzio, M.; Reda, F.; Diella, G.; Di Simone, E.; Novelli, L.; D'Atri, A.; Giannini, A.; De Gennaro, L. Not only a Problem of Fatigue and Sleepiness: Changes in Psychomotor Performance in Italian Nurses across 8-h Rapidly Rotating Shifts. *J. Clin. Med.* **2019**, *8*, 47. [CrossRef]
20. Di Muzio, M.; Dionisi, S.; Di Simone, E.; Cianfrocca, C.; Di Muzio, F.; Fabbian, F.; Barbiero, G.; Tartaglini, D.; Giannetta, N. Can nurses' shift work jeopardize the patient safety? A systematic review. *Eur. Rev. Med. Pharmacol. Sci.* **2019**, *23*, 4507–4519.
21. Barclay, N.L.; Myachykov, A. Sustained wakefulness and visual attention: Moderation by chronotype. *Exp. Brain. Res.* **2017**, *235*, 57–68. [CrossRef]

22. Weaver, A.L.; Stutzman, S.E.; Supnet, C.; Olson, D.M. Sleep quality, but not quantity, is associated with self-perceived minor error rates among emergency department nurses. *Int. Emerg. Nurs.* **2016**, *25*, 48–52. [CrossRef]

23. Reske, M.; Rosenberg, J.; Plapp, S.; Kellermann, T.; Shah, N.J. fMRI identifies chronotype-specific brain activation associated with attention to motion–why we need to know when subjects go to bed. *Euroimage* **2015**, *111*, 602–610. [CrossRef]

24. Weaver, M.D.; Vetter, C.; Rajaratnam, S.M.W.; O'Brien, C.S.; Qadri, S.; Benca, R.M.; Rogers, A.E.; Leary, E.B.; Walsh, J.K.; Czeisler, C.A.; et al. Sleep disorders, depression and anxiety are associated with adverse safety outcomes in healthcare workers: A prospective cohort study. *J. Sleep. Res.* **2018**, *27*, e12722. [CrossRef]

25. Rydz, E.; Hall, A.L.; Peters, C.E. Prevalence and recent trends in exposure to night shiftwork in Canada. *Ann. Work Expo. Health* **2020**, *64*, 270–281. [CrossRef]

26. Matheson, A.; O'Brien, L.; Reid, J.A. Women's experience of shiftwork in nursing whilst caring for children: A juggling act. *J. Clin. Nurs.* **2019**, *28*, 3817–3826. [CrossRef] [PubMed]

27. Verma, A.; Kishore, J.; Gusain, S. A comparative study of shift work effects and injuries among nurses working in rotating night and day shifts in a tertiary care hospital of North India. *Iran J. Nurs. Midwifery Res.* **2018**, *23*, 51–56. [CrossRef]

28. Khastar, H.; Mirrezaie, S.M.; Chashmi, N.A.; Jahanfar, S. Sleep improvement effect on sexual life quality among rotating female shift workers: A randomized controlled trial. *J. Sex. Med.* **2020**, *17*, 1467–1475. [CrossRef] [PubMed]

29. Querstret, D.; O'Brien, K.; Skene, D.J.; Maben, J. Improving fatigue risk management in healthcare: A systematic scoping review of sleep-related/fatigue-management interventions for nurses and midwives. *Int. J. Nurs. Stud.* **2019**, *106*, 103513. [CrossRef]

30. Arbour, M.; Tanner, T.; Hensley, J.; Beardsley, J.; Wika, J.; Garvan, C. Factors that contribute to excessive sleepiness in midwives practicing in the United States. *J. Midwifery Women Health* **2019**, *64*, 179–185. [CrossRef]

31. McCarthy, E.; Mazza, D. Cost and effectiveness of using Facebook advertising to recruit young women for research: PREFER (Contraceptive Preferences Study) Experience. *J. Med. Internet Res.* **2019**, *21*, e15869. [CrossRef] [PubMed]

32. Shaver, L.G.; Khawer, A.; Yi, Y.; Aubrey-Bassler, K.; Etchegary, H.; Roebothan, B.; Asghari, S.; Wang, P.P. Using Facebook advertising to recruit representative samples: Feasibility assessment of a cross-sectional survey. *J. Med. Internet. Res.* **2019**, *21*, e14021. [CrossRef]

33. Smeulers, M.; Verweij, L.; Maaskant, J.M.; de Boer, M.; Krediet, C.T.; Nieveen van Dijkum, E.J.; Vermeulen, H. Quality indicators for safe medication preparation and administration: A systematic review. *PLoS ONE* **2015**, *10*, e0122695. [CrossRef]

34. Kessels-Habraken, M.; Van der Schaaf, T.; De Jonge, J.; Rutte, C. Defining near misses: Towards a sharpened definition based on empirical data about error handling processes. *Soc. Sci. Med.* **2010**, *70*, 1301–1308. [CrossRef] [PubMed]

35. Chen, X.Q.; Jiang, X.M.; Zheng, Q.X.; Zheng, J.; He, H.G.; Pan, Y.Q.; Liu, G.H. Factors associated with workplace fatigue among midwives in southern China: A multi-centre cross-sectional study. *J. Nurs. Manag.* **2020**. [CrossRef]

36. Suclupe, S.; Martinez-Zapata, M.J.; Mancebo, J.; Font-Vaquer, A.; Castillo-Masa, A.M.; Viñolas, I.; Morán, I.; Robleda, G. Medication errors in prescription and administration in critically ill patients. *J. Adv. Nurs.* **2020**, *76*, 1192–1200. [CrossRef]

37. Cappadona, R.; Di Simone, E.; De Giorgi, A.; Zucchi, B.; Fabbian, F.; Manfredini, R. Biological rhythms, health, and gender-specific differences. *Ital. J. Gender-Specific. Med.* **2020**, in press.

38. Santhi, N.; Lazar, A.S.; McCabe, P.J.; Lo, J.C.; Groeger, J.A.; Dijk, D.J. Sex differences in the circadian regulation of sleep and waking cognition in humans. *Proc. Natl. Acad. Sci. USA* **2016**, *113*, E2730–E2739. [CrossRef] [PubMed]

39. Gowen, R.; Filipowicz, A.; Ingram, K.K. Chronotype mediates gender differences in risk propensity and risk-taking. *PLoS ONE* **2019**, *14*, e0216619. [CrossRef] [PubMed]

40. Correa, A.; Molina, E.; Sanabria, D. Effects of chronotype and time of day on the vigilance decrement during simulated driving. *Accid. Anal. Prev.* **2014**, *67*, 113–118. [CrossRef]

41. Khan, W.A.A.; Conduit, R.; Kennedy, G.A.; Jackson, M.L. The relationship between shift-work, sleep, and mental health among paramedics in Australia. *Sleep Health* **2020**, *6*, 330–337. [CrossRef]
42. Levandoski, R.; Sasso, E.; Hidalgo, M.P. Chronotype: A review of the advances, limits and applicability of the main instruments used in the literature to assess human phenotype. *Trends Psychiatry Psychother.* **2013**, *35*, 3–11. [CrossRef]
43. Sheikhtaheri, A. Near misses and their importance for improving patient safety. *Iran. J. Public. Health* **2014**, *43*, 853–854.
44. Happell, B.; Reid-Searl, K.; Dwyer, T.; Caperchione, C.M.; Gaskin, C.J.; Burke, K.J. How nurses cope with occupational stress outside their workplaces. *Collegian* **2013**, *20*, 195–199. [CrossRef] [PubMed]
45. Lamont, S.; Brunero, S.; Perry, L.; Duffield, C.; Sibbritt, D.; Gallagher, R.; Nicholls, R. 'Mental health day' sickness absence amongst nurses and midwives: Workplace, workforce, psychosocial and health characteristics. *J. Adv. Nurs.* **2017**, *73*, 1172–1181. [CrossRef] [PubMed]
46. Manfredini, R.; Cappadona, R.; Fabbian, F. Nurses, shift work, and diabetes: Should late chronotype be considered as a risk factor? *BMJ* **2019**, *364*, 1178. [CrossRef] [PubMed]
47. Zion, N.; Shochat, T. Let them sleep: The effects of a scheduled nap during the night shift on sleepiness and cognition in hospital nurses. *J. Adv. Nurs.* **2019**, *75*, 2603–2615. [CrossRef] [PubMed]
48. Di Simone, E.; Giannetta, N.; Auddino, F.; Cicotto, A.; Grilli, D.; Di Muzio, M. Medication errors in the emergency department: Knowledge, attitude, behavior and training needs of nurses. *Indian J. Crit. Care Med.* **2018**, *22*, 46–352.

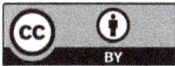

International Journal of
*Environmental Research
and Public Health*

MDPI

Article

Nursing Students' Experiences of Clinical Practices in Emergency and Intensive Care Units

María González-García [1,2,3], **Alberto Lana** [2,3,*], **Paula Zurrón-Madera** [2,3,4], **Yolanda Valcárcel-Álvarez** [1,2,3] **and Ana Fernández-Feito** [2,3]

[1] Health Care Service of Asturias, Central University Hospital of Asturias, Avda. Roma, s/n, 33011 Oviedo, Spain; maguig87@hotmail.com (M.G.-G.); yolanda.valcarcel@sespa.es (Y.V.-Á.)

[2] Department of Medicine, School of Medicine and Health Sciences, University of Oviedo, Avda. Julián Clavería, s/n, 33006 Oviedo, Spain; zurronpaula@uniovi.es (P.Z.-M.); fernandezfana@uniovi.es (A.F.-F.)

[3] Healthcare Research Area, Health Research Institute of Asturias (ISPA), Avda. Roma, s/n, 33011 Oviedo, Spain

[4] Mental Health Center of La Corredoria, Health Care Service of Asturias (Spain), C. Alfredo Blanco, s/n, 33011 Oviedo, Spain

* Correspondence: lanaalberto@uniovi.es

Received: 4 July 2020; Accepted: 3 August 2020; Published: 6 August 2020

check for updates

Abstract: Clinical practices are key environments for skill acquisition during the education of nursing students, where it is important to encourage reflective learning. This study sought to explore the experience of final year nursing students during their clinical placement in emergency and intensive care units and to identify whether differences exist between female and male students. Using qualitative methodology, a documentary analysis of 28 reflective learning journals was carried out at a public university in Northern Spain. Four themes were identified: "an intense emotional experience", "the importance of attitudes over and above techniques", "identifying with nurses who dominate their environment and are close to the patient in complex and dehumanized units" and "how to improve care in critically ill patients and how to support their families". The female students displayed a more emotional and reflective experience, with a strong focus on patient care, whereas male students identified more with individual aspects of learning and the organization and quality of the units. Both male and female students experienced intense emotions, improved their learning in complex environments and acquired attitudes linked to the humanization of care. However, the experience of these clinical rotations was different between female and male students.

Keywords: clinical placements; emergency hospital service; intensive care units; nursing care; nursing education research; nursing students; nursing

1. Introduction

During undergraduate nursing studies, the acquisition of competencies, in a broad sense, is essential. In addition to theoretical and practical learning and the development of nursing attitudes, it is important to establish transversal competencies, such as leadership, communication, or interpersonal skills, as well as competencies for adequate personal and professional development. To achieve these transversal competencies, it is important to encourage reflection [1].

Clinical practices are an essential element of learning for nursing students [2,3], as they enable the application of theoretical knowledge in a real environment, the training of technical skills through interaction with patients and health workers and the development of nursing attitudes [4]. In addition, this is an ideal opportunity for students to reflect on their learning. Emergency departments and intensive care units (ICU) are clinical environments that encourage competence development; however, they also pose a challenge for students and teachers. These units are very complex, with high pressure to care for serious patients, which can negatively influence the students' experience [5]. Careful planning, with guidance and follow-up by an instructor, are central elements in their development [6].

2. Background

Significant learning is not possible without reflection [7]. The reflective analysis of lived experiences or problems faced during professional practice can serve as a stimulus for learning [8]. A reflective attitude can be even more useful than technical mastery when dealing with changing situations in professional practice. During nursing training, reflective learning can take place through a reflective learning journal (RLJ). The RLJ is a written document in which students carefully analyze their thoughts, actions or interactions with others over a period of time [3,7]. Several studies have documented the usefulness of RLJs in enhancing the learning experience during clinical practice [9–11], stimulating professional development [12] and even personal development in the process of becoming a nurse [13–15]. In this way, RLJ can be used as an additional tool for teachers to assess students' acquisition of nursing competencies during clinical education but also to learn about students' personal experiences, including their coping strategies, thoughts, emotions and feelings [4,7,13].

Addressing emotions during clinical practice is very important [3,10,13]. When students are asked to keep an RLJ, they are voicing emotions experienced during clinical placements that are usually relegated to the context of individual students [10]. In addition, writing and reflecting on their feelings and emotions can also be therapeutic for students, since it allows them to stop and externalize their experiences [9,16], which increases their confidence in their ability to face future difficulties [13,17] and increases their capacity to empathize with patients and their families [18,19].

In addition, RLJs provide a "snapshot" of the daily reality on the clinical level (e.g., characteristics of services, type of patients, quality of nursing care, etc.) and the teaching process (e.g., student–nurse interaction, clinical practice schedules, etc.). Knowing the day to day life of emergency department and ICU from the perspective of students can be an enriching way to identify areas of improvement in these two nursing dimensions: clinical practice and teaching activity.

There is some prior research on the experience of students during the first year of clinical practice training [2,3,17,19,20]; however, there are fewer approaches to the experience of clinical placements in senior year students and in complex care settings, even though these may be more representative of how students will cope with the impending start of their professional development. In addition, we were unable to find any papers that compared clinical practice experiences by gender. Only a few studies include the student's gender in the verbatim, without establishing a comparative analysis [9]. This is relevant because previous research has documented differences between male and female nursing students in relation to professional values [21], personal values [22], career choice and post-graduation outcomes [23]. In addition, socially constructed traditional gender norms can determine expected behaviors and attitudes in both male and female students in the context of a traditionally female profession [24]. During clinical practice, and through the RLJ, it is possible to observe whether there are differences in the preference or rejection of some activities based on gender—for example, whether men feel more attracted to management and coordination aspects or whether women identify more with the humanization of care, empathy with patients, etc., both of which are situations that are dictated by gender roles.

The aim of our study was to explore the experience of final year nursing students during their clinical practices in emergency department and ICU and to examine how this experience is interpreted by both female and male students.

3. Materials and Methods

3.1. Design

A qualitative study using documentary analysis of RLJs written by nursing students in their senior year during their clinical practices.

3.2. Participants and Setting

In Spain, the Degree in Nursing is a four-year university degree with 240 credits (in accordance with the European Credit Transfer and Accumulation System, ECTS). During the final year, students at the University of Oviedo (Spain) take a specific course on clinical practices in the emergency department and ICU (12 ECTS credits). All students must perform at least two clinical rotations, one in the emergency department and another in ICU, to complete 230 h of training. In addition, students must submit a clinical case study and an RLJ of the subject, which accounts for 10% of the final grade. During the 2017/2018 academic year, 78 students studied this course at the University of Oviedo (Spain). Twenty-eight RLJs were selected from the students (15 from women and 13 from men) who obtained the highest grades in the January 2018 evaluation.

Clinical practices took place in the emergency department and ICU of six public hospitals. The center where the largest number of students performed clinical practices ($n = 20$) was a level 3 public university hospital (1000 beds), where around 300 patients are seen daily in the emergency department and which has 75 ICU boxes. The remaining hospitals that received students were level 2 (<500 beds).

3.3. Research Team

The research team consisted of five nurses (four women and one man) from the University of Oviedo. The principal investigator had two years' experience in critical care. She was a doctor, associate professor in nursing and the head of the clinical practicum subject. Three of the nurses had professional experience in emergency department and ICU and teaching experience in the Degree of Nursing. One researcher was also the teacher of the "Research in Nursing" subject at the University of Oviedo. The students knew the researchers through their participation in other subjects during the nursing degree.

3.4. Instruments

In this course, students are required to complete a compulsory portfolio on clinical practices. The portfolio consists of two sections. The first was a descriptive section with administrative and clinical data on the clinical practices, including data on the hospital and the practice unit, type of pathologies and nursing activities performed. The second was a reflective part (RLJ) on the contributions of the placements to their learning, on the level of satisfaction with the clinical practicum and suggestions for improvement. Specifically, students are strongly required to reflect on the following competencies achieved in three areas (knowledge, skills and attitude): (1) providing nursing care to critically ill patients; (2) correctly performing the most common techniques in emergency department and ICU; (3) respecting ethical values related to privacy, confidentiality and respect for patients; (4) meeting the information and communication needs of patients and families. This is delivered by email at the end of students' clinical practice training in a text document of unlimited length. At the beginning of the course, there is a two-hour face-to-face information session at the university on how to perform the RLJ, emphasizing its reflective nature, which must be more than just a description of the activities performed. Students were asked to engage in a reflective exercise concerning their daily actions [8] and to only record in their RLJ those aspects that were most relevant. They were given instructions on how to record each reflection, including the actions taken, the context, their emotions and how they could improve. In addition, several examples were provided. They were also encouraged to reflect on how the same activity could be done differently depending on the unit and the nurse carrying it out—for example, communication with a sedated patient.

3.5. Data Analysis

According to the methodology proposed by other authors [25,26], a three-phase content analysis of the RLJs was carried out. In the first phase, the texts were prepared for analysis. Within each journal, the sections "Identification of contributions to learning", "Description of the competencies acquired (knowledge, skills and attitudes)" and "Suggestions for improvement" were selected. In the second phase, the information was organized and the actual content analysis was carried out [27]. The meaning units identified in the reports were assigned codes. The codes were then grouped and gathered into subcategories and categories. Finally, the main themes that summarized the students' experience were formulated. According to the format of the RLJ, a previous thematic category, "knowledge, skills and attitudes competencies", was used as a starting point; however, the remaining topics emerged after the documentary analysis. In the third "reporting" phase, the results were presented. The complete analysis process was presented (codes, subcategories, categories and themes) as well as the description or storyline of the results.

The analyses were carried out without the use of software. The analyses were conducted independently by two researchers and, after pooling the analyses, they were triangulated with the participation of another researcher from the group.

3.6. Ethical Considerations

All students provided informed consent to the use of their journal for research purposes. Each participant was assigned a code to maintain anonymity, which was identified using "W" for women and "M" for men. Participation in this study had no influence on the grade assigned in their evaluation since this investigation was initiated months after the students completed the course. Our study was exempt from ethics committee approval, although it was conducted in accordance with the ethical standards set out in the original Declaration of Helsinki and its subsequent amendments.

4. Results

4.1. Experience of Nursing Students in Emergency Department and Intensive Care Units

Overall, the student experience reflected in the RLJs was positive in terms of learning, although a high emotional burden related to attendance at these units was noted. Most students perceived a high degree of coordination in these units and the importance of nurse/medical collaboration.

During the analysis, four themes were identified from the students' reflection on the competencies (Figure 1). The first referred to the student's feelings of undergoing "an intense emotional experience" and the second referred to the skills and attitudes achieved "the importance of attitudes over and above techniques." The third theme was related to nursing professionals and some characteristics of clinical practice units "to identify with nurses who dominate their environment and are close to the patient in complex and dehumanized units". Finally, the fourth theme referred to patients and their families: "how to improve care for critically ill patients and support their families."

4.1.1. Intense Emotional Experience

For all the students, these clinical placements involved intense emotions. Prior to the clinical practices, negative emotions predominated, as the previous confrontation of female and male students was characterized by fear, pressure, emotional block, etc. However, during the clinical training, they experienced emotional ambivalence. Thus, they experienced positive feelings, especially linked to the patient's favorable evolution and identification with the nursing profession. Concurrently, they also experienced negative emotions, associated with facing the care of patients in very serious clinical situations and death, causing them to reflect on life (Table 1).

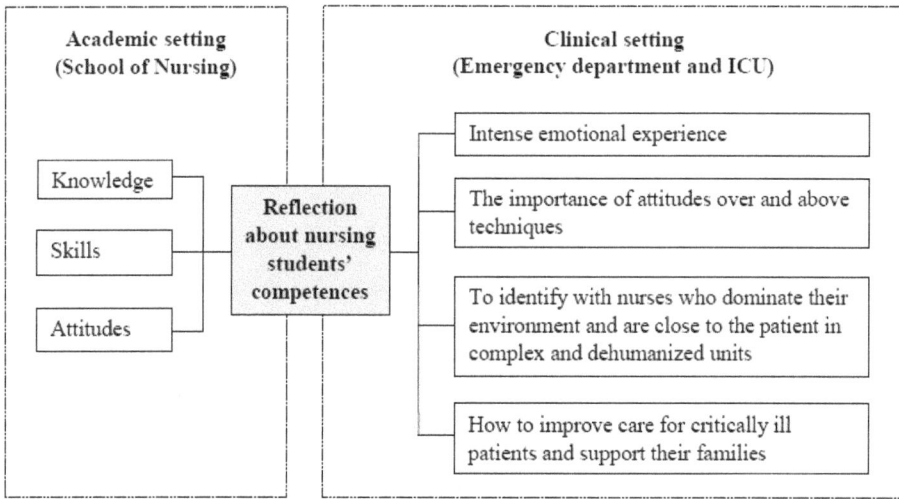

Figure 1. Experience of nursing students in emergency department and ICU during clinical practices.

Table 1. Main categories, sub-categories and codes about the theme "intense emotional experience".

Main Codes	Sub-Categories	Categories
Fear of the unknown Pressure Nervousness Emotional blockage	Previous expectations	
Identification of severe young patients Tough experience Fatigue Impotence of not being able to communicate Feeling lucky	Intense experience	Feelings
Insecurity in complex patients Fear of making mistakes Helplessness lack of time Helplessness poor patient evolution Satisfaction for good patient progress Gratification humanizing care Progressive safety/self-monitoring	Emotions during clinical practices	
Feeling like a nurse Professional and personal enrichment Awareness of the importance of the nursing profession Satisfaction with correct performance of techniques Gratification of professional collaboration	Identification with the nursing profession	Thoughts
Feeling overwhelmed Fine line life/death Inexperience in facing death	Difficulty coping with death	
Irreversible change in a second Valuing what matters Temporality of human life	Reflecting on life	

As for the previous expectations, there were no great differences between girls and boys, in both groups, and feelings of fear, pressure, being "frozen" or blocked, etc. predominated. During the clinical practices, positive feelings of satisfaction and personal growth were expressed.

"These clinical practices have been a turning point in my career as I have been able to grow as a person and as a future nursing professional." W4

"In this clinical module I have shown myself how right I have been in choosing a profession like this, how close one is to the patient and how much chance one has of, with very little, improving the condition of the patient and his or her family." M10

Both the female and male students showed progressive confidence as the clinical practicum progressed, facing these with greater ease and feeling more satisfied if the patients progressed well.

Some acknowledged their difficulty in coping with death, either because of inexperience or because they felt overwhelmed by the situation.

4.1.2. Importance of Attitudes over and above Techniques

The acquired competencies were articulated in three areas: knowledge, skills and attitudes (Table 2).

Table 2. Main categories, sub-categories and codes about the theme "importance of attitudes over and above techniques".

Main Codes	Sub-Categories	Categories
Identify situations of risk Prioritizing by triage	How to act	
New and specific knowledge Distribution of work/tasks according to professional profile Integrating theoretical knowledge Getting to know other cultures	Expanding knowledge	Knowledge
Performing new techniques Specific techniques Refinement of already known techniques Care linked to infection prevention Rapid action Performing under pressure	Technical skills	
Only one aspect of care Relative importance Observation	Emphasis on techniques	Skills
Responsibility Autonomy Confidentiality Teamwork Accepting errors Adapting to a changing environment Keeping calm Humanizing care	Acquired attitudes	
Empathy Guaranteeing privacy Paying attention to patient's emotions Importance of talking and listening Respect	Regaining human values	Attitudes

In terms of theoretical knowledge, some categories common to both sexes were learning how to handle critically ill patients or how to prioritize emergency care through triage. They also recognized learning new and specific knowledge, required in these units.

Regarding the competencies linked to skills or abilities, all mentioned the handling of devices and the refinement of new techniques as well as the improvement of other already known techniques. They also learned to act quickly, adjusting to the urgency of the moment.

Attitude-related competencies were extensively analyzed as they constituted a very large section within the RLJs. Two themes were appreciated: firstly, in relation to their personal experience as students where the acquired responsibility or autonomy stands out; secondly, almost all referred to learning related to the humanization of care, based on respect for the patient, empathy and accompaniment.

"I have learned that many times there is no need to speak or, rather, "fill the silences" with words, we should simply be there, giving company and human touch if necessary." W12

"When the intubated patients were thirsty I would dip a gauze in water and place it between their lips and they would thank me. I also, for example, put the radio on for a patient because it's quite tedious for everyone, I suppose, to be in bed all day without any entertainment." M12

In addition, students mentioned acquiring cultural competencies in dealing with people with social problems and patients from other countries/ethnicities.

"On the other hand, I have been in contact with people who are drug addicts as a result of a serious social problem and with a major underlying mental illness." W4

"Respecting the patients' beliefs and cultures, always seeking their integration in the hospital." M7

4.1.3. Identifying with Nurses Who Dominate Their Environment and Are Close to the Patient in Complex and Dehumanized Units

The perceptions of nursing professionals in the context of the emergency department and ICU are presented in Table 3. All the students appreciated the warm welcome to the units, the involvement of the nurses who taught them and their "willingness to teach".

Table 3. Main categories, sub-categories and codes about the theme "identify with nurses who dominate their environment and are close to the patient in complex and dehumanized units".

Main Codes	Sub-Categories	Categories
A warm welcome Motivation for teaching Integration of students into the team	Attitude of nurses towards students	Attitude of the nurses
Control of complex environment Autonomy/initiative Not overwhelmed Acting calmly in emergencies High pressure to provide care	Nursing activity work environment	Nurses' Actions
Reassuring attitude Informational role Close ties to the patient and family	Attending to patients	
Identifying nurses who are humane Learning by imitation of good practice Identifying each professional's style	Professional Identification: I want to be	Nurses as models
Contempt towards patients Poor education	Professional rejection: I don't want to be	
Highly technical services High complexity High care pressure (emergencies) Depersonalized services	Complex and dehumanized services	Characteristics of services
Paying attention to pain Listening more to patients Quieter and less noisy environment Improving communication Emotional support Improve use of the emergency service Limiting mobile phone use	As it should be	

"I've discovered a part of nursing that's exciting and that, if there's one thing professionals have in this service, it's passion and drive." W1

In addition, the students were grateful for the nurses' attitudes.

"On a day-to-day basis in the special services, doubts and learning opportunities arose in which the nurses were always willing to help and explain things to me." M6

Both female and male students identified the emergency department and ICU as highly technical and labor-intensive environments. They also appreciated that nurses in these units worked more independently and autonomously than their colleagues in other units, e.g., inpatient units, and that they fulfill an important role in informing and reassuring patients:

"They are in control of the complexity of the situation at all times, always preventing it from overwhelming them." W3

"Nurses are not only the professionals who know how to inject, administer medication or put a bandage on. The most important thing is to know how to listen and be close to their patients, who at certain times only need someone close by, to feel their support and understanding." M7

4.1.4. How to Improve Care in Critically Ill Patients and How to Support the Families

Both female and male students recognized that patients in these units presented very specific pathologies, which involved advanced practice care. They also understood the importance of informing and explaining the techniques to the patients in advance, as a measure to reassure them and avoid conflicts, especially due to long waits in the emergency department (Table 4). In this overall context, the students identified a certain depersonalization in patient care and proposed a more humane treatment, with simple verbal and non-verbal communication actions, such as calling each patient by their name or holding their hand.

Table 4. Main categories, sub-categories and codes about the theme "how to improve care for critically ill patients and support their families".

Main Codes	Sub-Categories	Categories
Highly complex patients Severity	Patient characteristics	Negative patient experience
Concerned Nervous	Negative emotions	
Informing appropriately Favorable environment Conveying reassurance Making the effort to listen	Professional care	Necessary actions with patients
Humanization Facilitate rest and comfort Guaranteeing privacy	Humanized care	
Offering trust and support Reassuring Providing information Stressful situation	Support for families	Actions with families
Interaction with professionals/students Facilitating a pleasant environment Strong emotional impact	Visit	

Regarding the families, all stressed the importance of adequately addressing their needs, creating a climate of trust and support, as they are under great pressure. The information that they receive plays an important role in this relationship as it can help to reassure them (Table 4). Both female and male students identified the importance of visiting times and how students and professionals should act during these encounters.

"Always showing them that we are there and that they can trust us to take care of their relatives." W3

"From my point of view I think it is important that the moment of family visits be as comfortable as possible for the relatives and the patient." M1

Lastly, several male and female students stressed the importance of reinforcing training on humanization in care before the start of the placements.

4.2. Differences in the Experiences of Clinical Practices in Critical Services by Gender

Female students reflected on a much more intense and negative emotional experience, linked to the environment of critical care practices with critically ill patients or by identification with young patients. Personal gratification after providing emotional care to patients was also common, as was concern for ensuring the best care:

"I have realized that if you treat them with affection and try to help them in any way you can, not only are they very grateful to you, but you also go home with a good feeling, and knowing that your work has served a purpose." W10

"Since we also usually have to make decisions or act very quickly which sometimes made me nervous because it can lead to confusion very easily." W13

However, for male students, perceived satisfaction was related to the identification of emergency department and ICU as an employment option.

"I must admit that it was the rotation that I enjoyed by far the most, especially in the area of emergencies, so I am seriously considering continuing to study to work in this type of care area in the future." M2

"The student's autonomy has to take a step forward in order to prepare for the professional world." M8

In relation to competencies, the majority of female students stated that the techniques were not the most important aspect but rather the provision of basic care, such as those related to comfort, rest or pain relief.

"Anyone with training can channel a venous line or perform an electrocardiogram. As a nurse, you are there to support that person, reassure them, and accompany them in their distress. Sometimes the best cure is a smile, a hand on the shoulder or an "I'm there for you."" W15

"Here, I learned how to take care of a patient, to keep an eye on him all the time, to wash him, to comb his hair, to take care of his nails... things that are less technical and more humane." W8

However, the male students gave importance to specific knowledge, such as how to change shifts properly or how to adapt to changing environments. The importance of teamwork was mentioned by virtually all male students.

"I see it as very important to be able to give shift changes in a proper manner. I have paid a lot of attention to those who, in my opinion, perform good shift changes and I have tried to assimilate this way of working." M3

"Teamwork, the willingness to always help one's partner is one of the attitudes that I have encouraged during the rotation, there is no "so-and-so's patient", we are all there for everyone and we help each other with everything." M10

In terms of identifying with the nurses and the environment in these units, several female students reflected on attitudes that caused them to feel rejection and that they did not want to imitate.

"I have learned how I do not want to work in terms of how some health professionals describe and treat patients, not respecting their privacy, making value judgments and talking about patients in a derogatory way." W7

Finally, in relation to patients, the female students outlined the negative feelings perceived in patients with great detail (e.g., fear, nervousness, stress, worry) and the importance of ensuring intimacy.

"People who are conscious, in addition to their illness, are afraid and isolated and alone." W7

"From my point of view and according to what I have been able to learn while I was there, we can and must guarantee assistance, always respecting the patient's physical and emotional intimacy." W3

5. Discussion

According to the results of our study, for the nursing students, clinical practice in the emergency department and ICU implied an intense emotional experience, demanding the importance of attitudes towards the techniques. The profile of the nurses highlighted their human nature and their role as a reference for students in these complex units with high care demands. They also identified the need to adequately inform and support critical patients and their families. Differences were detected between female and male students regarding the experience during this clinical training.

RLJs have been a useful tool for learning more about the experience of nursing students in complex units. Some authors [3,8] had already reflected on the usefulness of the journal as a method for venting and expressing feelings and for stimulating personal growth during the process of becoming a nurse [13,28]. Moreover, writing can be considered a therapeutic tool, in the same way as it is for patients admitted to ICU [29], and it can be useful for nursing students facing stressful situations such the emergency department and ICU [30,31].

The expectation surrounding these placements was very similar to that described by other authors: nervousness and worry before facing a new post, the need to apply knowledge and techniques previously explained in theory and progressive confidence and security over time [32]. In our case, this transition could be affected by the complexity and severity of the patients in specific services, which could accentuate the expression of negative feelings, which became evident during a very intense emotional experience [3,17,28].

The students expressed the same feelings that the patients displayed: nerves, fear, freezing up in urgent situations, etc. [32,33], as if they were acting as a mirror reflecting the same negative emotional reaction, whereas the nurses assumed a reassuring and controlling role in the situation, as identified by both male and female students.

Student autonomy in complex services is limited [5], thus generating greater dependence on the nursing preceptor and greater observation of his/her clinical performance. The students in our study, as in other reports [34], have felt supported by the nurses during their clinical practices, who have integrated them into the team. During the process of becoming a nurse, which is more complex than simply having practical knowledge or skills [19,35], it is very important for students to have models and feel supported and accompanied during the mentoring process. The importance of this mentoring should be emphasized, not only through the nurse preceptors in the practice units but also on behalf of the university faculty, accompanying the students throughout the process, especially during the senior year [13]. To achieve this objective, it could be very useful to integrate this reflexive student learning into the creation of an environment of mutual trust and growth between teacher and student [10,12]. It is also important to consider the working conditions in these units, where high care loads and staff shortages can make it difficult for nurses to teach [36].

Both through the attitudes learned and the nursing care observed in the units, the humanization of care was essential. The students assigned great importance to respecting patients and the need to attend to their feelings and demonstrate empathy. Indeed, developing an empathic attitude is one of the fundamental pillars of the relationship between health professionals and patients/families [37]. Sensitivity to patient suffering was increased in our study since they were in a hostile environment, where patients were vulnerable, separated from their families and almost entirely dependent on the health professional, from making a rapid and effective diagnosis in the emergency unit to covering a human being's basic needs in the ICU. Most of the plans for the ICU integrate the elements proposed by students, which is positive since it shows a growing awareness among future nursing professionals to improve the environment in these units [38].

In general, our results coincide with research conducted in Spain on RLJs as an assessment tool during the learning process of nursing students [11]. Many of the journals included reflections on the techniques but also frequently addressed patient and family related care, interactions with the team and the nurse preceptor and even death. Moreover, this study mentions very interesting aspects, such as the importance of providing clear guidelines for the implementation of these journals, the figure of the teacher as a guide in the process of reflection within the framework of a relationship of trust and the importance of assigning importance to the evaluation, in the understanding that, if it is proposed as a voluntary activity, students generally fail to participate.

In our study, a different experience was found among female and male students. The female students described their negative feelings in more detail during the clinical training and showed a more reflective attitude. This reality could be related to a greater ease of expressing emotions among the women, whereas the men may have had similar experiences or thoughts, although they may have ultimately decided not to include them in the journal or not to delve into the experience.

Regarding the competences achieved, female students focused more on the humanization of care whereas male students more frequently mentioned aspects linked to their individual learning or organizational aspects in these units. This different approach by gender coincides with the results observed in nurses working in the ICU [39]. Further research is necessary to better understand these differences and to assess whether students may be imitating or reproducing the model identified by the nurse preceptors.

Female students were also more concerned about poor patient progression or fear of making mistakes, which is consistent with the study by Fernandez-Feito et al., [21] where female students considered it more important to seek help when they could not meet patient needs.

5.1. Implications for Clinical Practice

Enhancing the use of these reflective tools can contribute to a better understanding of the experience of nursing students during their clinical placements and encourage personal and professional growth, which is difficult to achieve through theoretical training. In addition, it would be important to encourage male students to share their experience and their personal feelings. After being aware of this experience, it would be appropriate to design interventions to reduce the associated emotional impact and provide the students with strategies (e.g., coping styles) to reduce anxiety or negative feelings.

In turn, teachers and nurse preceptors play a key role in accompanying the student in the process of "becoming" a nurse, and, in this process, creating and sharing a reflective narrative (student–preceptor–teacher) can be very helpful.

5.2. Limitations

In our study, the RLJ represented a percentage of the final grade. It would be very interesting to comment on the narratives with the students in a session not only aimed at modifying the assigned grade but also analyzing the overall experience in these services, as a group. The differences found according to gender should be interpreted with caution since the analysis was not performed blinded to the students' genders, which may have biased the interpretation of the results. The results obtained were not subjected to the process of triangulation with other techniques, such as individual interviews or focus groups with students; this will be addressed in future research.

6. Conclusions

For nursing students, clinical practices in emergency department and ICU represent an intense emotional experience that allows them to improve their learning and cope with complex environments. In addition to acquiring new knowledge and refining already learned techniques, these clinical practices allow students to acquire attitudes clearly linked to the humanization of care. Female and male students experienced these clinical rotations from different viewpoints. Female students were more emotionally and reflectively focused on patient care, whereas male students identified more with individual aspects of learning and the organization and quality of the units.

Author Contributions: Conceptualization, M.G.-G. and A.F.-F.; methodology, M.G.-G., A.L. and A.F.-F.; formal analysis, M.G.-G., Y.V.-Á. and A.F.-F.; data collection, P.Z.-M., Y.V.-Á. and A.F.-F.; writing—original draft preparation, M.G.-G., A.L., Y.V.-Á., P.Z.-M. and A.F.-F.; writing—review and editing, A.L. and A.F.-F. All authors have read and agreed to the published version of the manuscript.

Funding: This research was supported by grants from the Instituto de Salud Carlos III, Spanish State Secretary of R+D+I, Fondo Europeo de Desarrollo Regional (FEDER) and Fondo Social Europeo (FSE) (grant number PI18/00086) and the Health Research Institute of Asturias (ISPA). The study funders had no role in the study design or in the collection, analysis or interpretation of data, and the authors have sole responsibility for the manuscript content.

Acknowledgments: We would like to thank all the senior nursing students for their reflections and the nurse preceptors at the emergency department and ICU for their contribution to the training of these students.

Conflicts of Interest: The authors declare no conflict of interest.

References

1. Kajander-Unkuri, S.; Salminen, L.; Saarikoski, M.; Suhonen, R.; Leino-Kilpi, H. Competence Areas of Nursing Students in Europe. *Nurse Educ. Today* **2013**, *33*, 625–632. [CrossRef]
2. Levett-Jones, T.; Pitt, V.; Courtney-Pratt, H.; Harbrow, G.; Rossiter, R. What are the primary concerns of nursing students as they prepare for and contemplate their first clinical placement experience? *Nurse Educ. Pract.* **2015**, *15*, 304–309. [CrossRef] [PubMed]
3. Mlinar Reljić, N.; Pajnkihar, M.; Fekonja, Z. Self-reflection during first clinical practice: The experiences of nursing students. *Nurse Educ. Today* **2019**, *72*, 61–66. [CrossRef] [PubMed]
4. Mahlanze, H.T.; Sibiya, M.N. Perceptions of student nurses on the writing of reflective journals as a means for personal, professional and clinical learning development. *Health SA Gesondheid.* **2017**, *22*, 79–86. [CrossRef]
5. Vatansever, N.; Akansel, N. Intensive Care Unit Experience of Nursing Students during their Clinical Placements: A Qualitative Study. *Int. J. Caring Sci.* **2016**, *9*, 1040–1048.
6. Bongar, M.V.V.; Pangan, F.C.; Macindo, J.R.B. Characteristics of a critical care clinical placement programme affecting critical care nursing competency of baccalaureate nursing students: A structural equation modelling. *J. Clin. Nurs.* **2019**, *28*, 1760–1770. [CrossRef]
7. Fernández-Peña, R.; Fuentes-Pumarola, C.; Malagón-Aguilera, M.C.; Bonmatí-Tomàs, A.; Bosch-Farré, C.; Ballester-Ferrando, D. The evaluation of reflective learning from the nursing student's point of view: A mixed method approach. *Nurse Educ. Today* **2016**, *44*, 59–65. [CrossRef]
8. Schön, D.A. *La Formación de Profesionales Reflexivos: Hacia un Nuevo Diseño de la Formación y el Aprendizaje en las Profesiones*; Ediciones Paidós: Madrid, Spain, 1992.
9. Bagnato, S.; Valerio, D.; Lorenza, G. The reflective journal: A tool for enhancing experience- based learning in nursing students in clinical practice. *J. Nurs. Educ. Pract.* **2013**, *3*, 102–111. [CrossRef]

10. Ruiz-López, M.; Rodríguez-García, M.; Villanueva, P.G.; Márquez-Cava, M.; García-Mateos, M.; Ruiz-Ruiz, B.; Herrera-Sánchez, E. The use of reflective journaling as a learning strategy during the clinical rotations of students from the faculty of health sciences: An action-research study. *Nurse Educ. Today* **2015**, *35*, e26–e31. [CrossRef]

11. San Rafael Gutiérrez, S. El Diario de Prácticas Clínicas Como Herramienta de Evaluación de los Procesos de Enseñanza Aprendizaje de los Alumnos de Enfermería. Ph.D. Thesis, Universidad de Alicante, Alicante, Spain, 2016.

12. Dahl, H.; Eriksen, K.Å. Students' and teachers' experiences of participating in the reflection process "THiNK". *Nurse Educ. Today* **2016**, *36*, 401–406. [CrossRef]

13. Bjerkvik, L.K.; Hilli, Y. Reflective writing in undergraduate clinical nursing education: A literature review. *Nurse Educ. Pract.* **2019**, *35*, 32–41. [CrossRef] [PubMed]

14. Rodriguez García, M.; Ruiz López, M.; González Sanz, P.; Fernandez Trinidad, M.; De Blas Gómez, I. Experiencias y vivencias del estudiante de 4° de enfermería en el practicum. *Cult. Cuid.* **2014**, *18*, 25–33. [CrossRef]

15. García-Carpintero Blas, E.; Siles-González, J.; Martínez-Roche, E. Percepciones de los estudiantes sobre sus vivencias en las prácticas clínicas. *Enferm. Univ.* **2019**, *16*, 259–268.

16. Naber, J.; Markley, L. A guide to nursing students' written reflections for students and educators. *Nurse Educ. Pract.* **2017**, *25*, 1–4. [CrossRef] [PubMed]

17. Sun, F.K.; Long, A.; Tseng, Y.S.; Huang, H.M.; You, J.H.; Chiang, C.Y. Undergraduate student nurses' lived experiences of anxiety during their first clinical practicum: A phenomenological study. *Nurse Educ. Today* **2016**, *37*, 21–26. [CrossRef]

18. Reis, S.P.; Wald, H.S.; Monroe, A.D.; Borkan, J.M. Begin the BEGAN (The Brown Educational Guide to the Analysis of Narrative)—A framework for enhancing educational impact of faculty feedback to students' reflective writing. *Patient Educ. Couns.* **2010**, *80*, 253–259. [CrossRef]

19. Teskereci, G.; Boz, İ. "I try to act like a nurse": A phenomenological qualitative study. *Nurse Educ. Pract.* **2019**, *37*, 39–44. [CrossRef]

20. Westin, L.; Sundler, A.J.; Berglund, M. Students' experiences of learning in relation to didactic strategies during the first year of a nursing programme: A qualitative study. *BMC Med. Educ.* **2015**, *15*, 1–8. [CrossRef]

21. Fernández-Feito, A.; Basurto Hoyuelos, S.; Palmeiro Longo, M.G.D.V. Differences in professional values between nurses and nursing students: A gender perspective. *Int. Nurs. Rev.* **2019**, *66*, 577–589. [CrossRef]

22. Luciani, M.; Rampoldi, G.; Ardenghi, S.; Bani, M.; Merati, S.; Ausili, D.; Strepparava, M.G.; Di Mauro, S. Personal values among undergraduate nursing students: A cross-sectional study. *Nurs. Ethics* **2020**. [CrossRef]

23. Hoffart, N.; McCoy, T.P.; Lewallen, L.P.; Thorpe, S. Differences in Gender-related Profile Characteristics, Perceptions, and Outcomes of Accelerated Second Degree Nursing Students. *J. Prof. Nurs.* **2019**, *35*, 93–100. [CrossRef] [PubMed]

24. McDonald, J. Conforming to and Resisting Dominant Gender Norms: How Male and Female Nursing Students Do and Undo Gender. *Gend. Work Organ.* **2013**, *20*, 561–579. [CrossRef]

25. Elo, S.; Kyngäs, H. The qualitative content analysis process. *J. Adv. Nurs.* **2008**, *62*, 107–115. [CrossRef] [PubMed]

26. Vaismoradi, M.; Turunen, H.; Bondas, T. Content analysis and thematic analysis: Implications for conducting a qualitative descriptive study. *Nurs. Health Sci.* **2013**, *15*, 398–405. [CrossRef]

27. Graneheim, U.H.; Lundman, B. Qualitative content analysis in nursing research: Concepts, procedures and measures to achieve trustworthiness. *Nurse Educ. Today* **2004**, *24*, 105–112. [CrossRef]

28. Siles González, J.; Solano Ruiz, M.C.; Noreña Peña, A.; Gabán Gutiérrez, A.; Gil Estevan, M.D.; Martínez Sabater, A.; Núñez del Castillo, M.; Ferrer Hernández, M.E.; Rocamora Salort, F.; Fernández Molina, M.A.; et al. *XII Jornadas de Redes de Investigación en Docencia Universitaria: El reconocimiento Docente: Innovar e Investigar con Criterios de Calidad*; Percepción de los alumnos de enfermería de las unidades especiales a través de sus diarios; Universidad de Alicante: Alicante, Spain, 2014; pp. 510–525.

29. Nydahl, P.; Fischill, M.; Deffner, T.; Neudeck, V.; Heindl, P. Diaries for intensive care unit patients reduce the risk for psychological sequelae: Systematic literature review and meta-analysis. *Med. Klin. Intensivmed. Notfmed.* **2019**, *114*, 68–76. [CrossRef]

30. Walton, J.A.; Lindsay, N.; Hales, C.; Rook, H. Glimpses into the transition world: New graduate nurses' written reflections. *Nurse Educ. Today* **2018**, *60*, 62–66. [CrossRef]

31. Alteren, J. Narratives in student nurses' knowledge development: A hermeneutical research study. *Nurse Educ. Today* **2019**, *76*, 51–55. [CrossRef]

32. Alonso-Ovies, Á.; La Calle, G.H. Icu: A branch of hell? *Intensive Care Med.* **2016**, *42*, 591–592. [CrossRef]

33. Johnson, C.C.; Suchyta, M.R.; Darowski, E.S.; Collar, E.M.; Kiehl, A.L.; Van, J.; Jackson, J.C.; Hopkins, R.O. Psychological Sequelae in Family Caregivers of Critically Ill Intensive Care Unit Patients. A Systematic Review. *Ann. Am. Thorac. Soc.* **2019**, *16*, 894–909. [CrossRef]

34. Álvarez Teruel, J.D.; Tortosa Ybánez, M.T.; Pellín Buades, N. *Investigación y Propuestas Innovadoras de Redes Universidad de Alicante Para la Mejora Docente*; El diario de prácticas clínicas en la unidad de cuidados intensivos; Universidad de Alicante: Alicante, Spain, 2015; pp. 1665–1676.

35. Sandvik, A.H.; Eriksson, K.; Hilli, Y. Becoming a caring nurse—A Nordic study on students' learning and development in clinical education. *Nurse Educ. Pract.* **2014**, *14*, 286–292. [CrossRef]

36. Rodríguez García, M.C. Percepción de los estudiantes del Grado en Enfermería sobre su entorno de prácticas clínicas: Un estudio fenomenológico. *Enferm. Clin.* **2019**, *29*, 264–270. [CrossRef] [PubMed]

37. Moreto, G.; González Blasco, P.; Piñero, A. Reflections on dehumanisation in medical education: Empathy, emotions, and possible pedagogical resources for the emotional education of the medical student. *Educ. Med.* **2018**, *19*, 172–177. [CrossRef]

38. Rojas, V. Humanización de los cuidados intensivos. *Rev. Méd. Clín. Condes* **2019**, *30*, 120–125. [CrossRef]

39. Via Clavero, G.; Sanjuán Naváis, M.; Martínez Mesas, M.; Pena Alfaro, M.; Utrilla Antolín, C.; Zarragoikoetxea Jáuregui, I. Identidad de género y cuidados intensivos: Influencia de la masculinidad y la feminidad en la percepción de los cuidados enfermeros. *Enferm. Intensiva* **2010**, *21*, 104–112. [CrossRef] [PubMed]

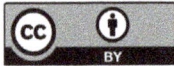

International Journal of
*Environmental Research
and Public Health*

MDPI

Article

Experiences of Nursing Students during the Abrupt Change from Face-to-Face to e-Learning Education during the First Month of Confinement Due to COVID-19 in Spain

Antonio Jesús Ramos-Morcillo [1], César Leal-Costa [1,*], José Enrique Moral-García [2,*]
and María Ruzafa-Martínez [1]

[1] Faculty of Nursing, University of Murcia, 30100 Murcia, Spain; ajramos@um.es (A.J.R.-M.);
    maruzafa@um.es (M.R.-M.)
[2] Physical Activity and Sports Sciences, Faculty of Education, Pontifical University of Salamanca,
    Street Henry Collet, 52-70, 37007 Salamanca, Spain
* Correspondence: cleal@um.es (C.L.-C.); jemoralga@upsa.es (J.E.M.-G.)

check for
updates

Received: 4 July 2020; Accepted: 29 July 2020; Published: 30 July 2020

Abstract: The current state of alarm due to the COVID-19 pandemic has led to the urgent change in the education of nursing students from traditional to distance learning. The objective of this study was to discover the learning experiences and the expectations about the changes in education, in light of the abrupt change from face-to-face to e-learning education, of nursing students enrolled in the Bachelor's and Master's degree of two public Spanish universities during the first month of confinement due to the COVID-19 pandemic. Qualitative study was conducted during the first month of the state of alarm in Spain (from 25 March–20 April 2020). Semi-structured interviews were given to students enrolled in every academic year of the Nursing Degree, and nurses who were enrolled in the Master's programs at two public universities. A maximum variation sampling was performed, and an inductive thematic analysis was conducted. The study was reported according with COREQ checklist. Thirty-two students aged from 18 to 50 years old participated in the study. The interviews lasted from 17 to 51 min. Six major themes were defined: (1) practicing care; (2) uncertainty; (3) time; (4) teaching methodologies; (5) context of confinement and added difficulties; (6) face-to-face win. The imposition of e-learning sets limitations for older students, those who live in rural areas, with work and family responsibilities and with limited electronic resources. Online education goes beyond a continuation of the face-to-face classes. Work should be done about this for the next academic year as we face an uncertain future in the short-term control of COVID-19.

Keywords: COVID-19; pandemics; students; nursing; teaching; education; distance; schools; Life Changing Events; qualitative research

1. Introduction

The fast propagation of the severe acute respiratory syndrome coronavirus 2 (SARS-CoV-2) led to its definition as a pandemic on 13 March 2020 by the WHO [1], as it met the epidemiological criteria and had infected more than 100,000 people in 100 countries [2–4]. The main public health recommendation was to remain at home and stay safe within it [5]. The world, in a globalized manner, is facing an extraordinary public health emergency in which the nurses are, as always, on the front line. Challenges are even greater in this period of pandemic [6,7], and nurses have the knowledge and aptitudes for providing the care necessary in the different clinical scenarios [5] that are emerging.

However, this pandemic is not only affecting the area of health. A great part of the nursing activity is affected as well. In Spain, as well as in other countries, the presence of nursing students in health care centers has been suspended [5]. It has been observed how, at great speeds, schools and universities have closed in the world, affecting more than 1.570 million students in 191 countries [8]. It has been necessary to decide how to continue the education of future nurses, and multiple education solutions have been deployed, all of which are based on distance learning. The professors, experts in the subjects and knowledgeable about the didactics of traditional classes, have found themselves compelled to deal with e-learning overnight, although not all of them were prepared. The same has occurred with the students, who have had to change from a model based on obligations and face-to-face learning, to a model in which the students will have to freely and voluntarily become involved in their learning [9]. All of this aside from finding themselves in a context of expectation and uncertainty.

Nursing educators (teachers, managers) must guarantee that the students meet the academic requirements, and at the same time, recognize the current conditions faced by the health services and the needs of simultaneously satisfying the demands from students, parents, brothers, partners, and the multiple roles every individual play in their day-to-day lives. Internationally and locally, a great variety of criteria for learning and evaluation, etc., have appeared, which are adapted to their national, work and social contexts. For example, and with respect to evaluation, in Berkeley (California, USA), a pass/fail grading has been proposed [10], and in Spain, the Association of Spanish Universities (CRUE) has recommended adapting the evaluation tests utilizing distance learning evaluation procedures [11].

Understanding the experiences and expectations of the students when faced with this important change, is necessary for helping the education and teaching authorities to assign sufficient resources and re-orient university education for nursing students. To be able to manage this situation in an imminent future, it is necessary to learn from these experiences and to define the strong and weak points. The objective of this study was to discover the learning experiences and the expectations about the changes in education of nursing students enrolled in the Bachelor's and Master's nursing degrees in two Spanish public universities, when faced with the abrupt change from face-to-face to e-learning education during the first month of confinement due to the COVID-19 pandemic.

2. Materials and Methods

2.1. Study Design

A qualitative approach was utilized, and an inductive thematic analysis [12] was conducted to understand the experiences and expectations of the participants.

2.2. Settings and Participants

This research study was conducted in its entirety during the first month of the state of alarm in Spain (which began on 14 March 2020). The state of alarm implied the confinement of the entire population, the closing of all the schools and universities, closing of non-essential businesses, closing of borders and ceasing all non-essential activities. The people were only allowed to go out to the street for essential matters: shopping of food, going to pharmacies, banks, and to care for older people who were dependent, etc.

In Spain, Bachelor's degree in Nursing has a duration of four years (240 European Credit Transfer System, ECTS) and it is common for a Master's degree to have a duration of one year (60 ECTS). The reference population in this study was students from every academic year in the Bachelor's degree in Nursing, or nurses who were conducting their Master's studies, enrolled in universities in Murcia and Granada (Spain). The participants were selected through the use of a maximum variation sampling strategy [13] to obtain heterogeneous and rich information that represented the main sociodemographic variables: gender, age, academic year, rural/urban, children, Bachelor's/Master's, university of Murcia and Granada. The maximum variation strategy is utilized to find the greatest diversity of discourses possible to identify and analyze the largest volume possible of expressions/presentation of the phenomenon studied to explain conditions/contexts where each one of them takes place.

If one did not answer the request, the students themselves proposed a replacement with another participant with similar characteristics. None of the students contacted disagreed to participate.

The students were invited to participate through the Student Delegation at the university, utilizing snowball sampling. This technique allowed us to build the sample by asking each interviewee for suggestions of people who had a similar or different perspective. This is an approach for locating information-rich key informants [13]. The saturation criterion was applied to establish the number of informants needed, an accepted method to estimate the sample size [14].

2.3. Data Collection

Semi-structured interviews were conducted to obtain the information. The semi-structured interview is normally based on a script, where the subject matter and part of the questions have been planned before starting, but it also offers the possibility of changing or adding new questions as the interview and/or the research study moves forward, with new interviews conducted. It is the most common type of interview utilized in qualitative research on health. Data were collected from 25 March to 20 April 2020. This was done in the first month as it the period of time with the greatest cognitive and social impact on learning and to obtain results that could be used to support, or not, the education measures that were utilized. All the interviews were individual and were performed online through electronic resources after agreeing on a day and time. The interviews were recorded and notes were made after each interview. All the interviews were conducted by researchers who had sufficient training and experience in semi-structured interviews (A.J.R.-M., M.R.-M.). The interviewers did not have an academic relationship with the informants. The interview followed a script which shifted from general to specific matters, and dealt with general aspects of the confinement, teaching methodologies utilized, learning and expectations (Table A1). A prior pilot study of the script was conducted [15].

2.4. Data Analysis

The 6 phases proposed for the thematic analysis were followed [16]: (1) Familiarizing yourself with your data; (2) Generating initial codes; (3) Searching for themes; (4) Reviewing themes; (5) Defining and naming themes; (6) Producing the report. The recorded interviews were transcribed verbatim. Once transcribed, the interviews were imported to the MAXQDA 12 program for its posterior analysis. A.J.R.-M., M.R.-M., C.L.-C. and J.E.M.-G. coded the data. The transcriptions, coding and themes-subthemes were discussed by the research team for their verification. Finally, participants provided feedback on the findings. The study was reported according to the Consolidated Criteria for Reporting Qualitative Research (COREQ) [15].

2.5. Ethical Considerations

This research study was approved by the Research Ethics Commission from the University of Murcia (ID: 2800/2020). All the participants received an informational electronic document about the purpose and research process, which they later kept. They were advised that their participation was voluntary. They could ask and reflect prior to the interview. Each participant was given a code to maintain anonymity.

3. Results

A total of 32 interviews were conducted, and they lasted between 17 and 51 min. The shortest interviews corresponded to the more advanced academic years (3rd and 4th year students). Of these participants, 75% were women and 25% men. The age of the participants oscillated between 18–50 years old, with an average age of 25.3, and with a participation rate of 69% for the students from the University of Murcia, and 21.8% for the University of Granada students. The sample was composed by 18.75% of the students enrolled in their 1st or 2nd academic year or in the Master's program, which accounted for about 57% of the sample, and 21.8% from the 3rd and 4th academic years, for a total of about 43%. Of those interviewed, 21.8% had children and 21.8% lived in a rural setting. Some of the characteristics of the participants are found in Table 1.

Table 1. Characteristics of the participants and duration of the interviews.

N°	Gender	Age	University	Degree Year	Working	Interview Duration
1	Woman	20	Murcia	2	No	39 min
2	Woman	19	Murcia	2	No	50 min
3	Woman	21	Murcia	4	No	20 min
4	Woman	21	Murcia	4	No	20 min
5	Woman	28	Granada	1	Yes	38 min
6	Man	21	Granada	3	No	20 min
7	Woman	19	Granada	1	No	36 min
8	Woman	41	Murcia	1	Yes	38 min
9	Woman	50	Murcia	3	No	35 min
10	Woman	21	Granada	4	No	23 min
11	Woman	20	Murcia	2	No	51 min
12	Man	32	Murcia	4	Yes	23 min
13	Woman	19	Granada	2	No	37 min
14	Woman	22	Granada	4	No	19 min
15	Man	21	Murcia	4	No	17 min
16	Woman	20	Granada	1	No	28 min
17	Woman	46	Murcia	2	No	40 min
18	Woman	25	Murcia	3	No	31 min
19	Woman	20	Murcia	3	No	31 min
20	Woman	25	Murcia	1	Yes	29 min
21	Woman	26	Murcia	4	No	18 min
22	Man	24	Murcia	Master	Yes	25 min
23	Woman	23	Granada	Master	Yes	28 min
24	Man	22	Granada	Master	No	29 min
25	Woman	18	Murcia	1	No	33 min
26	Man	42	Murcia	3	No	29 min
27	Man	26	Murcia	3	No	30 min
28	Woman	24	Murcia	Master	Yes	30 min
29	Man	26	Murcia	3	No	30 min
30	Woman	20	Murcia	2	No	35 min
31	Woman	24	Granada	Master	No	26 min
32	Woman	26	Murcia	Master	No	36 min

Six major themes were defined: (1) practicing the nursing care; (2) uncertainty; (3) time; (4) teaching methodologies; (5) the context of confinement and the added difficulties; (6) face-to-face education win. A detailed description of the themes and sub-themes can be found in Table 2.

Table 2. Themes and subthemes.

Themes	Subthemes
Practicing the nursing care	The value of clinical training
	To help
Uncertainty	-
Time	Phases: 1st shock and 2nd normalization
	Time management
	The future
Teaching methodologies	Videoconference
	The rest of the methodologies
	Use profile of the methodologies by the professors
	Interaction with the teachers
The context of confinement and the added difficulties	-
Face-to-face win	Face-to-face is better … for everything
	Older and female: face-to-face is better

3.1. Practicing Nursing Care

The outstandingly practical component of care in nursing education was the most emotional aspect for the students. The experiences found were differentiated according to the group of students, depending if they had or not practice-based subjects during the education period affected by the state of alarm, the proximity to ending their training as nurses, or if they were health professionals who were conducting post-graduate studies.

3.1.1. The Value of Clinical Training

For 1st and 2nd year students, the learning is normally done with courses that are eminently theoretical or theory/practical. The informants indicated that this transitory e-learning will not have a special influence on their training, as long as all the clinical training on health care institutions is present:

> *"In think that it's not something that will affect us excessively for good or bad. In my year [1st]. In other years it will, because they have clinical training" P5*

By contrast, 3rd and 4th year students whose coursework is mainly based on clinical training in health care institutions placed value on clinical training. They linked it with the acquisition of competences and referred to it as being an essential part of health sciences degrees:

> *"My education would not be good if clinical training was missing" P15; "without the clinical training, we can't acquire competences" P19; "Especially in our degree, the clinical training … " P21*

Clinical training provides them with security in the learning of nursing care in health care services. Part of the students in their last year (4th year) indicated that they would rather not graduate in July to do all the clinical training, therefore graduating later:

> *"I don't feel prepared. My Erasmus in Italy was really bad because I was a nursing student and a foreigner. At the hospital, I don't feel confident" P10; "Some of us prefer not to graduate in June and to do the clinical training" P14*

The Master's students indicated that not being able to do the clinical training implied the loss of job opportunities:

> *"If you cannot do the clinical training, you will lose job opportunities" P22*

3.1.2. To Help

All the participants expressed their wish to help during the pandemic. They expressed their desire to be nurses to help. At the University of Granada, a list of volunteers in their 4th year was even created. The expectation was present that the government could mobilize them in case of need. Independently of the academic year, for all the students, this crisis re-enforced their wishes to become nurses:

"I wish I already had my degree" P17; "I wish to be a nurse already, too bad I wasn't in 4th year so I could go" P16; "If this happens in the future, I would like to be helping" P25; "I feel like left out, I can't be in the battlefield helping" P21; "Now I really feel like being a nurse. It is a shame that we cannot help. In Granada there is a list of volunteers. I really feel like helping" P14

Master's students who work feel satisfied to be able to help (aside from being satisfied because they can work):

"I feel very well with myself because I can help, even though is very difficult ... " P23; "I really feel like being in the middle of it and help. I've seen that help is really needed, it is very important work, although not very much appreciated." P24

3.2. Uncertainty

The lack of concretion about the different aspects related with their studies is mentioned by all the interviewees. This uncertainty is accompanied by unpleasant situations due to the possible outcomes. They are mainly related with matters that could not be resolved relatively fast, such as the clinical practice and the adaptation of evaluation processes:

"We don't know how they are going to evaluate us. They will for sure evaluate what we have done in the last month of clinical practices" P6; "We don't know what's going to happen. I hope they don't give a general pass. I want to take the exams and the other things. I don't want them to evaluate me with just one work submitted" P5; "Not knowing how things will be done. Not getting the grades I want to get because of these circumstances" P16

This is especially important for the 4th-year students, who reported a great feeling of wasting time. They cannot go to the clinical practices and they only have, as well, one subject: the final project (TFG). One of the alternatives to not waste time completely and that is being done by the participants is to prepare for the access exam for clinical nurse specialist training (national post-graduate residency program, EIR). Some of the participants indicated that preparing for the EIR exam was a means of escape from a situation of wasting time and total paralysis:

"It takes my motivation away, and (finishing my degree) is getting really hard, because I don't see the end of it" P10; "I am not taking advantage of the time" P3; "I'm preparing for the EIR exam at the academy as a means of escape. With the only the TFG ... I need something else. Right now all my time is TFG and the subjects from the EIR" P4

The 3rd-year students find themselves in the same situation but without any subjects:

"The 3rd years clinical training has been abandoned. They don't know if we are going to recover them" P6

The Masters' students have a different point of view. The differences are many. The Masters' degree can provide job opportunities, the change from traditional education to e-learning practically affects an entire trimester (half of the Master's program), and in their discourse, they have fewer demands and less pressure for obtaining the degree. At the same time, they are the only ones who speak about the teaching guidelines, indicating that they are truly being followed. In comparison, only one Bachelor's degree student referred to the teaching guidelines:

"If the clinical training cannot be done, you miss job opportunities" P22; "I don't know how the teaching guidelines have changed" P16; "The clinical training have been postponed until September, and it bothers me some because it interferes with the summer contract for working as a nurse" P24

3.3. Time

Time is a determinant transversal aspect. Two differentiated phases are observed as the state of alarm moved forward (1st shock and 2nd normalization). Besides, participants reflected regarding a necessary time management and the influence in the future.

3.3.1. Phases: 1st Shock and 2nd Normalization

Two well-differentiated phases are distinguished in the timeline. On the first days, the shock phase appears (1st phase), within which we find "disorientation". This first phase lasts between 7–10 days. During this first week, it is observed that mental performance decreases, along with the ability to concentrate. This is a subtle expectant phase, where the situations are not well defined:

"You think that the first week is for you, for resting, you take care of unfinished business and uncertainty increases" P11; "The first week was not assimilated, I didn't have routines" P19; "During the first week, I had less concentration and studies less" P5; "The timetable is different, it's more chaotic" P21

After the first phase, the students enter a normalization phase (2nd phase) in which they acquire new routines, attend online classes and seminars. The conditions of confinement start to be assimilated and the new everyday life is normalized:

"Now I do more things than before, I take more notes. It is very different from the first week, now it is easier" P25; "Now I have the habits. Before I didn't do anything, and now I do everything, it is as if I'm getting used to it" P28

The first phase, as well as the second phase also coincide with the period in which the university ensured that the online tools were fully functioning and instructions were given to the professors about how to continue with their teaching tasks:

"Only 2 out of 5 teachers give online classes, the rest upload presentations that we have to understand" P13; "The teachers do not agree with each other. One says one thing and another something else" P6

3.3.2. Time Management

The 1st and 2nd year students, as well as the Masters' students, have classes. This forces them to manage their time differently. The 1st and 2nd year students interviewed indicated that time management was necessary. They indicated that this was beneficial for having good "mental health", and that having due dates helped them with managing their time:

"Having self-discipline and a timetable. Not rigid, but saying that the mornings were for University and the afternoons for watching T.V. series or exercising. If you don't organize your time, work accumulates" P20; "My planning is Monday to Friday mornings for work, and the afternoon for group work or leisure. I rest on the weekends. Having due dates has helped me organize" P13; "The homework is good, because they help with following the course" P11

All of the participants, except for the ones who worked, indicated that they had changed their sleep schedule and go to bed much later, between 1:30 and 3 a.m. The main reason mentioned was that the lack of activity did not make them tired, although this argument was ambivalent, as they went to bed later and got up later as well, so they slept the same number of hours:

"It takes me longer to fall sleep. I'm not tired because I don't do anything during the day" P11; "I go to bed later and I get up later. I go to bed at 2–2:30 a.m. and I get up at 10" P5; "I fall sleep very late. At 2:00 a.m. The hours have changed, you sleep when you shouldn't" P19

3.3.3. The Future

The participants indicate that this situation affects their future plans and expectations related with obtaining their degree and work. They believe that they can be singled out for being the promotion with missing education, their international training is paralyzed, and they are afraid. Their professional expectations are also affected:

> *"I'm afraid of having bad training and that the work exchange says that this year's promotion from the University of Granada do not have the competences necessary" P6; "The plans for earning money to go to an Erasmus program are cancelled ... " P13; "The practices have been postponed to September, and yes, it bothers me because it interferes with the summer contract for working as a nurse" P24*

3.4. Teaching Methodologies

The participants indicate that as for the teachers, different teaching methodologies are being utilized: real-time videoconferences (including chats), lessons recorded on video and uploaded to the e-learning platform, audio podcast, chat (exclusively), homework and uploading of documents (Word, PPT, PDF). They also mention that as time goes on, the teacher's adaptation to the online resources continuously improve.

3.4.1. Videoconference

It is without a doubt the best evaluated. This is because they think it is the most similar to a traditional class (face-to-face), and allow interaction with the professor, and provides them with nearness. Another aspect they indicate as being valuable is that this methodology helps with the teacher's explanation of the subject that is more comprehensible as compared to other methodologies. The interaction is also valued, as it allows them to say that something has not been understood and that it should be explained in another way. Lastly, they would like all the videoconferences to be recorded so they could be watched again whenever needed. This last aspect was pointed out by the students who were also working:

> *"The interaction in the videoconferences is not the same, because the questions are written and it is not the same to write something than when you talk" P26; "The videoconference is where we receive feedback. You can say that you don't understand something and if it could be explained once again" P16; "It is a way to stay in touch. Doubts emerge and the teacher can resolve them" P7*

The Master's students indicate that on some occasions, the duration of the videoconference classes is excessive. It is interesting to highlight that the Bachelor's students did not state this at any time:

> *"We've had videoconferences that lasted 5 h. This can be done better. We had one who did a good summary and it lasted 2 h. This is more relaxing, and then you broaden the knowledge with the documents provided" P24*

Despite the value of the videoconferences, the discourse is ambivalent, as negative aspects are identified, especially related with the quality of interaction with the professor. The traditional classwork contributes fundamental elements in the quality of communication, and this how it is felt by the participants.

> *"It is worse. When the teacher sees you asking about a doubt, she/he knows where you are coming from. This is lost with e-learning. Information is lost and the student does not obtain the same information as in the face-to-face class. The teacher doesn't see your face." P24; "I'm much more in favor of traditional classes. I always obtain more information in them and I'm more comfortable." P24*

3.4.2. The Rest of the Methodologies

Except for the recorded lessons, the rest of the methodologies are catalogued as sub-standard. The chats (exclusively) and the homework are not attractive, although they value them as positive aspects because it lets them stay connected with the subject and the university:

"The worse thing is when they only upload class notes, no one forces you to read them" P25; "In the homework, there are questions because they are not easy to understand, with the explanation it is easy, but when you are going to do it, it is more difficult" P25

Among the limitations, they point out that in some asynchronous methodologies and with a rigid format, limited learning is obtained, interaction is needed for explanation, and a certain amount of pressure is needed. Another limitation is the lack of feedback with the homework:

"We are going to learn the minimum, but not all, because they don't explain it to you, they don't explain it in different ways. The text [from the documents] is only written in one way ... " P7; "the works that don't have feedback give you half the knowledge" P13; "If you only upload notes, no one is forcing you to read them. It is very easy to fall into laziness when they only upload notes" P25

A limitation of e-learning that was pointed out by all the participants was that everything that was practice-related could not be learned. They identified this as a great limitation, and point out that in nursing, practice was vital:

"Many things are not understood through the computer. For example, the basic care laboratories have to be observed and practiced" P7; "The practical things not, but the theoretical yes. They can make a video, but it's not the same. They can tell us how to give a bath on a bed, but if you don't do it ... " P5; "It is impossible to learn the practical part. Until you are not in that role, it is impossible to learn" P24

The students are not able to propose other methodologies that are distinct from the ones offered. Two students pointed out that it could be completed with gamification (kahoot):

"Gamification would be good, for example when calculating the dose" P19

3.4.3. Use Profile of the Methodologies by the Teachers

Within the methodologies, it was found that the least complex, for example, providing Word, PPT or PDF documents, were related to the older teachers. The videoconferences and recorded classes were given by younger teachers in general. At the same time, they indicated that teachers from other non-nursing departments utilized the least complex methodologies:

"It depends on the difficulty of the course. Physiology has only uploaded documents" P16; For example, Pharmacology is a very dense and complicated subject, and you need someone to explain it to you, and until now, we have not received anything, only notes. I don't think it's enough, they are too schematic and hard to understand". P1; "The younger ones (teachers) feel like doing more things" P19; "It is more difficult for some teacher, especially those who are older" P5

3.4.4. Interaction with the Teachers

They pointed out that it is good in the videoconferences. An inconvenience is that sometimes the teacher is not aware of the doubts posted on the chat if there are too many messages. In the chat, the interaction is good, but the interruptions, even though they may be short, makes it impossible to follow it. Lastly, the students are surprised about how fast the teachers answers the e-mails:

"The chat, if you miss 5 min, you get lost" P22; "There is a good reception by the teacher for communicating" P11; "[tutoring] they are good, the answer sooner. They have improved" P21

3.5. The Context of Confinement and the Added Difficulties

The context of confinement has created some limitations for following e-learning education. These are related with internet access, access to electronic devices, and work and family responsibilities.

In rural environments, situations exist where internet access is lacking, which creates problems with being up to date with the classes. Another problem indicated is that not all had internet at home, and situations exist in which a person only has the limited amount of data available from a smartphone:

"Some people do not have all the means" P25; "I don't have internet at home, I only have data from the smartphone" P27 "I live here in the countryside, and the internet does not always work well, and if my kids are connected, then I can't do anything" P17

The confinement has obliged working from home whenever possible. This implies that it is possible for a family with three children to need an internet connection at the same time and the availability of five electronic devices simultaneously to be able to work and follow the classes. This availability is not very common. Another limitation that was pointed out was working in the presence of children/siblings at home:

"With the children at home, things cannot be done [mothers]" P25; "Studying at home when the entire family is at home, it is very hard to concentrate sometimes, they make noise, I can't print, etc." P25

Part of the students pointed out that is inconvenient, as they are used to studying in public libraries and have had to study at home:

"I always study at the library, not at home" P19; "I used to go to the library to study or do homework. No one bothers me there. At home, I set the washer, put on my pajamas and go to sleep" P28

Another difficulty added by the confinement is that one is not "trained" for shifting to e-learning. One has experience with an education system that has never been 100% online and where the traditional class is the learning stage. With respect to online exams, they do not feel secure either:

"We are used to traditional classes. This has been difficult for everyone, and more for the bachelor students than the Masters ones" P23; "I supposed they will give multiple-choice exams in a short time. It is the first time it will be online and one could be tense" P13; "If I hear it from the teacher beforehand, I understand it better, and now it's different. You take notes and then you have to understand them . . . " P16

3.6. Face-to-Face Win

3.6.1. Face-to-Face is Better . . . for Everything

The participants clearly preferred face-to-face to e-learning education. When faced with the possibility that some percentage of online classes will be provided along with traditional classes in future academic years, they do not think it is an option that will contribute much or needed. An exception is provided by students who have family or work responsibilities, who, exclusively for the theoretical classes, prefer them to be online and recorded, in order to be able to watch them at any time. Another aspect that was underlined was that the traditional system of education is the one they know and are used to, and changing it is difficult:

"Face-to-face is better . . . for everything" P17; "The University of Murcia is traditional, and we come from the same type of learning. It takes some time to adapt" P22; "Face-to-face is better in every aspect. For example, you learn the lesson and the teacher can provide examples, it can go further than the PowerPoint presentation. It is better to be face-to-face with the professor than through a screen" P23

3.6.2. Older and Female: Face-to-Face is Better

The older students seem to be the most vulnerable group, and various problems are observed. On the one hand, they have to tend to their children now that they are all at home, they have more responsibilities at home, plus certain digital competences that they have yet to incorporate. The management of their time is a great problem, which is influenced by the use of time, space and the electronic devices by the rest of the family, to which they grant them priority without being aware:

"For me the chat is not good, because I can't write that fast. I see the limitation in me. I miss the traditional classes. Face-to-face classes are better . . . for everything" P17; "You have to be very alert

with the online classroom, that you do not ignore the messages. Yesterday there was a class, and did not know" P9; "Some classmates are much older, and this is difficult. They write to the group [WhatsApp] sending pictures, and asking "What do I do? Where should I click?"" P25; "I'm much more in favor of face-to-face classes. I always obtain more information in them and I'm more comfortable" P24

4. Discussions

It is necessary to underline that all the results and discussion are centered on the first month of confinement after the start of the state of alarm, and this brings with it very specific cognitive and social states that are needed for the proper understanding of the discussion of the present research study.

Although the sample included a greater number of students from the University of Murcia as compared to those from the University of Granada, and different percentages of men and women of different ages, we believe that the main sociodemographic variables were well represented through the use of maximum variation sampling.

The nurses usually become nurses due to their desire to help other people to recover and maintain optimal health, and here we find ourselves in a situation in which not many options are available to help those who are severely sick due to COVID-19 [5]. Vocation is a determinant factor for those who decided to study nursing, and the main drive is the opportunity to care for others [17]. Our results support these two ideas in two ways: (1) they indicate that this attitude towards their professional life is still true in the new generations, with the remarkable fact that all the participants are so committed and wishing to help. (2) the pandemic has positively re-enforced their wishes to become nurses, obtaining similar results as other authors [18]. Although, the state of alarm decree includes the possible mobilization of students in their last year at university, their mobilization was principally needed in a small scale in Madrid and Catalonia, the areas greatly affected by COVID-19 [19].

The fast shift to e-learning education has not ceased to be a continuation of teaching and education through online resources, although it has not been clearly planned and adapted for e-learning [10]. Our results clearly present various relevant ideas related to this. In first place, and related with the clinical training, the health science degrees and more specifically the nursing degree have an essential need to be developed in clinical context. This element clearly cannot be substituted, and is perceived by all the students as being essential. Nevertheless, at present, a discussion exists about how high-fidelity clinical simulation could substitute the clinical training in real-world environments [20,21]. This methodology, which facilitates an intermediate learning between the theoretical dimension and the practical dimension, is proposed, aspiring to construct a real environment. However, and despite it being a type of learning established and known by the student body at the University of Murcia as well as the Granada, it is striking that this type of learning has not been described as an alternative. We interpret this finding as the clinical training being indispensable for the students.

Also, it forces us to reflect if this is the new reality of health care, and if the future nursing professionals should learn how to navigate in these conditions. The debate regarding the return of the nursing students to clinical environments is open and some recommendation has been provided [22]. The question now for the universities and nursing educators is that if as soon as the resources are provided and an adequate organization and adaptation occurs, the students should return to the health care services, what is the balance between the potential risk for the students and the importance of the clinical training? In second place, and related with the teaching of theory, the students prefer face-to-face teaching as opposed to the e-learning. They believe that the interaction is higher in quality and learning is greater. At present, another debate is open, as shown by two systematic reviews that do not provide concluding results on the existence of the greater learning linked to e-learning education of health professionals and students, highlighting the poor quality of existing studies and the importance of contextual factors [23,24]. Perhaps due to these reasons, the videoconference, distance learning, but synchronous and bi-directional, is the best assessed.

Another critical aspect is that the change to the online methodology was not chosen by the students, and the expectations they have with respect to their studies have been clearly disrupted.

Their entire academic life has been marked by a specific style of teaching, and they have become organized to continue with it, but the pandemic has imposed a different one with which they do not feel comfortable yet, thereby creating uncertainty and little security. This worries a great part of the Health Science academics [25]. It therefore absolutely necessary to start to work on the adaptation to e-learning that takes into account the previously-mentioned aspects so that the student's uncertainty decreases, especially in light of the evaluations. Academics have already expressed awareness of the students' concerns that are centered on their future degree and career progression [25]. The university counted with a technological infrastructure that has been able to deal with a drastic and fast change to distance teaching. However, the urgency of adapting this type of teaching has highlighted some situations of disadvantage. Thus, the older students, as compared to the younger ones, and in great part women and mothers, do not possess the most basic digital competences. This finding is robust, as the older students themselves, as well as the younger ones, are able to point this out in agreement with each other. They also point out that there is a small percentage of students who do not have the electronic resources or a connection to the internet necessary for adequately following the teaching.

Universities are trying to provide answers to some of these problems. It could be said that the phases of shock and normalization described by the students coincided with the period of reaction and acts of implementation by the institutions. There are activities that allow for fast implementation. For example, the Universities of Murcia and Granada freely loaned laptop computers with software to 100% of the students who requested them [26], with this number being more than 300 students in Murcia alone, as well as mobile internet-access devices [27]. However, the implementation of activities related with the evaluation has required conscientious reflection and consensus that has forced their implementation later in time [11].

In any case, once this first stage has been overcome, and faced with the absence of permanent solutions for this pandemic in the short term, it is necessary to propose distance learning strategies with a robust design, with the time necessary to create study plans that are well thought-out and durable [10,28]. We should be aware that we are currently undergoing an "emergency" education, a temporary shift of instructional delivery to an alternate delivery mode due to crisis circumstances [29]. The reality is that this transition to e-learning under these circumstances has nothing to do with a design that takes the maximum advantage and possibilities of the online format. We should reflect on the differences in the rhythm, the student-instructor relationship, pedagogy, the role of the instructor, the role of the student, the synchronicity of online communication, the role of online evaluations, and the source of feedback [30].

Limitations

Among the limitations of the study, we find that a thorough discussion and comparison with the opinions of other authors has not been possible, given the novel and exceptional situation we are currently living in. On the other hand, we should be aware that the sample studied cannot be representative of the reference population, and this can evidently affect the generalization of the results.

5. Conclusions

After the first week of adaptation to the conditions of confinement and the establishment of new online teaching systems, the students begin a new normality. The imposition of e-learning brings more limitations to students who are older, with work and family responsibilities, living in a rural environment and with limited electronic resources. Online teaching has allowed substituting the teaching of theory, although face-to-face teaching is preferred, at the same time it has shown that clinical practices are indispensable for the training of the nursing students. Online education goes beyond the online continuation of the classes. The parties responsible should already be working on this for the next academic year, in light of the uncertain future of a short-term control of COVID-19.

Author Contributions: Conceptualization, A.J.R.-M., J.E.M.-G. and M.R.-M.; Data curation, A.J.R.-M.; Formal analysis, A.J.R.-M., C.L.-C. and M.R.-M.; Investigation, A.J.R.-M., C.L.-C.and M.R.-M.; Methodology, A.J.R.-M.,

C.L.-C., J.E.M.-G. and M.R.-M.; Project administration, A.J.R.-M.; Supervision, A.J.R.-M.; Validation, A.J.R.-M.; Writing—original draft, A.J.R.-M. and M.R.-M.; Writing—review & editing, A.J.R.-M., C.L.-C., J.E.M.-G. and M.R.-M. All authors have read and agreed to the published version of the manuscript.

Funding: This research received no external funding.

Acknowledgments: Our most sincere thanks to the people who agreed to participate in this research.

Conflicts of Interest: The authors declare no conflict of interest.

Appendix A

Table A1. Interviews Guide.

Introductory questions. How is your … ?	- Leisure - Sleep - Rest - Diet - Exercise - Interrelation - Information about COVID19, where they are informed, if they have reviewed notes of any subject (handwashing, concept of prevalence, incidence…).
Online teaching methodology	- M1 Do you think that the university is providing an adequate response to the situation related to teaching? - M2 What types of tools are being proposed to you. - M3 Which one do you like best, describe advantages and disadvantages. - M4 What things/competencies cannot be learned (teaching limitations). - M5 Is it difficult to adapt to the communication channels that are used right now? - M6 Is the content given in class adequately adapted to online teaching methodologies? - M7 How is your interaction with other participants different from face-to-face? - M8 How is your interaction with the teacher? - M9 Tasks
Learning	- A1 How is time organized with this imposition - A2 Has your ability to concentrate and/or study been affected? - A3 What are the differences when studying in this manner? - A4 Do you think that this manner of learning forces a different type of learning management? Is it necessary to have more self-management? - A5 Is it possible to achieve learning in the same way as face-to-face learning, better, worse… - A6 What modalities, online methodologies do you propose for improving your online learning?
Expectations	- E1 Expectations about grades - E2 What influence do you think this way of teaching during this time will have on your training as a nurse. - E3 Do you think that after this online teaching a greater part of it will be necessary when everything returns to normal? Why? - E4 Are students prepared for this type of teaching? - E5 Do you think it is necessary to go one step further? Should this type of teaching go further?

Table A1. *Cont.*

4th year students	- AA1 What is going to happen? - AA2 What are you afraid of? - AA3 What do you think will happen with the practice? - AA4 What do you think will happen to your degree? - AA5 If you miss a practicum how good is your training?
Life expectancy	- How does the situation caused by the crisis in the professional field affect your desire to become a nurse?

References

1. World Health Organization. WHO Director-General's Opening Remarks at the Media Briefing on COVID-19-11 March 2020. Available online: https://www.who.int/dg/speeches/detail/who-director-general-s-opening-remarks-at-the-media-briefing-on-covid-19---11-march-2020 (accessed on 15 May 2020).
2. Remuzzi, A.; Remuzzi, G. COVID-19 and Italy: What next? *Lancet* **2020**, *395*, 1225–1228. [CrossRef]
3. Torri, E.; Sbrogiò, L.G.; Di Rosa, E.; Cinquetti, S.; Francia, F.; Ferro, A. Italian Public Health Response to the COVID-19 Pandemic: Case Report from the Field, Insights and Challenges for the Department of Prevention. *Int. J. Environ. Res. Public Health* **2020**, *17*, 3666. [CrossRef]
4. Choi, H.; Cho, W.; Kim, M.-H.; Hur, J.-Y. Public Health Emergency and Crisis Management: Case Study of SARS-CoV-2 Outbreak. *Int. J. Environ. Res. Public Health* **2020**, *17*, 3984. [CrossRef] [PubMed]
5. Jackson, D.; Bradbury-Jones, C.; Baptiste, D.; Gelling, L.; Morin, K.; Neville, S.; Smith, G.D. Life in the pandemic: Some reflections on nursing in the context of COVID-19. *J. Clin. Nurs.* **2020**. [CrossRef] [PubMed]
6. Tsai, J.; Wilson, M. COVID-19: A potential public health problem for homeless populations. *Lancet Public Health* **2020**, *5*, e186–e187. [CrossRef]
7. Nurchis, M.C.; Pascucci, D.; Sapienza, M.; Villani, L.; D'Ambrosio, F.; Castrini, F.; Specchia, M.L.; Laurenti, P.; Damiani, G. Impact of the Burden of COVID-19 in Italy: Results of Disability-Adjusted Life Years (DALYs) and Productivity Loss. *Int. J. Environ. Res. Public Health* **2020**, *17*, 4233. [CrossRef] [PubMed]
8. UNESCO & IESALC COVID-19 and higher education: Today and tomorrow. In *Impact Analysis, Policy Responses and Recommendations*; UNESCO: Paris, France, 2020.
9. Diez de la Cortina, S. Teaching in Times of Pandemic [Enseñar en Tiempos de Pandemia]. Available online: https://www.educaweb.com/noticia/2020/04/21/ensenar-tiempos-pandemia-19145/ (accessed on 15 May 2020).
10. Morin, K.H. Nursing Education After COVID-19: Same or Different? *J. Clin. Nurs.* **2020**. [CrossRef] [PubMed]
11. CRUE Universidades Españolas. Available online: http://www.crue.org/Documentos%20compartidos/Informes%20y%20Posicionamientos/Informe%20procedimientos%20evaluacio%CC%81n%20no%20presencial.pdf (accessed on 15 May 2020).
12. Braun, V.; Clarke, V. Using thematic analysis in psychology. *Qual. Res. Psychol.* **2006**, *3*, 77–101. [CrossRef]
13. Patton, M.Q. *Qualitative Evaluation and Research Methods*, 4th ed.; SAGE: Thousand Oaks, CA, USA, 2015; ISBN 978-1-4129-7212-3.
14. Morse, J.M. The Significance of Saturation. *Qual. Health Res.* **1995**, *5*, 147–149. [CrossRef]
15. Tong, A.; Sainsbury, P.; Craig, J. Consolidated criteria for reporting qualitative research (COREQ): A 32-item checklist for interviews and focus groups. *Int. J. Qual. Health Care* **2007**, *19*, 349–357. [CrossRef] [PubMed]
16. Kiger, M.E.; Varpio, L. Thematic analysis of qualitative data: AMEE Guide No. 131. *Med. Teach.* **2020**, 1–9. [CrossRef] [PubMed]
17. Eley, D.; Eley, R.; Bertello, M.; Rogers-Clark, C. Why did I become a nurse? Personality traits and reasons for entering nursing. *J. Adv. Nurs.* **2012**, *68*, 1546–1555. [CrossRef] [PubMed]
18. Swift, A.; Banks, L.; Baleswaran, A.; Cooke, N.; Little, C.; McGrath, L.; Meechan-Rogers, R.; Neve, A.; Rees, H.; Tomlinson, A.; et al. COVID-19 and student nurses: A view from England. *J. Clin. Nurs.* **2020**. [CrossRef] [PubMed]

19. Rodríguez Veiga, D. Nursing Students are Already Risking Their Lives Against Covid-19 with Precarious Contracts [Las Estudiantes de Enfermería ya se Juegan la Vida Contra el Covid-19 con Contratos Precarios]. Available online: https://www.elespanol.com/sociedad/20200331/estudiantes-enfermeria-juegan-vida-covid-19-contratos-basura/478703443_0.html (accessed on 23 May 2020).

20. Sullivan, N.; Swoboda, S.M.; Breymier, T.; Lucas, L.; Sarasnick, J.; Rutherford-Hemming, T.; Budhathoki, C.; Kardong-Edgren, S. (Suzie) Emerging Evidence Toward a 2:1 Clinical to Simulation Ratio: A Study Comparing the Traditional Clinical and Simulation Settings. *Clin. Simul. Nurs.* **2019**, *30*, 34–41. [CrossRef]

21. Hayden, J.K.; Smiley, R.A.; Gross, L. Simulation in Nursing Education: Current Regulations and Practices. *J. Nurs. Regul.* **2014**, *5*, 25–30. [CrossRef]

22. Hayter, M.; Jackson, D. Pre-registration undergraduate nurses and the COVID-19 pandemic: Students or workers? *J. Clin. Nurs.* **2020**. [CrossRef] [PubMed]

23. Fontaine, G.; Cossette, S.; Maheu-Cadotte, M.-A.; Mailhot, T.; Deschênes, M.-F.; Mathieu-Dupuis, G.; Côté, J.; Gagnon, M.-P.; Dubé, V. Efficacy of adaptive e-learning for health professionals and students: A systematic review and meta-analysis. *BMJ Open* **2019**, *9*, e025252. [CrossRef] [PubMed]

24. Voutilainen, A.; Saaranen, T.; Sormunen, M. Conventional vs. e-learning in nursing education: A systematic review and meta-analysis. *Nurse Educ. Today* **2017**, *50*, 97–103. [CrossRef] [PubMed]

25. Pather, N.; Blyth, P.; Chapman, J.A.; Dayal, M.R.; Flack, N.A.M.S.; Fogg, Q.A.; Green, R.A.; Hulme, A.K.; Johnson, I.P.; Meyer, A.J.; et al. Forced Disruption of Anatomy Education in Australia and New Zealand: An Acute Response to the Covid-19 Pandemic. *Anat. Sci. Educ.* **2020**, *13*, 284–300. [CrossRef] [PubMed]

26. University of Murcia The Notica. Newsletter of ÁTICA of the University of Murcia [La Notica. *Boletín informativo de ÁTICA de la Universidad de Murcia*]. Available online: https://www.um.es/notica/boletin14/prestamo.htm (accessed on 29 May 2020).

27. University of Granada 1,000 Internet Connection Lines for Students Who Have Difficulty Connecting [1.000 Líneas de Conexión a Internet Para los Estudiantes con Dificultades Para Conectarse]. Available online: https://covid19.ugr.es/noticias/1000-lineas-conexion-internet-estudiantes-dificultades (accessed on 29 May 2020).

28. McCormack, B. What value nursing knowledge in a time of crisis? *J. Clin. Nurs.* **2020**. [CrossRef] [PubMed]

29. Hodges, C.; Moore, S.; Lockee, B.; Trust, T.; Bond, A. The Difference Between Emergency Remote Teaching and Online Learning. Available online: https://er.educause.edu/articles/2020/3/the-difference-between-emergency-remote-teaching-and-online-learning (accessed on 13 May 2020).

30. Means, B.; Bakia, M.; Murphy, R. *Learning Online: What Research Tells Us about Whether, When and How*; Routledge: New York, NY, USA, 2014.

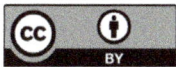

International Journal of
*Environmental Research
and Public Health*

MDPI

Article

Relief Alternatives during Resuscitation: Instructions to Teach Bystanders. A Randomized Control Trial

María José Pujalte-Jesús [1], César Leal-Costa [2,*], María Ruzafa-Martínez [2,*], Antonio Jesús Ramos-Morcillo [2,*] and José Luis Díaz Agea [3]

[1]   Faculty of Nursing, Universidad Católica de Murcia UCAM, 30107 Murcia, Spain; mjpujalte@ucam.edu
[2]   Faculty of Nursing, University of Murcia, 30107 Murcia, Spain
[3]   Faculty of Nursing, Catholic University of Murcia, 30107 Murcia, Spain; jluis@ucam.edu
*   Correspondence: cleal@um.es (C.L.-C.); maruzafa@um.es (M.R.-M.); ajramos@um.es (A.J.R.-M.)

Received: 30 June 2020; Accepted: 26 July 2020; Published: 30 July 2020

check for
updates

Abstract: To analyze the quality of resuscitation (CPR) performed by individuals without training after receiving a set of instructions (structured and unstructured/intuitive) from an expert in a simulated context, the specific objective was to design a simple and structured CPR learning method on-site. An experimental study was designed, consisting of two random groups with a post-intervention measurement in which the experimental group (EG) received standardized instructions, and the control group (CG) received intuitive or non-standardized instructions, in a public area simulated scenario. Statistically significant differences were found ($p < 0.0001$) between the EG and the CG for variables: time needed to give orders, pauses between chest compressions and ventilations, depth, overall score, chest compression score, and chest recoil. The average depth of the EG was 51.1 mm (SD 7.94) and 42.2 mm (SD 12.04) for the CG. The chest recoil median was 86.32% (IQR 62.36, 98.87) for the EG, and 58.3% (IQR 27.46, 84.33) in the CG. The use of a sequence of simple, short and specific orders, together with observation-based learning makes possible the execution of chest compression maneuvers that are very similar to those performed by rescuers, and allows the teaching of the basic notions of ventilation. The structured order method was shown to be an on-site learning opportunity when faced with the need to maintain high-quality CPR in the presence of an expert resuscitator until the arrival of emergency services.

Keywords: cardiopulmonary resuscitation; chest compression; method; experiential learning; observation; CPR

---

1. Introduction

The out-of-hospital cardiorespiratory arrest (OHCA) is a frequent health problem in developed countries, and only a small percentage of the victims receive cardiopulmonary resuscitation (CPR) by the bystanders [1]. Early and high-quality resuscitation maneuvers can double, or even quadruple, survival [2], however, CPR training of the general population is scarce. The current protocols differ depending if they are directed towards professionals or laypersons, and the health services continue exploring alternatives to improve bystander CPR rates when witnessing out-of-hospital cardiorespiratory arrests. Among these alternatives, we find mass training and telephone-based CPR, to such an extent that in 2015, the European resuscitation guidelines [3] recognized the important role of dispatcher-assisted CPR in the diagnosis and providing of telephone-assisted, early cardiopulmonary resuscitation.

From that point on, the attempts to combine standardized communication in CPR have increased [4,5], with supporters [6] and critics [7] until 2019, when the International Liaison Committee on Resuscitation (ILCOR) [8] recommended that the dispatchers provide instructions to the bystanders.

From that point on, many research studies provided information about the increased survival rate [9,10], and affirmed that the provision of dispatch cardiopulmonary resuscitation instructions, instead of no instructions at all, improved the results from cardiopulmonary arrest [11].

However, all of these studies suggest that the clinical results after out-of-hospital cardiac arrest have a greater possibility of improving when dispatcher assistance is available; the scientific societies identify, in their knowledge gap, the preferred CPR instruction sequence for Dispatcher-Assisted Cardiopulmonary Resuscitation (DA-CPR) [8], because an optimal sequence of orders is not yet available for those who are limited to receiving instructions from emergency services personnel. At present, the ILCOR is still seeking the best evidence through the Consensus on Science with Treatment Recommendations (CoSTR) [12].

Between the CPR observed by an expert and telephone-based CPR, we find real-life situations where only one expert/healthcare worker performs resuscitation maneuvers surrounded by people without training, but who could play an important role in maintaining high-quality CPR if they could learn how to do so on-site. These possible scenarios would need to have certain essential elements, described by Bandura [13,14], when learning a skill through observation: attention and motivation. If motivated people were available who are willing to relieve the expert resuscitator, then this expert could provide the necessary instructions to teach CPR to the bystanders for the benefit of the patient. The exhaustion of a single resuscitator could reduce the possibilities of maintaining high-quality CPR until the arrival of the emergency services.

Recent studies back the use of standardized communication in resuscitation maneuvers to improve the communication and care of the patient during life-support maneuvers [15], and other research studies have associated the use of "action-linked phrases" such as "shock delivered, start compressions" with a decreased start time of the chest compressions [16].

The general objective of our study was to analyze the quality of the CPR, performed by individuals who had no prior knowledge on resuscitation, after receiving a set of instructions (structured and unstructured/intuitive) from an expert within a context of simulated CPR. The specific objective was to design a simple and structured method for the fast learning of CPR on-site.

2. Materials and Methods

2.1. Study Design and Settings

A post-intervention two-group post-test-only randomized experiment [17–20] was designed, in which the experimental group (EG) received standardized instructions, and the control group (CG) received intuitive, unstructured instructions. This is one of the simplest experimental designs [21]. The groups (experimental and control) were randomly assigned. One group received the training; the other group did not receive the training, and was used for comparison. A previous trial was not required for this design, as participants were randomly assigned to the groups, and thus it was assumed that both groups were statistically equivalent. In this design, the objective was to determine whether differences existed between the two groups after the training program. Therefore, a prior trial was not considered for this study design. Although this test could have been used to determine whether the groups were comparable before the experiment, this was not done, to avoid the possible negative effects entailed by the trail to the internal validity, which could be detrimental for the participants' learning. On the other hand, the participants were randomly assigned to the groups and the experimental conditions, ensuring that the groups were equivalent (they had the same socio-demographic characteristics, particularly not having any previous training or prior knowledge about resuscitation).

2.2. Selection of Participants

The target population was the university population from the Region of Murcia (Spain); volunteers were solicited through announcements in the virtual campus among the students from the Catholic

University of Murcia. The collection of data was performed between the months of November 2019 and February 2020.

The study included all the volunteer participants older than 18 who had signed the informed consent form and who did not comply with the exclusion criteria. These exclusion criteria were: physical limitation that could impede them from performing chest compressions and ventilation for 2 min, intellectual limitation that could impede them from following and performing the orders, refusing to participate in the study, being a healthcare worker or a healthcare student, and having received CPR training at least 5 years prior. The participants were informed about the purpose of the study to evaluate the efficacy of a method to teach CPR on-site in the least amount of time. The participants were not informed about the results of their intervention until the end of the study. The expert resuscitators were selected from clinical simulation teaching staff volunteers at the university. The inclusion criteria were: being an instructor in basic life support (BLS) and automated external defibrillation (AED) accredited by the European Resuscitation Council (ERC), and/or being a CPR professor for more than 2 years. Ultimately, this group was comprised of eight experts, of which six were women and two were men.

2.3. Intervention

After complying with the eligibility criteria to participate in the study, the participants were randomly assigned to the experimental group "structured orders" or to the control group "unstructured orders". This assignment was performed using a random assignment tool (sealedenvelope.com, London, UK). Likewise, once assigned to a group, the roles of ventilation (VR) or chest compression (CR) were randomly assigned. Participants were blinded to the allocation until randomization. For performing the mouth-to-mouth ventilations, face protection devices (Laerdal® Face Shield, Laerdal Medical Corporation, Stavanger, Norway) were made available to the participants. When the research was conducted, knowledge about the COVID-19 pandemic was unknown in Spain.

A total of 138 individuals comprised the final sample. Of these, 12 were excluded because they had received CPR training in the last 5 years. Of the remaining 126 participants, 64 were randomly assigned to the structured orders group (experimental group, EG) and 62 to the unstructured orders group (control group, CG). Of the 64 EG participants, 32 were assigned the ventilation role (VR) and 32 to the chest compression role (CR); after the randomization, two VR participants were excluded when they refused to perform mouth-to-mouth ventilation, one CR participant was excluded for fatigue which impeded concluding the trial, and one participant was excluded due to loss of data. From the 62 participants in the GC group, 30 were assigned to the VR group and 32 to the CR group; after the randomization, two CR participants were excluded due to fatigue that impeded them from finishing the trial. Lastly, the 120 remaining participants received the training planned, and the results were analyzed. A CONSORT study flow diagram is shown in Figure 1.

2.4. Experimental Group: Structured Orders

Before starting, the participants were told that they were dealing with a simulated scenario on the street, and that they were witnessing how an expert performed CPR on a person in OHCA. They were told that the expert would ask for their help after two cycles of 30 compressions/2 ventilations (30:2) after their arrival. After this period, they would receive a series of orders that they had to follow to provide CPR for the next 2 min.

Only compressions were performed during the time the expert gave orders. The orders provided (adapted from the main guides in CPR terminology) [16,22–25] to the participants with the chest compressions role (CR) were:

1. "Kneel in front of me".
2. "Interlock your hands, one over the other, and straighten your arms".

3. "When I count to three, you have to place your hand in the middle of the chest and compress "hard and fast" [25] 30 times".
4. "Have you understood?" (If the participant answered "NO" to this question, the order would be repeated again without any changes).
5. "1, 2, 3, now!"

The orders provided to the participants with the ventilation role (VR) were given, while the CR participants performed the first chest compressions. These orders were:

1. "Put your hand on the forehead".
2. "Put the other hand on the chin and lift".
3. "Cover the nose and blow two times when your partner reaches 30".

In this sequence of instructions, to warn the rest of the participants and the resuscitators that the end of the compressions was near and to minimize the interruptions, the expert had the added requisite of counting the last five compressions aloud.

The expert who participated in the experimental group was trained in the structured learning method, and had previously practiced in simulation. The expert was the same for the completely experimental group.

2.5. Control Group: Structured Orders

To conduct the trial with the unstructured orders group (CG), the expert and the participants were informed about the same simulation scenario. The experts were told that they could ask for help after two cycles of 30:2, and they were asked to give the sequence of orders they thought to be faster and more opportune, following their intuition and previous knowledge, in order for the participants to relieve them in the following 2 min.

To eliminate the learning effect [13], meaning the familiarization of the experts with the procedure, and therefore improving the results in later trials, the pretest trials were dispensed with [26], and eight different experts were selected to interact with the CG participants, so that they were not allowed to repeat the trial more than four times. The experts were not study participants, and they did not have prior knowledge of the structured orders utilized with the EG or the hypothesis of the study.

Comments, corrections, or explanations were not allowed in any of the two groups once the orders were given and the CPR started by the participants.

2.6. Analysis Parameters

The main result of the study was the time needed for giving orders (seconds). The secondary result variables were: pauses between compression and ventilation (seconds), depth (mm), rate (compressions/minute), effective rate of ventilation (% between 500–600 mL), rate of chest recoil (%), positioning of the hands (% of success with respect to the center of the chest), scores reached in the mannequin (compression score (0–100), of ventilation (0–100), total/final (0–100)), age (years), sex (male/female), weight (kg), height (meters), and body mass index (BMI) (kg/m2).

2.7. Measurements

The demographic data were collected in questionnaires after the informed consent. For collecting the data relative to the quality of the CPR, the Resusci Anne QCPR® manikin (Laerdal Medical Corporation, Stavanger, Norway) was utilized, which was calibrated and checked before conducting the experiment, and periodically during the experimental phase.

2.8. Analysis

The continuous variables with a normal distribution were expressed as mean and standard deviation (SD); the data without a normal distribution were described as median and interquartile range (IQR). A difference in means analysis was performed for independent samples with the Student's *t* test or the Mann–Whitney U test, according to the distribution of the data. The categorical variables were described as frequencies and percentages (%). The results were considered statistically significant at $p < 0.05$. The data were reported according to the CONSORT guidelines [27]. The processing and analysis of the data were conducted with the statistical package IBM SPSS® for Windows version 22.0 (IBM Corporation, Armonk, DA, USA).

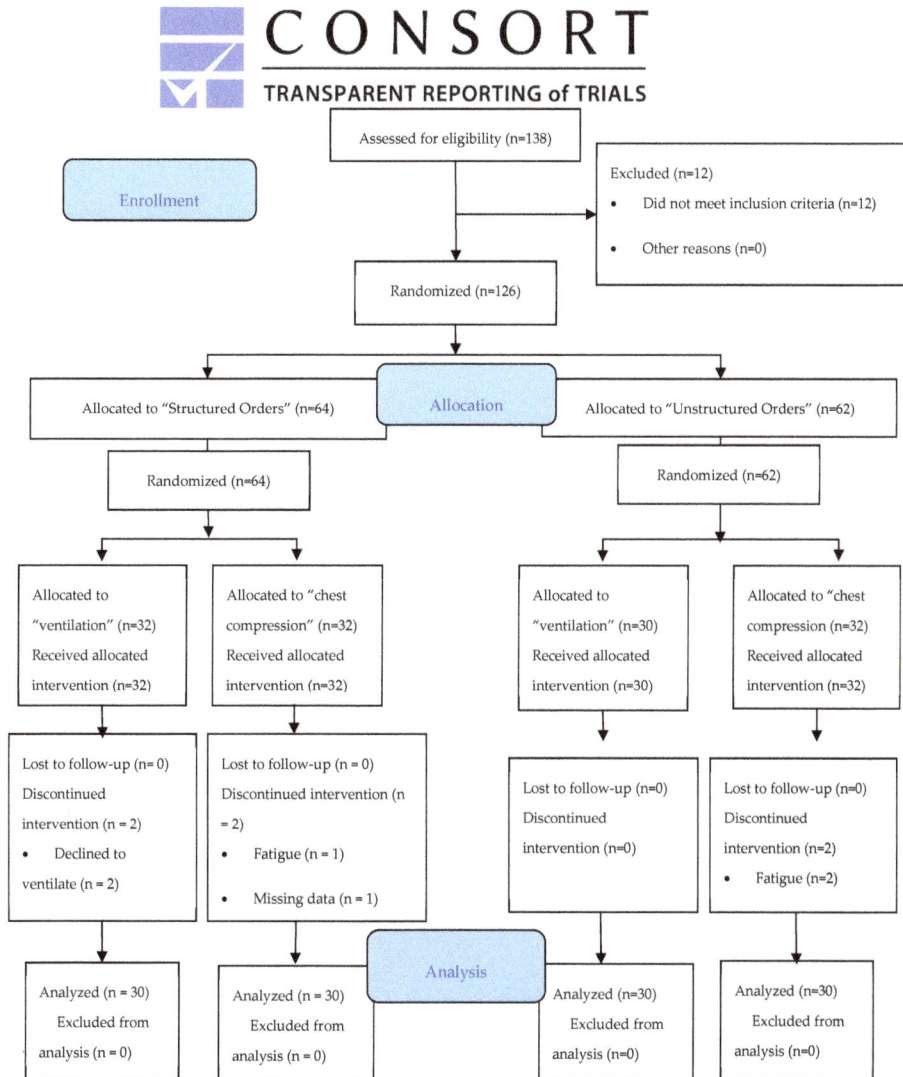

Figure 1. Study CONSORT flow diagram.

2.9. Ethical Considerations

All the participants gave their informed consent for inclusion before participating in the study. The study was conducted in accordance with the Declaration of Helsinki, and the protocol was approved by the Ethics Committee of Catholic University of Murcia (CE031901).

3. Results

The mean age of the participants was 21 years old (SD 4.75), the mean height was 1.71 m (SD 0.08), the mean weight was 66.1 kg (SD 12.14), and the mean BMI was 22.5 kg/m^2 (SD 2.92). Of these, 60% (n = 72/120) of the participants were women. Table 1 shows the demographic data according to groups (CG and EG).

Table 1. Baseline demographics (n = 120).

Demographic Variables	Unstructured Orders Group (n = 60)	Structured Orders Group (n = 60)	*p*-Value
Age (years)—mean (SD)	21 (5.07)	21 (3.78)	0.669
Sex (% female)	36 (60)	36 (60)	0.574
Height (m)—mean (SD)	1.72 (0.09)	1.70 (0.09)	0.31
Weight (kg)—mean (SD)	67.3 (13.46)	64.3 (11.68)	0.209
BMI (kg/m^2)—mean (SD)	22.7 (3.20)	22.1 (2.77)	0.236

Statistically significant differences were obtained (*p* < 0.0001) between the EG and CG for the variables: time needed to give orders (Figure 2A), pauses between chest compressions and ventilations (Figure 2B), depth, overall score, chest compression score, and chest recoil.

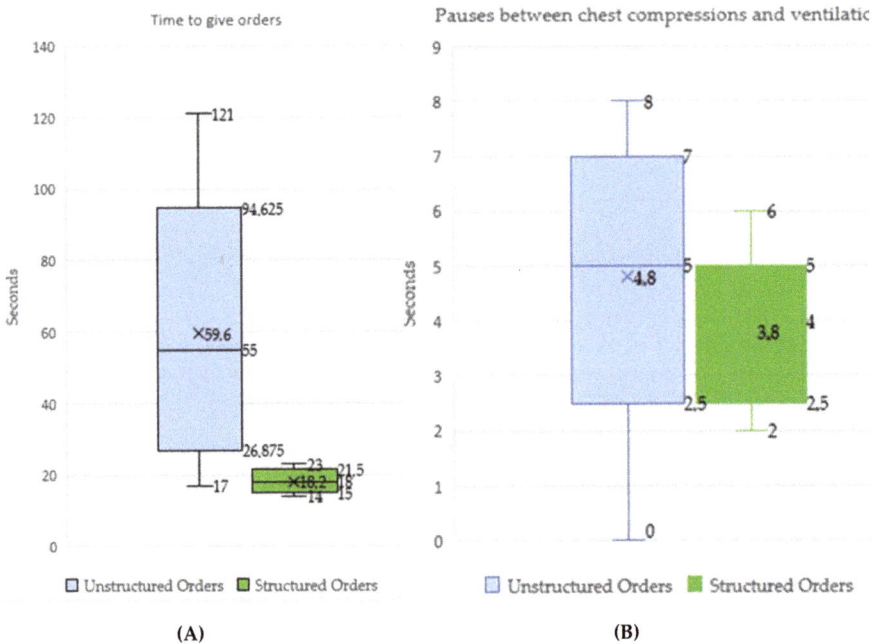

Figure 2. (**A**) Time needed to give orders. (**B**) Pauses between chest compressions and ventilations.

The mean depth was 51.1 mm (SD 7.94) for EG, and 42.2 mm (SD 12.04) for the CG (Table 2).

The median of the variable rate for the EG was 121 compressions per minute (IQR 110, 130), and 121 compressions per minute (IQR 113, 132) for the CG. The median of effective ventilation (% between 500–600 mL) was 20% (IQR 5, 50) for the EG, and 40% (IQR 0, 60.42) for the CG. The median for chest recoil was 86.32% (IQR 62.36, 98.87) for the EG, and 58.3% (IQR 27.46, 84.33) for the CG. From the participants, 83.3% (25/30) correctly positioned their hands in the EG, and 80% (24/30) in the CG (Table 2).

No statistically significant differences were found according to sex, age, height, weight, or BMI between the CG and the EG, or the VR or CR groups.

As for the scores achieved (Figure 3), the means/medians obtained were: 67 points (IQR 49, 83) for the EG, and 65 points (IQR 34, 81.5) for the CG in ventilation; 78.5 points (IQR 61.5, 87.25) for the EG, and 53 points (IQR 37.25, 61) for the CG in compression; 73 points (SD 14.5) for the EG, and 45 points (SD 22.47) for the CG in the overall CPR score.

Table 2. Study outcome data.

Variables of Study	Unstructured Orders	Structured Orders	t-Test/Mann–Whitney U	p-Value
Time needed to give orders (seconds)—mean (SD)	55.3 (26.09)	17.9 (2.34)	t = 7.813	<0.001
Pauses between chest compressions and ventilations (seconds)—median (IQR)	5 (5, 6)	4 (3, 4)	U = 152	<0.001
Depth (mm)—mean (SD)	42.2 (12.04)	51.1 (7.94)	t = 3.38	0.001
Rate (comp/min)—median (IQR)	121 (113, 132)	121 (110, 130)	U = 443.5	0.923
Overall score (0–100)—mean (SD)	45.03 (22.5)	73 (14.5)	t = 5.73	<0.001
Ventilation score (0–100) [a]—median (IQR)	65 (34, 81.5)	67 (49, 83)	U = 370.5	0.437
Chest compression score (0–100)—median (IQR)	53 (37.25, 61)	78.5 (61.5, 87.25)	U = 171	<0.001
Hands position—median (IQR)	100 (100, 100)	100 (100, 100)	U = 437.5	0.784
% Effective ventilation (500–600 mL) [a]—median (IQR)	40 (0, 60.42)	20 (5, 50)	U = 394.5	0.682
% Chest recoil—median (IQR)	58.3 (27.46, 84.33)	86.32 (62.36, 98.87)	U = 263.5	0.006

[a] Two cases with missing data.

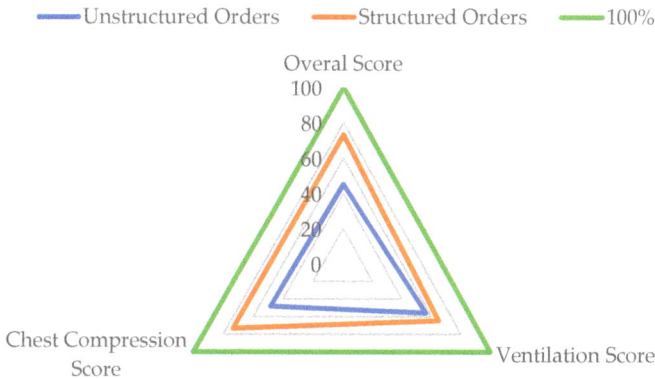

Figure 3. Comparison of the scores reached by each group, with respect to the maximum score.

As for ventilation, 40% (12/30) of the CG participants correctly performed the head-tilt/chin-lift maneuver to ventilate. In the EG, this maneuver was performed by 66.67% (20/30) of the participants. Statistically significant differences were found in effective ventilation after performing the head-tilt/chin-lift maneuver ($p < 0.0001$).

4. Discussion

Increasing the rates of resuscitation when witnessing cardiorespiratory arrests is still a challenge in Spain [28]. This study intended to demonstrate the efficiency of a fast and structured method of communication on-site for situations in which an expert is performing CPR in the presence of bystanders who are willing to provide relief, either in the compression, or in ventilation maneuvers.

Observation-based, vicarious, or through-demonstration learning [13] are some one of the most-commonly utilized methods for learning motor skills [29]. Diverse studies have suggested that visual orientation can accelerate the acquisition of complex motor skills [30]. In our case, we believe that this visual guide offered advantages over instructions that were not provided in person (such as through the phone, for example). We also believe that observational learning had effects (in both the experimental groups as well as the control group) on the quality of resuscitation; this is the reason why the co-variation of the results attributed to the independent variable (structure method) is even more powerful, as this observational learning was found in both groups (experimental and control). Therefore, it is thought that there could be a causal attribution of the structured method towards the improvement of CPR. Thus, it can be concluded that the use of structured orders results in the better performance of CPR, compared to intuitive or unstructured orders of individuals without prior knowledge of CPR.

The main finding of our study consisted of the statistically significant decrease in the time needed to provide the orders that allowed relieving the expert and performing high-quality CPR. The time invested by the expert in the experimental group was significantly less compared to the unstructured orders group. The pauses between compressions and ventilations also decreased. In addition, an improvement was registered in the mean depth and the chest recoil, compared to the set of unstructured orders.

From our point of view, the decrease in these times could be related to the simplicity of the orders, in agreement with the results from Hunt et al. [16], insofar as it was suggested that there was a greater chance that the appropriate action could occur when short, easy, and specific phrases were utilized. The pauses between compression and ventilation were significantly reduced in the experimental group, with this result possibly due to the implementation of improvements proposed by Lauridsen et al. [15], such as the use of backwards counting before the relief, or counting out loud of the last five compressions.

The simplification of the orders can also improve the quality of the chest compressions [31]. This could help in the understanding and discussion of the results from other studies [32] that suggest that non-trained bystanders are not useful during CPR.

As for ventilation, achieving the volunteer's relief of the compression expert relies on a margin of 30 compressions (between 15–17 s) for the ventilation volunteer to receive the indications correctly. The participants who performed the head-tilt/chin-lift maneuver performed effective ventilations (500–600 mL) that were significantly better than those who did not. However, for the ventilation skills, no significant differences were found between the groups; in fact, the scores reached by the unstructured orders group were higher. Thus, it seems possible that although a layperson resuscitator performs the head-tilt/chin-lift maneuver correctly, this does not ensure proper ventilation, but could result in mistakes in the volume ventilated (hyperventilation or hypoventilation).

This makes us believe that on the one hand, ventilation is a skill that requires more training time compared to compression, and on the other hand, that compression-only CPR in the presence of an expert is also a valid alternative; not only for those people who are reticent about performing mouth-to-mouth ventilation [33], but also for the notable public interest in learning CPR [34]. All of these improvements resulted in higher scores, provided by the simulator, of the experimental group than the control group.

The variables rate and hand positioning did not show significant differences between both groups, and were within the range accepted by scientific societies [35].

Our study was conducted with the aim of assessing the effectiveness of providing orders. However, this method has an added benefit, in that in a real-life situation in which the expert has to be relieved, a layperson could be properly corrected fast. Thus, during the resuscitation procedure, the strong points could be emphasized, and the weak points improved, in order to provide high quality CPR until the arrival of the emergency services. This advantage is shown in studies, such as those from González-Salvado et al. [36], which affirms that practical learning guided by an instructor provides better results.

In conclusion, the learning of technical skills seems to be greatly simplified when the layperson or beginner is allowed to observe an expert, as pointed out in other studies [37,38], which associate a greater ability of response and performance of the layperson after viewing ultra-brief videos.

Limitations

Among the main limitations of the study, we find the extrapolation of the results due to the characteristics of the sample and the type of experiment. The external validity could be improved with a representative sample of a real population, not only with a healthy university population. In the second place, we believe that the validity of the experiments with simulation is limited, as it does not occur in a real-life context, and other variables, such as stress or the interference from other spectators, could not be taken into account. Another limitation that should be mentioned is the lack of a pre-test to assess the resuscitation skills of the participants, beyond their statement of being a layperson. In this case, the design of the study would have been more complex. Thus, this was not done, to avoid the threat to the internal validity known as learning. However, if properly managed, it could have provided a greater internal validity of the study, which could have helped establish, with greater precision, if the groups were homogeneous for their comparison.

5. Conclusions

The use of a sequence of simple, short and specific orders, together with observation-based learning, makes possible the execution of chest compression maneuvers that are very similar to those performed by rescuers, and allows the teaching of the basic notions of ventilation.

Improvements were identified in the variables "time needed to give orders", "pauses between chest compressions and ventilations", and "chest recoil" when CPR was performed by laypersons in the experimental group.

The method of structured orders was shown to provide an on-site learning opportunity when faced with the need to maintain high-quality CPR in the presence of an expert resuscitator before the arrival of emergency services, and after their arrival, in case further help is needed.

More research studies are needed to assess these findings in a non-university population, and to measure other variables that could have an influence on the results, such as the role of the layperson's stress when facing this situation in a non-simulation context.

Author Contributions: Conceptualization: M.J.P.-J. and C.L.-C.; formal analysis: M.J.P.-J., C.L.-C., M.R.-M., A.J.R.-M., and J.L.D.A.; investigation: C.L.-C and J.L.D.A.; methodology: C.L.-C., M.R.-M., A.J.R.-M., and J.L.D.-A.; project administration: C.L.-C. and J.L.D.-A.; resources: M.J.P.-J.; supervision: J.L.D.A.; validation: C.L.-C., M.R.-M., and J.L.D.A.; writing—original draft: M.J.P.-J.; writing—review and editing: M.J.P.-J., C.L.-C., M.R.-M., A.J.R.-M., and J.L.D.A. All authors have read and agreed to the published version of the manuscript.

Funding: This research received no external funding.

Acknowledgments: Our most sincere thanks to the people who agreed to participate in this research.

Conflicts of Interest: The authors declare no conflict of interest.

References

1. Hawkes, C.; Booth, S.; Ji, C.; Brace-McDonnell, S.J.; Whittington, A.; Mapstone, J.; Cooke, M.W.; Deakin, C.D.; Gale, C.P.; Fothergill, R.; et al. Epidemiology and outcomes from out-of-hospital cardiac arrests in England. *Resuscitation* **2017**, *110*, 133–140. [CrossRef] [PubMed]
2. Hasselqvist-Ax, I.; Riva, G.; Herlitz, J.; Rosenqvist, M.; Hollenberg, J.; Nordberg, P.; Ringh, M.; Jonsson, M.; Axelsson, C.; Lindqvist, J.; et al. Early Cardiopulmonary Resuscitation in Out-of-Hospital Cardiac Arrest. *N. Engl. J. Med.* **2015**, *372*, 2307–2315. [CrossRef]
3. Zideman, D.A.; De Buck, E.D.J.; Singletary, E.M.; Cassan, P.; Chalkias, A.F.; Evans, T.R.; Hafner, C.M.; Handley, A.J.; Meyran, D.; Schunder-Tatzber, S.; et al. European Resuscitation Council Guidelines for Resuscitation 2015 First aid. *Resuscitation* **2015**, *95*, 278–287. [CrossRef] [PubMed]
4. Pek, J.H.; de Korne, D.F.; Hannawa, A.F.; Leong, B.S.H.; Ng, Y.Y.; Arulanandam, S.; Tham, L.P.; Ong, M.E.H.; Ong, G.Y.-K. Dispatcher-assisted cardiopulmonary resuscitation for paediatric out-of-hospital cardiac arrest: A structured evaluation of communication issues using the SACCIA® safe communication typology. *Resuscitation* **2019**, *139*, 144–151. [CrossRef] [PubMed]

5. Yamada, N.; Fuerch, J.; Halamek, L. Impact of Standardized Communication Techniques on Errors during Simulated Neonatal Resuscitation. *Am. J. Perinatol.* **2015**, *33*, 385–392. [PubMed]
6. Yamada, N.K.; Halamek, L.P. On the Need for Precise, Concise Communication during Resuscitation: A Proposed Solution. *J. Pediatrics* **2015**, *166*, 184–187. [CrossRef]
7. Wu, Z.; Panczyk, M.; Spaite, D.W.; Hu, C.; Fukushima, H.; Langlais, B.; Sutter, J.; Bobrow, B.J. Telephone cardiopulmonary resuscitation is independently associated with improved survival and improved functional outcome after out-of-hospital cardiac arrest. *Resuscitation* **2018**, *122*, 135–140. [CrossRef]
8. Soar, J.; Maconochie, I.; Wyckoff, M.H.; Olasveengen, T.M.; Singletary, E.M.; Greif, R.; Aickin, R.; Bhanji, F.; Donnino, M.W.; Mancini, M.E.; et al. 2019 International Consensus on Cardiopulmonary Resuscitation and Emergency Cardiovascular Care Science with Treatment Recommendations: Summary From the Basic Life Support; Advanced Life Support; Pediatric Life Support; Neonatal Life Support; Education, Implementation, and Teams; and First Aid Task Forces. *Circulation* **2019**, *140*. [CrossRef]
9. Ro, Y.S.; Shin, S.D.; Song, K.J.; Hong, K.J.; Ahn, K.O.; Kim, D.K.; Kwak, Y.H. Effects of Dispatcher-assisted Cardiopulmonary Resuscitation on Survival Outcomes in Infants, Children, and Adolescents with Out-of-hospital Cardiac Arrests. *Resuscitation* **2016**, *108*, 20–26. [CrossRef]
10. Goto, Y.; Maeda, T.; Goto, Y. Impact of Dispatcher-Assisted Bystander Cardiopulmonary Resuscitation on Neurological Outcomes in Children with Out-of-Hospital Cardiac Arrests: A Prospective, Nationwide, Population-Based Cohort Study. *J. Am. Heart Assoc.* **2014**, *3*, e000499. [CrossRef]
11. Bohm, K.; Vaillancourt, C.; Charette, M.L.; Dunford, J.; Castrén, M. In patients with out-of-hospital cardiac arrest, does the provision of dispatch cardiopulmonary resuscitation instructions as opposed to no instructions improve outcome: A systematic review of the literature. *Resuscitation* **2011**, *82*, 1490–1495. [CrossRef] [PubMed]
12. Olasveengen, T.M.; Mancini, M.E.; Vaillancourt, C.; Brooks, S.C.; Castren, M.; Chung, S.P.; Couper, K.; Dainty, K.N.; Escalante, R.; Gazmuri, R.J.; et al. Emergency Care: Dispatcher Instruction in CPR: Systematic Review. Available online: https://costr.ilcor.org/document/emergency-care-dispatcherinstruction-in-cpr (accessed on 25 February 2019).
13. Lyons, P.; Bandura, R.P. Case-based modeling for learning: Socially constructed skill development. *Educ.+ Train.* **2018**, *60*, 139–154. [CrossRef]
14. Domjan, M. *Principios de Aprendizaje y Conducta*; Paraninfo: Madrid, Spain, 2007; ISBN 9788497325844.
15. Lauridsen, K.G.; Watanabe, I.; Løfgren, B.; Cheng, A.; Duval-Arnould, J.; Hunt, E.A.; Good, G.L.; Niles, D.; Berg, R.A.; Nishisaki, A.; et al. Standardising communication to improve in-hospital cardiopulmonary resuscitation. *Resuscitation* **2020**, *147*, 73–80. [CrossRef] [PubMed]
16. Hunt, E.A.; Cruz-Eng, H.; Bradshaw, J.H.; Hodge, M.; Bortner, T.; Mulvey, C.L.; McMillan, K.N.; Galvan, H.; Duval-Arnould, J.M.; Jones, K.; et al. A novel approach to life support training using "action-linked phrases". *Resuscitation* **2015**, *86*, 1–5. [CrossRef]
17. Research Methods Knowledge Base. Available online: http://anatomyfacts.com/Research/ResearchMethodsKnowledgeBase.pdf (accessed on 25 February 2019).
18. Salazar, L.F.; Crosby, R.A.; DiClemente, R.J. *Research Methods in Health Promotion*; John Wiley & Sons: Hoboken, NJ, USA, 2015.
19. Experimental Research Designs. Available online: https://psycnet.apa.org/record/2015-10205-005 (accessed on 25 February 2019).
20. Allen, M. *The SAGE Encyclopedia of Communication Research Methods*; Sage Publications: Southend Oaks, CA, USA, 2017.
21. Trochim, W.M.K.; Donnelly, J.P. *Research Methods Knowledge Base*, 3rd ed.; Atomic Dog: New York, NY, USA, 2020.
22. Painter, I.; Chavez, D.E.; Ike, B.R.; Yip, M.P.; Tu, S.P.; Bradley, S.M.; Rea, T.D.; Meischke, H. Changes to DA-CPR instructions: Can we reduce time to first compression and improve quality of bystander CPR? *Resuscitation* **2014**, *85*, 1169–1173. [CrossRef]
23. Chen, K.-Y.; Ko, Y.-C.; Hsieh, M.-J.; Chiang, W.-C.; Ma, M.H.-M. Interventions to improve the quality of bystander cardiopulmonary resuscitation: A systematic review. *PLoS ONE* **2019**, *14*, e0211792. [CrossRef]

24. García del Águila, J.; López-Messa, J.; Rosell-Ortiz, F.; de Elías Hernández, R.; Martínez del Valle, M.; Sánchez-Santos, L.; López-Herce, J.; Cerdà-Vila, M.; Roza-Alonso, C.L.; Bernardez-Otero, M. Recomendaciones para el soporte telefónico a la reanimación por testigos desde los centros de coordinación de urgencias y emergencias. *Med. Intensiva* **2015**, *39*, 298–302. [CrossRef]

25. Trethewey, S.P.; Vyas, H.; Evans, S.; Hall, M.; Melody, T.; Perkins, G.D.; Couper, K. The impact of resuscitation guideline terminology on quality of dispatcher-assisted cardiopulmonary resuscitation: A randomised controlled manikin study. *Resuscitation* **2019**, *142*, 91–96. [CrossRef]

26. Fontes, S.; García-Gallego, C.; Quintanilla, L.; Rodríguez, R.; Rubio, P.; Sarriá, E. Fundamentos de investigación en psicología. In *Diseños y Estrategias*; UNED: Madrid, Spain, 2010.

27. Schulz, K.F.; Altman, D.G.; Moher, D. CONSORT 2010 Statement: Updated guidelines for reporting parallel group randomised trials. *BMJ* **2010**, *340*. [CrossRef]

28. Ortiz, F.R.; Roig, F.E.; Navalpotro Pascual, J.M.; Iglesias Vázquez, J.A.; Sucunza, A.E.; Cordero Torres, J.A.; Cobos, E.; del Valle, M.M.; Rozalen, I.C.; martín Sánchez, E.; et al. Out-of-Hospital Spanish Cardiac Arrest Registry (OHSCAR). Results of the first year. *Resuscitation* **2015**, *96*, 100. [CrossRef]

29. Williams, A.M.; Hodges, N.J. Practice, instruction and skill acquisition in soccer: Challenging tradition. *J. Sports Sci.* **2005**, *23*, 637–650. [CrossRef] [PubMed]

30. D'Innocenzo, G.; Gonzalez, C.C.; Williams, A.M.; Bishop, D.T. Looking to Learn: The Effects of Visual Guidance on Observational Learning of the Golf Swing. *PLoS ONE* **2016**, *11*, e0155442. [CrossRef] [PubMed]

31. Rodriguez, S.A.; Sutton, R.M.; Berg, M.D.; Nishisaki, A.; Maltese, M.; Meaney, P.A.; Niles, D.E.; Leffelman, J.; Berg, R.A.; Nadkarni, V.M. Simplified dispatcher instructions improve bystander chest compression quality during simulated pediatric resuscitation. *Resuscitation* **2014**, *85*, 119–123. [CrossRef] [PubMed]

32. Li, S.; Kan, T.; Guo, Z.; Chen, C.; Gui, L. Assessing the quality of CPR performed by a single lifeguard, two lifeguards and a lifeguard with a bystander after water rescue: A quasi-experimental trial. *Emerg. Med. J.* **2020**. [CrossRef] [PubMed]

33. Taniguchi, T.; Sato, K.; Fujita, T.; Okajima, M.; Takamura, M. Attitudes to Bystander Cardiopulmonary Resuscitation in Japan in 2010. *Circ. J.* **2012**, *76*, 1130–1135. [CrossRef]

34. Chang, M.P.; Gent, L.M.; Sweet, M.; Potts, J.; Ahtone, J.; Idris, A.H. A novel educational outreach approach to teach Hands-Only Cardiopulmonary Resuscitation to the public. *Resuscitation* **2017**, *116*, 22–26. [CrossRef]

35. Olasveengen, T.M.; de Caen, A.R.; Mancini, M.E.; Maconochie, I.K.; Aickin, R.; Atkins, D.L.; Berg, R.A.; Bingham, R.M.; Brooks, S.C.; Castrén, M.; et al. 2017 International Consensus on Cardiopulmonary Resuscitation and Emergency Cardiovascular Care Science with Treatment Recommendations Summary. *Circulation* **2017**, *136*, e424–e440. [CrossRef]

36. González-Salvado, V.; Rodríguez-Ruiz, E.; Abelairas-Gómez, C.; Ruano-Raviña, A.; Peña-Gil, C.; González-Juanatey, J.R.; Rodríguez-Núñez, A. Training adult laypeople in basic life support. A systematic review. *Revista Española de Cardiología (Engl. Ed.)* **2020**, *73*, 53–68. [CrossRef]

37. Beskind, D.L.; Stolz, U.; Thiede, R.; Hoyer, R.; Robertson, W.; Brown, J.; Ludgate, M.; Tiutan, T.; Shane, R.; McMorrow, D.; et al. Viewing an ultra-brief chest compression only video improves some measures of bystander CPR performance and responsiveness at a mass gathering event. *Resuscitation* **2017**, *118*, 96–100. [CrossRef]

38. Benoit, J.L.; Vogele, J.; Hart, K.W.; Lindsell, C.J.; McMullan, J.T. Passive ultra-brief video training improves performance of compression-only cardiopulmonary resuscitation. *Resuscitation* **2017**, *115*, 116–119. [CrossRef]

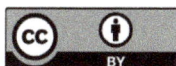

International Journal of
*Environmental Research
and Public Health*

MDPI

Article

Increase in Video Consultations During the COVID-19 Pandemic: Healthcare Professionals' Perceptions about Their Implementation and Adequate Management

Diana Jiménez-Rodríguez [1,*], Azucena Santillán García [2], Jesús Montoro Robles [3], María del Mar Rodríguez Salvador [4], Francisco José Muñoz Ronda [4] and Oscar Arrogante [5,*]

[1] Department of Nursing, Physiotherapy and Medicine, University of Almeria, 04120 Almeria, Spain

[2] Department of Cardiology, Burgos University Hospital, 09006 Burgos, Spain; ebevidencia@gmail.com

[3] Teaching Unit, Nursing Subcommittee, Primary Care District Poniente of Almeria, 04746 Almeria, Spain; jenrique.montoro.sspa@juntadeandalucia.es

[4] Knowledge and Research Management Department, Primary Care District of Almeria, 04007 Almeria, Spain; mariam.rodriguez.salvador.sspa@juntadeandalucia.es (M.d.M.R.S.); rondalia@gmail.com (F.J.M.R.)

[5] University Centre of Health Sciences San Rafael, San Juan de Dios Foundation, Nebrija University, 28036 Madrid, Spain

* Correspondence: d.jimenez@ual.es (D.J.-R.); oarrogan@nebrija.es (O.A.)

Received: 16 June 2020; Accepted: 12 July 2020; Published: 15 July 2020

check for updates

Abstract: In response to the COVID-19 pandemic, health care modalities such as video consultations have been rapidly developed to provide safe health care and to minimize the risk of spread. The purpose of our study is to explore Spanish healthcare professionals' perceptions about the implementation of video consultations. Based on the testimonies of 53 professionals, different categories emerged related to the four identified themes: benefits of video consultations (for professionals, patients, and the health system, and compared to phone calls), negative aspects (inherent to new technologies and the risk of a perceived distancing from the professional), difficulties associated with the implementation of video consultations (technological difficulties, lack of technical skills and refusal to use video consultation among professionals and patients), and the need for training (technological, nontechnical, and social-emotional skills, and adaptation of technical skills). Additionally, the interviewees indicated that this new modality of health care may be extended to a broader variety of patients and clinical settings. Therefore, since video consultations are becoming more widespread, it would be advisable for health policies and systems to support this modality of health care, promoting their implementation and guaranteeing their operability, equal access and quality.

Keywords: clinical skills; COVID-19; healthcare providers; implementation; interpersonal skills; perception; qualitative research; telemedicine; training; video consultation

---

1. Introduction

Telemedicine is the use of telecommunication systems to provide health care from a distance [1]. This modality comes in different variations: online consultations, by telephone or videoconference, telemonitoring/screening with devices that monitor a patient's vital signs, sensors with GPS trackers, and chatbots for recommendations [2]. However, the most commonly used are video consultations [1,3]. The main medical conditions that require video consultations are hypertension, diabetes, heart failure, asthma, chronic obstructive pulmonary disease and the care of elderly patients [3]. Therefore, video consultations have been widely used with patients who have common chronic conditions [4] and primary care needs [5]; these types of consultations are even considered the future of healthcare [6]. More specifically, nursing professionals have used video consultations in follow-up care for patients after surgery, patients with chronic diseases, families of children with cancer and premature newborns [7]. Telemedicine has demonstrated similar health outcomes and patient/healthcare professional satisfaction compared with in-person healthcare consultations, and has improved access to health care services [1,8]. In addition, some cost-utility and cost-effectiveness studies have demonstrated that telemedicine can reduce costs [1,8,9].

On March 11, 2020, the World Health Organization declared the novel coronavirus disease 2019 (COVID-19) outbreak as a pandemic. Most positive cases are asymptomatic or self-limiting, but the clinical spectrum of the disease extends to severe progressive pneumonia with acute respiratory distress syndrome (ARDS), which is a life-threatening condition requiring mechanical ventilation and intensive care support [10]. The symptomatology of COVID-19 infection is not specific, which makes it clinically indistinguishable from other viral respiratory illnesses [11]. According to recent systematic reviews, the most common disease-related symptoms are fever, cough, muscle aches and/or fatigue, dyspnea, headache, sore throat, and gastrointestinal symptoms [11] and skin lesions with different clinical characteristics [12]. In addition, there is evidence that COVID-19 may exacerbate certain cardiovascular symptoms and lead to cardiovascular complications [13]. Finally, some mental disorders have even been aggravated during this pandemic [14]. In this sense, nurses are central to COVID-19 prevention and the care of infected patients. Nurses are not only providing frontline care in severe COVID-19 cases that require hospitalization, but are also monitoring outpatients in community settings, and providing education to patients and the general public about the outbreak [15]. However, the rapid progression of COVID-19 around the world has become a real challenge for health organizations and policies, exemplified by the implementation of social distancing measures, such as quarantine periods [16]. As all healthcare professionals are at risk of contagion, new modalities of care are emerging in order to avoid face-to-face contact with patients and to ensure that patients receive the care they need [17,18]. Furthermore, as governments have been promoting social distancing, the creation of safe medical settings has become a priority [19] in order to avoid the risk of spreading the disease [20]. For instance, in Spain, 24.1% of positive COVID-19 cases have been reported among healthcare professionals [21].

In this sense, video consultations are considered the perfect solution during this worldwide pandemic [18], mitigating its impact on the population's health and the use of health resources, and are being promoted, especially in the United Kingdom and the United States of America [22]. In addition, the population's interest in telehealth and the number of telemedicine visits have dramatically increased during the pandemic, owing to restrictions on in-person clinical encounters [23,24]. Moreover, telemedicine platforms are ideal for responding to global infectious disease outbreaks and preventing overcrowding in emergency departments in hospitals, primary care clinics and emergency services [25]. Consequently, many governments have been forced to adapt to the sudden implementation of telemedicine to promote safety for low-acuity patients, their family members and healthcare professionals, and to avoid delays in the provision of health care that may result in more health problems or complicate existing clinical situations, jeopardizing patients' future health [19]. For instance, online mental health services have been promoted within the context of COVID-19 [20]. Therefore, this pandemic is a call to action in countries without integrated telemedicine in their national health system [22].

In Spain, 100% of the population has access to the public health system. In response to the COVID-19 pandemic, the Spanish health authorities implemented follow-up systems at the primary care level, mainly consisting of phone calls [2]. In addition, some private health providers offered video consultations for the general public free of charge. Consequently, some Spanish health authorities are currently strengthening the use of teleconsultations and telemedicine as a public health policy for the reorganization and normalization of health care services.

However, studies have paid surprisingly little attention to the perception of telemedicine among healthcare professionals, mainly focusing rather on barriers to and difficulties with this modality of healthcare [3]. Thus, when a new approach is implemented, it is important to examine how it is perceived by healthcare professionals, as this could influence its usefulness and effectiveness. Furthermore, introducing video consultations to healthcare services is far more difficult than healthcare professionals assume, as they need to change their routines and the manner in which they care for patients [17]. Healthcare professionals need to understand that interactions during video consultations are different from face-to-face consultations, and thus, they need to be ready to deal with certain challenges: establishing a connection and starting a video consultation, dealing with disruption to the conversational flow, breakdowns of video consultation platforms and latency in the conversation [26]. Although at present health authorities are racing to implement virtual health-care technologies as fast as they can, and healthcare professionals are motivated to use them to reduce the spread of COVID-19 [27], their perceptions about this new modality of healthcare provision must be examined in order to ensure and improve its effectiveness.

For this reason, the purpose of our study is to explore Spanish healthcare professionals' perceptions about the implementation of video consultations and its management in the provision of high-quality health care.

2. Materials and Methods

2.1. Study Design

A descriptive observational study was carried out using a qualitative methodology. This methodology is the most suited to achieving a deep understanding of the phenomenon of interest [28], such as the emerging implementation of a modality for the provision of health care that has an impact on the professionals who have to manage it. In this way, understanding their perception regarding video consultations may help us to understand this phenomenon and make more informed decisions regarding future courses of action. In addition, to ensure the quality and transparency of our research, The Consolidated Criteria for Reporting Qualitative Research (COREQ checklist proposed by Tong et al. [29]) was followed.

2.2. Sample and Setting

Although the sample size was not selected a priori, qualitative data were collected following two precepts: the data saturation precept proposed by Morse [30] (interviews continue until new elements of discourse are no longer collected) and the novelty precept proposed by Mayan [31] (data is collected until it is considered that something important and novel could be derived therefrom about the phenomenon of interest).

All study informants were working healthcare professionals in the public health system in the same Spanish region. Consequently, biases related to different organizational and care environments were avoided.

According to the recommendations for sample selection proposed by Patton [32], our purpose was to use selected participants (healthcare professionals with or without experience in video consultation) to obtain the greatest quantity of information in order to understand the phenomenon under study in depth. In this way, snowball or chain sampling was carried out, identifying relevant participants with the collaboration of key informants (training and research managers in healthcare departments) who nominated good candidates for our study.

Ultimately, the study included a total of 53 healthcare professionals. The study was carried out between 02 April 2020 and 25 May 2020.

2.3. Data Collection

A structured interview, comprising four closed-ended and four open-ended questions, was used to collect sociodemographic data and to facilitate in-depth discussion of all relevant topics (see the interview outline in Table 1). All participants were interviewed online (using the Google Meet™ video platform (Google, Mountain View, CA, USA)) due to social distancing restrictions during the COVID-19 pandemic. The interviews lasted 15 min on average and were carried out by a researcher with extensive experience in qualitative research, who had no working relationship with any healthcare professional and strictly followed the interview outline, thus ensuring objectivity and avoiding possible biases. The entire content of the interviews was recorded with the participants' consent.

Table 1. Interview outline.

Aspects Addressed	Questions
Sociodemographic data	Age Sex Professional category Work experience (years) Workplace (primary health or hospital services)
Closed-ended questions about general aspects of video consultations	Do you consider video consultations to be an appropriate means by which to provide health care? If your answer was affirmative, which patients do you consider would mainly benefit from this modality of health care? If you have already held a video consultation, indicate the approximate number of video consultations you have held. Do you consider that healthcare professionals need to be trained in this modality of health care?
Open-ended questions about specific aspects about video consultations	Indicate the benefits and positive aspects associated with the use of video consultations. Indicate the negative aspects associated with the use of video consultations. Indicate the difficulties in implementing video consultations. To properly hold a video consultation, which skills do you consider are relevant and should be taught?

2.4. Data Analysis

The mean and standard deviation (SD) were calculated to analyze sociodemographic data and responses to closed-ended questions. Qualitative data were obtained from the healthcare professionals' responses to the four proposed open-ended questions. All perceptions and opinions from the healthcare professionals were transcribed and reviewed by two different members of the research team who were experts on qualitative methodologies. A content analysis of the qualitative data was performed; this allowed us to discover the views of each health professional by analyzing their responses and perceptions about the phenomenon of interest [33]. The themes identified were aligned with the four proposed open-ended questions.

Subsequently, qualitative data were analyzed to identify reiterated words, sentences, or ideas that were finally codified into different categories and grouped into the identified themes [31]. Firstly, an initial reading of the discourses was performed to analyze the categories. Then, the emerging categories were codified through the consensus and refinement reached by the two researchers [31].

All data were stored, managed, classified, and organized using the qualitative data analytical software, ATLAS.ti 8 Windows (Scientific Software Development GmbH, Berlin, Germany).

2.5. Ethical Considerations

This study was approved by the Research and Ethics Board of the Department of Nursing, Physiotherapy, and Medicine at the university (n° EFM 75/2020), and was carried out following the ethical principles for medical research of the international Declaration of Helsinki [34]. All participants received information about the study, participated voluntarily, and provided their written consent. In addition, and to ensure anonymity, the participants were numerically labeled in chronological order according to the date of the interview, preceded by the letter "S" (subject).

3. Results

The quantitative data collected from the closed-ended questions showed that 96.2% of the healthcare professionals considered videoconference consultations to be an adequate option for providing health care, indicating which patients would most benefit from this modality. The types of patients that were mentioned most often, i.e., in 14 to 7 informant responses, were chronic patients, patients who required medical follow-ups and examinations, difficulties in movement (either due to physical disability or geographical dispersion, or work reasons), and administrative petitions (such as prescriptions, work leaves due to illness or accident, etc.). However, the types of patients that were mentioned least often, i.e., in 4 to 2 responses, were resolutions of medical questions (from patients, caregivers, mothers, etc.), any type of medical condition that did not require physical examinations, on-demand consultations such as screening to evaluate in-person assistance or not, health education, mental health disorders, common, minor diseases, and dermatology. Furthermore, most interviewed professionals had not provided health care via videoconference ($n = 44$; 83%). Conversely, the number of video conferences among healthcare professionals who had used this modality ranged from 1 to 5 (mean = 2.66; SD = 1.322). Lastly, 90.6% of participants considered it necessary to train and educate professionals in this modality of healthcare. It should be noted that no differences were found based on gender or professional category in any quantitative data collected.

As for the qualitative data, results were obtained after analyzing the contents of the open-ended questions. During this content analysis, possible divergence in the participants' discourse according to their professional category and workplace (primary care or hospital services) was taken into account, although these factors did not affect the majority of the categories identified, with a few exceptions, as described in the corresponding category, presented below and grouped into four main themes (aligned with the four open-ended questions) and the categories that emerged from the participants' narratives and that were strongly supported by them (see also Table 2).

Table 2. Comprehensive list of themes and categories identified after thematic analysis.

Healthcare Professionals' Perceptions about Video Consultations' Implementation	Theme 1. Benefits of Video Consultations	Theme 2. Negative Aspects	Theme 3. Difficulties in the Implementation of Video Consultations	Theme 4. Skills Needed to Hold a Video Consultation and Training is Needed
Categories	Benefits of video consultations for both healthcare professionals and patients	Negative aspects inherent to new technologies	Technological difficulties	Technological skill
	Benefits for the health system	Risk of perceived distancing from professional	Lack of technical skills among professionals and patients	Nontechnical and social-emotional skills
	Benefits of video consultations compared to phone calls		Refusal to use video consultations by healthcare professionals and patients	Adaptation of technical skills

3.1. Theme 1. Benefits of Video Consultations

Within the context of the COVID-19 pandemic, where interviews were conducted, the clear benefit of avoiding spreading the disease was confirmed by healthcare professionals. In addition, they considered that video consultations may provide numerous benefits, with no significant differences according to their professional category or workplace. In this way, the categories that emerged, in order of repetition frequency, are as follows:

3.1.1. Benefits of Video Consultations for Both Healthcare Professionals and Patients

Our healthcare professionals referred to avoiding movement that may be unnecessary (both for patients who do not have to visit to health centers in person and healthcare professionals who do not have to travel to patients' homes). This benefit was repeated in the discourse of most healthcare professionals.

"It avoids the patient's travels to health centers" (S39)

"You can solve their problems without having to travel and they see you, which is important for them" (S42)

"To avoid the loss of working hours in patients when the medical consultation coincides with their working time, avoiding the time required to the movement from their works centers to the health centers and the waiting for their turn" (S7)

"The management of time, of the patient and the professional, convenience, flexibility, less bureaucracy" (S43)

3.1.2. Benefits for the Health System

This category includes benefits such as efficient consultations, avoiding agglomerations and waiting lists, quick resolutions of common, minor diseases, a decrease in workload at healthcare centers, and cost reduction. In this sense, our healthcare professionals perceived that the implementation of video consultations may have direct benefits for the health system.

"It favors accessibility and immediacy, and serves as an efficient filter for in-person consultation". (S2)

"in specific situations, it can decrease the waitlist time" (S10)

"(...) less crowds in waiting rooms, streamlining of banal diseases" (S11)

3.1.3. Benefits of Video Consultations Compared to Phone Calls

The informants indicated benefits of video consultations compared to phone calls, which is currently the most used modality of telemedicine in Spain. In this sense, informants perceived as beneficial the possibility of assessing patients' physical aspect, in contrast to phone consultations. Since the interaction is direct, contact with the patient is ensured, allowing both verbal and nonverbal communication to occur.

"You can see the patient's face (...) you can assess aspects of non-verbal communication" (S3)

"I have provided care on the phone with information via *Telematics, although I think that the video consultation goes beyond, because it allows you to assess the expression and transmit more to the patient, re-enforcing communication"* (S21)

"A faithful contact with the patient is maintained, dedicating the time needed without interruptions" (S49)

3.2. Theme 2. Negative Aspects

Two quite different categories emerged: the first was consistent among the interviewed professionals, while the second was almost anecdotal.

3.2.1. Negative Aspects Inherent to New Technologies

Obviously, since it is a technology that does not require physical contact, there are some medical procedures that are impossible. Our healthcare professionals highlighted two main issues: the impossibility of physical examinations or procedural techniques during video consultations, and its management and/or technological difficulties, such as a lack of access for both professionals and patients (especially for the elderly). In this case, general practitioners mainly indicated the impossibility of performing physical examinations as a major drawback. Although our informants considered some negative aspects of this modality, they did not propose any solutions to address them.

"There is a lack of examination if it was needed" (S38)

"The elder population and those who are not so old, for them to have the tools necessary to conduct it, and the knowledge, and this is relevant to some professionals" (S43)

"For some patients, it use could be complex. For those who are older, they need the necessary support to be able to use this means of communication" (S50)

3.2.2. Risk of Perception of Distancing From Professional

Healthcare professionals were concerned that their patients may perceive the use of video consultations as a form of distancing from the health professional. In this sense, healthcare professionals were concerned that relationships with their patients may deteriorate and/or the internet connection required to hold a video consultation may create an environment of mistrust for patients.

"The perception of some patients of distancing" (S33)

"Mistrust in the use of technology, difficulties for older people, who do not have the devices, the relationship can be seen as more distant" (S34)

3.3. Theme 3. Difficulties in the Implementation of Video Consultations

The difficulties that emerged from the informants' discourse were inherent to the use of new technologies, which may be unfamiliar or challenging. The needs to provide resources to healthcare professionals so that they could hold a video consultation, and the need to train and shape them for the adequate use of this new modality, were underlined.

3.3.1. Technological Difficulties

In anticipation of the future implementation of this healthcare modality, technology was a re-emphasized issue, related to certain patients having access to the required resources and technological difficulties for both professionals and patients, with particular emphasis on the elderly.

"Not all the patients, especially the older ones, have access to these technologies or they don't know how to handle them" (S12)

"Lack of use by the professionals and the older patients" (S20)

"Computer problems and the older patients who do not know how they work" (S38)

3.3.2. Lack of Technical Skills Among Professionals and Patients

Another difficulty for the implementation of this healthcare resource is the lack of technical suitability of both professionals and patients, mainly regarding the elderly.

"It needs more time and adequate technical skills from both parties" (S2)

"Perhaps at first, until the population is familiarized with this technique" (S26)

"Difficulty of older people to adapt to this method" (S50)

3.3.3. Refusal to Use Video Consultations by Healthcare Professionals and Patients

This issue emerged in a handful of the analyzed discourses. Our informants were concerned about the possible refusal to use this new modality by professionals and/or patients.

"Technical difficulties. Rejection of specific patients/doctors to this type of distance care" (S7)

"Mistrust, resistance from both parties towards the use of the technology" (S34)

3.4. Theme 4. Skills Needed to Hold a Video Consultation and the Need for Training

Within in this theme, technological skills appeared once again to be the main issue, while nontechnical and social-emotional skills were second. To a lesser extent, the need emerged to adapt the technical skills that are required for this modality.

3.4.1. Technological Skill

This is related to the need to adequately manage the software or application used and the technological requirements.

"Handling of telematics tools" (S20)

"Correctly use the technology" (S29)

"Use of the informatics tools or applications" (S34)

3.4.2. Nontechnical and Social-Emotional Skills

Informants emphasized a wide variety of skills, since they were concerned that such skills may not be adequately managed using a modality without physical proximity. In this way, they indicated the following skills in order of importance: effective communication (the most repeated), empathy and patience, verbal and nonverbal language, skills required for structured and guided clinical interviews, assertiveness, and conflict resolution.

"Communication skills (active listening, empathy, emotional support), motivation, creativity, conflict resolution, patience" (S35)

"Active listening, communication and clinical interview skills, deferred conflict resolution, fomenting trust through this medium" (S48)

3.4.3. Adaptation of Technical Skills

This is related to the need to find a substitute for physical contact. Although the interviewees raised this concern, they did not propose any solutions.

"Probability of guiding a self-examination" (S16)

"Assess clinical aspects that can replace the clinical examination in part" (S32)

4. Discussion

Our results show that even though 83% of the interviewed informants had not conducted a video consultation, they considered it to be an adequate option for health care (96.2%). Most of our participants had not used this modality because the most common form of telemedicine in Spain is the phone call, although the Spanish health system is currently encouraging the use of video consultation as a public health policy for the reorganization and normalization of healthcare services [2]. Taking into account that video consultations are currently considered a necessary tool, the present study was proposed to explore Spanish healthcare professionals' perceptions about their future implementation and adequate management in this country; it is very important to gauge health care providers' perceptions of this approach, given that the they are the ones who will conduct such consultations, and therefore, the quality of this modality will be dependent on them. These perceptions have not been investigated to date, although recent studies have focused on the general population, indicating a growing interest in telehealth, as it is a highly-demanded modality of health care during the pandemic [24].

In addition, the interviewed professionals indicated numerous clinical situations and diseases where video consultations may be used (for both chronic and acute disease conditions). In this sense, they are in agreement with the reviewed evidence, in that this technology could be useful in cases such as chronic diseases, medical follow-ups, and mental health or dermatology examinations [7,35]. However, the interviewed healthcare professionals extended video consultation use to almost all patients who had access to this technology, as also indicated by new research on this growing field [36–38].

Furthermore, as this modality of healthcare may be complex, the healthcare professionals interviewed considered that training was needed (90.6%). This is because the most-utilized modality of telehealth in Spain is still the phone call [2]. However, it should be taken into account that the implementation of an effective program in telemedicine takes time [18], so it is logical that training and education would be needed. In this sense, this finding is consistent with the study by Portnoy et al. [39], who stated that healthcare professionals may be trained and shaped to be "telefacilitators".

Telemedicine has been shown to be an ideal response to the COVID-19 pandemic, with its use having been greatly extended in recent months [25]. This was shown by healthcare professionals themselves, who indicated the avoidance of infection and spread as a clear benefit of video consultations. Also, many other benefits for both patients and healthcare professionals were noted, e.g., avoiding travel, wider availability, its immediate nature, saving time, ease of use and consequent increased efficacy [40]. In this way, video consultations improve accessibility, and can be used to opportunely tend to urgent concerns. Regarding time-saving, Calton et al. [40] stated that video consultations saved "windshield time" for home-visiting general practitioners.

Additionally, the healthcare professionals interviewed considered that video consultations offered efficient screening for consultations, avoiding crowds and waiting lists, allowing for quick resolutions of common, minor diseases, and decreasing workloads and costs in healthcare centers, as shown by other studies [1,8,9,25].

In contrast, our informants considered as negative the improper use of the technology and the inability to perform physical examinations. However, there are current platforms, applications, and medical devices that may compensate for the need to perform such examination at patients' homes, so medical procedures or techniques may be adapted to some patients [41,42]. In this sense, it is important to ensure that remote healthcare professionals are able to see that the patients are performing the examination correctly [41].

The difficulties identified by our informants regarding the implementation of video consultations were consistent with those of other studies [1,3,8,39,41]. Technological difficulties are the most worrisome issue among healthcare professionals. In addition, it should be noted that the refusal to use video consultations may be solved by performing preliminary trials, which often improve attitudes towards technology [40]. However, problems may arise among patients of advanced age, who may have reduced cognitive abilities [3]. Conversely, the barriers perceived by patients for the implementation of video consultations should also be taken into account. In this study, the perception of patients was not addressed. In this sense, a previous study indicated that although patients were willing to use them, they will likely go back to in-person consultations, as they may prefer to be attended to by their usual healthcare provider, or they may even ignore video consultations if they do not know how to use them [39]. There is no doubt that video consultations are needed in different health systems; therefore, this pandemic is a call to action in countries without such an option already integrated into their health systems [22]. However, most countries have not created a regulatory framework to authorize and integrate telemedicine into their national health systems, including during emergency and outbreak situations [22]. Although our informants did not indicate any ethical issues related to the use of video consultations, previous studies have raised concerns that exchanging health information and providing care electronically could create new risks regarding the quality of healthcare, safety, privacy and confidentiality [43,44]. As for the skills needed to hold a video consultation, the healthcare professionals perceived that they needed to be trained to improve their technological skills. This is congruent with other studies that identified the need for staffing qualified professionals in this modality of healthcare [45]. In addition, our informants indicated the need for training regarding both nontechnical and social-emotional skills, such as effective communication, empathy, patience, nonverbal and verbal language, skills required for a structured and guided clinical interview, assertiveness, and conflict resolution. They emphasized a wide variety of skills which they felt may not be adequately managed using this healthcare modality. Although social-emotional skills related to video consultations have not been analyzed in depth, Humphreys et al. [46] stated that the interaction between patients and health care providers during video consultation care was substantially different from in-person care, mainly in cases of palliative care or cancer patients. However, other studies indicated that both types of care may be similar if the internet connection is of high-quality [40,41]. In this way, patients and healthcare providers tend to communicate in the same manner as in in-person consultations. Minor technical breakdowns have been demonstrated not to cause major disruptions to clinical interactions [41]. In fact, video consultations have been considered an effective modality in the provision of health care to cancer and palliative patients and their relatives [40,47,48], for whom nontechnical and social-emotional skills are essential. Therefore, training regarding video consultation, to facilitate its adequate adaptation in the provision of high-quality care, is needed [46]. Furthermore, our informants perceived that they should be trained in adapting medical procedures and techniques, although this is more complex, as specific devices may sometimes be required at patients' homes [41].

Video consultations were considered as a promising tool before the COVID-19 pandemic [49], and at present, are being used around the world [1,3] due to the need to avoid the spread of the virus [17,18]; therefore increased training and research in this field are required to ensure that high-quality health care is being provided. However, patients will also need to be provided with the devices required to adequately perform video consultations [41,44].

Lastly, as we carried out a small-scale qualitative study, there could be limitations related to the transferability of our findings. Nonetheless, this study aimed to address healthcare professionals' perceptions about the immediate implementation of video consultations in their daily clinical practice, and this objective was achieved. In this sense, it should be noted that most interviewed informants had never held a video consultation, so their perceptions may change when they use this modality of health care. In addition, video consultations may differ according to the platform, software, or devices used. Consequently, more research on this topic is recommended. Lastly, it would be advisable to study the barriers perceived by patients related to the implementation of video consultations.

5. Conclusions

For the effective implementation of video consultations as a modality of health care within a health system, it is important to examine how it is perceived by healthcare professionals, as this could have an impact on its effectiveness. Our informants identified the positive and negative aspects related to video consultations, the difficulties associated with its implementation, and the skills required for its management; they also acknowledged that training is required. During the COVID-19 pandemic, the implementation of video consultations may yield information on the future of telemedicine with the goal of providing healthcare not only to chronic patients, but also to those with acute diseases. They have been shown to be useful in a broader sense, and so should not be stopped when the pandemic is mitigated. As our informants indicated, the use of video consultations may be extended to a wide variety of patients and clinical situations. It would be advisable to implement health policies and systems to support this modality of health care, promoting its implementation and guaranteeing its operability, equal access and quality of healthcare.

Author Contributions: Conceptualization, D.J.-R., M.d.M.R.S., F.J.M.R. and O.A.; data curation, D.J.-R.; formal analysis, D.J.-R. and F.J.M.R.; investigation, D.J.-R., M.d.M.R.S., J.M.R., F.J.M.R. and O.A.; methodology, D.J.-R., M.d.M.R.S., F.J.M.R. and O.A.; project administration, D.J.-R.; supervision, D.J.-R.; validation, D.J.-R.; visualization, O.A.; writing—original draft, D.J.-R., A.S.G. and O.A.; writing—review & editing, D.J.-R., A.S.G., J.M.R., M.d.M.R.S., F.J.M.R. and O.A. All authors have read and agreed to the published version of the manuscript.

Funding: This research received no external funding.

Acknowledgments: We wish to publicly recognize our gratitude to the Provincial Headquarters of the Foundation for Biosanitary Research of Eastern Andalusia (FIBAO, in Spanish) in Almería, for their invaluable collaboration in the strategic and methodological organization of this study.

Conflicts of Interest: The authors declare no conflict of interest.

References

1. Flodgren, G.; Rachas, A.; Farmer, A.J.; Inzitari, M.; Shepperd, S. Interactive telemedicine: Effects on professional practice and health care outcomes. *Cochrane Database Syst. Rev.* **2015**, *2015*, CD002098. [CrossRef] [PubMed]

2. Vidal-Alaball, J.; Acosta-Roja, R.; Hernández, N.P.; Luque, U.S.; Morrison, D.; Pérez, S.N.; Llano, J.P.; Vèrges, A.S.; Seguí, F.L.; Pastor, N.; et al. Telemedicine in the face of the COVID-19 pandemic. *Atención Primaria* **2020**, *52*, 418–422. [CrossRef] [PubMed]

3. Bertoncello, C.; Colucci, M.; Baldovin, T.; Buja, A.; Baldo, V. How does it work? Factors involved in telemedicine home-interventions effectiveness: A review of reviews. *PLoS ONE* **2018**, *13*, e0207332. [CrossRef] [PubMed]

4. Mallow, J.A.; Petitte, T.; Narsavage, G.; Barnes, E.R.; Theeke, E.; Mallow, B.K.; Theeke, L.A. The use of video conferencing for persons with chronic conditions: A systematic review. *E-Health Telecommun. Syst. Netw.* **2016**, *5*, 39–56. [CrossRef]

5. Peters, L.; Greenfield, G.; Majeed, A.; Hayhoe, B. The impact of private online video consulting in primary care. *J. R. Soc. Med.* **2018**, *111*, 162–166. [CrossRef]

6. Spence, D. Bad medicine: The future is video consulting. *Br. J. Gen. Pr.* **2018**, *68*, 437. [CrossRef]

7. Nordtug, B.; Brataas, H.V.; Rygg, L. The use of videoconferencing in nursing for people in their homes. *Nurs. Rep.* **2018**. [CrossRef]

8. Ignatowicz, A.; Atherton, H.; Bernstein, C.J.; Bryce, C.; Court, R.; Sturt, J.; Griffiths, F. Internet videoconferencing for patient–clinician consultations in long-term conditions: A review of reviews and applications in line with guidelines and recommendations. *Digit. Health* **2019**, *5*. [CrossRef]

9. Díez, I.D.L.T.; López-Coronado, M.; Vaca, C.; Sáez-Aguado, J.; De Castro, C. Cost-utility and cost-effectiveness studies of telemedicine, electronic, and mobile health systems in the literature: A systematic review. *Telemed. e-Health* **2015**, *21*, 81–85. [CrossRef]

10. Meini, S.; Pagotto, A.; Longo, B.; Vendramin, I.; Pecori, D.; Tascini, C. Role of lopinavir/Ritonavir in the treatment of COVID-19: A review of current evidence, guideline recommendations, and perspectives. A review of current evidence, guideline recommendations, and perspectives. *J. Clin. Med.* **2020**, *9*, 2050. [CrossRef]

11. Nascimento, I.J.B.D.; Cacic, N.; Abdulazeem, H.M.; Von Groote, T.C.; Jayarajah, U.; Weerasekara, I.; Esfahani, M.A.; Civile, V.T.; Marušić, A.; Jeroncic, A.; et al. Novel coronavirus infection (COVID-19) in humans: A scoping review and meta-analysis. *J. Clin. Med.* **2020**, *9*, 941. [CrossRef] [PubMed]

12. Kaya, G.; Kaya, A.; Saurat, J.-H. Clinical and histopathological features and potential pathological mechanisms of skin lesions in COVID-19: Review of the literature. *Dermatopathology* **2020**, *7*, 2. [CrossRef] [PubMed]

13. Aboughdir, M.; Kirwin, T.; Khader, A.A.; Wang, B. Prognostic value of cardiovascular biomarkers in COVID-19: A review. *Viruses* **2020**, *12*, 527. [CrossRef]

14. Tanhan, A.; Yavuz, K.F.; Young, J.S.; Nalbant, A.; Arslan, G.; Yıldırım, M.; Ulusoy, S.; Genç, E.; Uğur, E.; Çiçek, I. A proposed framework based on literature review of online contextual mental health services to enhance wellbeing and address psychopathology during COVID-19. *Electron. J. Gen. Med.* **2020**, *17*, em254. [CrossRef]

15. Choi, K.R.; Jeffers, K.S.; Logsdon, M.C. Nursing and the novel coronavirus: Risks and responsibilities in a global outbreak. *J. Adv. Nurs.* **2020**, *76*, 1486–1487. [CrossRef] [PubMed]

16. Nafees, M.; Khan, F. Pakistan's response to COVID-19 pandemic and efficacy of quarantine and partial lockdown: A review. *Electron. J. Gen. Med.* **2020**, *17*, em240. [CrossRef]

17. Greenhalgh, T.; Wherton, J.; Shaw, S.; Morrison, C. Video consultations for COVID-19. *BMJ* **2020**, *368*, m998. [CrossRef]

18. Hollander, J.E.; Carr, B.G. Virtually perfect? Telemedicine for COVID-19. *N. Engl. J. Med.* **2020**, *382*, 1679–1681. [CrossRef]

19. Smith, W.R.; Atala, A.J.; Terlecki, R.P.; Kelly, E.E.; Matthews, C.A. Implementation guide for rapid integration of an outpatient telemedicine program during the COVID-19 pandemic. *J. Am. Coll. Surg.* **2020**. [CrossRef]

20. Hagge, D.; Knopf, A.; Hofauer, B. Telemedicine in the fight against SARS-COV-2-opportunities and possible applications in otorhinolaryngology: Narrative review. *HNO* **2020**, *68*, 433–439. [CrossRef]

21. Análisis de los casos de COVID-19 en personal sanitario notificados a la RENAVE hasta el 10 de mayo en España. Fecha del informe: 29-05-2020. Available online: https://www.isciii.es/QueHacemos/Servicios/VigilanciaSaludPublicaRENAVE/EnfermedadesTransmisibles/Paginas/InformesCOVID-19.aspx (accessed on 30 May 2020).

22. Wu, C.; Liu, Y.; Ohannessian, R.; Duong, T.; Odone, A. Global telemedicine implementation and integration within health systems to fight the COVID-19 pandemic: A call to action. *JMIR Public Health Surveill.* **2020**, *6*, e18810.

23. Contreras, C.M.; Metzger, G.A.; Beane, J.D.; Dedhia, P.H.; Ejaz, A.; Pawlik, T.M. Telemedicine: Patient-provider clinical engagement during the COVID-19 pandemic and beyond. *J. Gastrointest. Surg.* **2020**, *8*, 1–6. [CrossRef] [PubMed]

24. Hong, Y.R.; Lawrence, J.; Williams, D., Jr.; Mainous III, A. Population-level interest and telehealth capacity of us hospitals in response to COVID-19: Cross-sectional analysis of google search and national hospital survey data. *JMIR Public Health Surveill.* **2020**, *6*, e18961. [CrossRef] [PubMed]

25. Rockwell, K.L.; Gilroy, A.S. Incorporating telemedicine as part of COVID-19 outbreak response systems. *Am. J. Manag. Care* **2020**, *26*, 147–148.

26. Shaw, S.; Seuren, L.M.; Wherton, J.; Cameron, D.; A'Court, C.; Vijayaraghavan, S.; Morris, J.; Bhattacharya, S.; Greenhalgh, T. Video consultations between patients and clinicians in diabetes, cancer, and heart failure services: Linguistic ethnographic study of video-mediated interaction. *J. Med. Internet Res.* **2020**, *22*, e18378. [CrossRef]

27. Webster, P. Virtual health care in the era of COVID-19. *Lancet* **2020**, *395*, 1180–1181. [CrossRef]

28. Martínez-Salgado, C. El muestreo en investigación cualitativa. Principios básicos y algunas controversias. *Ciência Saúde Coletiva* **2012**, *17*, 613–619. [CrossRef]

29. Tong, A.; Sainsbury, P.; Craig, J.C. Consolidated criteria for reporting qualitative research (COREQ): A 32-item checklist for interviews and focus groups. *Int. J. Qual. Health Care* **2007**, *19*, 349–357. [CrossRef]

30. Patton, M. *Qualitative Research and Evaluation Methods*, 3rd ed.; Sage: Thousand Oaks, CA, USA, 2002.

31. Morse, J.M. The significance of saturation. *Qual. Health Res.* **1995**, *5*, 147–149. [CrossRef]

32. Mayan, M.J. *Essentials of Qualitative Inquiry*; Informa UK Limited: London, UK, 2016.

33. Piñuel Raigada, J.L. Epistemología, metodología y técnicas del análisis de contenido [Epistemology, methodology and content analysis techniques]. *Estud. Sociolingüística* **2002**, *3*, 1–42.

34. World Medical Association. World Medical Association declaration of Helsinki: Ethical principles for medical research involving human subjects. *JAMA* **2013**, *310*, 2191–2194. [CrossRef] [PubMed]

35. Lee, J.J.; English, J.C. Teledermatology: A review and update. *Am. J. Clin. Dermatol.* **2017**, *19*, 253–260. [CrossRef] [PubMed]

36. Shokri, T.; Lighthall, J.G. Telemedicine in the era of the COVID-19 pandemic: Implications in facial plastic surgery. *Facial Plast. Surg. Aesthetic Med.* **2020**, *22*, 155–156. [CrossRef] [PubMed]

37. De Marchi, F.; Cantello, R.; Ambrosini, S.; Mazzini, L. On behalf of the CANPALS study group telemedicine and technological devices for amyotrophic lateral sclerosis in the era of COVID-19. *Neurol. Sci.* **2020**, *41*, 1–3. [CrossRef]

38. Szmuda, T.; Ali, S.; Słoniewski, P.; NSurg Wl Group. Telemedicine in neurosurgery during the novel coronavirus (COVID-19) pandemic. *Neurol. Neurochir. Pol.* **2020**, *54*, 207–208. [PubMed]

39. Portnoy, J.M.; Waller, M.; Elliott, T. Telemedicine in the era of COVID-19. *J. Allergy Clin. Immunol. Pr.* **2020**, *8*, 1489–1491. [CrossRef]

40. Calton, B.A.; Rabow, M.W.; Branagan, L.; Dionne-Odom, J.N.; Oliver, D.P.; Bakitas, M.A.; Fratkin, M.D.; Lustbader, D.; Jones, C.A.; Ritchie, C.S. Top ten tips palliative care clinicians should know about telepalliative care. *J. Palliat. Med.* **2019**, *22*, 981–985. [CrossRef]

41. Video Consultations: A Guide for Practice. Available online: https://bjgplife.com/2020/03/18/video-consultations-guide-for-practice/ (accessed on 29 May 2020).

42. Peyret, A.S.; Durón, R.M.; Díaz, M.A.S.; Meléndez, D.C.; Ventura, S.G.; González, E.B.; Rito, Y.; Juárez, I.E.M. Herramientas de salud digital para superar la brecha de atención en epilepsia antes, durante y después de la pandemia de COVID-19 [E-health tools to overcome the gap in epilepsy care before, during and after COVID-19 pandemics]. *Rev. Neurol.* **2020**, *70*, 323–328.

43. Hall, J.L.; McGraw, D. For telehealth to succeed, privacy and security risks must be identified and addressed. *Health Aff.* **2014**, *33*, 216–221. [CrossRef]

44. Chaet, D.; Clearfield, R.; Sabin, J.E.; Skimming, K. Council on ethical and judicial affairs American Medical Association. Ethical practice in telehealth and telemedicine. *J. Gen. Intern. Med.* **2017**, *32*, 1136–1140. [CrossRef]

45. Patel, U.K.; Malik, P.; Demasi, M.; Lunagariya, A.; Jani, V.B. Multidisciplinary approach and outcomes of Tele-neurology: A review. *Cureus* **2019**, *11*, e4410. [CrossRef] [PubMed]

46. Humphreys, J.; Schoenherr, L.; Elia, G.; Saks, N.T.; Brown, C.; Barbour, S.; Pantilat, S.Z. Rapid implementation of inpatient telepalliative medicine consultations during COVID-19 pandemic. *J. Pain Symptom Manag.* **2020**, *60*, e54–e59. [CrossRef] [PubMed]

47. Svendsen, C.O.; Vestergaard, L.V.; Dieperink, K.B.; Danbjørg, D.; Alpert, J.; Mohammadzadeh, N.; Østervang, C. Patient rounds with video-consulted relatives: Qualitative study on possibilities and barriers from the perspective of healthcare providers. *J. Med. Internet Res.* **2019**, *21*, e12584.

48. Perrone, G.; Zerbo, S.; Bilotta, C.; Malta, G.; Argo, A. Telemedicine during COVID-19 pandemic: Advantage or critical issue? *Medico-Legal J.* **2020**. [CrossRef] [PubMed]

49. Jess, M.; Timm, H.; Dieperink, K.B. Video consultations in palliative care: A systematic integrative review. *Palliat. Med.* **2019**, *33*, 942–958. [CrossRef]

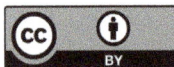

International Journal of
Environmental Research and Public Health

MDPI

Article

Use of the Barthel Index to Assess Activities of Daily Living before and after SARS-COVID 19 Infection of Institutionalized Nursing Home Patients

Bibiana Trevissón-Redondo [1], Daniel López-López [2], Eduardo Pérez-Boal [3], Pilar Marqués-Sánchez [1], Cristina Liébana-Presa [1], Emmanuel Navarro-Flores [4], Raquel Jiménez-Fernández [5], Inmaculada Corral-Liria [5], Marta Losa-Iglesias [5,*] and Ricardo Becerro-de-Bengoa-Vallejo [6]

1   SALBIS Research Group, Faculty of Health Sciences, Universidad de León, 24071 León, Spain; btrer@unileon.es (B.T.-R.); pilar.marques@unileon.es (P.M.-S.); cliep@unileon.es (C.L.-P.)
2   Research, Health and Podiatry Unit, Department of Health Sciences, Faculty of Nursing and Podiatry, Universidade da Coruña, 15403 Ferrol, Spain; daniellopez@udc.es
3   Faculty of Health Sciences, Universidad de León, 24071 León, Spain; epereb@unileon.es
4   Frailty Research Organizaded Group (FROG), Department of Nursing, Faculty of Nursing and Podiatry, University of Valencia, 46010 Valencia, Spain; emmanuel.navarro@uv.es
5   Faculty of Health Sciences, Universidad Rey Juan Carlos, 28933 Madrid, Spain; raquel.jimenez@urjc.es (R.J.-F.); inmaculada.corral.liria@urjc.es (I.C.-L.)
6   Facultad de Enfermería, Fisioterapia y Podología, Universidad Complutense de Madrid, 28040 Madrid, Spain; ribebeva@ucm.es
*   Correspondence: marta.losa@urjc.es; Tel.: +34-616962413

Citation: Trevissón-Redondo, B.; López-López, D.; Pérez-Boal, E.; Marqués-Sánchez, P.; Liébana-Presa, C.; Navarro-Flores, E.; Jiménez-Fernández, R.; Corral-Liria, I.; Losa-Iglesias, M.; Becerro-de-Bengoa-Vallejo, R. Use of the Barthel Index to Assess Activities of Daily Living before and after SARS-COVID 19 Infection of Institutionalized Nursing Home Patients. *Int. J. Environ. Res. Public Health* **2021**, *18*, 7258. https://doi.org/10.3390/ijerph18147258

Academic Editor: Robbert Huijsman

Received: 25 May 2021
Accepted: 5 July 2021
Published: 7 July 2021

Abstract: The objective of the present study was to evaluate the activities of daily living (ADLs) using the Barthel Index before and after infection with the severe acute respiratory syndrome coronavirus 2 (SARS-CoV-2) and also to determine whether or not the results varied according to gender. The ADLs of 68 cohabiting geriatric patients, 34 men and 34 women, in two nursing homes were measured before and after SARS-CoV-2 (Coronavirus 2019 (COVID-19)) infection. COVID-19 infection was found to affect the performance of ADLs in institutionalized elderly in nursing homes, especially in the more elderly subjects, regardless of sex. The COVID-19 pandemic, in addition to having claimed many victims, especially in the elderly population, has led to a reduction in the abilities of these people to perform their ADLs and caused considerable worsening of their quality of life even after recovering from the disease.

Keywords: activities of daily living; Barthel index; SARS-CoV-2

1. Introduction

Coronavirus 2 (severe acute respiratory syndrome coronavirus 2 (SARS-CoV-2)) is an infectious disease that causes a severe acute respiratory syndrome. This virus belongs to the family of positive-sense enveloped RNA beta coronaviruses that emerged in Wuhan, China, in December 2019 [1]. It is the cause of the clinical disease known as COVID-19, which has caused more than 50 million infections and more than 1.25 million deaths according to the World Health Organization (WHO) [2].

In Spain, 5417 nursing homes exist, with 690 of these in Castilla y León, of which 71% are private [3].

According to the recent monographic report on Spain from the ltccovid.org portal, a site that belongs to the International Long-Term Care Policy Network, which is a network managed by the London School of Economics (LSE), data updated on May 28 indicate that 237,906 people have been infected by COVID-19 in Spain and 27,119 have died from this disease. Deaths in nursing homes have risen to 19,194, which is 70% of the total number of deaths, with 2449 in Castilla y León [4].

In a disease as infectious as COVID-19, host factors are the key to determining the severity and progression of the disease [5]. For severe COVID-19 disease, the main risk factors include age, male gender, obesity, smoking, and comorbid chronic diseases, such as hypertension, type 2 diabetes mellitus, and others [6–8].

Symptoms that are presented by COVID-19-infected patients vary from one person to another and can mimic symptoms present in other common infections. The most frequently found symptoms are fever, cough, myalgia, fatigue, dyspnea, anosmia, and ageusia [9,10]. Sometimes, these patients report having increased sputum production, headache, hemoptysis, diarrhea, and myalgia [11–16], although it is believed that approximately 20% of patients do not present any type of symptom [17]. The average recovery time in someone with mild illness is two weeks, while in severe illness, it can be 3–6 weeks [18]. After several weeks of convalescence, rehabilitation is essential to recover functionality as soon as possible, especially in the elderly population. The goal of rehabilitation in patients with COVID-19 infection is to facilitate improvements in the sensation of dyspnea, relieve anxiety and depression, reduce virus-associated complications, improve functionality, preserve pre-existing functions, and improve the quality of life by helping these patients to regain the same level of physical and functional independence that they had before contracting the disease.

After resolution of the acute phase, physical, emotional, and psychological impairments can often persist for a prolonged period and contribute to complex and multi-factorial disabilities that require continuous care and rehabilitative multimodal management [19–21]. As part of the rehabilitative therapy of these patients, evaluation of several factors that can affect these individuals once they have recovered from the virus is recommended: (1) deterioration of general functionality, (2) deterioration in the ability to carry out activities of daily living (ADLs), and (3) social disadvantages, which are evaluated using scales such as the Performance Status, the Barthel index, and the Functional Independence Measure [22].

In a community dwelling, screening of older people and assessing their abilities to conduct ADLs, such as getting out of bed, toileting, bathing, dressing, grooming, and eating, are frequently used as indicators of the functional status of an individual. These measures are applied to detect early onset of disability and are key factors for care management [23].

Geriatric assessment using the Barthel index is very important when aiming to optimize the care of elderly patients during a new epidemic outbreak. Therefore, the goal of this study was to evaluate ADLs in residents before and after contracting COVID-19 by establishing a period of time in which no underlying disease or prompt rehabilitation could invalidate the results. The Barthel index was selected as the assessment tool to verify if an individual's ADLs decreased after overcoming the infection, which activities were most affected, and whether or not the gender of the elderly person affected the results.

2. Materials and Methods

The clinical study was designed as a longitudinal prospective cohort study. This study was approved by the ethics committee of the San Carlos Clinical Hospital of Madrid with internal code 21/251-E. Authorization was requested from the management of the two geriatric residences under study, and all patients provided informed consent before enrolling in the study. From March 2020 to December 2020, 68 residents contracted and overcame the SARS-CoV-2 virus, with different degrees and affectations.

For the sample size, we based our calculations on previous results obtained by Masanori Okamoto et al. [24] in which they analyzed the Barthel index in patients who had been diagnosed with benign tumors and then underwent surgery. They then compared these patients to the patients diagnosed with atypical lipomatous tumors who were surgically treated and obtained results of 98.01 ± 0.62 and 97.08 ± 2.49, respectively. For a two-tailed test with an α level of 0.05 and 95% confidence interval (CI) and a statistical analysis of the desired power of 80% (error $\beta = 20\%$), a minimum sample size of 59 people was obtained, and after estimating a 15% dropout rate, a total of 68 people was needed.

Int. J. Environ. Res. Public Health **2021**, *18*, 7258

The ADLs were evaluated in the residents periodically by the nurse using the Barthel index. The Barthel index (or Barthel scale) is an instrument used in medicine for the functional assessment of a patient.

In the homes for the elderly in Spain, more specifically in those of Castilla y León, the community in which our study was conducted, the ADLs of residents were evaluated in order to establish the degree of dependency, a scale established by Royal Decree 504/2007 of 20 April for determining the dependency situation established by the Law 39/2006, of 14 December. This decree addresses the promotion of personal autonomy and care for people who are in a dependent situation. Based on this decree, it is mandatory for nursing homes to conduct at least two determinations of the Barthel index in these types of residences annually; therefore, based on this regional law and the Barthel Index, which has a track record of being used in numerous studies and is still widely used today as a simple method to assess ADL for various diseases [25], we decided that this index would be a good indicator for evaluating the impact that the pandemic had had on our institutionalized elders.

This scale is used to measure the ability of a person to perform 10 basic ADLs; in this way, a quantitative estimate of their degree of independence can be obtained. The scale is also known as the Maryland Disability Index. The patient is questioned with respect to different activities, and their abilities to perform each of the corresponding activities is assigned a score according to their ability to perform the activity.

In the case of washing and grooming, if a patient can perform it without any complication, a maximum score of 5 points is given; however, if a patient cannot perform the activity, they are assigned a score of 0. The activities of eating, dressing, stooling, urinating, using the toilet, and climbing steps can have maximum score of 10 points if an individual can successfully perform the activity; however, if they need help with the activity, 5 points are given; if they are unable to perform it, a score of 0 is assigned. Finally, moving and walking carry maximum scores of 15 points each. If a person needs a minimal amount of help to carry out the activity, the person receives a score of 10 points, whereas if the person needs more help, they will be awarded 5 points. If the person is completely dependent on help, a score of 0 is assigned.

Once all of the scores are obtained, the sum is organized in such a way that the totally independent residents will have a score of 100, the residents with mild dependency will have a score of 91 to 99 points, moderate dependency is established with a score of 61 to 90, severe dependence entails scores ranging from 21 to 60 points, and total dependence is considered as a score of 20 points or less [25,26]. The Barthel index values obtained at a maximum of three months before the disease was contracted were used as the reference values. Indices were obtained at a maximum of three months after overcoming the infection and being discharged by the medical team in order to assess whether the infection had changed the status of the ADLs and therefore the degree of dependence had changed.

All of the individual Barthel scores were collected in an Excel table after scores were collected in the morning to ensure that the tiredness derived from the daily activity was not a factor that would have altered the results.

All of the results were added to determine the score by item and the total score.

The facilities used in the sample are among those with the greatest number of elderly people, and they are the residences that have more control over the ADLs. Among these places, some of them are arranged (indicating that part of the care derived from living in the residence receives public funding) in which the administration performs a very exhaustive monitoring of the places. This type of residence conducts Barthel assessments every three months; thus, when the pandemic affected these facilities, all of the elderly residents had been tested with the index, at most, three months prior to the start of the pandemic. After taking into account that SARS-CoV-2 was contracted by residents in the facility, affecting almost all them in a short period of time, we were able to obtain the Barthel index values in the survivors immediately after contracting the virus up to a maximum post-exposure time of three months, thus assessing the pure effects of the virus without the possibility of improvement after rehabilitation, derived diseases, and complications.

The ability to eat in the dining room of the residence hall or in the resident's room was evaluated, the ability to dress was assessed in the resident's room and always with their usual clothes, and the ability to go to the toilet and pass urine and stool was evaluated in their own toilet so as not to change the usual conditions under which the elderly perform these activities. The ability to climb stairs and wander was evaluated in the presence of the physiotherapist and at places that the elderly residents usually walked.

Based on the information from medical records, we analyzed the following factors: (1) age, (2) sex, (3) height, (4) weight, and (5) body mass index (BMI).

All residents belonged to two nursing homes in the province of León, Castilla y León, Spain. The study population was Caucasian and Spanish-speaking, with a medium–low sociocultural level and a medium economic level. Regarding the religion of the elderly, they were Catholic and the level of education in the majority was basic.

This index has been described by many authors as the most widely used index for evaluating ADL in chronically ill patients and periodically evaluating their progression [27–29]. The reliability of the test according to Cronbach's alpha is 0.86–0.92 for the original version and 0.90–0.92 for the version proposed by Shah et al. [28].

A sample of 68 residents was taken. These people were divided into two groups according to gender (men and women). The inclusion criteria dictated that the patients were older than 65 years [30], that they lived together in the nursing home, and that they had a clinical diagnosis of COVID-19 infection.

The elderly who had contracted and recovered from SARS-CoV-2 were recruited into the study.

The follow-up period was defined as the time that had elapsed from prior to the SARS-CoV-2 infection until recovery. The Barthel index was evaluated over a maximum time frame of six months, a maximum of three months before contracting COVID-19 and a maximum of three months post-infection using the score obtained before infection and after recovery in a certain period of time to evaluate only the impact on the ADL caused by the COVID-19 infection and not the possible events that could happen a posteriori or the improvements derived from rehabilitation.

The protocols used for assessing the elderly were followed at all times according to the guidelines established by the health authorities. Controls were evaluated by polymerase chain reaction (PCR) and antigen tests administered to detect when the virus went into remission and when the patients were transferred to what was called the "clean zone" (the residences had to carry out isolation protocols and divide the buildings into clean and dirty zones, depending on whether the resident had an active infection). Therefore, once the residents obtained a negative result on the tests, they were transferred to the clean zone, free of SARS-CoV-2, and the Barthel assessment was performed. It should be noted that the elderly who went to the COVID-19-free zone had substantially improved their situation and were well enough to be able to resume their pre-infection life, although the majority had limitations.

Indeed, most of the elderly in this study were polymedicated and presented a variety of pathologies. It is true that comorbidities could affect ADL in a manner similar to lung infections suffered in winter (flu, pneumonia, catarrhal processes), which could cause an elderly person to become bed-ridden for days or even weeks. However, the virulence of this infection is devastating, not only for the lives it has claimed, but for the substantial loss of independence for an elderly patient.

Of course, during the days of convalescence, the elderly stopped their physical activities, as happens with other seasonal or bacterial infections, but no infection had caused a loss of muscle function or energy in patients in such a short time as did the COVID-19-induced virus.

The residence was divided into zones, which were delineated by floors, so that residents could move around on the floor on which they were located. Dining and living rooms were doubled so that the elderly could maintain their normal activities as much as possible, but it is true that during the most acute days, as in other infections, the elderly patients remained bedridden.

The habits of the elderly were effectively suspended since the entire operation of the facilities was forced to switch to contingency plans and most types of activities were suspended, which is one reason that the ADLs of the elderly were not the same, but this would not explain such a marked loss in such a short period of time in the ADLs of these patients.

Regarding the issue of comorbidities, we could have conducted a study on whether the comorbidities of the patients studied were a decisive factor in causing the loss of independence when performing ADLs, whether any of the administered medications caused confusion in these patients, or how much the elderly regained their independence in their ADLs once rehabilitation was initiated (it must be taken into account that the elderly began rehabilitation with physiotherapy and occupational therapy after the convalescent period and once discharged with negative PCR results) but the Barthel assessment was administered before rehabilitation to accurately determine the impact of the virus on our participants.

Statistical Analysis

A descriptive analysis of the characteristics of the participants from both groups was performed. Continuous variables were reported using the mean and standard deviation (SD) and confidence interval 95% (IC95%). The normality of the data was tested using the Shapiro–Wilk test.

For parametric data, paired T-tests were used to determine differences within the same group, and an independent T-test was used between groups.

The differences between before and after COVID-19 were analyzed using one-way repeated-measures analysis of variance (ANOVA). The age, weight, height, and BMI were analyzed as quantitative covariates to test within-subjects effects, and sex was analyzed as a categorical variable to test between-subjects factors, followed by pairwise comparisons using the Bonferroni correction.

For demonstrating the effect size of the comparisons, the Cohen's d coefficient was calculated. Cohen's d effect size can be interpreted as described previously: (1) values ≤ 0.20 indicate slight effects, (2) values between 0.20 and 0.49 indicate fair effects, (3) values between 0.50 and 0.79 indicate moderate effects, and (4) values >0.79 indicate large effects [31].

For all analyses, a value of $p < 0.05$ was considered statistically significant. The data were analyzed using SPSS software for Mac (Version 22; IBM Corp, Armonk, NY, USA).

3. Results

All of the variables showed a normal distribution ($p > 0.05$). A significant difference between the ages, heights, and weights of the group of men with respect to the group of women was found; however, for BMI, no significant difference was noted. All data are shown in Table 1.

As can be seen in Table 2, the results of the Barthel index, pre- and post-COVID-19 infection, present significant differences for all evaluated and for the total score.

As can be seen in Table 3, the pre-COVID-19 results of the Barthel index based on gender were compared. Significant results were obtained for both the transfers and ambulation of women compared to men with women, who obtained lower scores for both items; however, after recovering from the COVID-19 infection, the difference in ambulation was still significant between genders. In this case, men obtained worse scores than women, while in transfers, a significant difference did not exist. Urination appeared to be significantly different between men and women, with the latter obtaining the worst scoring, whereas before contracting the infection, differences were insignificant.

Table 1. Demographic and descriptive data of the sample population according to male and female groups.

Demographic and Descriptive Data	Total Group N = 68 Mean ± SD (IC95%)	Male Group N = 34 Mean ± SD (IC95%)	Female Group N = 34 Mean ± SD (IC95%)	p-Value
Age (years)	85.86 ± 6.42 (84.03–87.69)	84.00 ± 6.06 (81.49–86.50)	87.72 ± 6.34 (85.09–90.34)	0.039
Weight (Kg)	68.52 ± 14.84 (64.30–72.74)	72.76 ± 13.97 (66.99–78.52)	64.28 ± 14.74 (58.19–70.36)	0.042
Height (cm)	168.32 ± 10.85 (165.24–171.40)	175.52 ± 9.04 (171.78–179.25)	161.12 ± 7.11 (158.18–164.05)	0.001
BMI (Kg/m^2)	24.07 ± 4.21 (22.87–25.27)	23.54 ± 3.69 (22.01–25.07)	24.59 ± 4.68 (22.65–26.52)	0.384

Abbreviations: BMI, body mass index; SD: standard deviation; IC95%: confidence interval; independent T-tests were used. $p > 0.05$ (with a 95% confidence interval) was considered statistically significant.

Table 2. Pre- and post-Coronavirus 2019 (COVID-19) results based on the Barthel index.

Variables	Before COVID-19 N = 68 Mean ± DS (IC95%)	After COVID-19 N = 68 Mean ± DS (IC95%)	p-Value	Cohen's d
Eat	10.00 ± 0.00 (10.00–10.00)	8.60 ± 2.48 (7.89–9.31)	<0.001 *	0.37
Wash up	3.00 ± 2.67 (2.24–3.76)	1.00 ± 2.02 (0.43–1.57)	<0.001 *	0.38
Dress	8.10 ± 3.18 (7.20–9.00)	4.48 ± 4.04 (3.65–5.95)	0.407 *	0.44
Get ready	4.10 ± 1.94 (3.55–4.65)	3.10 ± 2.45 (2.40–3.80)	0.490 *	0.22
Deposition	9.60 ± 1.37 (9.21–9.99)	7.90 ± 3.51 (6.90–8.90)	<0.001 *	0.30
Urination	8.30 ± 2.60 (7.56–9.04)	5.70 ± 3.91 (4.59–6.81)	0.552 *	0.36
Toilet	7.70 ± 4.07 (6.54–8.86)	4.30 ± 4.17 (3.12–5.48)	0.600 *	0.38
Transfers	14.50 ± 1.82 (13.98–15.02)	9.00 ± 6.14 (7.25–10.75)	<0.001 *	0.51
Ambulation	14.50 ± 1.52 (14.07–14.93)	6.60 ± 4.99 (5.18–8.02)	<0.001 *	0.73
Steps	3.30 ± 4.36 (2.06–4.54)	0.40 ± 1.98 (0.16–0.96)	<0.001 *	0.39
Total score	83.20 ± 15.20 (78.7–87.67)	52.30 ± 27.22 (44.56–60.04)	<0.001 *	0.57

Abbreviations: DS: standard deviation; IC95%: confidence interval; * one-way repeated-measures analysis of variance (ANOVA) was used. $p < 0.05$ (with a 95% confidence interval) was considered statistically significant.

Table 3. Pre- and post-COVID-19 results based on the Barthel index by gender.

| Variables | Before COVID-19 N = 68 | | | | After COVID-19 N = 68 | | | |
	Mean ± DS (IC95%)				Mean ± DS (IC95%)			
	Female	Male	*p*-Value	Cohen's d	Female	Male	*p*-Value	Cohen's d
Eat	10.00 ± 0.00 (10.00–10.00)	10.00 ± 0.00 (10.00–10.00)	1.00	NA	8.60 ± 2.29 (7.65–9.54)	8.60 ± 2.70 (7.48–9.71)	0.500	0.00
Wash up	2.60 ± 2.54 (1.54–3.65)	3.4 ± 2.78 (2.25–4.54)	0.147	0.13	1.20 ± 2.17 (7.65–9.54)	0.80 ± 1.87 (0.02–1.57)	0.244	0.09
Dress	8.00 ± 2.22 (6.66–9.33)	8.20 ± 3.18 (6.88–9.51)	0.413	0.03	5.00 ± 4.08 (3.31–6.68)	4.60 ± 4.06 (2.92–6.27)	0.364	0.04
Get ready	4.20 ± 1.87 (3.42–4.97)	4.00 ± 2.04 (3.15–4.84)	0.359	0.05	3.00 ± 2.50 (1.96–4.03)	3.20 ± 2.44 (2.18–4.21)	0.388	0.04
Defecation	9.40 ± 1.65 (8.71–10.08)	9.80 ± 1.00 (9.38–10.21)	0.153	0.14	7.60 ± 3.85 (6.01–9.18)	8.20 ± 3.18 (6.88–9.51)	0.275	0.08
Urination	8.00 ± 2.50 (6.96–9.03)	8.60 ± 2.70 (7.48–9.71)	0.209	0.11	4.6 ± 3.79 (3.03–6.16)	6.80 ± 3.78 (5.23–8.36)	0.022 *	0.27
Toilet	7.40 ± 4.11 (5.70–9.09)	8.00 ± 4.08 (6.31–9.68)	0.303	0.07	4.00 ± 4.33 (2.21–5.78)	4.60 ± 4.06 (2.92–6.27)	0.307	0.07
Transfers	14.00 ± 2.50 (12.96–15.03)	14.96 ± 0.20 (14.87–15.04)	0.031 *	0.26	9.20 ± 5.71 (6.84–11.55)	8.80 ± 6.65 (6.06–11.54)	0.410	0.03
Ambulation	14.00 ± 2.04 (13.15–14.84)	14.96 ± 0.20 (14.87–15.04)	0.012 *	0.31	8.40 ± 4.72 (4.44–10.35)	4.80 ± 4.67 (2.87–6.72)	0.004 *	0.35
Steps	3.00 ± 4.08 (1.31–4.68)	3.60 ± 4.68 (1.66–5.53)	0.315	0.07	0.80 ± 2.76 (−0.3–1.94)	0.00 ± 0.00 (0.00–0.00)	0.077	0.20
Total score	80.80 ± 16.18 (74.12–87.47)	85.60 ± 15.22 (79.31–91.88)	0.142	0.15	53.00 ± 28.43 (41.26–64.73)	51.60 ± 26.52 (40.65–62.54)	0.428	0.02

Abbreviations: DS: standard deviation; IC95%: confidence interval; NA: not applicable; * independent T-tests were used. *p* < 0.05 (with a 95% confidence interval) was considered statistically significant.

4. Discussion

In this study, using the Barthel index, the ADLs of patients who had contracted the SARS-CoV-2 infection were evaluated. The Barthel index was applied to evaluate 10 items of ADL in two to four stages; its efficacy is widely accepted for this type of assessment [29,32,33]. The Barthel index has been used to assess functional impairment resulting from multiple sclerosis, cerebrovascular accidents, physical disabilities in the elderly, and many other neurological diseases [29,34,35].

At the end of 2019, a new coronavirus, SARS-CoV-2, began to spread rapidly throughout the world, endangering the health of people around the planet [36]. This new disease causes serious sequelae in 20% of affected patients, and admission to the intensive care unit (ICU) is often necessary due to the respiratory problems; it can even cause death [16].

Muscle weakness is one of the most frequent problems in patients with long bedtime periods and in patients seen in ICUs [37,38]. Critical illness survivors experience marked disability and deficits in physical and cognitive function that can even persist for years after their initial ICU stay [39].

Disability acquired after ICU is associated with reduced health-related quality of life and worse ADL [40].

Our study suggests that ADLs could be reduced after contracting COVID-19. In a study by Iwashyna et al., it was concluded that the elderly, after suffering with severe septicemia, present cognitive impairment and substantial disability that worsens their ability to perform ADLs [41]. Our study shows that COVID-19 infection causes a significant deterioration in all basic ADLs, including eating, washing, dress, getting ready, defecation, urination, using the toilet, transfers, ambulation, and steps, if the results of institutionalized elderly patients with respect to the results of ADL pre- and post-COVID-19 are compared.

Gender and age are the main risk factors for contracting COVID-19 disease [42]. A study found that in similar age groups, the infection was more serious for men than for women [43], and it was men who had the highest mortality rates [44]. These data could explain why, after contracting COVID-19, men obtained worse ADL scores than women despite having a lower average age.

However, the results before contracting the infection were worse for women, a finding that could be explained because aging is the main cause of deterioration [45]. The women in this study had an average age of 87.72 years, which was greater than that of the men; it should be noted that studies conclude that it is from the age of 80 and upward when the death rate of >95% is more significant [46].

The state of emergency resulting from the COVID-19 pandemic, which has had a greater impact on older people, especially with respect to those in institutions, has been minimally studied in terms of the quality of post COVID-19 ADL. Few reports evaluate the relationship between the Barthel index and COVID-19-derived sequelae. We found that the Barthel index, which is a simple and widely used method for assessing ADL, showed a significant correlation with the sequelae suffered by institutionalized patients who had contracted COVID-19, and the total results of the Barthel index could potentially be used to predict the related quality of life after recovering from COVID-19. We believe that the Barthel index is a useful tool for classifying and quantifying impairment in ADLs.

This study has a limitation with respect to the number of participants, but due to the unpredictability of the pandemic, not many elderly people who had undergone a Barthel assessment three months before contracting the COVID-19 infection could be found, regardless of the dramatic mortality caused by the infection (>94%). This situation made it even more difficult to increase the study sample number since it was important to perform the Barthel assessment in a short time frame and ensure that other aspects, such as emerging diseases or improvements due to the rehabilitation of these subjects, did not influence our results.

5. Conclusions

Of course, the pandemic has completely taken the worldwide population out of their normal lives, especially the older institutionalized population. It is important to develop maintenance programs for ADLs in situations of this type; perhaps it would be interesting to develop an early rehabilitation plan so that a patient suffering from the infection could continue to undergo rehabilitation despite continuing to test positive on the PCR test in order not to lose ADL capability. This could apply not only to this infection but to all types of illnesses. Promoting the autonomy of patients despite suffering from infection in order to prevent deterioration should be carried out. These pandemic situations must be addressed in order to be prepared and minimize the impact that they may cause on the elderly population.

In summary, this study shows a significant reduction in the quality of ADLs among the elderly institutionalized population in two nursing homes immediately before contracting and after recovering from the COVID-19 infection as measured by the Barthel index.

It appeared that the infection induced by SARS-CoV-2 caused a deterioration in the ADLs more in men than in women and that undoubtedly age was closely related to the loss of the ability to carry out ADLs. Elderly men, especially, saw their abilities diminish more than women, who, although their capacities diminished, did so to a lesser extent.

All of these findings should be taken into account to alleviate the impact that this infection is having not only on the health of our elders and the consequential health expenses that this situation will have but also in terms of the barrier to personal autonomy in the day to day lives of patients. It should be highlighted that the results of this study were not altered by the possible improvement derived from early rehabilitation or the worsening caused by an emerging disease. Data that substantiate our results would be of vital importance for a multidisciplinary team in order to evaluate the deterioration of the ADLs of the surviving elderly people, in order to establish an immediate and personalized rehabilitation plan, not only to preserve their health but also to preserve the quality of life of these people after they recover from this disease.

Author Contributions: Data curation, B.T.-R.; Formal analysis, B.T.-R. and R.B.-d.-B.-V.; Investigation, B.T.-R. and C.L.-P.; Methodology, B.T.-R., M.L.-I. and R.B.-d.-B.-V.; Project administration, R.B.-d.-B.-V.; Resources, E.P.-B.; Supervision, D.L.-L., P.M.-S. and R.B.-d.-B.-V.; Validation, E.P.-B., E.N.-F., R.J.-F., I.C.-L. and M.L.-I.; Visualization, D.L.-L., M.L.-I. and R.B.-d.-B.-V.; Writing—original draft, B.T.-R.; Writing—review & editing, D.L.-L., E.P.-B., P.M.-S., C.L.-P., E.N.-F., R.J.-F., I.C.-L., M.L.-I. and R.B.-d.-B.-V. All authors have read and agreed to the published version of the manuscript.

Funding: This research received no external funding.

Institutional Review Board Statement: The study was conducted according to the guidelines of the Declaration of Helsinki, and approved by the Ethics Committee of Hospital Clínico San Carlos (protocol code 21/251-E and 7 April 2021.

Informed Consent Statement: Informed consent was obtained from all subjects involved in the study.

Data Availability Statement: The dataset supporting the conclusions of this article is available in the marta.losa@urjc.es in the Faculty of Health Sciences, Universidad Rey Juan Carlos, 28933 Madrid, Spain.

Acknowledgments: The authors thank to all the people for their participation in this study.

Conflicts of Interest: The authors declare no conflict of interest.

References

1. Lu, R.; Zhao, X.; Li, J.; Niu, P.; Yang, B.; Wu, H.; Wang, W.; Song, H.; Huang, B.; Zhu, N.; et al. Genomic characterisation and epidemiology of 2019 novel coronavirus: Implications for virus origins and receptor binding. *Lancet* **2020**, *395*, 565–574. [CrossRef]
2. Coronavirus Disease (COVID-19). Available online: https://www.who.int/emergencies/diseases/novel-coronavirus-2019?gclid=CjwKCAiA9vOABhBfEiwATCi7GK5w2uwLUcdq2R727fbXua9MPX7WsTpyO3PVYgzFqCPmK2M7X3S3iRoCwgQQAvD_BwE (accessed on 5 February 2021).
3. Abellán, G.A.; Aceituno, N.P.; Ramiro, F.D. Estadísticas Sobre Residencias: Distribución de Centros y Plazas Residenciales Por Provincia. Datos de Abril de 2019. Available online: http://envejecimiento.csic.es/documentos/documentos/enred-estadisticasresidencias2019.pdf (accessed on 30 March 2021).
4. Zalakain, J.; Davey, V.; Suárez-González, A. The COVID-19 on Users of Long-Term Care Services in Spain. In *International Long-Term Care Policy Network*; CPEC-LSE: Barcelona, Catalonia, May 2020.
5. Wiersinga, W.J.; Rhodes, A.; Cheng, A.C.; Peacock, S.J.; Prescott, H.C. Pathophysiology, Transmission, Diagnosis, and Treatment of Coronavirus Disease 2019 (COVID-19): A Review. *JAMA* **2020**, *324*, 782–793. [CrossRef] [PubMed]
6. Wu, C.; Chen, X.; Cai, Y.; Xia, J.; Zhou, X.; Xu, S.; Huang, H.; Zhang, L.; Zhou, X.; Du, C.; et al. Risk Factors Associated With Acute Respiratory Distress Syndrome and Death in Patients With Coronavirus Disease 2019 Pneumonia in Wuhan, China Supplemental content. *JAMA* **2020**, *180*, 934–943. [CrossRef] [PubMed]
7. Zhou, F.; Yu, T.; Du, R.; Fan, G.; Liu, Y.; Liu, Z.; Xiang, J.; Wang, Y.; Song, B.; Gu, X.; et al. Clinical course and risk factors for mortality of adult inpatients with COVID-19 in Wuhan, China: A retrospective cohort study. *Lancet* **2020**, *395*, 1054–1062. [CrossRef]
8. Garibaldi, B.T.; Fiksel, J.; Muschelli, J.; Robinson, M.L.; Rouhizadeh, M.; Perin, J.; Schumock, G.; Nagy, P.; Gray, J.H.; Malapati, H.; et al. Patient Trajectories Among Persons Hospitalized for COVID-19. *Ann. Intern. Med.* **2021**, *174*, 33–41. [CrossRef] [PubMed]
9. Hornuss, D.; Lange, B.; Schröter, N.; Rieg, S.; Kern, W.V.; Wagner, D. Anosmia in COVID-19 Patients. *Clin. Microbiol. Infect.* **2020**, *10*, 1426–1427. [CrossRef]
10. Vaira, L.A.; Salzano, G.; Deiana, G.; De Riu, G. Anosmia and Ageusia: Common Findings in COVID-19 Patients. *Laryngoscope* **2020**, *130*, 1787. [CrossRef]
11. Huang, C.; Wang, Y.; Li, X.; Ren, L.; Zhao, J.; Hu, Y.; Zhang, L.; Fan, G.; Xu, J.; Gu, X.; et al. Clinical features of patients infected with 2019 novel coronavirus in Wuhan, China. *Lancet* **2020**, *395*, 497–506. [CrossRef]
12. Chen, N.; Zhou, M.; Dong, X.; Qu, J.; Gong, F.; Han, Y.; Qiu, Y.; Wang, J.; Liu, Y.; Wei, Y.; et al. Epidemiological and clinical characteristics of 99 cases of 2019 novel coronavirus pneumonia in Wuhan, China: A descriptive study. *Lancet* **2020**, *395*, 507–513. [CrossRef]
13. Wang, D.; Hu, B.; Hu, C.; Zhu, F.; Liu, X.; Zhang, J.; Wang, B.; Xiang, H.; Cheng, Z.; Xiong, Y.; et al. Clinical Characteristics of 138 Hospitalized Patients with 2019 Novel Coronavirus-Infected Pneumonia in Wuhan, China. *JAMA* **2020**, *323*, 1061–1069. [CrossRef]
14. Li, L.; Chen, D.; Wang, C.; Yuan, N.; Wang, Y.; He, L.; Yang, Y.; Chen, L.; Liu, G.; Li, X.; et al. Autologous platelet-rich gel for treatment of diabetic chronic refractory cutaneous ulcers: A prospective, randomized clinical trial. *Wound Repair Regen.* **2015**, *23*, 495–505. [CrossRef] [PubMed]

15. Richardson, S.; Hirsch, J.S.; Narasimhan, M.; Crawford, J.M.; McGinn, T.; Davidson, K.W.; Richardson, S.; Hirsch, J.S.; Narasimhan, M.; Crawford, J.M.; et al. Presenting Characteristics, Comorbidities, and Outcomes among 5700 Patients Hospitalized with COVID-19 in the New York City Area. *JAMA* **2020**, *323*, 2052–2059. [CrossRef] [PubMed]

16. Chen, G.; Wu, D.; Guo, W.; Cao, Y.; Huang, D.; Wang, H.; Wang, T.; Zhang, X.; Chen, H.; Yu, H.; et al. Clinical and immunological features of severe and moderate coronavirus disease 2019. *J. Clin. Investig.* **2020**, *130*, 2620–2629. [CrossRef] [PubMed]

17. Buitrago-Garcia, D.; Egli-Gany, D.; Counotte, M.J.; Hossmann, S.; Imeri, H.; Ipekci, A.M.; Georgia, S.; Nicola, L. Occurrence and transmission potential of asymptomatic and presymptomatic SARSCoV-2 infections: A living systematic review and meta-analysis. *PLoS Med.* **2020**, *17*, e1003346. [CrossRef]

18. Lovato, A.; De Filippis, C. Scholarly Review Clinical Presentation of COVID-19: A Systematic Review Focusing on Upper Airway Symptoms. Available online: https://us.sagepub.com/en-us/nam/open-access-at-sage (accessed on 5 February 2021).

19. Ceravolo, M.G.; De Sire, A.; Andrenelli, E.; Negrini, F.; Negrini, S. Systematic rapid "living" review on rehabilitation needs due to COVID-19: Update to March 31st, 2020. *Eur. J. Phys. Rehabil. Med. Ed. Minerva Med.* **2020**, *56*, 347–353.

20. Li, J. Rehabilitation management of patients with COVID-19: Lessons learned from the first experience in China. *Am. J. Phys. Med. Rehabil. Med.* **2020**, *56*, 335–338.

21. Lew, H.L.; Oh-Park, M.; Cifu, D.X. The War on COVID-19 Pandemic: Role of Rehabilitation Professionals and Hospitals. *Am. J. Phys. Med. Rehabil.* **2020**, *99*, 571–572. [CrossRef]

22. Keith, R.A.; Granger, C.V.; Hamilton, B.B.; Sherwin, F.S. The functional independence measure: A new tool for rehabilitation. *Adv. Clin. Rehabil.* **1987**, *1*, 6–18. [PubMed]

23. Gill, T.M. Assessment of function and disability in longitudinal studies Journal of the American Geriatrics Society. *NIH Public Access* **2010**, *58*, 308.

24. Okamoto, M.; Kito, M.; Yoshimura, Y.; Aoki, K.; Suzuki, S.; Tanaka, A.; Takazawa, A.; Yoshida, K.; Ido, Y.; Ishida, T.; et al. Using the Barthel Index to Assess Activities of Daily Living after Musculoskeletal Tumour Surgery: A Single-centre Observational Study. *Prog. Rehabil. Med.* **2019**, *4*, 20190010. [CrossRef]

25. Mahoney, F.I.; Barthel, D.W. Functional evaluation: The barthel index. *Md. State Med. J.* **1965**, *14*, 61–65. [PubMed]

26. Gresham, G.E.; Phillips, T.F.; Labi, M.L.C. ADL status in stroke: Relative merits of three standard indexes. *Arch. Phys. Med. Rehabil.* **1980**, *61*, 355–358. [PubMed]

27. Moncayo-Hernández, B.A.; Herrera-Guerrero, J.A.; Vinazco, S.; Ocampo-Chaparro, J.M.; Reyes-Ortiz, C.A. Sarcopenic dysphagia in institutionalised older adults. *Endocrinol Diabetes Nutr.* **2021**, *21*, 00146-4.

28. Shah, S.; Vanclay, F.; Cooper, B. Improving the sensitivity of the Barthel Index for stroke rehabilitation. *J. Clin. Epidemiol.* **1989**, *42*, 703–709. [CrossRef]

29. Wade, D.T.; Collin, C. The barthel ADL index: A standard measure of physical disability? *Disabil. Rehabil.* **1988**, *10*, 64–67. [CrossRef]

30. WHO. *Proposed Working Definition of an Older Person in Africa for the MDS Project*; WHO: Geneva, Switzerland, 2016.

31. Cohen, J. A power primer. *Psychol. Bull.* **1992**, *112*, 155–159. [CrossRef]

32. Collin, C.; Wade, D.T.; Davies, S.; Horne, V. The barthel ADL index: A reliability study. *Disabil. Rehabil.* **1988**, *10*, 1061–1063. [CrossRef]

33. Cohen, M.E.; Marino, R.J. The tools of disability outcomes research functional status measures. *Arch. Phys. Med. Rehabil.* **2000**, *81*, 21–29. [CrossRef]

34. Green, J.; Young, J. A test-retest reliability study of the Barthel Index, the Rivermead Mobility Index, the Nottingham Extended Activities of Daily Living Scale and the Frenchay Activities Index in stroke patients. *Disabil. Rehabil.* **2001**, *23*, 670–676. [CrossRef] [PubMed]

35. Van Der Putten, J.J.M.F.; Hobart, J.C.; Freeman, J.A.; Thompson, A.J. Measuring change in disability after inpatient rehabilitation: Comparison of the responsiveness of the Barthel Index and the Functional Independence Measure. *J. Neurol. Neurosurg. Psychiatry* **1999**, *66*, 480–484. [CrossRef] [PubMed]

36. Guan, W.; Ni, Z.; Hu, Y.; Liang, W.; Ou, C.; He, J.; Liu, L.; Shan, H.; Lei, C.; Hui, D.S.; et al. Clinical Characteristics of Coronavirus Disease 2019 in China. *N. Engl. J. Med.* **2020**, *382*, 1708–1720. [CrossRef]

37. Fan, E.; Cheek, F.; Chlan, L.; Gosselink, R.; Hart, N.; Herridge, M.S.; Hopkins, R.O.; Hough, C.L.; Kress, J.P.; Latronico, N.; et al. An official american thoracic society clinical practice guideline: The diagnosis of intensive care unit-acquired weakness in adults. *Am. J. Respir. Crit. Care. Med.* **2014**, *190*, 1437–1446. [CrossRef] [PubMed]

38. Brugliera, L.; Spina, A.; Castellazzi, P.; Cimino, P.; Tettamanti, A.; Houdayer, E.; Arcuri, P.; Alemanno, F.; Mortini, P.; Iannaccone, S. Rehabilitation of COVID-19 Patients. *J. Rehabil. Med.* **2020**, *52*, jrm00046. [CrossRef] [PubMed]

39. Ohtake, P.J.; Lee, A.C.; Scott, J.C.; Hinman, R.S.; Ali, N.A.; Hinkson, C.R.; Needham, D.M.; Shutter, L.; Smith-Gabai, H.; Spires, M.C.; et al. *Physical Impairments Associated with Post-intensive Care Syndrome: Systematic Review Based on the World Health Organization's International Classification of Functioning, Disability and Health Framework Physical Therapy*; Oxford University Press: Oxford, UK, 2018; Volume 98, pp. 631–645.

40. Hermans, G.; Van den Berghe, G. Clinical review: Intensive care unit acquired weakness. *Crit Care.* **2015**, *19*, 274. [CrossRef] [PubMed]

41. Iwashyna, T.J.; Ely, E.W.; Smith, D.M.; Langa, K.M. Long-term cognitive impairment and functional disability among survivors of severe sepsis. *JAMA* **2010**, *304*, 1787–1794. [CrossRef] [PubMed]

42. Rokni, M.; Ghasemi, V.; Tavakoli, Z. Immune responses and pathogenesis of SARS-CoV-2 during an outbreak in Iran: Comparison with SARS and MERS. *Rev. Med. Virol.* **2020**, *30*, e2107. [CrossRef]
43. Singh, S.; Chowdhry, M.; Chatterjee, A.; Khan, A. Gender-Based Disparities in COVID-19 Patient Outcomes: A Propensity-matched Analysis. *medRxiv* **2020**. [CrossRef]
44. Wenham, C.; Smith, J.; Morgan, R. COVID-19: The gendered impacts of the outbreak. *Lancet* **2020**, *395*, 846–848. [CrossRef]
45. Martín, I.; Vrotsou, K.; Vergara, I.; Bueno, A. Análisis factorial exploratorio del cuestionario VIDA de valoración de actividades instrumentales de la vida diaria. *Aten. Primaria* **2014**, *46*, 317–319. [CrossRef]
46. Curtis, J.R.; Kross, E.K.; Stapleton, R.D. The Importance of Addressing Advance Care Planning and Decisions about Do-Not-Resuscitate Orders during Novel Coronavirus 2019 (COVID-19). *JAMA* **2020**, *323*, 1771–1772. [CrossRef]

International Journal of
*Environmental Research
and Public Health*

MDPI

Article

Association between Health Problems and Turnover Intention in Shift Work Nurses: Health Problem Clustering

Jison Ki [1], Jaegeum Ryu [2], Jihyun Baek [2], Iksoo Huh [1,2] and Smi Choi-Kwon [1,2,*]

[1] College of Nursing, Seoul National University, 103, Daehak-ro, Jongno-gu, Seoul 03080, Korea; candy8@snu.ac.kr (J.K.); huhixoo@gmail.com (I.H.)
[2] The Research Institute of Nursing Science, Seoul National University, 103, Daehak-ro, Jongno-gu, Seoul 03080, Korea; jgryu21@gmail.com (J.R.); jihyunoctober@gmail.com (J.B.)
* Correspondence: smi@snu.ac.kr; Tel.: +82-2-740-8830

Received: 1 June 2020; Accepted: 21 June 2020; Published: 24 June 2020

check for updates

Abstract: Shift work nurses experience multiple health problems due to irregular shifts and heavy job demands. However, the comorbidity patterns of nurses' health problems and the association between health problems and turnover intention have rarely been studied. This study aimed to identify and cluster shift work nurses' health problems and to reveal the associations between health problems and turnover intention. In this cross-sectional study, we analyzed data from 500 nurses who worked at two tertiary hospitals in Seoul, South Korea. Data, including turnover intention and nine types of health issues, were collected between March 2018 and April 2019. Hierarchical clustering and multiple ordinal logistic regressions were used for the data analysis. Among the participants, 22.2% expressed turnover intention and the mean number of health problems was 4.5 (range 0–9). Using multiple ordinal logistic regressions analysis, it was shown that sleep disturbance, depression, fatigue, a gastrointestinal disorder, and leg or foot discomfort as a single health problem significantly increased turnover intention. After clustering the health problems, four clusters were identified and only the neuropsychological cluster—sleep disturbance, fatigue, and depression—significantly increased turnover intention. We propose that health problems within the neuropsychological cluster must receive close attention and be addressed simultaneously to decrease nurse's turnover intentions.

Keywords: nurses; turnover intention; hierarchical clustering; fatigue; sleep

1. Introduction

Nurses often work irregular shifts and bear high physical and psychological job demands that may, in turn, jeopardize their health status. Specifically, shift work may cause a variety of physical and mental health problems [1]. The deterioration of nurses' health status could not only lead to a decline in their quality of life but could also affect the quality of care provided by them [2]. In addition, health problems may affect nurses' turnover, which is a serious issue worldwide [3]. The high turnover rate of nurses has led to an increase in both direct and indirect costs in the health system and could further protract the shortage of nurses that has lasted for the past several years [4]. A recent survey of Korean nurses reported that about 10% of shift work nurses cited health problems as their main reason for resigning [5].

Prior studies also show that nurses complained of two or more health problems simultaneously, which may be interrelated [2,6–8]. Musculoskeletal pain in nurses has been reported in many studies [9,10], and poor dietary habits due to irregular shift work were reported to cause gastrointestinal disorders [11,12]. Sleep disturbance, which is most frequently reported in studies of shift nurses, could lead to mood disorders, such as depression, both of which lead to chronic fatigue [13–15].

Although nurses experience various health problems, there is relatively little research on the relationships between complex health problems in nurses [2]. Moreover, few studies have investigated the relationship between concomitant health problems and turnover intention.

Because the burden may vary depending on the number and the kind of health problems shift work nurses have [16], it may be important to identify specific comorbidity patterns of nurses' health problems through clustering and determine which clusters most affect turnover intention, where a cluster-that is, a comorbid pattern of health problems—can be defined as a group of concurrent or related health problems that can be distinguished from other clusters [17].

Therefore, the purpose of this study was to first characterize shift work nurses' health problems. We then determined the pattern of symptom modalities by clustering the health problems through the hierarchical clustering method. Lastly, we identified the impact of health problem clusters on turnover intention.

2. Materials and Methods

2.1. Study Design and Participants

This cross-sectional study was part of the Shift Work Nurses' Health and Turnover (SWNHT) study, which is a prospective cohort study designed to investigate the longitudinal relationships between shift work nurses' health and turnover. It was supported by the National Research Foundation of Korea (NRF) grant funded by the Korea Ministry of Science and Information and Communications Technologies and approved by the Institutional Review Board (IRB) at two tertiary hospitals in Seoul, South Korea. Data collection was performed from March 2018 until April 2020. In the SWNHT study, we recruited 594 female nurses (294 novice nurses who had no exposure to rotating shift work, and 300 nurses with exposure to 8-hour rotating work, including night shifts, for at least 1 month) (Figure 1). Because health problems can vary according to sex [18,19] and the SWNHT study included a survey of nurses' menstrual and gynecological symptoms, the SWNHT study was limited to female nurses. Data were collected three times for novice nurses: before exposure to shift work (novice registered nurse (NRN) T0, $n = 294$), after six months of work (NRN T1, $n = 204$), and 12 months after T1 (NRN T2, $n = 204$). For experienced registered nurses, data were collected twice: baseline (experienced registered nurse (ERN) T1, $n = 300$) and 12 months after T1 (ERN T2, $n = 269$; see details in Section 2.2 Data Collection).

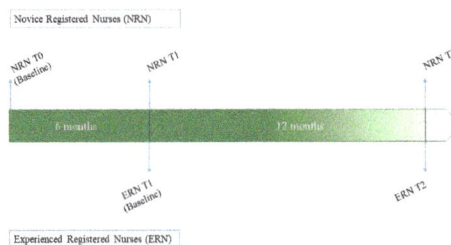

Figure 1. Schematic overview of the Shift Work Nurses' Health and Turnover (SWNHT) study.

In this study, we used data collected from October 2018 to January 2019 (NRN T1, $n = 204$) and from March 2018 to May 2018 (ERN T1, $n = 300$) to analyze the association between health problems and turnover intention among shift work nurses. In this analysis, we defined shift work as a combination of day, evening, and night shifts; therefore, we excluded four nurses, including three nurses who worked only daytime hours and one nurse who worked from midday to 8 p.m.

2.2. Data Collection

The primary purpose of the SWNHT study was to investigate health problems, presenteeism, and turnover intention in shift work nurses. To enroll novice nurses without shift work experience, we distributed and collected survey envelope packages that included survey instructions, consent forms, and a questionnaire on the third day of their work orientation before ward placement. To enroll experienced shift work nurses, we attached a recruitment notice to the ward bulletin boards, and nurses who wished to participate in the study voluntarily contacted the research team. We maximized voluntary participation by protecting confidentiality, ensuring anonymity, and no hospital-associated researchers took part in the data collection process. We collected the follow-up data through an online survey program; their response rates were 69.4% (NRN T1, NRN T2) and 89.7% (ERN T1). The SWNHT study questionnaire included questions regarding general and job-related characteristics, health-related variables (e.g., dietary habits, menstrual symptoms, exposure to blood and body fluid, sleep, fatigue, depression, physical activity, etc.), occupational stress, presenteeism, and turnover intention. To objectively verify the sleep scale data, we also obtained actigraphy data from the subjects who consented to wear the actigraphy.

2.3. Measurements

2.3.1. Demographic and Job-Related Characteristics

The examined demographic characteristics included age (years), education (bachelor's degree or lower/master's degree or higher), marital status (single/married), having children (yes/no), and body mass index (kg/m^2). The examined job-related characteristics included work unit (general ward, intensive care unit, delivery room, and emergency room), months of shift work experience, and the average number of night shifts per month.

2.3.2. Turnover Intention

We measured turnover intention since it is the most predictive measure of actual turnover [20]. In a longitudinal study in Europe, nurses who had turnover intentions were more likely to leave their jobs [21]. In this study, the subjects were asked to choose one of four options (strongly agree, agree, disagree, or strongly disagree) to answer the question: "I plan on staying for the next year" [22].

2.3.3. Health Problems

The nine health problems in this study were selected by two professors at a nursing college and two nurses in a research team, and were based on reviews of the literature about shift work nurses' health problems [10,18,23–27]. These were (1) upper musculoskeletal pain (including neck, shoulder, and back pain), (2) leg or foot discomfort, (3) sleep disturbance, (4) fatigue, (5) depression, (6) menstrual disorders (including dysmenorrhea and menopause symptoms), (7) gynecological disorders (including disease of the uterus or ovary), (8) headaches (including migraine, dizziness, and chronic headaches), and (9) gastrointestinal disorders (including gastric ulcer, diarrhea, constipation, and stomachache).

Among the nine health problem categories, sleep disturbance, fatigue, and depression were measured using the instruments described below. For the other six health problem categories, the subjects were asked to indicate the health problems they experienced during the last month with "yes" or "no."

Sleep Disturbance

To assess the quality of sleep, we used the Korean version of the Insomnia Severity Index (ISI), which was developed by Morin and translated by the Korean Sleep Research Society. The insomnia severity scale consists of seven questions related to sleep disorders measured on a 5-point scale (0–4 points) for each item. The score ranges from 0 to 28; higher scores indicate a lower quality of sleep. A score above 10 indicates sleep disturbance [28]. The Cronbach's alpha value of the Korean version of ISI was 0.928 in our study.

Fatigue

Fatigue was measured using the Fatigue Severity Scale (FSS). The FSS consists of nine questions about the degree of fatigue during the past week and is scored from 1 (strongly disagree) to 7 (strongly agree). A higher average score indicates higher fatigue. The criterion for fatigue is more than four points on average [29]. The Cronbach's alpha value of the FSS was 0.917 in our study.

Depression

We measured depression using the shortened Center for Epidemiological Studies Depression Scale (CES-D). The shortened CES-D consists of 10 questions about depressive feelings and thoughts during the past week and is scored from 0 (less than 1 day) to 3 (about 5–7 days). Higher total scores indicate more depressive symptoms. A total score of 10 or above indicates depression [30]. The Cronbach's alpha value of the shortened CES-D was 0.877 in our study.

2.4. Statistical Analysis

All analyses were performed using SAS version 9.4 (SAS Institute Inc., Cary, NC, USA) and R Project for Statistical Computing software version 3.4.4 (CRAN, Soule, Korea). We confirmed that there were no missing data. The descriptive statistics (frequency, percentage, mean, and standard deviation) for the demographic characteristics were analyzed. Pearson's chi-squared test, Fisher's exact test, and an analysis of variance were used to identify general characteristics associated with turnover intention. Hierarchical clustering was used to group the health problems reported by participants. Hierarchical clustering is a statistical method for grouping objects or variables according to the similarity between clusters using a bottom-up approach. In the field of nursing, this technique has been used mainly for symptom clustering of cancer patients; however, it has recently become more widely used in various studies [31]. The method used for measuring the distance between variables was the squared Euclidean distance and the linkage method used for measuring the distance between clusters was the average linkage. The number of final clusters is usually determined by the researchers by taking into account clinical suitability [32]. Multiple ordinal logistic regressions that included covariates, such as education, marital status, having children, body mass index (kg/m^2), work unit, months of shift work experience, and the number of night shifts per month, was used to investigate the association of single health problems and clusters of health problems with turnover intention. The four categories of "strongly agree," "agree," "disagree," and "strongly disagree" used for the turnover intention variable satisfied the proportional odds assumption at $p > 0.050$ with the covariates and variables of interest.

2.5. Ethical Consideration

This study was approved by the Institutional Review Board (IRB) at Seoul National University Hospital (IRB No. H-1712-094-907) and the Samsung Medical center (IRB No. 2017-12-075-002). After agreeing to participate in the study, all nurse participants signed a consent form and completed the baseline questionnaire.

3. Results

3.1. Demographic and Job-Related Characteristics

The participants were 500 female nurses working shifts, including night shifts. The nurses' mean age was 26.7 years (standard deviation (SD) = 4.20), and 19.8% were over 30 years old. There were no differences in demographic and job-related characteristics between the participants in the two tertiary hospitals. Most nurses were single (88.2%) and had no children (94.0%). The average body mass index (BMI) was 20.19 kg/m^2; 22.8% of the subjects were underweight and only one subject was obese. The shift work length was 35 months on average, which was highly correlated with age (r = 0.92, $p < 0.001$). Therefore, we excluded age from the covariates of the multiple ordinal logistic regressions (Table 1).

Table 1. Demographic and job-related characteristics by turnover intention ($n = 500$).

Variables	Categories	Total ($n = 500$, 100.0%) n (%) or M ± SD	Strong Intent to Stay ($n = 53$, 10.5%) n (%) or M ± SD	Intent to Stay ($n = 336$, 67.2%) n (%) or M ± SD	Intent to Leave ($n = 99$, 19.9%) n (%) or M ± SD	Strong Intent to Leave ($n = 12$, 2.4%) n (%) or M ± SD	χ^2 or F	p
Age (years)		26.72 ± 4.20	28.77 ± 5.68	26.29 ± 3.87	27.08 ± 4.31	26.58 ± 2.35	5.70	0.001 *
Education	≤BSN	459 (91.8)	48 (90.6)	310 (92.3)	89 (89.9)	12 (100.0)	1.74	0.626
	≥MSN	41 (8.2)	5 (9.4)	26 (7.7)	10 (10.1)	0 (0.0)		
Marital Status	Single	441 (88.2)	42 (79.3)	303 (90.2)	85 (85.9)	11 (91.7)	6.00	0.108
	Married	59 (11.8)	11 (20.7)	33 (9.8)	14 (14.1)	1 (8.3)		
Having Children	Yes	30 (6.0)	8 (15.1)	15 (4.5)	7 (7.1)	0 (0.0)	10.14	0.030 *
	No	470 (94.0)	45 (84.9)	321 (95.5)	92 (92.9)	12 (100.0)		
Body Mass Index (kg/m²)		20.19 ± 2.24	20.96 ± 2.36	20.19 ± 2.19	19.92 ± 2.34	18.77 ± 1.22	4.24	0.006 *
Work Unit	Ward	366 (73.2)	41 (77.4)	239 (71.1)	76 (76.8)	10 (83.3)	4.61	0.673
	ICU	109 (21.8)	8 (15.1)	79 (23.5)	20 (20.2)	2 (16.7)		
	DR, ER	25 (5.0)	4 (7.5)	18 (5.4)	3 (3.0)	0 (0.0)		
Shift Work Experience (months)		34.93 ± 42.94	58.66 ± 59.97	30.84 ± 40.01	37.03 ± 39.38	27.58 ± 27.80	6.83	<0.001 *
Average Number of Nights Per Month (days)		6.00 ± 1.26	5.62 ± 1.48	5.98 ± 1.37	6.06 ± 1.16	6.13 ± 0.78	1.45	0.228

BSN-Bachelor of Science in Nursing, MSN-Master of Science in Nursing, ICU-Intensive Care Unit, DR-delivery room, ER-emergency room; * $p < 0.05$.

One hundred and eleven nurses (22.2%) had a turnover intention and 12 nurses (2.4%) strongly intended to leave. The turnover intention was statistically higher in subjects who were younger (F = 5.70, p = 0.001), had no children (χ^2 = 10.14, p = 0.030), had a lower BMI (F = 4.24, p = 0.006), and had shorter periods of shift work (F = 6.83, p < 0.001).

3.2. Prevalence and Association between Single Health Problems and Turnover Intention

The mean number of health problems was 4.5 (range 0–9), with 95.2% (n = 476) of participants having more than two health problems. The most frequently reported health problem was upper musculoskeletal pain (82.4%), followed by leg or foot discomfort (67.8%), fatigue (65.0%), and sleep disturbance (62.4%). The associations between single health problems and turnover intention using multiple ordinal logistic regressions are provided in Table 2. Fatigue (odds ratio (OR) = 3.4, 95% confidence interval (CI) = 2.21–5.24), depression (OR = 1.79, 95% CI = 1.22–2.62), leg or foot discomfort (OR = 1.69, 95% CI = 1.12–2.56), sleep disturbance (OR = 1.61, 95% CI = 1.10–2.37), and a gastrointestinal disorder (OR = 1.51, 95% CI = 1.03–2.19) were significantly related to turnover intention.

Table 2. Association between single health problems and turnover intention using a multiple ordinal logistic regression.

Variables	Total (n = 500, 100.0%) n (%)	Adjusted [1] Odds Ratio	95% CI	p
Upper Musculoskeletal Pain	412 (82.4)	1.07	0.65–1.74	0.775
Leg or Foot Discomfort	339 (67.8)	1.69	1.12–2.56	0.012 *
Sleep Disturbance	312 (62.4)	1.61	1.10–2.37	0.013 *
Fatigue	325 (65.0)	3.4	2.21–5.24	<0.001 *
Depression	207 (41.4)	1.79	1.22–2.62	0.002 *
Menstrual Disorder	194 (38.8)	1.26	0.86–1.85	0.229
Gynecological Disorder	36 (7.2)	0.98	0.47–2.01	0.959
Headache	195 (39.0)	1.2	0.82–1.75	0.343
Gastrointestinal Disorder	222 (44.4)	1.51	1.03–2.19	0.031 *

[1] Adjusted for education, marital status, having children, body mass index (kg/m^2), work unit, shift work experience (months), and the number of nights per month (days) in multiple ordinal logistic regression model; * p < 0.05.

3.3. Hierarchical Clustering of Health Problems

Based on the hierarchical clustering analysis, four clusters were identified (Figure 2): the pain cluster (upper musculoskeletal pain and leg or foot discomfort), the neuropsychological cluster (depression, sleep disturbance, and fatigue), the gynecological cluster (menstrual disorder and gynecological disorder), and the gastrointestinal cluster (headache and gastrointestinal disorder).

3.4. Prevalence and Association between Clusters of Health Problems and Turnover Intention

As a result of our multiple ordinal logistic regression analyses, only the neuropsychological cluster (depression, sleep disturbance, and fatigue) was found to be significantly related to turnover intention. In the neuropsychological cluster, if the participant had only one health problem, it did not relate to turnover intention. If the participant experienced two (OR = 3.35, 95% CI = 1.90–5.92) or three (OR = 5.73, 95% CI = 3.17–10.33) health problems in the cluster simultaneously, the odds ratio of the turnover intention increased linearly, which was statistically significant (F = 5.84, p < 0.001; Table 3).

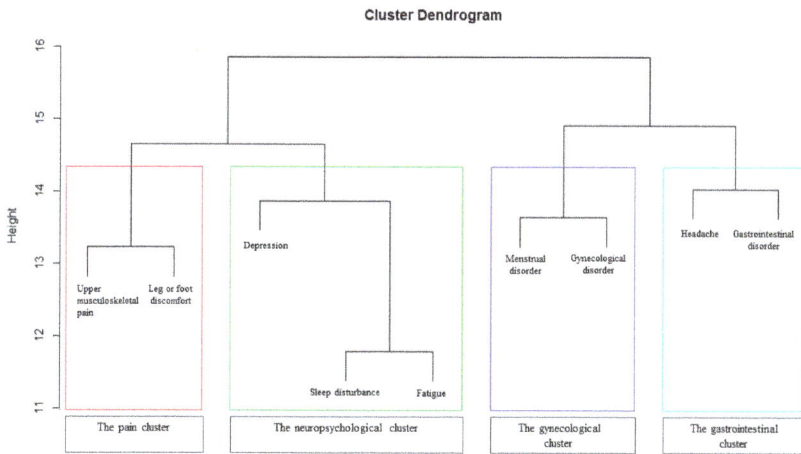

Figure 2. Dendrogram of the health problem clusters.

Table 3. Association between clusters of health problems and turnover intention using multiple ordinal logistic regressions.

Cluster	Health Problem				Adjusted [1]	
	Contents	Number	n (%)	Odds Ratio	95% CI	p
Pain Cluster	Upper musculoskeletal pain + Leg or foot discomfort	0	37 (7.4)	1.00		
		1	175 (35.0)	0.57	0.27–1.23	0.155
		2	288 (57.6)	1.11	0.54–2.30	0.763
Neuropsychological Cluster	Sleep disturbance + Fatigue + Depression	0	99 (19.8)	1.00		
		1	97 (19.4)	1.59	0.85–2.97	0.141
		2	165 (33.0)	3.35	1.90–5.92	<0.001 *
		3	139 (27.8)	5.73	3.17–10.33	<0.001 *
Gynecological Cluster	Menstrual disorder + Gynecological disorder	0	292 (58.4)	1.00		
		1	186 (37.2)	1.22	0.83–1.81	0.298
		2	22 (4.4)	1.21	0.48–3.05	0.676
Gastrointestinal Cluster	Headache + Gastrointestinal disorder	0	193 (38.6)	1.00		
		1	197 (39.4)	1.43	0.94–2.19	0.092
		2	110 (22.0)	1.60	0.98–2.64	0.060

[1] Adjusted for education, marital status, having children, body mass index (kg/m²), work unit, shift work experience (months), and the number of nights per month (days) in multiple ordinal logistic regression model; * $p < 0.05$.

4. Discussion

We investigated the prevalence of shift work nurses' health problems and characterized the patterns of symptom modalities by clustering health problems. We then investigated the association of single health problems and clusters of health problems with turnover intentions. We found that most shift work nurses experienced multiple health problems at the same time. We also found that having more than two health problems in the neuropsychological cluster was significantly related to turnover intention. This study was the first to attempt the clustering of nurses' health problems and explore the relationship between the clusters and turnover intention in shift work nurses.

We found that 22.2% of nurses had turnover intention. In previous studies, turnover intention varied from 4% to 54% [33–35]. The first reason for the difference in turnover intention between existing studies and our study could have been the different measurement tools used in each study. While our study asked about future plans regarding turnover, such as "I plan on staying for the next year," other studies asked how often they thought about turnover in the past [36,37]. Some studies measured turnover intention with various questions, such as whether they were seeking another job or whether they thought about leaving the nursing profession forever [33,38]. The second reason that turnover intention in our study was higher than in previous studies may be due to different hospital environments. The hospitals where our study was performed were tertiary hospitals in Seoul, which had a higher patient severity and higher nurse labor intensity than other hospitals in Korea. Third, we measured turnover intention and not actual turnover, which is reported to be higher than actual turnover rates [21]. In 2018, the annual average nurse turnover rate was 13.9% in Korea [5].

We found that fatigue was common in our subjects, highly related to turnover intention, and had the highest odds ratio (OR = 3.4, 95% CI = 2.21–5.24). Our results were consistent with a previous study that reported a positive correlation between fatigue and turnover intention [39]. Although we could not determine with certainty how long they had suffered from fatigue, it appeared that fatigue was one of the common disabling health problems that lead to turnover intention. Fatigue may exert a direct effect on turnover intention since nurses' fatigue has been reported to interfere with work efficiency and concentration and increase the risk of medical error and injury [40,41]. Although the direction of causality was not identified, nurses' fatigue was reported to be related to sleep disturbance, poor health, and depression [18,25].

Not surprisingly, we found that about 50% of nurses complained of fatigue and sleep disturbance at the same time and sleep disturbance was associated with turnover intention as a single health problem (OR = 1.61, 95% CI = 1.10–2.37). Sleep disturbance has received the most attention as a cause of turnover intention among nurses' health problems [42,43]. Irregular and insufficient sleep time due to shift work may often cause sleep disturbance, which may affect nurses' physical and mental health [1]. Another finding of interest was that about 28% of nurses had all three interrelated symptoms of fatigue, sleep disturbances, and depression; this was associated with turnover intention as a single health problem (OR = 1.79, 95% CI = 1.22–2.62). Depression in nurses is prevalent in many studies, and in one study, the prevalence of depression among nurses was almost twice as high as in other professions [26,44,45]. Depression may decrease concentration, which reduces the productivity of nursing and affects nurses' judgment, thus increasing occupational injury and turnover intention [26,43].

Our study revealed that fatigue, sleep disturbance, and depression may play important roles in increasing turnover intention as a cluster and as individual symptoms. Approximately one-third of nurses experienced all three health problems; these findings suggest fatigue, sleep disturbance, and depression in the neuropsychological cluster were correlated with each other. Despite the fact that biological and behavioral mechanisms in the development of depression, fatigue, and sleep disturbances are unknown, several studies have reported that these three health problems are related and co-occur [46,47]. Most importantly, 80% of nurses experienced one or more health problems in the neuropsychological cluster and this cluster was associated with turnover intention. Moreover, their odds ratio of turnover intention increased linearly as the number of health problems increased within this cluster. Future studies should probe the comorbidity of sleep disturbance, depression, and fatigue of shift work nurses and develop comprehensive health promotion to alleviate these three health problems.

We found that having a gastrointestinal disorder was another common health problem, which was consistent with the result of a previous study of 20,000 Korean nurses [12]. This high prevalence of gastrointestinal disorders among shift work nurses may, first, be due to disturbed circadian rhythm. The gastrointestinal system, like sleep, has a circadian rhythm, which controls bowel movement and the secretion of gastric juices [48]. Second, it might be due to irregular meal times and skipped meals [49]. Although not shown in the result, most of the nurses in our study reported eating irregularly (92.8%) and they ate breakfast twice a week, which was lower than the average number of times Korean adults eat breakfast [50]. The most common reason for skipped meals in our study was irregular work times (64.8%). Considering that having a gastrointestinal disorder was common among shift work nurses and was a single health problem that increased turnover intention, special attention needs to be paid to having regular and sufficient mealtimes as much as possible.

In our results, gastrointestinal disorders and headaches formed the gastrointestinal cluster. This connection could be explained by the association between the brain and the stomach through neural, endocrine, and immune pathways and the high prevalence of headaches in patients with a gastrointestinal disorder [51,52]. However, the gastrointestinal cluster was not related to turnover intention. It is possible that headaches, as an individual health problem, had no significant association with turnover intention, which could have decreased the effect of the cluster. Furthermore, we presume that headaches as a single health problem were not shown to be associated with turnover intention because headaches are often easily relieved by medication and may not have been as severe as a gastrointestinal disorder.

Upper musculoskeletal pain, which had the highest prevalence, formed a pain cluster with leg or foot discomfort. Nurses work most of the time in a standing position, walking an average of 8747 steps (4.1 miles) per shift [53], and high physical demands have been associated with musculoskeletal problems in nurses [54]. Additionally, multi-site musculoskeletal pain has been shown to be more common than single-site pain, especially in women [55]. Unexpectedly, this cluster was not related to turnover intention, although leg or foot discomfort was related to turnover intention. This might be because most nurses (82%) suffered upper musculoskeletal pain regardless of turnover intention and, similar to the gastrointestinal cluster, the association of the pain cluster with turnover intention was reduced by the effect of upper musculoskeletal pain. Although the pain cluster did not relate to turnover intention, given that these health problems in the pain cluster had a high prevalence and cause sickness and absence from work and decreased work productivity [24], there is a need to investigate the prevalence of musculoskeletal disorders in nurses by workplace and to provide appropriate prevention and treatment programs.

Although our study provides a new perspective on nurses' health problems, it has some limitations. First, this study relied on self-report measures of health problems, except for three health problems (sleep disturbance, depression, and fatigue). Second, we surveyed only the presence of health problems, but not the severity; however, as the participants were nurses with medical knowledge, their judgment of the presence of health problems might be more reliable than that of the general public [56], which would partially compensate for the fact that some health problems were not assessed with standardized tools. Third, we could not infer the causal relationship from the cross-sectional design of the study. The fourth significant limitation is that this study did not measure how many nurses actually leave their job; therefore, the findings of our study may not apply to actual turnover, as turnover intention does not always lead to actual turnover. Fifth, the shift work nurses who participated were all female and from two tertiary hospitals in Seoul in Korea. Therefore, the generalizability of the results is limited. Future studies on the comorbidity of sleep disturbance, depression, and fatigue in shift work nurses from various hospitals in various regions, along with the inclusion of male nurses, are recommended.

5. Conclusions

In this study, the association of single health problems and clusters of health problems with turnover intention differed. Although fatigue, sleep disturbance, depression, gastrointestinal disorders, and leg or foot discomfort were related to turnover intention as single health problems, after clustering, only the neuropsychological cluster—including fatigue, sleep disturbance, and depression—was related to turnover intention. Given that nurses had more than two health problems and turnover intention increased linearly within the neuropsychological cluster, these problems must receive close attention and be addressed to decrease the nurse turnover rate. Future studies should implement longitudinal research to determine the effect of the neuropsychological cluster on turnover.

Author Contributions: J.K. developed the concept of this manuscript, analyzed the data, and prepared this manuscript. J.R. and J.B. were responsible for the data collection and contributed to the manuscript revision. I.H. developed the study protocol and advised on the data analysis. S.C.-K. developed the study protocol and concept, and revised this manuscript to its final version. All authors have read and agreed to the published version of the manuscript.

Funding: This work was supported by the National Research Foundation of Korea (NRF) grant funded by the Korea Ministry of Science and ICT (No. NRF-2017R1A2B2002652).

Conflicts of Interest: The authors declare no conflict of interest.

References

1. Kecklund, G.; Axelsson, J. Health consequences of shift work and insufficient sleep. *BMJ* **2016**, *355*, i5210. [CrossRef] [PubMed]
2. Letvak, S. We cannot ignore nurses' health anymore: A synthesis of the literature on evidence-based strategies to improve nurse health. *Nurs. Adm. Q.* **2013**, *37*, 295–308. [CrossRef] [PubMed]
3. Hayward, D.; Bungay, V.; Wolff, A.C.; MacDonald, V. A qualitative study of experienced nurses' voluntary turnover: Learning from their perspectives. *J. Clin. Nurs.* **2016**, *25*, 1336–1345. [CrossRef]
4. Duffield, C.M.; Roche, M.A.; Homer, C.; Buchan, J.; Dimitrelis, S. A comparative review of nurse turnover rates and costs across countries. *J. Adv. Nurs.* **2014**, *70*, 2703–2712. [CrossRef]
5. Korea Hospital Nurse Association. *Survey on the Status of Hospital Nursing Staffing*; Korea Hospital Nurse Association: Seoul, Korea, 2018.
6. Yeom, E.Y.; Jeong, G.S.; Kim, K.A. Influencing Factors on Presenteeism of Clinical Nurses. *Korean J. Occup. Health Nurs.* **2015**, *24*, 302–312. [CrossRef]
7. Lee, Y.; Jung, M. Presenteeism and absenteeism according to health problems on nurses. *J. Korean Acad. Community Health Nurs.* **2008**, *19*, 459–468.
8. Yoshida, M.; Miki, A. Factors Related to Presenteeism in Young and Middle-aged Nurses. *J. Occup. Health* **2018**, *60*, 31–40. [CrossRef]
9. Yassi, A.; Lockhart, K. Work-relatedness of low back pain in nursing personnel: A systematic review. *Int. J. Occup. Environ. Health* **2013**, *19*, 223–244. [CrossRef]
10. Abdul Rahman, H.; Abdul-Mumin, K.; Naing, L. Psychosocial Work Stressors, Work Fatigue, and Musculoskeletal Disorders: Comparison between Emergency and Critical Care Nurses in Brunei Public Hospitals. *Asian Nurs. Res.* **2017**, *11*, 13–18. [CrossRef]
11. Wong, H.; Wong, M.C.S.; Wong, S.Y.S.; Lee, A. The association between shift duty and abnormal eating behavior among nurses working in a major hospital: A cross-sectional study. *Int. J. Nurs. Stud.* **2010**, *47*, 1021–1027. [CrossRef]
12. Kim, O.; Ahn, Y.; Lee, H.Y.; Jang, H.J.; Kim, S.; Lee, J.E.; Jung, H.; Cho, E.; Lim, J.Y.; Kim, M.J.; et al. The Korea Nurses' Health Study: A Prospective Cohort Study. *J. Women's Health* **2017**, *26*, 892–899. [CrossRef] [PubMed]
13. Zhai, L.; Zhang, H.; Zhang, D. Sleep Duration and Depression among Adults: A Meta-Analysis of Prospective Studies. *Depress. Anxiety* **2015**, *32*, 664–670. [CrossRef] [PubMed]
14. Caruso, C.C. Negative Impacts of Shiftwork and Long Work Hours. *Rehabil. Nurs.* **2014**, *39*, 16–25. [CrossRef] [PubMed]
15. Ferri, P.; Guadi, M.; Marcheselli, L.; Balduzzi, S.; Magnani, D.; Di Lorenzo, R. The impact of shift work on the psychological and physical health of nurses in a general hospital: A comparison between rotating night shifts and day shifts. *Risk Manag. Healthc. Policy* **2016**, *9*, 203–211. [CrossRef] [PubMed]
16. Kim, H.-J.; McGuire, D.B.; Tulman, L.; Barsevick, A.M. Symptom clusters: Concept analysis and clinical implications for cancer nursing. *Cancer Nurs.* **2005**, *28*, 270–282. [CrossRef]
17. Barsevick, A. Defining the Symptom Cluster: How Far Have We Come? *Semin. Oncol. Nurs.* **2016**, *32*, 334–350. [CrossRef]
18. Oyane, N.M.F.; Pallesen, S.; Moen, B.E.; Akerstedt, T.; Bjorvatn, B. Associations Between Night Work and Anxiety, Depression, Insomnia, Sleepiness and Fatigue in a Sample of Norwegian Nurses. *PLoS ONE* **2013**, *8*, e70228. [CrossRef]
19. Tuckett, A.; Henwood, T.; Oliffe, J.L.; Kolbe-Alexander, T.L.; Kim, J.R. A Comparative Study of Australian and New Zealand Male and Female Nurses' Health. *Am. J. Men's Health* **2016**, *10*, 450–458. [CrossRef]
20. Meeusen, V.C.; Van Dam, K.; Brown-Mahoney, C.; Van Zundert, A.A.; Knape, H.T. Understanding nurse anesthetists' intention to leave their job: How burnout and job satisfaction mediate the impact of personality and workplace characteristics. *Health Care Manag. Rev.* **2011**, *36*, 155–163. [CrossRef]

21. Estryn-Behar, D.; van der Heijden, B.; Fry, C.; Hasselhorn, H. Longitudinal Analysis of Personal and Work-Related Factors Associated With Turnover Among Nurses. *Nurs. Res.* **2010**, *59*, 166–177. [CrossRef]

22. Han, K.; Trinkoff, A.M.; Gurses, A.P. Work-related factors, job satisfaction and intent to leave the current job among United States nurses. *J. Clin. Nurs.* **2015**, *24*, 3224–3232. [CrossRef] [PubMed]

23. Turpin, R.S.; Ozminkowski, R.J.; Sharda, C.E.; Collins, J.J.; Berger, M.L.; Billotti, G.M.; Baase, C.M.; Olson, M.J.; Nicholson, S. Reliability and validity of the Stanford Presenteeism Scale. *J. Occup. Environ. Med.* **2004**, *46*, 1123–1133. [CrossRef] [PubMed]

24. Stolt, M.; Suhonen, R.; Virolainen, P.; Leino-Kilpi, H. Lower extremity musculoskeletal disorders in nurses: A narrative literature review. *Scand. J. Public Health* **2016**, *44*, 106–115. [CrossRef]

25. Cai, S.; Lin, H.; Hu, X.; Cai, Y.; Chen, K.; Cai, W. High fatigue and its associations with health and work related factors among female medical personnel at 54 hospitals in Zhuhai, China. *Psychol. Health Med.* **2018**, *23*, 304–316. [CrossRef] [PubMed]

26. Brandford, A.A.; Reed, D.B. Depression in registered nurses: A state of the science. *Workplace Health Saf.* **2016**, *64*, 488–511. [CrossRef]

27. Kang, W.; Jang, K.-H.; Lim, H.-M.; Ahn, J.-S.; Park, W.-J. The menstrual cycle associated with insomnia in newly employed nurses performing shift work: A 12-month follow-up study. *Int. Arch. Occup. Environ. Health* **2019**, *92*, 227–235. [CrossRef]

28. Morin, C.M.; Belleville, G.; Bélanger, L.; Ivers, H. The Insomnia Severity Index: Psychometric indicators to detect insomnia cases and evaluate treatment response. *Sleep* **2011**, *34*, 601–608. [CrossRef]

29. Krupp, L.B.; LaRocca, N.G.; Muir-Nash, J.; Steinberg, A.D. The fatigue severity scale: Application to patients with multiple sclerosis and systemic lupus erythematosus. *Arch. Neurol.* **1989**, *46*, 1121–1123. [CrossRef]

30. Radloff, L.S. The CES-D Scale: A Self-Report Depression Scale for Research in the General Population. *Appl. Psychol. Meas.* **1977**, *1*, 385–401. [CrossRef]

31. Dunn, H.; Quinn, L.; Corbridge, S.J.; Eldeirawi, K.; Kapella, M.; Collins, E.G. Cluster analysis in nursing research: An introduction, historical perspective, and future directions. *West. J. Nurs. Res.* **2018**, *40*, 1658–1676. [CrossRef]

32. Clatworthy, J.; Buick, D.; Hankins, M.; Weinman, J.; Horne, R. The use and reporting of cluster analysis in health psychology: A review. *Br. J. Health Psychol.* **2005**, *10*, 329–358. [CrossRef] [PubMed]

33. Brooks, I.; Swailes, S. Analysis of the relationship between nurse influences over flexible working and commitment to nursing. *J. Adv. Nurs.* **2002**, *38*, 117–126. [CrossRef]

34. Milisen, K.; Abraham, I.; Siebens, K.; Darras, E.; Dierckx de Casterlé, B. Work environment and workforce problems: A cross-sectional questionnaire survey of hospital nurses in Belgium. *Int. J. Nurs. Stud.* **2006**, *43*, 745–754. [CrossRef] [PubMed]

35. Jiang, F.; Zhou, H.; Rakofsky, J.; Hu, L.; Liu, T.; Wu, S.; Liu, H.; Liu, Y.; Tang, Y. Intention to leave and associated factors among psychiatric nurses in China: A nationwide cross-sectional study. *Int. J. Nurs. Stud.* **2019**, *94*, 159–165. [CrossRef] [PubMed]

36. Camerino, D.; Conway, P.M.; Estryn-Béhar, M.; Costa, G.; Hasselhorn, H.-M. Age-dependent relationships between work ability, thinking of quitting the job, and actual leaving among Italian nurses: A longitudinal study. *Int. J. Nurs. Stud.* **2008**, *45*, 1645–1659. [CrossRef]

37. Estryn-Béhar, M.; Van der Heijden, B.I.; Ogińska, H.; Camerino, D.; Le Nézet, O.; Conway, P.M.; Fry, C.; Hasselhorn, H.-M. The impact of social work environment, teamwork characteristics, burnout, and personal factors upon intent to leave among European nurses. *Med. Care* **2007**, *45*, 939–950. [CrossRef] [PubMed]

38. Chang, C.S.; Du, P.L.; Huang, I.C. Nurses' perceptions of severe acute respiratory syndrome: Relationship between commitment and intention to leave nursing. *J. Adv. Nurs.* **2006**, *54*, 171–179. [CrossRef]

39. Liu, Y.; Wu, L.M.; Chou, P.L.; Chen, M.H.; Yang, L.C.; Hsu, H.T. The influence of work-related fatigue, work conditions, and personal characteristics on intent to leave among new nurses. *J. Nurs. Scholarsh.* **2016**, *48*, 66–73. [CrossRef]

40. Richter, K.; Acker, J.; Adam, S.; Niklewski, G. Prevention of fatigue and insomnia in shift workers-a review of non-pharmacological measures. *EPMA J.* **2016**, *7*, 16. [CrossRef]

41. Ferris, J. Nursing Fatigue: An Evidence-Based Practice Review for Oncology Nurses. *Clin. J. Oncol. Nurs.* **2015**, *19*, 662–664. [CrossRef]

42. Shimizu, T.; Eto, R.; Horiguchi, I.; Obata, Y.; Feng, Q.; Nagata, S. Relationship between Turnover and Periodic Health Check-Up Data among Japanese Hospital Nurses: A Three-Year Follow-Up Study. *J. Occup. Health* **2005**, *47*, 327–333. [CrossRef] [PubMed]

43. Lai, H.; Lin, Y.; Chang, H.; Wang, S.; Liu, Y.; Lee, H.; Peng, T.; Chang, F. Intensive care unit staff nurses: Predicting factors for career decisions. *J. Clin. Nurs.* **2008**, *17*, 1886–1896. [CrossRef]

44. Hsieh, M.L.; Li, Y.M.; Chang, E.T.; Lai, H.L.; Wang, W.H.; Wang, S.C. Sleep disorder in Taiwanese nurses: A random sample survey. *Nurs. Health Sci.* **2011**, *13*, 468–474. [CrossRef] [PubMed]

45. Sun, Q.; Ji, X.; Zhou, W.; Liu, J. Sleep problems in shift nurses: A brief review and recommendations at both individual and institutional levels. *J. Nurs. Manag.* **2019**, *27*, 10–18. [CrossRef]

46. Bower, J.E.; Ganz, P.A.; Irwin, M.R.; Kwan, L.; Breen, E.C.; Cole, S.W. Inflammation and behavioral symptoms after breast cancer treatment: Do fatigue, depression, and sleep disturbance share a common underlying mechanism? *J. Clin. Oncol. Off. J. Am. Soc. Clin. Oncol.* **2011**, *29*, 3517–3522. [CrossRef]

47. Ho, S.-Y.; Rohan, K.J.; Parent, J.; Tager, F.A.; McKinley, P.S. A longitudinal study of depression, fatigue, and sleep disturbances as a symptom cluster in women with breast cancer. *J. Pain Symptom Manag.* **2015**, *49*, 707–715. [CrossRef]

48. Knutsson, A.; Bøggild, H. Gastrointestinal disorders among shift workers. *Scand. J. Work. Environ. Health* **2010**, *36*, 85–95. [CrossRef]

49. Joung Kim, Y.; Ban, D.J. Prevalence of irritable bowel syndrome, influence of lifestyle factors and bowel habits in Korean college students. *Int. J. Nurs. Stud.* **2005**, *42*, 247–254. [CrossRef]

50. Cho, S.H.; Chun, H.; Lee, H.S.; Lee, S.W.; Shim, K.W.; Lee, J.Y.; Byun, A.R.; Lee, H.Y. The Relationship between Shared Breakfast and Skipping Breakfast with Depression and General Health State in Korean Adults: The 2014 Korea National Health and Nutrition Examination Survey. *Korean J. Fam. Pract.* **2018**, *8*, 441–447. [CrossRef]

51. Lee, S.; Lee, J.; Kwon, Y.; Kim, J.; Sohn, J. Clinical Implications of Associations between Headache and Gastrointestinal Disorders: A Study Using the Hallym Smart Clinical Data Warehouse. *Front. Neurol.* **2017**, *8*, 526. [CrossRef]

52. Aamodt, A.; Stovner, L.; Hagen, K.; Zwart, J. Comorbidity of Headache and Gastrointestinal Complaints. The Head-HUNT Study. *Cephalalgia* **2008**, *28*, 144–151. [PubMed]

53. Welton, J.M.; Decker, M.; Adam, J.; Zone-Smith, L. How far do nurses walk? *Medsurg Nurs.* **2006**, *15*, 213–216. [PubMed]

54. Trinkoff, A.M.; Lipscomb, J.A.; Geiger-Brown, J.; Storr, C.L.; Brady, B.A. Perceived physical demands and reported musculoskeletal problems in registered nurses. *Am. J. Prev. Med.* **2003**, *24*, 270–275. [CrossRef]

55. Carnes, D.; Parsons, S.; Ashby, D.; Breen, A.; Foster, N.; Pincus, T.; Vogel, S.; Underwood, M. Chronic musculoskeletal pain rarely presents in a single body site: Results from a UK population study. *Rheumatology* **2007**, *46*, 1168–1170. [CrossRef]

56. Colditz, G.A.; Hankinson, S.E. The Nurses' Health Study: Lifestyle and health among women. *Nat. Rev. Cancer* **2005**, *5*, 388–396. [CrossRef]

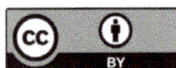

International Journal of
Environmental Research and Public Health

MDPI

Article

Association of Happiness and Nursing Work Environments with Job Crafting among Hospital Nurses in South Korea

Sujin Chang [1], Kihye Han [2,*] and Yongae Cho [2]

[1]   Department of Nursing, Seoul National University Bundang Hospital, Gyeonggi-do 13620, Korea; zzanga0520@naver.com
[2]   College of Nursing, Chung-Ang University, Seoul 06974, Korea; yacho2018@cau.ac.kr
*   Correspondence: hankihye@cau.ac.kr; Tel.: +82-2-820-5995

Received: 30 April 2020; Accepted: 2 June 2020; Published: 5 June 2020

check for
updates

Abstract: Nurses are key professionals in healthcare sectors, whose job attitude is closely associated with patient health outcomes and safety. Job crafting describes how workers shape their tasks to find a sense of meaning and value in their work. This study aimed to examine the associations of happiness at the individual level and nursing work environments at the organizational level with job crafting among hospital nurses in Korea. This cross-sectional study analyzed survey data from 220 nurses working in four Korean hospitals. Multiple linear regression modeling was used to examine associations among the study variables. Nurses who were satisfied with their lives were significantly more likely to exhibit higher levels of job crafting (B = 0.07, $p < 0.001$). Nursing work environments had no significant association with nurses' job crafting. In comparison with nurses working in general units, operating room nurses were significantly less likely to craft their job (B = −0.35, $p = 0.001$). Organizational support should be established to improve nurses' happiness and job crafting. Hospitals should provide various opportunities for education and training to strengthen job crafting.

Keywords: happiness; job crafting; nurses; work environment

1. Introduction

Due to rapid technological changes and an explosive increase in information volume and flexibility in the workplace, job descriptions in the healthcare sector require revision and updating frequently [1]. Job-centered human resource management has expanded granular job units and the roles of individuals, leading to organizational changes. Currently, it is considered that change cannot occur without workers who voluntarily immerse themselves in these organizational changes [2]. Individual autonomy, creativity and immersion have come to the fore in terms of workforce management because these characteristics positively affect the organization and help achieve organizational goals. In these contexts, job crafting has attracted increased attention. Job crafting is defined as the process of modifying tasks to make the work more meaningful [3]. Job crafting is related to workers' behaviors, i.e., their intention to find a sense of meaning and value in their work, and it also has a positive effect on both individuals and the organization. Previous research supports the positive results of job crafting, including job satisfaction and organizational commitment [4], psychological well-being [5] and productive job outcomes [6].

As nurses are the key professionals in healthcare sectors, their job attitudes are closely associated with patient health outcomes and safety [7]. In organizations where nurses deliver quality nursing care with positive attitudes toward their jobs, turnover and healthcare costs are reduced [8]. For these reasons, hospitals should understand factors associated with nurses' job crafting and encourage nurses to develop positive motivation for their work. The key determinants of job crafting have been reported as individual characteristics such as a high sense of vocation [3], self-directedness [9], high levels of psychological capital [10], intrinsic motivation for job performance [11] and extroversion [12]. Workers can achieve job crafting through self-directed behaviors; thus, the effect of the personal characteristics of the job crafters themselves would be greater than that of organizational characteristics [6].

On a personal level, happiness is the ultimate goal in life for nearly everyone. As workers spend most of their daily lives in workplace settings, their happiness is closely related to their working life [13]. People who often experience happiness are more likely to actively set new goals at work and try to realize them. These factors, in turn, can result in better job outcomes [14]. Nurses who are happy can become immersed in their professional nursing practice, perform their work creatively and have a positive effect on organizational performance [15]. Happiness—a positive emotion—and internal satisfaction with life can act as intrinsic motivators for nurses to craft their jobs.

In terms of human resource management for nurses, organizations should foster good work environments in which job crafting can be emphasized and facilitated [3]. Nurses provide frontline care to patients and collaborate with various professionals in hospitals, and thus require frequent emotional exchanges with coworkers [16]. Due to high nurse turnover rates and low staffing levels, it may not be feasible for hospital nurses to undertake new tasks or additional work during their shifts [17]. It is important to create working environments where nurses can find the true meaning of nursing practice and support them with policies that engender positive motivation for their work.

Individual and organizational factors have rarely been collectively included as potential factors for job crafting in studies involving Korean nurses. Therefore, our study aimed to examine the effects of happiness at the individual level and nursing work environments at the organizational level on the job crafting of hospital nurses in Korea. Our research question was whether happiness and nursing work environments may be associated with the job crafting of hospital nurses in Korea.

2. Materials and Methods

2.1. Design

This study employed a cross-sectional survey design.

2.2. Participants and Data Collection

We selected four hospitals based on variations in hospital characteristics, which included teaching status (2 teaching and 2 non-teaching) and location (2 in Seoul and 2 outside metropolitan areas). All hospitals had more than 500 beds. After obtaining approval from the Institutional Review Board of the study hospital, data were collected in April 2019. Nurses with more than 6 months of nursing experience were invited to participate in the study, and approximately 2900 nurses in the four hospitals met the inclusion criteria. As the study units were conveniently selected, the number of available nurses was estimated at 450. A structured questionnaire along with the recruiting notice and informed consent form were enclosed in an envelope. We distributed 240 data collection packages. After completing the consent form and questionnaire, the participants were asked to enclose the materials in a sealed envelope and return them to designated locations for collection by the research staff. To maximize voluntary participation, anonymity and confidentiality, no hospital associates were involved in data collection procedures. Of the 240 questionnaires, 231 were returned (a return rate of 96%). After excluding 11 nurses with missing information for key variables, we analyzed the data for 220 nurses. According to Cohen's (1988) formula for determining the appropriate sample size for multiple linear regression with an effect size of 0.15 (i.e., medium size), a power of 0.95 and an alpha of 0.05 with 12 explanatory variables, the study required a sample size of 184 [18]. Therefore, the sample size of our study was deemed sufficient.

2.3. Measures

Happiness was measured using the Korean happiness index, a culturally sensitive indicator developed by the Korean Psychological Association [19]. Happiness has different meanings according to an individual's view of life or values, and even the same person has a different point of view of happiness depending on his/her situation. The Korean happiness index is comprised of 3 subdomains: life satisfaction (the cognitive element of happiness, 3 items), positive affectivity (3 items) and negative affectivity (3 items). In this study, all items were rated on a Likert-type scale, ranging from strongly disagree (1) to strongly agree (7). Item scores were summated for each subdomain. The happiness score was calculated by subtracting the negative affectivity score from the combined score of life satisfaction and positive affectivity, which was then transformed into a 100-point scale. Higher scores in life satisfaction, positive affectivity and the overall happiness score indicated a better point of view of happiness, whereas higher scores in negative affectivity indicated an unpleasant emotion. Acceptable reliability and convergent and discriminative validity were demonstrated in a previous study [20]. This instrument was likewise determined to be reliable in our study (Cronbach's α = 0.75–0.92).

Nursing work environments were assessed using the Korean version of the Practice Environment Scale of the Nursing Work Index [20]. This instrument has been used globally to measure nursing practice environments. It consists of 29 items representing the following 5 subdomains: nurse participation in hospital affairs (9 items), nursing foundation for quality of care (9 items), nurse manager ability, leadership and support of nurses (4 items), staffing and resource adequacy (4 items) and collegial nurse-physician relationships (3 items). Each item has a 4-point Likert scale ranging from 1 (strongly disagree) to 4 (strongly agree). In this study, each subdomain score was calculated using the average score of the items. Higher scores indicated better perceived nursing work environments. Nursing practice environments can be classified as favorable (having 4–5 subdomains with scores higher than 2.5), mixed (having 2–3 subdomains with scores higher than 2.5) or unfavorable (having 0–1 subdomain with scores higher than 2.5) [21]. This scale was demonstrated to have satisfactory construct validity and reliability in a previous study [20]. A reliable internal consistency with Cronbach's α ranging from 0.67 to 0.83 was found in the present study.

Job crafting was measured using the Korean version of the job crafting questionnaire [22]. This instrument has 3 subdomains with 5 items in each: (1) task crafting, which refers to shaping the nature and scope of the work; (2) cognitive crafting, which involves redefining one's perception of the job; and (3) relationship crafting, which describes changing the type and nature of interactions with colleagues at work. Item responses range from 1 (strongly disagree) to 5 (strongly agree). Each subdomain was evaluated based on the mean of the item score, with higher scores indicating higher levels of job crafting. The instrument was reported to have concurrent, convergent and construct validity [22] and exhibited good reliability in our study (Cronbach's α = 0.78–0.85).

Additional participant data collected included demographic characteristics (age, gender, marital status and educational attainment) and job-related variables (years of experience working as a registered nurse, work units, work schedule, overtime, position and monthly income).

2.4. Data Analysis

Descriptive analysis involved frequencies and percentages for categorical variables and means and standard deviations for continuous variables. To compare job crafting according to personal and job-related characteristics, analysis of variance and t-test were performed. To examine the associations of happiness and nursing work environments with job crafting, we generated multiple linear regression models. The outcome variable, job crafting, was checked for normality using the Shapiro–Wilk test and was found to be normal ($p > 0.05$). The independent variables, happiness and nursing work environments, were treated as continuous variables. The statistical model was adjusted for potential confounding from personal and job-related characteristics with the exception of age (due to its strong correlation with years of registered nurse experience) and gender (few male nurses in the sample). Analyses were conducted using SPSS Statistics for Windows Version 25.0 (IBM Corp., Armonk, NY, USA).

The Institutional Review Board of Seoul National University Bundang Hospital reviewed and approved the study protocol (IRB NO: B-1903-528-301).

3. Results

The demographic characteristics of the participants are shown in Table 1. Nurses ranged in age from 23 to 56 years with an average age of 31 years. Almost all of them were female. Approximately two-thirds of the nurses were unmarried and held a bachelor's degree. The mean years of experience as a registered nurse was 7.5 years with a range of 0.5–25 years. Slightly more than half the participants were working in general wards.

Table 1. Demographic characteristics of study participants.

Variable	Categories	*n* (%)
Age, years	Mean (standard deviation)	30.91 (6.08)
	<30	109 (49.5)
	31–39	89 (40.5)
	≥40	22 (10.0)
Gender	Male	12 (5.5)
	Female	208 (94.5)
Marital status	Single	146 (66.4)
	Married	74 (33.6)
Educational (degree) attainment	Associate's	41 (18.6)
	Bachelor's	156 (70.9)
	Master's/Doctoral	23 (10.5)
Years of experience working as a registered nurse	Mean (standard deviation)	7.50 (5.84)
	<3	59 (26.8)
	≥3 and <5	36 (16.4)
	≥5 and <10	58 (26.4)
	≥10	67 (30.5)
Work units	General wards	118 (53.6)
	Intensive care unit, Emergency room	62 (28.2)
	Operating rooms	23 (10.5)
	Outpatients	17 (7.7)
Work schedule	Fixed	40 (18.2)
	Rotating	180 (81.8)
Overtime, hour(s) per day	<1	79 (35.9)
	≥1 and <2	116 (52.7)
	≥2	25 (11.4)
Position	Staff nurse	185 (84.1)
	Charge nurse	35 (15.9)
Monthly income, million won	<3	60 (27.3)
	≥3 and <3.5	108 (49.1)
	≥3.5	52 (23.6)

The mean happiness score was 56.8 out of a possible 100 (Table 2). Nurses rated their work environments as mixed (3 subdomains with scores higher than 2.5), with the highest score for nurse manager ability, leadership and support of nurses (2.8) and the lowest score for staffing and resource adequacy (2.0). The mean score of job crafting was 3.6, with cognitive crafting having the lowest score (3.5) and relationship crafting having the highest score (3.7).

Table 2. Descriptive findings of key variables.

Key Concept	Subdomain	Mean (SD)	Minimum	Maximum
Happiness	Total score	56.80 (15.49)	0	94.35
	Life satisfaction	14.48 (3.11)	3	21
	Positive affectivity	13.43 (3.54)	3	21
	Negative affectivity	12.21 (3.63)	3	21
Nursing work environments	Total score	2.51 (0.38)	1.24	3.79
	Nurse participation in hospital affairs	2.36 (0.47)	1.33	3.78
	Nursing foundation for quality of care	2.76 (0.35)	1.11	3.78
	Nurse manager ability, leadership and support of nurses	2.77 (0.58)	1	4
	Staffing and resource adequacy	1.96 (0.58)	1	3.75
	Collegial nurse–physician Relationships	2.56 (0.60)	1	4
Job crafting	Total score	3.59 (0.52)	2	4.93
	Task crafting	3.58 (0.56)	1.8	5
	Cognitive crafting	3.50 (0.71)	1	5
	Relationship crafting	3.68 (0.60)	1.8	5
SD—standard deviation				

Nurses who were satisfied with their lives were significantly more likely to exhibit higher levels of job crafting (B = 0.07, $p < 0.001$) (Table 3). Nursing work environments had no significant association with nurses' job crafting. In comparison with nurses working in general wards, operating room nurses were significantly less likely to craft their job (B = −0.35, $p = 0.001$).

Table 3. Associations of happiness and nursing work environments with job crafting among nurses.

Independent Variable	Categories	B	p
Happiness	Life satisfaction	0.07	<0.001
	Positive affectivity	−0.02	0.159
	Negative affectivity	−0.01	0.212
Nursing work environments	Nurse participation in hospital affairs	0.13	0.206
	Nursing foundation for quality of care	0.07	0.529
	Nurse manager ability, leadership and support Of nurses	0.02	0.737
	Staffing and resource adequacy	0.03	0.655
	Collegial nurse–physician relationships	0.09	0.108
Age, years	<30	0.21	0.213
	31–39	0.06	0.614
	≥40	reference	
Gender	Male	0.14	0.248
	Female	reference	
Marital status	Single	−0.14	0.081
	Married	reference	
Educational attainment	Associate's	−0.04	0.692
	Bachelor's	−0.12	0.259
	Master's/Doctoral	reference	
Years of experience working as a registered nurse	<3	−0.30	0.055
	≥3 and <5	−0.03	0.842
	≥5 and <10	0.07	0.505
	≥10	reference	

Table 3. *Cont.*

Independent Variable	Categories	B	*p*
Work units	Intensive care unit, Emergency room	0.08	0.260
	Operating rooms	−0.35	0.001
	Outpatients	0.08	0.587
	General wards	reference	
Work schedule	Fixed	0.10	0.344
	Rotating	reference	
Overtime, hour(s) per day	<1	−0.18	0.090
	≥1 and <2	−0.14	0.115
	≥2	reference	
Position	Staff nurse	0.07	0.440
	Vharge nurse	reference	
Monthly income, million won	<3	0.05	0.661
	≥3 and <3.5	−0.10	0.337
	≥3.5	reference	

4. Discussion

As job crafters, nurses value the nature of nursing as a profession (i.e., cognitive crafting), develop and use the expertise learned from work experience to improve their practice, embrace new work areas (i.e., task crafting), build intimate relationships with patients and caregivers and interact with colleagues through coaching and mentoring (i.e., relationship crafting) [23]. Our findings indicated that nurses who reported greater satisfaction with their lives were more likely to exhibit proactive attitudes toward crafting their job and roles at work. Life satisfaction is known to create psychological capital, which may facilitate an individual's ability to think about and interpret their daily lives and events at work in a positive light [24]. Furthermore, those satisfied with their lives could be self-motivated to redesign their jobs [25]. In this case, nurses' happiness would enhance self-esteem and passion for professional roles and quality job performance [26], which are all associated with job crafting.

Unexpectedly, nursing practice environments had no significant association with nurses' job crafting when controlling for individual-level happiness in a multivariate statistical model. This suggests that the effect of individual-level happiness on the outcome was stronger than that of organizational level characteristics. Consistent with our findings, job crafting among employees in large Korean corporations has been reported to be associated with individual-level characteristics such as personality, temperaments and autonomy rather than team environmental factors (e.g., team culture and leaders' leadership style) [27].

In comparison with nurses working in general wards, operating room nurses were less likely to craft their job. Due to the lack of research on job crafting among operating room nurses, the results could not be explained with evidence. Nevertheless, one possible explanation may be differences in job autonomy and decisional authority, which were reported to help workers redesign their job and exercise job crafting in nursing and other professions [28]. In the controlled environments of operating rooms, the scope of duties for nurses is more standardized and formalized; thus, job autonomy is lower. The delivery of regular job-crafting-related education and training programs to operating room nurses could address this issue. Increasing autonomy in a job creates intrinsic motivation due to the perception that one can control one's job performance [29]. Organizational cultures that establish nurses' own scope of duties by granting the nurses greater autonomy in independent decision making should be nurtured.

In terms of the job crafting subdomains, our nurses reported the lowest score in cognitive crafting. The cognitive change to solve problems at work can consequently result in a change in the task and relational aspects, which could affect nurses' organizational commitment and job satisfaction [3]. In order to enhance the value and meaning of nursing and improve task and relationship crafting, it is necessary to offer training programs that can provide directions for job crafting. Moreover, as the behaviors of the job crafting subdomains are interrelated in a complex manner, it is necessary to improve hospital nurses' job crafting from an integrated perspective of task, cognition and relationship crafting rather than focusing on specific areas alone.

The level of happiness among our study nurses was moderate, which was similar to the findings of a previous study involving Korean nurses [30]; however, it was lower than that observed in a general population of adults [19]. One of the well-known factors that can affect female workers' happiness is participation in leisure activities, which can relieve job stress and increase both job and life satisfaction [31]. Many organizations now offer leisure support such as reimbursement for cultural activity expenses, travel programs and social clubs. However, hospital nurses may be limited in their leisure activities because of irregular and/or rotating shift schedules and night shifts [32]. Therefore, strategies to increase happiness among nurses should be thoroughly explored. To ensure sufficient leisure time and increase nurses' happiness, hospital organizations should consider shortening nurses' working hours through improved staffing, flexible work schedules and reduced overtime.

Our findings should be interpreted with consideration of the study limitations. First, our nurses were recruited from four hospitals through a convenience sampling process; thus, there are concerns over generalizability. Second, our study was cross-sectional and could not demonstrate causal relationships among variables. Lastly, the self-reported data could be vulnerable to denial and social desirability bias.

5. Conclusions

Nurses who are job crafters have greater job satisfaction, provide better nursing care and help hospitals achieve organizational goals [4]. Our study demonstrated that happiness at the individual level rather than nursing practice environments at the organizational level was significantly associated with job crafting among nurses. To improve nurses' happiness and job crafting, organizational supports should be established, such as leisure activity programs and minimal overtime. In addition, organizations should identify the facilitators and barriers of nurses' job crafting across positions and unit types and provide various opportunities for education and training to promote job crafting. These organizational efforts could contribute to positive work motivation and create an environment where nurses can be happy especially when they have to be at the workplace for an extended period. Future studies should include larger sample sizes from multiple sites so that representative findings can be obtained. In addition, further studies should suggest evidence-based approaches for improving nurses' happiness and job crafting.

Author Contributions: S.C., K.H. and Y.C. conceived the study. S.C. and K.H. designed the research. S.C. collected and analyzed the data. S.C., K.H. and Y.C. wrote the initial manuscript and revised it for intellectual content. All authors have read and agreed to the published version of the manuscript.

Funding: This research was funded by the National Research Foundation of Korea (NRF) grant funded by the Korean government (MSIT) (No. 2019R1F1A1058862).

Conflicts of Interest: The authors declare no conflict of interest.

References

1. Lim, M.; Ha, Y.; Oh, D.; Sohn, Y. Validation of the Korean version of Job Crafting Questionnaire (JCQ-K). *Korean Corp. Manag. Rev.* **2014**, *21*, 181–206.
2. Herold, D.M.; Fedor, D.B.; Caldwell, S.; Liu, Y. The effects of transformational and change leadership on employees' commitment to a change: A multilevel study. *J. Appl. Psychol.* **2008**, *93*, 346. [CrossRef] [PubMed]
3. Wrzesniewski, A.; LoBuglio, N.; Dutton, J.E.; Berg, J.M. Job crafting and cultivating positive meaning and identity in work. In *Advances in Positive Organizational Psychology*; Bakker, A.B., Ed.; Emerald Group Publishing Limited: Bingley, UK, 2013; Volume 1, pp. 281–302.
4. Ghitulescu, B.E. Shaping Tasks and Relationships at Work: Examining the Antecedents and Consequences of Employee Job Crafting. Ph.D. Thesis, University of Pittsburgh, Pittsburgh, PA, USA, 2007.

5.   Berg, J.M.; Grant, A.M.; Johnson, V. When callings are calling: Crafting work and leisure in pursuit of unanswered occupational callings. *Organ. Sci.* **2010**, *21*, 973–994. [CrossRef]

6.   Tims, M.; Bakker, A.B.; Derks, D. The impact of job crafting on job demands, job resources, and well-being. *J. Occup. Health Psychol.* **2013**, *18*, 230. [CrossRef]

7.   Ko, J.-O. Influence of clinical nurses' emotional labor on happiness in workplace. *J. Korea Contents Assoc.* **2013**, *13*, 250–261. [CrossRef]

8.   Shusha, A. The effects of job crafting on organizational citizenship behavior: Evidence from Egyptian medical centers. *Int. Bus. Res.* **2014**, *7*, 140. [CrossRef]

9.   Tims, M.; Bakker, A.B. Job crafting: Towards a new model of individual job redesign. *SA J. Indus. Psychol.* **2010**, *36*, 1–9. [CrossRef]

10. Luthans, F.; Youssef, C.M.; Avolio, B.J. *Psychological Capital: Developing the Human Competitive Edge*; Oxford University Press: New York, NY, USA, 2007; p. 256.

11. Slemp, G.R.; Kern, M.L.; Vella-Brodrick, D.A. Workplace well-being: The role of job crafting and autonomy support. *Psychol. Wellbeing* **2015**, *5*, 7. [CrossRef]

12. Sharma, D. Factors affecting employee engagement: A brief review of literature. *Int. J. Manag. Soc. Sci.* **2016**, *4*, 240–246.

13. Fisher, C.D. Happiness at work. *Int. J. Manag. Rev.* **2010**, *12*, 384–412. [CrossRef]

14. Fredrickson, B.L. The role of positive emotions in positive psychology: The broaden-and-build theory of positive emotions. *Am. Psychol.* **2001**, *56*, 218. [CrossRef] [PubMed]

15. Loukzadeh, Z.; Bafrooi, N.M. Association of coping style and psychological well-being in hospital nurses. *J. Caring Sci.* **2013**, *2*, 313. [PubMed]

16. Baylina, P.; Barros, C.; Fonte, C.; Alves, S.; Rocha, Á. Healthcare workers: Occupational health promotion and patient safety. *J. Med. Syst.* **2018**, *42*, 159. [CrossRef] [PubMed]

17. Tims, M.; Bakker, A.B.; Derks, D. Development and validation of the job crafting scale. *J. Vocat. Behav.* **2012**, *80*, 173–186. [CrossRef]

18. Cohen, J. A power primer. *Psychol. Bull.* **1992**, *112*, 155–159. [CrossRef]

19. Suh, E.K.; Koo, J.S. A concise measure of subjective well-being (COMOSWB): Scale development and validation. *Korean J. Soc. Pers. Psychol.* **2011**, *25*, 95–113.

20. Cho, E.H.; Cho, M.N.; Kim, E.Y.; Yoo, I.Y.; Lee, N.J. Construct validity and reliability of the Korean version of the Practice Environment Scale of Nursing Work Index for Korean Nurses. *J. Korean Acad. Nurs.* **2011**, *41*, 325–332. [CrossRef]

21. Lake, E.T.; Friese, C.R. Variations in nursing practice environments: Relation to staffing and hospital characteristics. *Nurs. Res.* **2006**, *55*, 1–9. [CrossRef]

22. Slemp, G.R.; Vella-Brodrick, D.A. The Job Crafting Questionnaire: A new scale to measure the extent to which employees engage in job crafting. *Int. J. Wellbeing* **2013**, *3*, 126–146.

23. Wrzesniewski, A.; Dutton, J.E. Crafting a job: Revisioning employees as active crafters of their work. *Acad. Manag. Rev.* **2001**, *26*, 179–201. [CrossRef]

24. Duffy, R.D.; Dik, B.J.; Steger, M.F. Calling and work-related outcomes: Career commitment as a mediator. *J. Vocat. Behav.* **2011**, *78*, 210–218. [CrossRef]

25. Seligman, M.E.P.; Csikszentmihalyi, M. Positive psychology: An introduction. In *Flow and the Foundations of Positive Psychology*; Csikszentmihalyi, M., Ed.; Springer: Dordrecht, The Netherlands; Heidelberg, Germany, 2014; pp. 279–298.

26. Leigh, A.; Grant, A.M. *Eight Steps to Happiness: The Science of Getting Happy and How it Can Work for You*; Victory Books: Melbourne, MEL, Australia, 2010.

27. Park, H. The Hierarchical Linear Relationship among Job Crafting, Individual and Team Level Variables of Employees in Large Corporations. Ph.D. Thesis, Seoul National University, Gwanak-gu, Seoul, Korea, 2015.

28. Petrou, P.; Demerouti, E.; Peeters, M.C.; Schaufeli, W.B.; Hetland, J. Crafting a job on a daily basis: Contextual correlates and the link to work engagement. *J. Organ. Behav.* **2012**, *33*, 1120–1141. [CrossRef]

29. Katz, D.; Kahn, R.L. *The Social Psychology of Organizations*; Wiley: New York, NY, USA, 1978; p. 848.

30. Ju, E.J.; Kwon, Y.C.; Nam, M.H. Influence of clinical nurses' work environment and emotional labor on happiness index. *J. Korean Acad. Nurs. Admin.* **2015**, *21*, 212–222. [CrossRef]

31. Son, S.; Park, J.-Y.; Suh, K.-H. Relationships between gratitude disposition, subjective well-being, and feeling of happiness among female workers: Focused on mediating effects of job attitude. *Korean J. Stress. Res.* **2015**, *23*, 215–223. [CrossRef]

32. Lee, K.; Suh, Y. A phenomenological study on happiness experienced by career nurses. *J. Korean Acad. Nurs. Admin.* **2014**, *20*, 492–504. [CrossRef]

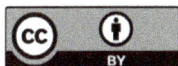

International Journal of
*Environmental Research
and Public Health*

MDPI

Review

Mishel's Model of Uncertainty Describing Categories and Subcategories in Fibromyalgia Patients, a Scoping Review

Ana Fernandez-Araque [1,*], Julia Gomez-Castro [1], Andrea Giaquinta-Aranda [1,2],
Zoraida Verde [3] and Clara Torres-Ortega [1,4]

1   Department of Nursing, Faculty of Health Sciences, University of Valladolid, 42004 Soria, Spain;
    juliamaria.gomez@uva.es (J.G.-C.); agaranda1993@hotmail.com (A.G.-A.); clara.torres@enf.uva.es (C.T.-O.)
2   Haemodialysis Service, Santa Bárbara Hospital, 42005 Soria; Spain
3   Department of Biochemistry, Molecular Biology and Physiology, University of Valladolid, 42004 Soria, Spain;
    zoraida.verde@uva.es
4   Emergency Service of the Hospital Santa Bárbara, 42005 Soria, Spain
*   Correspondence: anamaria.fernandez@uva.es; Tel.: +0034-975129514

check for
updates

Received: 21 April 2020; Accepted: 19 May 2020; Published: 26 May 2020

Abstract: The aim of this review was to demonstrate the presence of categories and subcategories of Mishel's model in the experiences of patients with fibromyalgia by reviewing qualitative studies. Uncertainty is defined as the inability to determine the meaning of disease-related events. A scoping review of qualitative studies was carried out. Twenty articles were included, with sample sizes ranging from 3 to 58 patients. Articles from different countries and continents were included. Three categories of the model and eight subcategories could be shown to be present in the experiences of fibromyalgia patients through the scoping review. The first category, concerning antecedents of uncertainty in patients with fibromyalgia, is constituted by the difficulty in coping with symptoms, uncertainty about the diagnosis and uncertainty about the complexity of the treatment. The second concerns the cognitive process of anxiety, stress, emotional disorder and social stigma. The third category refers to coping with the disease, through the management of social and family support and the relationship with health care professionals.

Keywords: fibromyalgia; stigma; illness uncertainty; scoping review; qualitative research

1. Introduction

Uncertainty characterizes the nature of fibromyalgia syndrome (FMS). FMS is associated with psychiatric comorbidity and coping problems [1,2]. FMS is a chronic pain condition, which has a global mean prevalence of 2.7% [3,4]. FMS is a chronic musculoskeletal disease which affects physical, mental and sexual health [5]. FMS affects 2.4% of the Spanish population [4]. The Committee of the American College of Rheumatology (ACR) formulated a construct of fibromyalgia 30 years ago in an attempt to rectify a situation of diagnostic confusion faced by patients presenting with widespread pain [6].

Fibromyalgia is a complex syndrome. Evidence-based interdisciplinary guidelines have suggested a comprehensive clinical assessment to avoid this diagnostic conundrum [7]. At diagnosis, most individuals have been experiencing symptoms and have been in the health care system for at least 5 to 8 years [8]. The profound symptomatic impact of FMS may be exacerbated by the perceived inauthenticity [9,10]. Its unpredictable course raises concerns about when and how symptoms will appear or progress, with uncertainty being one of the most characteristic emotions of this disease [11]. All this can have a negative emotional, psychological and socioeconomic impact, both on the patient and on the family [12]. Emphasis in FMS research has shifted over the past decade and in the last year [13].

The concept of uncertainty has been used in many disciplines including nursing, medicine, and health communication with slightly differing definitions, extensions, and applications. Nurses provide information that helps patients develop meaning from the illness experience by providing structure. Nurses help patients to manage chronic uncertainty by assisting with patients' reappraisal of uncertainty from stressful to hopeful in addition to providing relevant information [14,15].

The Uncertainty in Illness Theory and its reconceptualization are models derived from and for nursing practice [16]. Uncertainty in illness is defined as a cognitive state resulting from insufficient cues with which to form a cognitive schema or meaning of a situation or event. Mishel proposes that managing uncertainty is critical to adaptation during illness, and his theory explains how individuals cognitively process illness-associated events and construct meaning from them [17]. This theory is based on Warburton's information processing theories, the study of Budner's personality and is influenced in turn by the ideas of Lazarus and Folkman that relate uncertainty with stress and coping [18]. However, Mishel added uncertainty as a stressor in the context of the disease, which is valuable for nurses. This allows us to assess aspects categorized into complex diseases that the individual has to face [19]. The concepts of the theory are organized around three categories using what is known as Mishel's model of uncertainty in disease [16,17]: firstly, the antecedents of uncertainty refer to the form, composition and structure of the stimuli that the person perceives before some prominent subcategories such as difficulty coping with symptoms, uncertainty regarding diagnosis and uncertainty about the complexity of treatment; the second category is the cognitive appraisal of uncertainty, which can vary from person to person and depends on two main subcategories—uncertainty as a danger, and anxiety, stress expression, emotional disorder and stigma [20]; the final subcategory involves coping with uncertainty through social and family support, through health professionals and through support with peers [21].

Uncertainty affects almost every aspect of a person's life. In response to the confusion and disorder caused by a state of continuous uncertainty, the system has no choice but to change to survive. Ideally, under conditions of chronic uncertainty, the person should gradually move from a negative assessment of uncertainty to the adoption of a new way of seeing life that accepts this as part of its reality. This occurs through the cognitive assessment of uncertainty and coping with the uncertainty relating to the disease [22,23].

Therefore, we consider it relevant to show how the three basic categories of Mishel's model for uncertainty about the disease may be present in qualitative studies carried out in patients with fibromyalgia due to its high potential for uncertainty and high emotional demands. Although the studies analyzed in this article are not based on this model, we intend to demonstrate the presence of these categories and be able to detect them, and to show professionals how and where to act, based on the experiences of the patients themselves through the review of qualitative studies. This makes it possible to determine at which moment of the disease process are nursing interventions most time-effective and beneficial for the positive adaptation of the person to their experience of fibromyalgia [24].

The aim of this review was to demonstrate the presence of categories and subcategories of Mishel's model in the experiences of patients with FMS by reviewing qualitative studies.

2. Materials and Methods

A scoping review was carried out, considering qualitative studies with methodological rigor. We selected original articles that explored the experiences of patients with fibromyalgia in order to detect the existence of the three categories present in Mishel's theory of uncertainty about the disease.

2.1. Search

The inclusion criteria for the selection of studies were qualitative designs on adult patients diagnosed with fibromyalgia syndrome, with individual or group intervention methods and verbal accounts of experiences, regardless of the use of the Mishel model as a theoretical framework. Studies selected were conducted within the last ten years, in any language, with free or private access; as we used the library database of the University of Valladolid, this provided us access to articles without free access.

Different search sources and databases were used, such as SCOPUS, CINAHL and PubMed. In the same way, we used descriptors from MESH, CINAHL/MeSH, subject. Headings and DeCS (for the Spanish Language) were employed, in addition to non-standardized terms. The English terms that we used were fibromyalgia, uncertainty, coping, and Mishel. The search was conducted from October 2019 to January 2020, including publications until 2020. We used the following search string for Scopu: fibromyalgia AND uncertainty AND Mishel. For the PubMed database, we used fibromyalgia OR fibro * [tiab] O fibromyalgia AND coping [tiab] O uncertainty [tiab] Mishel O experiences and qualitative investigation [mh]. For the CINAHL Boolean/Phrase, we used the terms fibromyalgia, uncertainty, and Mishel.

2.2. Critical Evaluation

First, we carried out a selection by the title and the abstract of the articles. Then, we discarded repeated articles and those that had no relation to our objective. The articles that we considered relevant, after reading the full text, were evaluated through a peer review. The model used to evaluate the methodological quality of the articles analyzed was the CASPe program for qualitative studies [25], eliminating those that did not meet the minimum established methodological criteria (Table S1). The assessment points included in this guide are "present", "doubtful" and "not registered". Therefore, some eligibility criteria were proposed: of the nine questions, when an article presented three negative responses or two negative responses and a doubtful one, this article was excluded for the review of this study. In total, three articles were excluded, which guarantied the methodological quality of this review.

2.3. Data Extraction

Subsequently, two authors performed an in-depth reading and extracted the data shown in Table 1. The first extraction consisted of obtaining the following data from each article, for a first analysis: relevant data (author/s, publication date and country); setting context design/model; aim of this study; age range; sample; gender of participants, method of data collection, type of interview.

For the review of the participants' experiences, the same two authors also proceeded to look for the existence in the discourses of aspects related to uncertainty about the disease itself—called antecedents of uncertainty—with a cognitive appraisal of uncertainty and coping with uncertainty.

The presence of the three categories of the Mishel model allowed us to go one step further by searching for subcategories within each category, which was intended to show real evidence in the verbal accounts of FMS patients with greater emphasis and clarity. Supplementary file 1 shows this review.

2.4. Process Followed to Determine the Categories and Subcategories of Uncertainty

We proceeded with two steps to extract and show the presence in the verbal accounts and experiences of patients with FMS of the categories and possible subcategories in each study: (1) we identified statements, responses, individual or group aspects related to uncertainty, cognitive processes and coping with the disease in each study and their coincidence or not with the rest of the studies reviewed; (2) after having identified the categories, we carried out a second in-depth reading that allowed us to obtain subcategories and classify them according to the Mishel model [19].

Table 1. Summary of studies included in the review.

Authors, Publication Date and Setting	Context	Design/Theory	Age Range	N/Sample Characteristic	Method of Data Collection	Type of Interview
Alameda et al., 2019 (Madrid, Spain) [26]	Community	Phenomenological	36-74	13/12 W-1 M	Life Story Interview	Individual
Boulton, 2018 (Canada, U.K.) [27]	Community	Narrative analysis	21-69	31/25 W-6 M	In-depth interviews	Individual
Briones et al., 2016 (Valencia, Spain) [28]	Association	Descriptive-exploratory	24-61	13/13 W	In-depth interviews	Individual
Briones et al., 2014 (Valencia, Spain) [29]	Primary care	Descriptive-exploratory	24-61	16/13 W-3 M	Semi-structured interview	Individual
Cedraschi et al., 2013 (Geneva, Switzerland) [22]	Primary care	Interpretative	33-76	56/56 W	Semi-structured interview	Individual
Cooper et al., 2017 (Johannesburg, South Africa) [30]	Community	Descriptive-exploratory	23-59	15/15 W	In-depth interviews and focal group	Individual and group
Escudero-Carretero et al., 2010 (Spain) [8]	Primary care	Interpretative	33-62	21/20 W-1 M	Focal group	Group
Humphrey et al., 2010 (EEUU, Germany, France) [31]	Primary care	Grounded Theory	25-79	40/20/5 M-15 W (EEUU) 10/5 M-5 W(Germany) 10/2 M-8 W (France)	Semi-structured interview	Individual
Juuso et al., 2011 (Sweden) [32]	Community	Phenomenological	38-64	13/13 W	Interview (Unspecified)	Individual
Matarín, 2017 (Spain) [33]	Association	Qualitative study with methodology using Gadamer's philosophical hermeneutics was carried out.	22-56	13/13 W	Focus group and semi-structured interviews	Individual and group
Miranda et al., 2016 (Brazil) [34]	Primary care	Grounded Theory		11/Unspecified	Semi-structured interviews Group dynamics and participant observation	Individual and group
Montesó-Curto et al., 2018 (Catalonia, Spain) [35]	Primary care	Phenomenological	53-69	44/43 W-1 M	Group Problem-Solving Therapy.	Group
Olive et al., 2013 (Cataluña, Spain) [36]	Community	Ethnographic narrative	49-56	3/2 W-1 M	Participant observation and In-depth interviews	Individual
Oliveira et al., 2019 (Río de Janeiro, Brasil) [37]	Community	Interpretative	33-73	12 W	Observation of group dynamics and semi-structured interview	Individual and group
Romero-Alcalá et al., 2019 (Spain, Chile) [38]	Association	Phenomenological and Gadamerian hermeneutics and the Roy adaptation theory	37-53	35 W and their partner	In-depth interviews and focal group	Individual and group
Sallinen et al., 2019 (Oslo, Norway) [39]	Community	Descriptive- exploratory	12-19	5/5 M	Life story interviews	Individual
Sorense et al., 2017 (Norway) [40]	Hospital	Hermeneutic analysis	18-64	Unspecified	In-depth interviews	Individual
Taylor et al., 2016 (Virginia, EEUU) [23]	Community	Interpretative	45-65	20/19 W-1 M and 20 control	Semi-structured interview	Individual
Triviño Martínez et al., 2016 (Alicante, España) [11]	Community	Phenomenological	36-66	14/14 W	Semi-structured interview	Individual
Wuytack et al., 2011 (Gante, Belgium) [41]	Hospital	Exploratory through Husserl's concept of transcendental subjectivity		6/6 W	Semi-structured interview	Individual

FMS: fibromyalgia; W: woman, M: men.

3. Results

Our search strategy resulted in a total of 20 final references after the selection process, as observed in Figure 1.

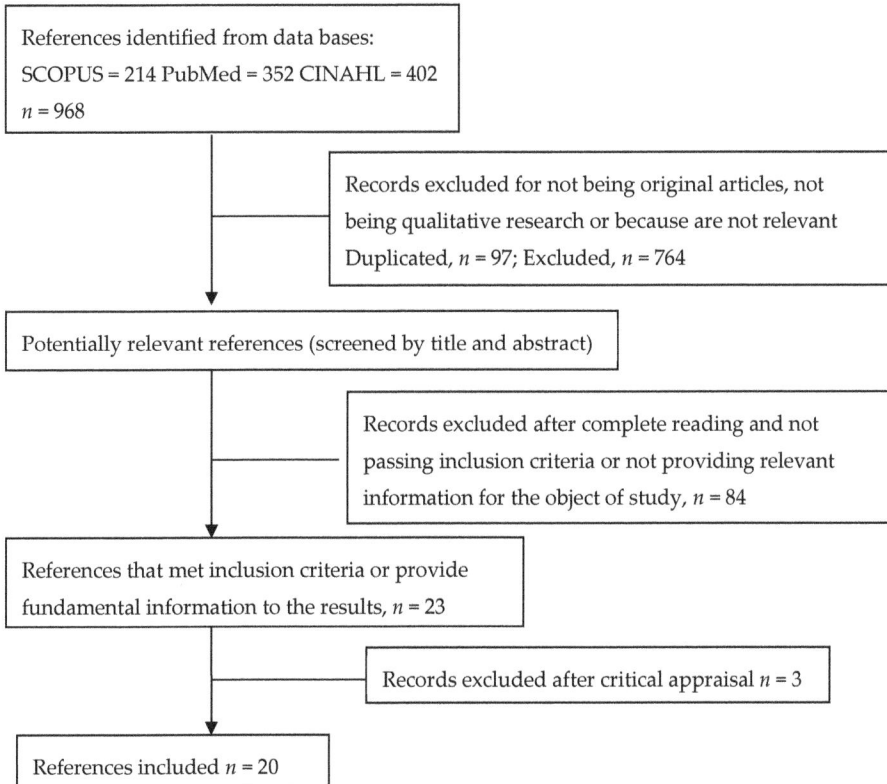

Figure 1. Flowchart of the study selection process.

Of the 20 studies that met the inclusion criteria, the sample sizes ranged from 3 to 58 participants. In all studies, the age range was 18 years old and over; the oldest subject was 90 years old. The predominant sex in the studies was female. In total, 45% of the studies reviewed were carried out with women only. Patients were from Canada, the United States, the United Kingdom, Spain, Germany, France, Belgium, Switzerland, Sweden, South Africa, Brazil and Chile (Table 1).

A review of the literature allowed us to identify the existence of categories related to the Mishel model on uncertainty regarding the disease and secondly to group the experiences of fibromyalgia patients by subcategories, obtaining eight relevant subcategories present in the discourses reviewed in the different studies (Table 2, Table S2).

In the first category—antecedents of uncertainty—we integrate the results related to the difficulty in coping with the symptoms, uncertainty about the diagnosis and uncertainty about the complexity of the treatment. The second category of Mishel's theory is cognitive assessment, which includes anxiety, stress, emotional disorder, and social stigma. The last category refers to coping with uncertainty about the disease. In this case, the subcategories detected in the different discourses and experiences of patients with FMS exhibited a reduction in uncertainty through effective coping due to the existence of subcategories related to the relationship between management and control by health professionals regarding the disease, as well as the support of the family and of peers (Table 2, Table S3).

Table 2. Categories and subcategories of Mishel's model of uncertainty in fibromyalgia syndrome identified in the experiences of patients with different qualitative studies.

Categories	1. Antecedents of Uncertainty			2. Cognitive Appraisal			3. Coping with Uncertainty	
Subcategories:	1.1. Difficulty with symptoms	1.2. Uncertainty regarding diagnosis	1.3. About complexity of treatment	2.1. As a danger Anxiety, stress expression, emotional disorder	2.2. Stigma	3.1. Coping with social and family support	3.2. Through health professionals	3.3. Through support with peers (e.g., associations)
Alameda et al., 2019 [26]	✓	✓	✓	✓			✓	
Boulton, et al., 2018 [27]	✓	✓					✓	
Briones et al., 2016 [28]	✓	✓	✓	✓	✓		✓	
Briones et al., 2014 [29]	✓	✓		✓	✓	✓		
Cedraschi et al., 2013 [22]	✓		✓	✓	✓		✓	✓
Cooper et al., 2017 [30]	✓	✓		✓				
Escudero-C.et al., 2010 [6]	✓	✓		✓		✓	✓	
Humphrey et al., 2010 [31]	✓	✓						
Juuso et al., 2011 [32]	✓	✓		✓	✓	✓	✓	✓
Matarin et al., 2017 [33]	✓					✓	✓	✓
Miranda et al., 2016 [34]	✓						✓	
Montesó-Curtó et al., 2018 [35]	✓	✓		✓	✓	✓	✓	✓
Olive et al., 2013 [36]	✓	✓	✓	✓		✓	✓	✓
Oliveira JPR et al., 2019 [37]	✓	✓		✓	✓	✓	✓	✓
Romero-A et al., 2019 [38]						✓	✓	
Sallimen et al., 2019 [39]	✓	✓	✓	✓	✓	✓	✓	
Sorense et al., 2017 [40]	✓		✓	✓		✓		✓
Taylor et al., 2016 [23]	✓	✓		✓	✓	✓		
Triviño Martínez et al., 2016 [11]		✓				✓		
Wuytack et al., 2011 [41]								

3.1. Antecedents of Uncertainty

3.1.1. Difficulty Coping with Symptoms

In total, 75% of the studies reviewed in our article agree that the unpredictable and changing nature of symptoms leads to a negative evaluation of physical symptoms. The most prominent factors are generalized chronic pain, fatigue, sleep disorders, memory problems, and the feeling of bloating. All these symptoms influence the perceived difficulty to cope with the disease and therefore to adapt to the disease [8,31,33,36]. As a result of the review within this category, we obtained a subcategory—difficulty in coping with symptoms—due to their severity and variability as a stressful factor in the disease process [16,22,28,30,37,40,42] which must be thoroughly evaluated to reduce uncertainty.

3.1.2. Uncertainty Regarding Diagnosis

Diagnosis occurs a last resort because there is no conclusive proven evidence of the disease, so it is considered an invisible disease [27,28]. From the time a patient begins contacting healthcare professionals until diagnosis, an average of approximately 7 years elapses [28,36,41]. During this time, patients are in a situation of uncertainty [40]. In total, 76.16% of the reviewed studies show—in the experiences of FMS patients—the need for a firm diagnosis as a turning point to develop coping strategies in the health–disease process and reduce anxiety. Therefore, it is the second subcategory identified in our results.

3.1.3. Uncertainty about Complexity of Treatment

This third subcategory—the complexity of the treatment of this syndrome—identified appears in the verbal accounts and experiences of 33.33% of the selected studies [27,28,33]. Patients with the highest degree of uncertainty about prognosis were those with the worst adherence to treatment [36]. Most of the participants in the different studies (Table 2) stated that health professionals lack information on the use of the various medications prescribed [40]; patients manifested unpleasant side effects of medications, which occasionally led them to avoid their use [23,28]. These patients then look for other therapy options such as non-pharmacological treatment and moderate physical exercise.

3.2. Cognitive Appraisal

In regard to the category of cognitive assessment, the presence of two subcategories is highlighted: the perception of danger by the presence of stress, anxiety and emotional disorders, and the cognitive perception and experience caused by the stigma of the disease [22,29,30,33,36,38,41].

3.2.1. Uncertainty as a Danger: Anxiety, Stress and Emotional Disorder

This disease is linked to psychopathology, stress, anxiety and depression. Chronic pain as a routine produces a great deal of suffering and limitations [37], and people affected by FMS feel imprisoned by pain [40]. Another method which some people use to try to confront the diagnosis is to approach religion or spirituality [16], which emerges as an emotional support. Faith in some superior being fills these people with motivation, relief, self-improvement, and strength.

Therefore, stressful and emotional factors may lead to a sense of danger that may constitute another subcategory drawn from the experiences of patients suffering from this disease. Depending on the individuals' own experiences, education and internal resources, the cognitive assessment of danger will differ from one patient to another.

3.2.2. Stigma

This subcategory was found in 38% of the selected articles (Table 2). Social stigma is the feeling of prejudice against people with FMS. On one hand, there is a stigma of the mental illness that surrounds this pathology; on the other hand, patients may feel morally offended by the supposed faking of their symptoms, when no obvious signs of illness are found [27,30,33]. Feeling believed by society and supported is a reinforcement of the mechanism of adaptation to FMS [40,41]. Many fibromyalgia patients, in addition to suffering discrimination and prejudice from others, also suffer from these feelings towards themselves.

Furthermore, we discovered another flaw within the social stigma, which we can label as a gender stigma: gender stigma appears as FMS mainly affects women, and there is a stereotype of a "woman who complains" [29]. In total, 14% of the articles analyzed identify gender self-stigma as the inability to fulfil feminine tasks imposed by society, which creates a feeling of remorse in women [29,35,36]. In men, fatigue is seen worse than in women, thus generating a feeling of helplessness and loss of virility [32].

3.3. Coping with Uncertainty

Coping strategies are the thoughts and behaviors that the person often uses to respond to stressful situations and lessen the perceived threat of experiencing chronic illness [19,20,41]. As a result of our review, we have identified important repetitions in the verbal accounts of the experiences of FMS patients that need to be reduced though effective coping mechanisms.

3.3.1. Coping with Social and Family Support

This subcategory was found in the review by means of three main verbal accounts: social support, family and work repercussion. In 16 of the articles included in this review (Table 2), the importance of sufferers having effective social relationships in their lives is expressed, because these relationships help them to overcome negative situations related to the disease. Pain and relapses can lead to the impossibility of making plans and social isolation, because patients cannot perform the same activities as before the disease [23]. In order not to be judged by people close to them, some patients avoid talking about the disease and the feelings that it entails, therefore avoiding the problem and developing a maladaptation to the situation [41].

Another aspect that many studies show is the great impact on work that the disease produces [32,35,37,40,42]. In environments where there is no public health system, patients may depend on parents or partners to pay for medical bills, leaving those without family support unprotected [31]. It is important to highlight among these results that people try to maintain personal and work roles, using energy dosing strategies to improve their self-concept [39]. The relationship with partners is especially affected because the physical discomfort of these patients leads to a negative mood. On the other hand, the disease involves a change in affectivity and sexual life that is not always well accepted in a couple [29,33,38]

3.3.2. Coping through Health Professionals

One of the subcategories identified and the one that most concerns us is that related to health professionals. This factor was highlighted by more than half of the studies analyzed (Table 2); it was found that a patient's lack of confidence in healthcare professionals is one of the factors that increases uncertainty. The relationship with healthcare professionals is controversial since there are those who believe in the disease and those who do not [25].

Participants demand credibility from healthcare professionals from the first moment they attend the consultation. Empathy is demanded, along with a comprehensive approach, taking into account expectations and the psychological dimension [22,30]. Most often, patients report that their doctors told them the name of their illness, but they were not informed about its possible physical and mental consequences, nor the possible treatments or therapies [27]. This discourse shows us a subcategory that requires the evaluation of our work as health professionals.

3.3.3. Coping through Peer Support (e.g., Associations)

In total, 38% of articles showed that patient associations can play an important role in finding information, especially when the health system is fragile. Patient associations provide peer support, relief, and shared experiences with others in the same situation. For this reason, in our results, this subcategory was detected as an element to contribute to adequate adaptation and an effective method of coping with FMS [40].

4. Discussion

The results of this review show the presence of the three main categories of Mishel's model about uncertainty in adults who suffer from FMS, which was the goal of our study, which was carried out through the revision of the verbal accounts of patients and their experiences in the 20 studies selected. The review included studies from different countries.

This theory has been applied to many chronic diseases, but few studies have been carried out in people with fibromyalgia [11]. However, the identification of uncertainty as a stressor and the ability to establish cognitive processes against stigma and coping through the use and availability of family resources, peers and healthcare professionals can be useful for comprehensive patient care. Furthermore, this can help us to evaluate and help patients to effectively deal with all the aspects related to uncertainty cause by their disease.

Assessing patients with FMS by these categories will allow us to understand the nature of the uncertainty for each patient individually and will help us to determine how to handle the uncertainty of patients with this disease as these are the most relevant aspects of their disease which concern the patients and interfere with the way they are coping with it [23].

The studies do not show differences in uncertainty regarding fibromyalgia between men and women, perhaps due to the lack of studies in men; only one study with men in this review met criteria for inclusion [39], and in those studies that involved men and women, there were a greater proportion of women than men, as can be seen in Table 1 [8,23,35]. Although one author concluded that FMS has a greater impact in men and it causes them to seek medical retirement earlier than women, this has not been proven with a significant sample size or in a qualitative study [43].

In regard of patient's age, the core sample were adults and mainly of intermediate age, which is similar to other studies showing the prevalence of FMS [42]. Patients of working age experience greater uncertainty.

We can affirm the existence of the first category of the Mishel model in the reviewed studies. The perception of patients with FMS, on the basis of initial experience, even before knowing the diagnosis, is similar [4,6,10,34,35,37,43,44], highlighting the difficulties that they have to understand the symptoms, their uncertainty with regard to the diagnosis and uncertainty about the complexity of treatment. It is important to consider the importance of the history of uncertainty in chronic diseases [15,45].

In half of the reviewed studies, we observed that patients mentioned feelings of uncertainty because of the symptoms, because of the pain and diagnosis complexity and because of the lack of adequate treatment [8,27,28,31–34,37,38,41]. Patients with more pain, who suffer more frequent relapses, have less resistance to stressors related to the disease, and therefore more uncertainty and consequently a worse adaptation [42,43]. All this provokes chronicity and hopelessness [22]. Being diagnosed with fibromyalgia caused mixed feelings in many of the participants [46], although it was a relief for them to have a name for their pain [8,27,30,47]. When patients find a meaning for their disease experience, they reduce their uncertainty or value the knowledge as providing a second chance. This indicates the need to act at this stage and to assess the subcategories of the diagnosis, the symptoms and the treatment, as well as to give information to the patients as nursing professionals and to be in closer contact with the patients, meeting their requirements and supporting them as necessary.

Other authors such as Boulton et al. [28] and Cedraschi et al. [22] warn that diagnosis does not suffice to reduce uncertainty due to the little knowledge that exists about the evolution of the disease and the prognosis; the feeling of the lack of knowledge of the disease and its treatment floods the affected people with despair. The diagnosis is a relief, although it is sometimes difficult to live with chronicity. The subcategory of the complexity of the treatment showed that those patients with the greatest degree of uncertainty about their prognosis were those with the worst adherence to treatment [36]. This is another important factor that nurses should understand about FMS patients.

The category of cognitive assessment was reflected in patients with FMS when they reported their experiences of fear and threat [36]. In total, 66% of the patients in the studies analyzed show feelings of vulnerability and fear without really accepting their new health–disease condition. This disease is linked to psychopathology, stress, anxiety and depression. Chronic pain as a routine produces a great deal of suffering and limitations [37], and people affected by FMS feel imprisoned by pain [40]. Another way in which some people try to confront the diagnosis is to approach religion or spirituality [16], which emerges as an emotional support. Faith in some superior being fills these people with motivation, relief, self-improvement, and strength.

Patients use different strategies to cope with the disease, which are family support, peer support, associations and support groups. Health professionals represent a main source of support.

In relation to health professionals, study participants value their credibility from the outset, including their comprehensive and individualized attention. They seek a good level of communication and understanding by professionals, and they need support in the search for effective solutions, considering this therapeutic support in itself [27,30,35]. Therefore, the coordination of different professionals is essential to understand the treatment prescribed, so multidisciplinary sessions would be necessary [27,38]. Multidisciplinary intervention allows the implementation of solutions for self-care, active listening, and reflection, leading to awareness and autonomy [38]. Health education in self-care, support and understanding empowers a person with FMS [32]. According to the search of Alameda et al. [27], the ultimate goal of nursing is to determine the vulnerability caused by the exclusion of these people.

Family members may also experience uncertainty about the illness of one of their relatives; if this occurs, care can be affected. Nurses should address the concerns of caregivers and provide information about the disease [42]. The stability of women improves with the physical and moral support of the partner and family [29].

Therefore, the three subcategories that have been detailed in Table 2 are present frequently in the discourses of the experiences of FMS patients, and these coincide with the most important aspects to assess in chronic and complex diseases [46]. This revision gives credence to these aspects in improving the management of uncertainty.

For some patients, beating FMS means being happy in difficult circumstances and finding small pleasures in daily life [41]. For others, it means clinging to fragments of their previous lives, whether through work or by continuing to pay attention to aspects of daily life. Taking this into consideration, we must continue to carry out studies and reviews that produce a benefit for a better nursing assessment and performance in these patients.

This review is not exempt from limitations. Even though the sources used in the search are pertinent, they might not give a full account of all the relevant studies in this subject. We must bear in mind that, although the databases used to search for the studies are relevant, not all the available studies were collected; therefore, there may be some missing relevant research in this area. We avoided the use of excessive databases to limit the number of repeated articles found; however, a large number of duplicate documents were discarded.

Finally, it would have been interesting to include studies with a more balanced sample of male and female patients and to have been able to review and analyze a gender comparison with more scientific evidence, as well as to have been able to identify possible gender differences and determine actions to further reduce the level of uncertainty and to increase the patients' ability to cope with the illness.

5. Conclusions

The approach to these categories in the assessment of FMS patients can be a valuable tool for a multidisciplinary team since it allows problems to be identified and interventions to be designed which aim to reducing uncertainty and improve patients' adaptation to the disease.

Uncertainty and FMS are closely linked due to a lack of knowledge about the pathophysiological mechanisms of the disease.

People diagnosed with FMS often perceive uncertainty as a danger or threat, which leads to situations of stress, anxiety and emotional disorder. The longer the uncertainty lasts in the context of the disease, the more unstable the person's mode of functioning will be.

This review demonstrates the presence of three categories and eight subcategories based on Mishel's model of uncertainty in disease. Addressing these categories can help patients find meaning in FMS, properly manage uncertainty and accept it as a natural part of a new life that makes sense despite the disease.

Practical Implication

The key message from the study findings for nurses is that they must be alert to potential risk factors for patients with FMS.

This review shows which aspects are most relevant to assess in FMS patients to reduce their uncertainty and face their disease with the best possible professional support.

Supplementary Materials: The following are available online at http://www.mdpi.com/1660-4601/17/11/3756/s1, Table S1: Results after a methodological evaluation using CASPe. Table S2: Analysis of the studies included in the review with the most relevant results for each. Table S3. Categories and subcategories of Mishel's model of Uncertainty in Fibromyalgia Syndrome, identified in the experiences of patients from different qualitative studies.

Author Contributions: Conceptualization, A.F.-A. and C.T.-O.; methodology, A.F.-A.; software, C.T.-O.; validation, A.F.-A., and A.G.-A.; formal analysis, C.T.-O.; investigation, A.F.-A.; resources, C.T.-O.; data curation, A.G.-A.; writing—original draft preparation, A.F.-A. and J.G.-C.; writing—review and editing, J.G.-C.; visualization, J.G.-C.; supervision, Z.V.; project administration, A.F.-A. All authors have read and agreed to the published version of the manuscript.

Funding: This review received no external funding.

Conflicts of Interest: The authors declare no conflict of interest.

References

1. Reich, J.W.; Johnson, L.M.; Zautra, A.J.; Davis, M.C. Uncertainty of illness relationships with mental health and coping processes in fibromyalgia patients. *J. Behav. Med.* **2006**, *29*, 307–316. [CrossRef] [PubMed]
2. Galvez-Sánchez, C.M.; Montoro, C.I.; Duschek, S.; Del Paso, G.A.R. Depression and trait-anxiety mediate the influence of clinical pain on health-related quality of life in fibromyalgia. *J. Affect. Disord.* **2020**, *265*, 486–495. [CrossRef] [PubMed]
3. Ashe, S.C.; Furness, P.J.; Taylor, S.J.; Haywood-Small, S.; Lawson, K. A qualitative exploration of the experiences of living with and being treated for fibromyalgia. *Health Psychol. Open* **2017**, *4*. [CrossRef] [PubMed]
4. Queiroz, L. Worldwide epidemiology of fibromyalgia. *Curr. Pain Headache Rep.* **2013**, *17*, 356. [CrossRef]
5. Levine, J.D.; Reichling, D.B. Fibromyalgia: The nerve of that disease. *J. Rheumatol.* **2005**, *32*, 29–37.
6. Long, T.C. The fibromyalgia dilemma. *J. Controv. Med. Claims* **2004**, *11*, 1–8.
7. Häuser, W.; Sarzi-Puttini, P.; Fitzcharles, M.A. Fibromyalgia syndrome: Under-, over- and misdiagnosis. *Clin. Exp. Rheumatol.* **2019**, *37*, 90–97.
8. Escudero, M.J.; García-Toyos, N.; Prieto Rodríguez, M.A.; Pérez Corral, O.; March Cerdá, J.C.; López Doblas, M. Fibromyalgia: patients' perception of their disease and the health system. Qualitative Research Study. *Reumatol. Clin.* **2010**, *6*, 16–22. [CrossRef]
9. Quintner, J.; Buchanan, D.; Cohen, M.; Taylor, A. Signification and Pain: A Semiotic Reading of Fibromyalgia. *Theor. Med. Bioeth.* **2003**, *24*, 345–354. [CrossRef]

10. Akkasilpa, S.; Goldman, D.; Magder, L.S.; Petri, M. Number of fibromyalgia tender points is associated with health status in patients with systemic lupus erythematosus. *J. Rheumatol.* **2005**, *32*, 48–50.

11. Triviño, A.; Solano, M.C.; Siles, J.; Ruiz, S. Application of an uncertainty theory for fibromyalgia. *Atten. Primaria* **2015**, *48*, 219–225.

12. Marcus, D.A.; Richards, K.L.; Chambers, J.F.; Bhowmick, A. Fibromyalgia family and relationship impact exploratory survey. *Musculoskelet. Care* **2013**, *11*, 125–134. [CrossRef] [PubMed]

13. Fitzcharles, M.A.; Yunus, M.B. The clinical concept of fibromyalgia as a changing paradigm in the past 20 years. *Pain Res. Treat.* **2012**, *2012*, 184835. [CrossRef] [PubMed]

14. Poindexter, K.H. Manejo de enfermería del síndrome de fibromialgia. *Medsurg Nurs.* **2017**, *26*, 349–352.

15. Peters, A.; McEwen, B.S.; Friston, K. Uncertainty and stress: Why it causes disease and how it is dominated by the brain. *Prog. Neurobiol.* **2017**, *156*, 164–188. [CrossRef]

16. Mishel, M. Reconceptualization of the uncertainty in illness theory. *J. Nurs. Scholarsh.* **1990**, *22*, 256–262. [CrossRef]

17. Mishel, M.H. Uncertainty in acute illness. *Annu. Rev. Nurs. Res.* **1997**, *15*, 57–80. [CrossRef]

18. Bailey, D.E., Jr.; Stewart, J.L. Uncertainty in Illness Theory. In *Nursing Theorists and Their Work*, 8th ed.; Alligood, M.R., Ed.; Elsevier Mosby: St. Louis, MO, USA, 2013; pp. 555–573.

19. Clayton, M.F.; Marleah, D.; Merle, M. Middle Range Theory for Nursing. In *Theories of Uncertainty in Illness*; Springer Publishing Company: New York, NY, USA, 2018; ISBN 978-0-8261-5991-5 49-88.

20. Kroencke, D.C. Coping with Multiple Sclerosis: The Impact of Uncertainty on Illness. Master's Thesis, University of Catalunya, Tarragona, Spain, 1999.

21. Malin, K.; Littlejohn, G.O. Personality and fibromyalgia syndrome. *Open Rheumatol. J.* **2012**, *6*, 273. [CrossRef]

22. Cedraschi, E.; Girard, C.; Luthy, M.; Kossovsky, J.; Desmeules, A.F. Primary attributions in women suffering fibromyalgia emphasize the perception of a disruptive onset for a long-lasting pain problem. *J. Psichosom. Res.* **2013**, *74*, 265–269. [CrossRef]

23. Taylor, A.G.; Adelstein, K.E.; Fischer-White, T.G.; Murugesan, M.; Anderson, J.G. Perspectives on Living with Fibromyalgia. *Glob. Qual. Nurs. Res.* **2016**, *3*. [CrossRef]

24. Cano, A.; González, T.; Cabello, J. Template to help you understand a qualitative study. In *CASPe Guidelines for Critical Reading of Medical Literature*; University of Alicante: Alicante, Spain, 2010.

25. Anema, C.; Johnson, M.; Zeller, J.M.; Fogg, L.; Zetterlund, J. Spiritual well-being in individuals with fibromyalgia syndrome: Relationships with symptom pattern variability, uncertainty, and psychosocial adaptation. *Res. Theory Nurs. Pract.* **2020**, *223*, 8–22. [CrossRef] [PubMed]

26. Alameda Cuesta, A.; Pazos Garciandía, Á.; Oter Quintana, C.; Losa Iglesias, M.E. Fibromyalgia, Chronic Fatigue Syndrome, and Multiple Chemical Sensitivity: Illness Experiences. *Clin. Nurs. Res.* **2019**. [CrossRef] [PubMed]

27. Boulton, T. Nothing and Everything: Fibromyalgia as a Diagnosis of Exclusion and Inclusion. *Qual. Health Res.* **2018**, *29*, 809–819. [CrossRef] [PubMed]

28. Briones-Vozmediano, B.; Tula, E.; Vives Cases, C.; Goicolea, I. "I'm not the woman I was": Women's perceptions of the effects of fibromyalgia on private life. *Health Care Women Int.* **2016**, *37*, 836–854. [CrossRef] [PubMed]

29. Briones-Vozmediano, E.; Ronda-Perez, E.; Vives-Cases, C. Perceptions of patients with fibromyalgia on the impact of the disease in the workplace. *Aten Primaria* **2014**, *47*, 205–212. [CrossRef]

30. Cooper, S.; Gilbert, L. An exploratory study of the experience of fibromyalgia diagnosis in South Africa. *Health* **2017**, *21*, 337–353. [CrossRef]

31. Humphrey, L.; Arbuckle, R.; Mease, P.; Williams, D.A.; Samsoe, B.D.; Gilbert, C. Fatigue in fibromyalgia: A conceptual model informed by patient interviews. *BMC Musculoskelet. Disord.* **2010**, *11*, 216. [CrossRef]

32. Juuso, P.; Skär, L.; Olsson, M.; Söderberg, S. Living with a double burden: Meanings of pain for women with fibromyalgia. *Int. J. Qual. Stud. Health Well-Being* **2011**, *6*. [CrossRef]

33. Matarín, T.M.; Fernández-Sola, C.; Hernández-Padilla, J.M.; Correa Casado, M.; Antequera Raynal, L.H.; Granero-Molina, J. Perceptions about the sexuality of women with fibromyalgia syndrome: A phenomenological study. *J. Adv. Nurs.* **2017**, *73*, 1646–1656. [CrossRef]

34. Miranda, N.A.C.G.; Berardinelli, L.M.M.; Saboia, V.M.; Brito, I.S.; Santos, R.S. Interdisciplinary care praxis in groups of people living with fibromyalgia. *Rev. Bras. Enferm.* **2016**, *69*, 1115–1123. [CrossRef]

35. Montesó-Curto, P.; García-Martinez, M.; Romaguera, S.; Mateu, M.L.; Cubí-Guillén, M.T.; Sarrió-Colas, L.; Panisello-Chavarria, M.L. Problems and solutions for patients with fibromyalgia: Building new helping relationships. *J. Adv. Nurs.* **2018**, *74*, 339–349. [CrossRef]

36. Olivé Ferrer, M.C.; Isla Pera, M.P. Experience of fibromyalgia. *Rev. Enferm.* **2013**, *36*, 48.

37. Oliveira, J.; Pereira Ramos, B.; Marcia Migueis, L.; Cavaliere, M.L.A.; Celi Alves, R.; Costa, L.P.D.; Barbosa, J.S.O. The routines of women with fibromyalgia and an interdisciplinary challenge to promote self-care. *Rev. Gaúcha Enferm.* **2019**, *40*, e20180411. Available online: http://www.scielo.br/scielo.php?script=sci_arttext&pid=S1983-14472019000100431&lng=en (accessed on 15 December 2019).

38. Romero-Alcalá, P.; Hernández-Padilla, J.M.; Fernández-Sola, C.; del Rosario Coín-Pérez-Carrasco, M.; Ramos-Rodríguez, C.; Ruiz-Fernández, M.D.; Granero-Molina, J. Sexuality in male partners of women with fibromyalgia syndrome: A qualitative study. *PLoS ONE* **2019**, *14*. [CrossRef] [PubMed]

39. Sallinen, M.; Mengshoel, A.M.; Solbrække, K. "I can't have it; I am a man. A young man!"—Men, fibromyalgia and masculinity in a Nordic context. *Int. J. Qual. Stud. Health Well-Being* **2019**, *14*, 1. [CrossRef] [PubMed]

40. Sorense, K.; Christianensen, B. Adolescents' experience of complex persistent pain. *Scand. J. Pain* **2017**, *15*, 106–112. [CrossRef] [PubMed]

41. Wuytack, F.; Miller, P. The lived experience of fibromyalgia in female patients, a phenomenological study. *Chiropr. Man. Ther.* **2011**, *19*, 22. [CrossRef]

42. Mas, A.J.; Carmona, L.; Valverde, M.; Ribas, B. Prevalence and impact of fibromyalgia on function and quality of life in individuals from the general population: Results from a nationwide study in Spain. *Clin. Exp. Rheumatol.* **2008**, *26*, 519.

43. Perez, I.R.; Linares, M.U.; Perez, M.B.; Brown, J.P.; Labry Lima, A.O.; Torres, E.H. Differences in characteristics sociodemographic, clinical and psychological men and women diagnosed with fibromyalgia. *Span. Clin. Mag.* **2007**, *207*, 433–439.

44. Clauw, D.J.; D'Arcy, Y.; Gebke, K.; Semel, D.; Pauer, L.; Kim, D. Jones Normalizing fibromyalgia as a chronic illness. *Postgrad. Med.* **2018**, *130*, 9–18. [CrossRef]

45. Råheim, M.; Håland, W. Lived experience of chronic pain and fibromyalgia: Women's stories from daily life. *Qual. Health Res.* **2006**, *16*, 741–761. [CrossRef]

46. Mannerkorpi, K.; Palstam, A.; Gard, G. Factors promoting sustainable work in women with fibromyalgia. *Disabil. Rehabil.* **2013**, *35*, 1622–1629.

47. Menzies, V. CE: Fibromyalgia Syndrome Current Considerations in Symptom Management. *Am. J. Nurs.* **2016**, *116*, 24–32. [CrossRef] [PubMed]

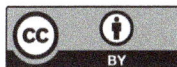

International Journal of
Environmental Research and Public Health

MDPI

Article

Prevalence of Comorbidities in Individuals Diagnosed and Undiagnosed with Alzheimer's Disease in León, Spain and a Proposal for Contingency Procedures to Follow in the Case of Emergencies Involving People with Alzheimer's Disease

Macrina Tortajada-Soler [1], Leticia Sánchez-Valdeón [2,*], Marta Blanco-Nistal [3],
José Alberto Benítez-Andrades [4], Cristina Liébana-Presa [2] and Enrique Bayón-Darkistade [2]

[1] Facultad de Ciencias de la Salud, Campus de Vegazana, Universidad de León, s/n, C.P. 24071 León, Spain; macrina-96@hotmail.com

[2] SALBIS Research Group, Facultad de Ciencias de la Salud, Campus de Ponferrada, Universidad de León, Avda/ Astorga s/n, C.P. 24402 Ponferrada (León), Spain; cristina.liebana@unileon.es (C.L.-P.); jebayd@unileon.es (E.B.-D.)

[3] Complejo Asistencial Universitario de León, C/ Altos de nava s/n, C.P. 24001 León, Spain; mblancon@saludcastillayleon.es

[4] SALBIS Research Group, Department of Electric, Systems and Automatics Engineering, University of León, s/n, 24071 León, Spain; jbena@unileon.es

* Correspondence: lsanv@unileon.es; Tel.: +34-646714103

Received: 23 April 2020; Accepted: 12 May 2020; Published: 13 May 2020

check for updates

Abstract: *Background:* Alzheimer's disease (AD) which is the most common type of dementia is characterized by mental or cognitive disorders. People suffering with this condition find it inherently difficult to communicate and describe symptoms. As a consequence, both detection and treatment of comorbidities associated with Alzheimer's disease are substantially impaired. Equally, action protocols in the case of emergencies must be clearly formulated and stated. *Methods:* We performed a bibliography search followed by an observational and cross-sectional study involving a thorough review of medical records. A group of AD patients was compared with a control group. Each group consisted of 100 people and were all León residents aged ≥65 years. *Results:* The following comorbidities were found to be associated with AD: cataracts, urinary incontinence, osteoarthritis, hearing loss, osteoporosis, and personality disorders. The most frequent comorbidities in the control group were the following: eye strain, stroke, vertigo, as well as circulatory and respiratory disorders. Comorbidities with a similar incidence in both groups included type 2 diabetes mellitus, glaucoma, depression, obesity, arthritis, and anxiety. We also reviewed emergency procedures employed in the case of an emergency involving an AD patient. *Conclusions:* Some comorbidities were present in both the AD and control groups, while others were found in the AD group and not in the control group, and vice versa.

Keywords: Alzheimer's disease; comorbidity; older adults; elderly

---

1. Introduction

A general increase in life expectancy has caused an aging population and a resulting rise in the incidence of diseases that were less prevalent a few years ago such as neurodegenerative disorders [1]. At present, Alzheimer's disease (AD) is the most common type of dementia [2–17]. It was first described in 1907 [9] by the German physician Alois Alzheimer [1], who diagnosed it in a 51-year-old woman. It was described as a disease characterized by an impaired memory, disorientation, and hallucinations leading to death [1]. Currently, AD is considered to be a neurodegenerative disease [1,9,11–13,15,17–20] that is progressive [4,11,12,17–20] and results in mental or cognitive dysfunctions [1,5,11,17].

AD has become a major world health problem affecting a continuously increasing number of people. In Spain, 500,000–800,000 people suffer from AD, a number expected to double by 2050 [2,3]. More specifically, it is calculated that 10% of the population aged ≥65 years and 50% of that ≥85 years will suffer from AD [18]. Aging, therefore, greatly increases the risk of AD [6,9,21], which by now has become a social and public health issue [1].

The main symptom of AD is the loss of episodic memory [4,9,10,14]. This is accompanied by other characteristic "warning signs" [4,6,9,20,22] namely:

1. Failures or memory loss, which make everyday activities difficult;
2. Difficulty to face and/or solve problems;
3. Disorientation;
4. Difficulty understanding visual images and spoken language;
5. Problems with oral and/or written language;
6. Placing objects out of place;
7. Diminished and absent capacity of judgment;
8. Loss of initiative;
9. Personality changes, including apathy and depression;
10. Higher anxiety levels, restlessness, and sleep disorders;
11. Development of a state of increased dependency.

1.1. Pathophysiology of AD

The pathophysiology of AD is characterized by the occurrence of neurofibrillary tangles and neuritic plaques [2,3,5,10,12,17]. Several theories try to explain its onset [2–5,7,8,12,16,23,24] as follows:

Amyloid theory The essential element of extracellular deposits is the protein β-amyloid, which forms fibrils that aggregate and cause the development of diffuse and neuritic plaques. The β-amyloid protein is produced by an abnormal cleavage of the amyloid precursor protein (APP). Normally, the product of secretase α action is a soluble peptide that can be easily removed from the body. In AD, the cleavage is performed by β- and γ-secretases producing insoluble peptides that are removed from neurons. Microglial cells unsuccessfully attempt their removal, and this results in inflammation and nerve damage.

Tau protein theory The tau protein is the main component of intracellular deposits in neurons. It is a microtubule-associated protein, with microtubules being cytoplasmic structures involved in the assembly and function of the cytoskeletal network of cells including neurons. Tau acts as a microtubule stabilizer. In AD, Tau hyper-phosphorylation prevents its binding to tubulin and results in autoaggregation and formation of neurotoxic intraneuronal precipitates.

Cholinergic theory A decrease in the levels of the neurotransmitter acetylcholine in patients with AD causes a diminished performance of neural connections.

In addition to the three theories mentioned above, several other hypotheses have attempted to explain the etiology of AD, such as oxidative stress and glutamate-mediated excitotoxicity [7,12].

1.2. Risk and Protective Factors

AD is associated with a series of risk and protective factors. A risk factor is understood as one that increases the probability that an individual will develop a health problem or disease; while a protective factor is one that reduces such probability. We present a list of such factors that are associated with AD as follows:

Risk factors [4,19,21,23,25–31]

- Non-modifiable factors include age, gender, genetics-related (karyotype alterations, gene mutations, etc.), parental education, family background;
- Modifiable factors include low educational or socioeconomic level, obesity, type II diabetes mellitus, cardiovascular diseases (hypertension, atherosclerosis, heart disease, atrial fibrillation, and dyslipidemia), smoking, stroke, depression, alcohol abuse, and pneumonia;
- Environmental factors [24] include aluminum, pesticides, pollution.

Protective factors [21]

- physical, educational, intellectual and social activities, moderate consumption of alcoholic beverages, and a Mediterranean diet.

Establishing which factors are protective or risk-linked for AD patients is made difficult by these patients' inherent inability to communicate consistently. One way to approach this problem is by detecting comorbidities associated with AD and developing possible action protocols to be employed in emergency cases. The present study compared the comorbidities in a population of individuals aged ≥65 years and diagnosed with AD with those in an undiagnosed (control) population of similar characteristics, in the city of León, during 2019. In brief, the objectives of this work are as follows:

- To compare the sociodemographic characteristics of the individuals in the two populations under scrutiny;
- To establish and compare the comorbidities associated with the individuals of each of the two populations;
- To know, if any, the protocols of action employed by the Alzheimer Center of León or the León University Hospital in emergency situations concerning people with AD.

The cognitive or mental impairment that people with Alzheimer's disease present increases the difficulty they have in expressing themselves and manifesting their symptoms. Therefore, there is a need to study the comorbidities associated with Alzheimer's, and to examine possible protocols for action in the case of an emergency with these patients who have difficulty with expression and communication. This proposal for action protocols would facilitate emergency situations (such as triage in the emergency department) for these patients with other people, despite their difficulty with expression and communication.

2. Materials and Methods

2.1. Population Study

We performed an observational and cross-sectional study of the medical records of the populations under comparison. This involved a preliminary search strategy from primary and secondary bibliographic sources. A total of 200 individuals were analyzed, 100 from each of the 2 populations.

A significance study was conducted using GPower software to estimate the sample size [32], then, two groups were established, i.e., control and AD, each consisting of 100 subjects, which provided a confidence level of 90%, on the basis of a total population with AD estimated in 7000 individuals, in the León region of Spain [33]. The Alzheimer's Center León register contains 370 patients, with a proportion of them diagnosed with dementias other than Alzheimer's (fluctuating percentage of about 20% diagnosed with other types of dementia, primarily frontotemporal dementia, Parkinson's, and Lewy body dementia).

Int. J. Environ. Res. Public Health **2020**, *17*, 3398

2.2. Literature Search

The bibliographic search connected with the present study included the PUBMED, WOS, and CUIDEN PLUS databases. A number of inclusion criteria were considered as follows:

- Publications from 2014 to 2019;
- Publications in English or Spanish;
- Data concerning the adult population aged ≥65 years diagnosed with AD;
- Both primary (original articles) and secondary (systematic reviews) sources;
- Full texts accessible through the University of León Library;
- Keywords employed (combined with Boolean operators AND and OR), in English included Alzheimer's disease, comorbidity, elderly, and aged and, in Spanish, "Enfermedad de Alzheimer", "comorbilidad", "adulto mayor", and "anciano".

2.3. Data Collection

The current study was complied with the rules of the Helsinki Declaration of 1975. It was approved by the Ethics Committee of León University Hospital according to Resolution #1929 of 26 February 2019.

The criteria for inclusion in the AD study group were:

- Alzheimer's disease diagnosis (this diagnosis has been previously identified by the Psychiatric Service of the León University Hospital);
- Age ≥65 years;
- Residency in the city of León, Spain;

The selection of subjects meeting these criteria was random.
The criteria for inclusion in the control group were:

- Not diagnosed with AD;
- Age ≥65 years;
- Residency in the city of León, Spain.

2.3.1. Alzheimer's Disease (AD) Group

Data were obtained from the Alzheimer's Comprehensive Care Center of León of the León Alzheimer Center. Each subject was identified by a code number to protect anonymity and confidentiality. This procedure was approved by the León Alzheimer Center and supported by signed agreements. Medical records were reviewed at random, reached the maximum number of individuals possible from the total number of people registered at the center, and met the inclusion criteria.

2.3.2. Control Group

Data corresponding to the undiagnosed population were collected from the León University Hospital.

Subjects who were undiagnosed in the general population with Alzheimer's disease, were randomly selected among those attending the Emergency Department of León University Hospital, for a few days, using the Gacela® computer program (León University Hospital, León, Spain), considering the following characteristics: age, sex, reason for admission, and medical history number. We used the Jimena® software (León University Hospital, León, Spain) to review and collect data, which included the pathologies suffered and the list of drugs taken by each individual. Each subject was identified by a code number to protect anonymity and confidentiality. This procedure was approved by the León Alzheimer Center and supported by signed agreements.

2.3.3. Data Processing

Data were stored and analyzed using an Office Excel® spreadsheet processor (2019 version) (University of León, Spain). The data analyzed for both groups included age, sex, comorbidities, and number of drugs taken. It is important to mention that diagnoses of comorbidities were uniformly identified by both primary care and continuing care physicians. They were entered into an SPSS version 24 computer statistical program (University of León, Spain), which was followed by analysis of the variables for each of the 2 populations to be compared with each other.

Additionally, action protocols to be used in the case of an emergency involving a patient with Alzheimer's disease were obtained.

2.4. Significance Studies

Data significance level was calculated with Pearson's Chi-square, and a value of $p \leq 0.1$ was considered to be satisfactory. As mentioned in Section 2.1., the 2 populations of 100 individual analyzed, in the present study, provided a confidence level of 90% and $p = 0.1$.

3. Results

3.1. Sociodemographics

3.1.1. Gender Distribution

The entire sample of 200 individuals comprising both the control and AD groups consisted of 61% women and 39% men. Figure 1 shows that the control group was composed of 47% males and 53% females; whereas the AD group consisted of 31% males and 69% females.

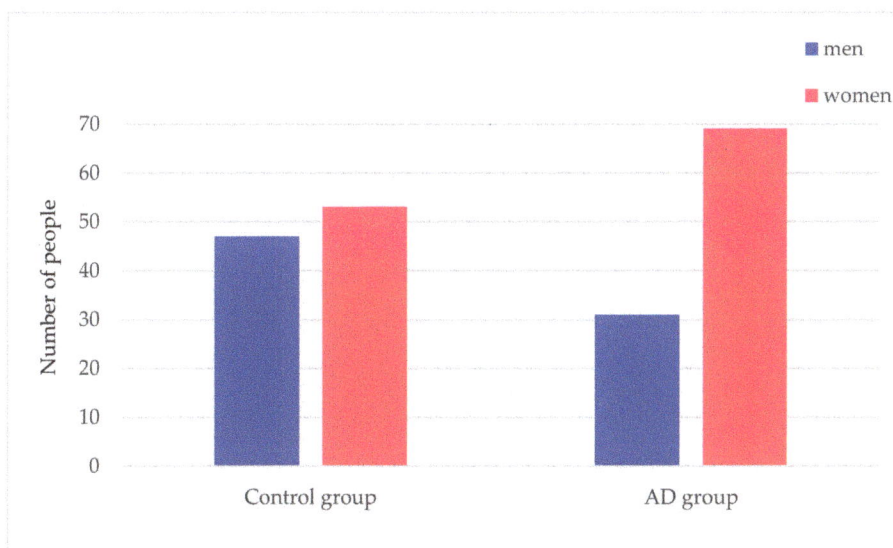

Figure 1. Alzheimer's disease and gender. This figure shows the number of men and women that make up both the control group and the Alzheimer's disease (AD) group.

3.1.2. Age Distribution

Figure 2 shows the comparative age analysis of the AD and control groups. This cohort study indicates that the number of subjects within the age interval 76–85 years is the largest in both groups. The age distribution of the AD and control groups clearly differs. The AD population shows an uneven pattern, with the >85 years group placed second after 76–85 years and a clearly smaller 66–75-year-old group. Instead, the distribution is rather symmetrical in the control population. In brief, the age interval in the AD group is shifted to older ages as compared with the control population.

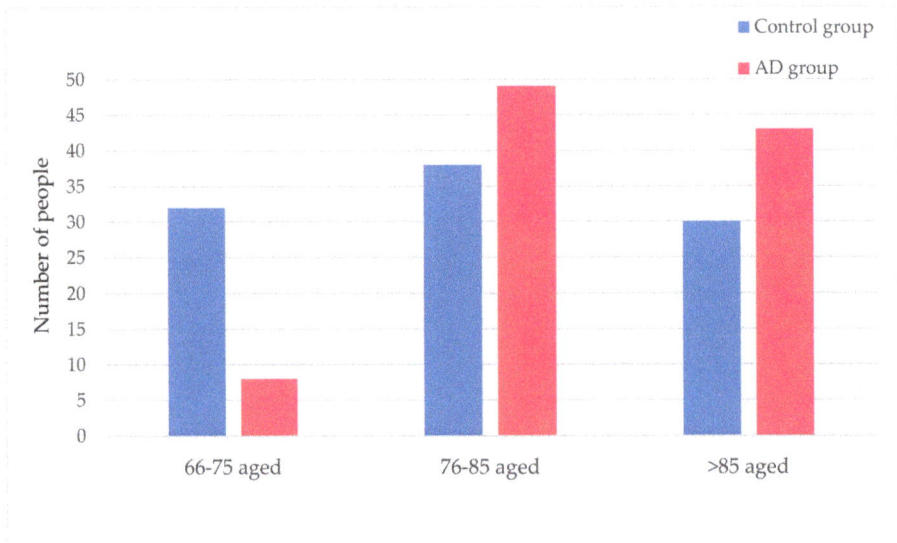

Figure 2. Age range distributions of the AD and controls. This figure shows the distribution of both the control group and the AD group, into three age range groups.

3.2. Pathologies

The comparison of the AD group with the control group and the analysis of the pathologies observed in the populations under study shows three clear age range groups according to their higher, similar, or lower incidence of pathologies.

3.2.1. Pathologies with a Higher Incidence in the AD Group

Table 1 shows the percentages of individuals with comorbidities more abundant in the AD group than in the controls. The pathologies in question are cataracts, urinary incontinence, vitamin D deficiency, osteoarthritis, hearing loss, osteoporosis, and personality disorders.

Table 1. Presence of comorbidities with higher incidence in the AD group.

	Control Group	AD Group
Medical condition	%	%
Cataract	12.0%	21.0%
Urinary incontinence	16.0%	38.0%
Vitamin D deficiency	5.0%	11.0%
Osteoarthritis	9.0%	26.0%
Hypoacusis	1.0%	13.0%
Osteoporosis	1.0%	20.0%
Personality disorders	1.0%	12.0%

The percentage of individuals not affected by these comorbidities are the remaining quantities up to 100, since in each group there are a total of 100 individuals.

Cataracts, urinary incontinence, and vitamin D deficiency affect 21%, 38%, and 11% of the individuals in the AD group, respectively, doubling the values observed in the control group, which are

12%, 16% and 5%, respectively. The difference is even more pronounced for osteoarthritis, which was present in 26% of the individuals in the AD group as compared with 9% in the control group. Strikingly, only 1% of individuals (one subject) was affected by hypoacusis, osteoporosis, or personality disorder in the control group, while the values were 13%, 20%, and 12% in the AD group, respectively.

In particular, emphasis is placed on the relationship between osteoporosis and gender.

Figure 3 shows the difference in prevalence of osteoporosis between men and women in the control and AD groups. As indicated in Table 1, 1% of women in the control group have osteoporosis while there are no cases of men. In the AD group, a total of 17% of women and 3% of men have osteoporosis.

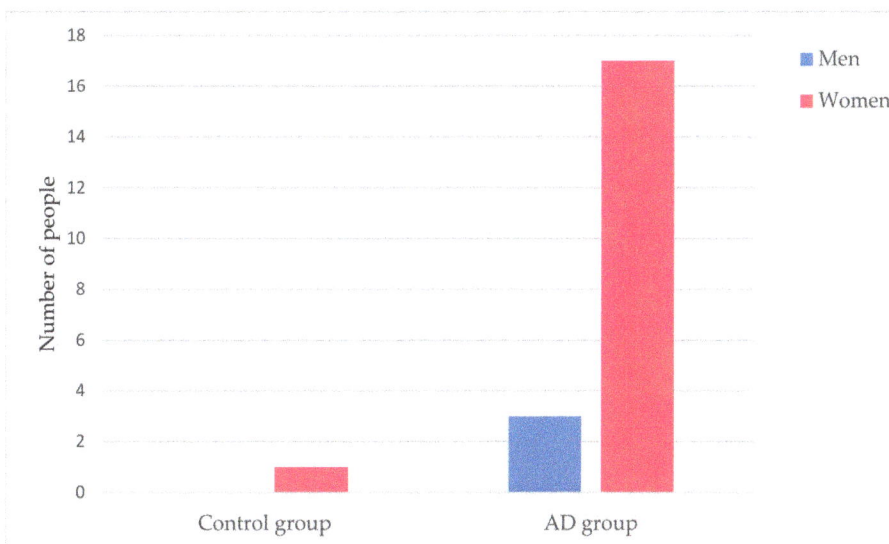

Figure 3. Osteoporosis' disease and gender. This figure shows the percentage of men and women who have osteoporosis, differentiated into the two groups under study.

Table 2 indicates the Pearson's Chi-square values and significance levels for the comorbidities shown in Table 1.

Table 2. Chi-square data and significance values for cataracts, urinary incontinence, vitamin D deficiency, osteoarthritis, hypoacusis, osteoporosis, and personality disorders.

Medical Condition	Chi-Square	df	Sig.
Cataracts	2.940	1	0.086 *
Urinary Incontinence	12.278	1	0.000 *
Vitamin D deficiency	2.446	1	0.118
Degenerative joint disease	10.009	1	0.002 *
Hearing loss	11.060	1	0.001 *
Osteoporosis	19.207	1	0.000 *
Personality disorders	9.955	1	0.002 *

* The Chi-square statistic is significant at the level 1.

The significance levels of cataracts, urinary incontinence, osteoarthritis, hypoacusis, osteoporosis, and personality disorders were 0.086, <0.00, 0.002, 0.001, <0.00, and 0.002, respectively. These values were lower than the p-value of 0.1. Instead, vitamin D deficiency showed a significance level value of 0.118, i.e., higher than the *p*-value. Therefore, we can say that the differences observed for the conditions listed on Table 2 are significant, except for vitamin D deficiency.

3.2.2. Pathologies with a Lower Incidence in the AD Group

Table 3 shows the percentages of individuals with comorbidities less abundant in the AD group as compared with the control group. The comorbidities which were analyzed included eye strain (increase in intraocular pressure), stroke, vertigo, hyperuricemia, circulatory insufficiency, atrial fibrillation, and respiratory insufficiency.

Table 3. Presence of comorbidities with lower incidence in the AD group.

	Control Group	AD Group
Medical condition	%	%
Eye strain	9.0%	2.0%
Ictus	5.0%	1.0%
Vertigo	11.0%	2.0%
Hyperuricemia	14.0%	9.0%
Circulatory insufficiency	34.0%	21.0%
Atrial fibrillation	11.0%	7.0%
Respiratory failure	25.0%	4.0%

The percentage of individuals not affected by these comorbidities are the remaining numbers up to 100, since in each group there is a total of 100 individuals.

The AD group shows 2%, 1%, and 2% of individuals affected by eye strain, stroke, and vertigo, respectively; whereas the values in the control group are higher, i.e., 5%, 11%, and 14%, respectively.

The percentages of control individuals affected by hyperuricemia (increased uric acid in the blood), circulatory failure, and atrial fibrillation are 14%, 34%, and 11%, respectively. In the AD group, those percentages are 9%, 21%, and 7%, respectively; all of them lower than in the undiagnosed population. The percentage of individuals with respiratory failure is 25% in the control and 4% in the AD group, indicating an incidence five times higher in the control group.

Table 4 shows the Pearson's Chi-square values corresponding to the comorbidities listed on Table 3.

Table 4. Chi-square data and significance values for eye strain, stroke, vertigo, hyperuricemia, circulatory failure, atrial fibrillation, and respiratory failure.

Medical Condition	Chi-Square	df	Sig.
Eye strain	4.714	1	0.030 *
Ictus	2.749	1	0.097 *b
Vertigo	6.664	1	0.010 *
Hyperuricemia	1.228	1	0.268
Circulatory insufficiency	4.238	1	0.040 *
Atrial fibrillation	0.977	1	0.323
Respiratory failure	17.786	1	0.000 *

* The Chi-square statistic is significant at the level 10. [b] More than 20% of the cells in this subtable had predicted cell counts less than 5. The Chi-square results may not be valid.

The significance levels of the comorbidities eye strain, stroke, dizziness, circulatory insufficiency, and respiratory insufficiency are all below the *p*-value of 0.10. In contrast, the comorbidities hyperuricemia and atrial fibrillation have a significance level of 0.268 and 0.323, respectively, i.e., higher than the *p*-value of 0.10. Thus, we can say that the differences observed for the conditions listed on Table 4 are significant except for hyperuricemia and atrial fibrillation.

3.2.3. Pathologies with a Similar Incidence in both Populations

Table 5 shows the comorbidities that do not show significant differences based on a comparison of the control and AD populations.

Table 5. Presence of comorbidities that do not show significant differences in both groups.

	Control Group	AD Group
Medical condition	%	%
Type 2 diabetes mellitus	20.0%	19.0%
Glaucoma	6.0%	6.0%
Depression	26.0%	27.0%
Obesity	7.0%	7.0%
Arthritis	9.0%	8.0%
High blood pressure	64.0%	51.0%
Dyslipidemia	39.0%	45.0%
Anxiety	12.0%	14.0%
Heart disease	26.0%	31.0%

The percentage of individuals not affected by these comorbidities are the remaining numbers up to 100, since in each group there is a total of 100 individuals.

The proportions of individuals affected by type 2 diabetes mellitus, glaucoma, depression, obesity, arthritis, anxiety, and heart disease in the AD group are 19%, 6%, 27%, 7%, 8%, 14%, and 31%, respectively. In the control group, these values are 20%, 6%, 26%, 7%, 9%, 12%, and 26%, respectively. The figures show a similar incidence of these comorbidities in both the AD and control groups. The comorbidities arterial hypertension and dyslipidemia present a relatively high incidence in both the control and AD groups; with values, in the AD group, of 51% and 45%, respectively and, in the control group, the corresponding percentages are 64% and 39%, respectively.

Table 6 shows the significance levels of the comorbidities type 2 diabetes mellitus, glaucoma, depression, obesity, arthritis, dyslipidemia, anxiety, and heart disease are all well above the *p*-value of 0.10. Instead, hypertension shows a significance level of 0.063, which is lower than the *p*-value of 0.10. Thus, we can say that only the differences observed for hypertension are significant.

Table 6. Chi-square data and significance values for type 2 diabetes mellitus, glaucoma, depression, obesity, arthritis, hypertension, dyslipidemia, anxiety, and heart disease.

Medical Condition	Chi-Square	df	Sig.
Type 2 diabetes mellitus	0.032	1	0.858
Glaucoma	0.000	1	1.000
Depression	0.026	1	0.873
Obesity	0.000	1	1.000
Arthritis	0.064	1	0.800
High blood pressure	3.458	1	0.063*
Dyslipidemia	0.739	1	0.390
Anxiety	0.177	1	0.674
Heart disease	0.613	1	0.434

* The Chi-square statistic is significant at the level, 10.

3.3. Medication

The number of medications taken by individuals from both study populations shows an average number of seven for each group, with the most abundant range being 6–10 medications.

Figure 4 shows that individuals in the control group took a larger number of drugs as compared with the AD group, with no one in the AD group taking >15 drugs. Nonetheless, the average number of drugs taken by each individual is the same (*n* = 7) in both groups.

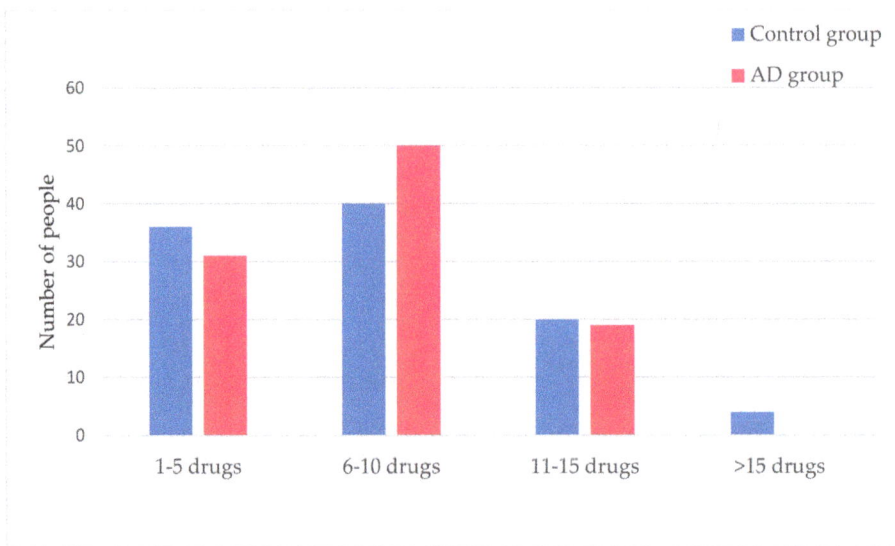

Figure 4. Number of medicines prescribed in the control and AD populations. This figure shows the amount of medication taken by subjects belonging to both the control and AD groups.

4. Operating Procedures in the Case of Emergencies

This section outlines the analyses of possible courses of action in the case of emergencies involving AD patients. We re-examined the standard operating procedures employed in the two centers from which the data presented here were collected, namely the Alzheimer's Comprehensive Care Center and the León University Hospital (León, Spain) (Table 7).

Table 7. Comparative table of the action protocols of León University Hospital and Alzheimer's Comprehensive Care Center of León.

	Comprehensive Care Center of León	León University Hospital
Target	Prevention and response in case of falls in patients with Alzheimer's disease	Activities to be performed by the nursing staff according to the different nursing diagnosis lists of the NANDA that the individual with Alzheimer's disease has
Coincidences	-Use of specific support measures for wandering, i.e., walking sticks or support rails -Specific protocol for physical restraint, if necessary, under medical order (with information to relatives) -Specific nursing care monitoring skin integrity or reassessment of the need for restraints -Increase environmental safety by avoiding slippery floors and architectural barriers, placing objects more easily accessible, positioning beds at a lower height and with handrails to prevent falls	
The differences	-Directed to all employees	-Directed only to the nursing staff
Key points	-The use of the J.H. Downton scale -It assesses the presence of certain intrinsic factors (age, drugs, or associated comorbidities) and extrinsic factors (of an environmental nature as inappropriate soil or equipment in each case) -There is an action protocol in case of falls -1st aid + 2nd reassures and secures the rest -Evaluate general condition and emergency equipment needs, report on the fall (questionnaire)	-Individualized protocol for the nursing staff
Lacks	-Lack of personalized care by the employees because there is a single protocol for all	-The J.H. Downton scale is not used -It does not take into account both intrinsic and extrinsic factors -There is no protocol for intervention in the event of a fall -Lack of protocols for the rest of the professional staff members working in the hospital

This table compares different points between the Protocol of the Alzheimer's Center León and the Protocol of the University Hospital of León

The protocol for the Alzheimer's Comprehensive Care Center regarding patients with Alzheimer's disease is focused on the prevention of falls and an action plan should a fall occur; whereas the protocol for the León University Hospital refers to the activities the nursing staff should perform according to the different nursing diagnosis lists of the NANDA (North American Nursing Diagnosis Association), for individuals with AD. The main difference between these two action protocols is that while that for the León University Hospital is exclusively directed to the nursing staff, the Alzheimer's Comprehensive Care Center's protocol is aimed at all its workers. Each of these approaches has different characteristics. A protocol of action, exclusively in the hands of the nursing staff, is based on their qualifications and competence to handle AD patients, and is standardized and excludes individual initiatives, thus, eliminating additional variables. An action plan aimed at all the workers dealing with AD patients has to be centered on the needs of such patients and must contemplate the fact that less qualified workers should seek professional advice whenever in doubt or when faced with unexpected events.

Fall prevention can require the physical restraint of AD patients, which must only be performed by medical order. In this respect, both centers have a specific protocol. When restraint requires the use of straps, the patient's skin integrity is first assessed. Importantly, the subjects in question and their relatives must be informed. Furthermore, the Alzheimer's Comprehensive Care Center's protocol contains a scale of evaluation of fall risks according to the J.H. Downton scale [34]. This evaluation has been applied to all the individuals in this center, who are professionally supervised depending on their individual risks. The reliability of the risk scale must be regularly reassessed. The León University Hospital's protocol does not use any scale to assess the risk of falls and simply considers the nature of the mental state alteration of each AD patient, for example, dementia, delirium, etc.

The Alzheimer Comprehensive Care Center also considers some intrinsic and extrinsic factors that affect fall risks. Classical intrinsic factors are age, medicines taken or associated comorbidities; while extrinsic factors are of an environmental nature, for example, inappropriate floor surfaces, lack of appropriate equipment, among others.

Procedures in the Event of a Fall

Intervention in the case of a fall is protocolized in the Alzheimer Comprehensive Care Center but not in the León University Hospital.

The first step of the intervention is to help the person who fell, as well as reassure other individuals in the vicinity who witnessed the event. The latter is essential since AD patients are particularly sensitive to traumatic situations even if not personally involved, and their behavior can be altered. The second step is a professionally conducted evaluation of the fallen patient's condition, with the help of an emergency team if necessary. It is extremely important to examine in detail why the fall occurred, in order to detect its possible causes, and therefore prevent other falls. It is equally important to consider the associated comorbidities of the patient, which may impinge on the action protocol to be used.

5. Discussion

The purpose of this work was to study the prevalence of comorbidities in an AD population as compared with a control population. First, we confirmed that the probability of developing AD is associated with an older population and is more frequent in females, in agreement with previous studies [26]. Presently, there is a debate as to whether AD is more prevalent among women due to genetic reasons or as a result of their longer life expectancy, which would make them more susceptible during later years.

Østergaard et al. (2015) [19] and Gallego and Guerrero (2017) [21] proposed that certain cardiovascular factors could facilitate the appearance of Alzheimer's disease. Among them, they mentioned high blood pressure, type 2 diabetes mellitus, heart disease, dyslipidemia, and obesity. This view was shared by Dugger et al. [25]. Our results do not fully support these suggestions. In fact, we detected a lower incidence of arterial hypertension in the AD group as compared with the control group, which was significant (Tables 5 and 6). No differences were observed between the AD group and the control group regarding the incidence of type 2 diabetes mellitus and obesity (Table 5). On the contrary, the incidence values for dyslipidemia and cardiopathy, although non-significant ($p \geq 0.1$), indicate a higher prevalence in the AD group.

In our study, the incidence of glaucoma, depression, anxiety, and arthritis was similar, though not significant, in both the AD and control populations. Xu et al. [35] claimed, in 2019, that the correlation between glaucoma and Alzheimer's disease was due to an enhanced susceptibility of AD patients to glaucoma. Depression and anxiety were described as AD predisposing factors by Ehrenberg et al., in 2019 [36]. Kao et al. [37] proposed that the correlation between arthritis and AD was actually an inverse relationship. According to our observations, there is a higher incidence of a history of stroke in the control group as compared with the AD group. The difference was significant and disagrees with previous studies by Nucera and Hachinski [27] and Hachinski [38], published in 2018, which showed that a previous history of stroke predisposed AD.

The comorbidities that we observed to be less prevalent in the AD group are ocular tension, vertigo, hyperuricemia, circulatory insufficiency, atrial fibrillation, and respiratory insufficiency. They are all significant except for hyperuricemia and atrial fibrillation. Lu et al. [39] reported, in 2017, a lack of a clear relationship between hyperuricemia and AD. No clear link between atrial fibrillation and AD was found by Ihara et al., in 2018 [40], while a positive correlation with AD was observed for vascular dementia.

The following comorbidities were found to be much more prevalent within the AD group as compared with the control group: cataracts, urinary incontinence, vitamin D deficiency, osteoarthritis, hearing loss, osteoporosis, and personality disorders. With the exception of vitamin D deficiency, their incidence values were all significant. In particular, in Figure 3 it is possible to see that there is a higher prevalence of osteoporosis in women than in men. This fact causes us to consider whether this comorbidity is associated with sex rather than a diagnosis of Alzheimer's disease. For this reason, it is necessary to go deeper into the relationship between osteoporosis and Alzheimer's disease and to see the factors that cause this comorbidity in patients with Alzheimer's. The vitamin D deficiency results, though not significant, agree with those of Annweiler et al. [41] and Chen et al. [42]. The latter also found, similar to our findings, that osteoporosis appears to be associated with Alzheimer's disease. Similarly, Lee et al. [43], Swords et al. [44], and Rouch et al. [45] reported the association of AD with urinary incontinence, hearing loss, and personality disorders. The fact that the AD group consists of more women (69%) than the control group (53%) may explain the higher incidence of osteoarthritis for the AD group [46]. Similarly, the fact that it is composed of an older population could also explain that this group of subjects has a greater number of associated comorbidities, not incidents in the same way as for the control group [46].

Altogether, our results show a satisfactory number of coincidences, as well as some discrepancies with those from other investigations. The discrepancies found could be due, among other possible aspects, to the difference between the sample size of our study with that of the other investigations or to the subjects chosen at random in one study or another.

6. Future Research

The observations reported, here, encourage further studies. First, an extension of the present research involving a greater number of patients and controls would be advisable. Secondly, longitudinal follow-up studies would allow the analysis of the existing and developing comorbidities of AD patients over long periods of time. As far as the Alzheimer's-free population is concerned, longitudinal studies would enable the detection of people that develop AD related to ageing. It would be possible to document whether the comorbidities they already suffered from were affected or not after the onset of AD, or whether the comorbidities were in any way related to the onset of AD itself. Such retrospective studies would obviously require a thorough analysis of medical records over long periods of time.

Int. J. Environ. Res. Public Health **2020**, *17*, 3398

Author Contributions: Conceptualization, M.T.-S., L.S.-V., M.B.-N., C.L.-P., and E.B.-D.; Formal analysis, M.T.-S., J.A.B.-A., and E.B.-D.; Investigation, M.T.-S., L.S.-V., M.B.-N., and C.L.-P.; Methodology, M.T.-S., L.S.-V, M.B.-N., J.A.B.-A., and C.L.-P.; Software, J.A.B.-A.; Supervision, E.B.-D.; Validation, M.T.-S. and L.S.-V.; Visualization, J.A.B.-A.; Writing—original draft, M.T.-S., L.S.-V., and E.B.-D.; Writing—review & editing, L.S.-V., J.A.B.-A., and E.B.-D. All authors have read and agreed to the published version of the manuscript.

Funding: This research received no external funding.

Acknowledgments: The authors would like to thank each of the people who participated in this project, all of them in a selfless way. Especially, Flor de Juan, Director, and Laura Fuentes, Neuropsychologist, both from the Alzheimer's Day Care Centre of León, for providing us access to the Centre and collecting data. To Beatriz Abad, nurse of the León University Hospital, who helped in the collection of data from the control group, and finally, to Rodolfo Garcia for the exhaustive review of the manuscript.

Conflicts of Interest: The authors declare no conflict of interest.

References

1. Custodio, N.; Montesinos, R. Enfermedad de Alzheimer Conociendo a la Enfermedad, que Llegó para Quedarse; 2015; p. 274. Available online: https://www.alzheimeruniversal.eu/wp-content/uploads/2015/09/libroenfermedaddealzheimer-150925020156-lva1-app7263.pdf (accessed on 23 April 2020).

2. Valenti, R.; Pantoni, L.; Markus, H.S. Treatment of vascular risk factors in patients with a diagnosis of Alzheimer's disease: A systematic review. *BMC Med.* **2014**, *12*, 160. [CrossRef] [PubMed]

3. Durazzo, T.C.; Mattsson-Carlgren, N.; Weiner, M.W.; Initiative, A.D.N. Smoking and increased Alzheimer's disease risk: A review of potential mechanisms. *Alzheimer's Dement.* **2014**, *10*, S122–S145. [CrossRef]

4. Alzheimer's Association; Chételat, G.; Villemagne, V.; Villain, N.; Jones, G.; Ellis, K.; Ames, D.; Martins, R.; Head, R.; Masters, C.; et al. Alzheimer's disease facts and figures. *Alzheimer's Dement.* **2011**, *7*, 208–244. [CrossRef]

5. Miranda, A.; Gómez-Gaete, C.; Mennickent, S. Dieta mediterránea y sus efectos benéficos en la prevención de la enfermedad de Alzheimer. *Revista Médica Chile* **2017**, *145*, 501–507. [CrossRef]

6. Cabrera-Pivaral, C.E.; Báez-Báez, M.G.L.; Rosa, A.D.J.C.-D.L. Mortalidad por enfermedad de Alzheimer en México de 1980 a 2014. *Gac. Med. Mex* **2018**, *154*, 550–554. [CrossRef] [PubMed]

7. Ashraf, G.M.; Tarasov, V.V.; Makhmutova, A.; Chubarev, V.N.; Avila-Rodriguez, M.; Bachurin, S.O.; Aliev, G. The Possibility of an Infectious Etiology of Alzheimer Disease. *Mol. Neurobiol.* **2018**, *56*, 4479–4491. [CrossRef]

8. Mancino, R.; Martucci, A.; Cesareo, M.; Giannini, C.; Corasaniti, M.T.; Bagetta, G.; Nucci, C. Glaucoma and Alzheimer Disease: One Age-Related Neurodegenerative Disease of the Brain. *Curr. Neuropharmacol.* **2018**, *16*, 971–977. [CrossRef]

9. Alzheimer's Association 2018 Alzheimer's disease facts and figures. *Alzheimer's Dement.* **2018**, *14*, 367–429. [CrossRef]

10. Garcez, M.L.; Falchetti, A.C.B.; Mina, F.; Budni, J. Alzheimer´s Disease associated with Psychiatric Comorbidities. *Anais Academia Brasileira Ciências* **2015**, *87*, 1461–1473. [CrossRef]

11. Haaksma, M.L.; Vilela, L.R.; Marengoni, A.; Calderón-Larrañaga, A.; Leoutsakos, J.-M.S.; Rikkert, M.G.M.O.; Melis, R.J.F. Comorbidity and progression of late onset Alzheimer's disease: A systematic review. *PLoS ONE* **2017**, *12*, e0177044. [CrossRef]

12. Butterfield, D.A.; Di Domenico, F.; Barone, E. Elevated risk of type 2 diabetes for development of Alzheimer disease: A key role for oxidative stress in brain. *Biochim. Biophys. Acta (BBA) Bioenerg.* **2014**, *1842*, 1693–1706. [CrossRef] [PubMed]

13. Richardson, J.; Roy, A.; Shalat, S.L.; Von Stein, R.T.; Hossain, M.M.; Buckley, B.; Gearing, M.; Levey, A.I.; German, D.C. Elevated serum pesticide levels and risk for Alzheimer disease. *JAMA Neurol.* **2014**, *71*, 284–290. [CrossRef] [PubMed]

14. Cervantes, C.M.; Mimenza, A.J.; Navarro, S.A.; Ávila, P.A.; Gutiérrez, L.G.; Arellano, S.J.; Avila-Funes, J.A. Factores asociados a la demencia mixta en comparación con demencia tipo Alzheimer en adultos mayores mexicanos. *Neurología* **2017**, *32*, 309–315. [CrossRef]

15. Monzani, F.; Pasqualetti, G.; Tognini, S.; Calsolaro, V.; Polini, A. Potential drug–drug interactions in Alzheimer patients with behavioral symptoms. *Clin. Interv. Aging* **2015**, *10*, 1457–1466. [CrossRef] [PubMed]

16. Yildiz, D.; Pekel, N.B.; Kiliç, A.K.; Tolgay, E.N.; Tufan, F. Malnutrition is associated with dementia severity and geriatric syndromes in patients with Alzheimer disease. *Turk. J. Med. Sci.* **2015**, *45*, 1078–1081. [CrossRef] [PubMed]

17. Podcasy, J.L.; Epperson, C.N. Considering sex and gender in Alzheimer disease and other dementias. *Dialog Clin. Neurosci.* **2016**, *18*, 437–446.

18. Borrell, F. Enfermedad de Alzheimer y Factores de Riesgo Ambientales|Armenteros Borrell|Revista Cubana de Enfermería. Available online: http://www.revenfermeria.sld.cu/index.php/enf/article/view/1024/239 (accessed on 21 April 2020).

19. Oosterveld, S.M.; Kessels, R.P.; Hamel, R.; Ramakers, I.H.G.B.; Aalten, P.; Verhey, F.R.J.; Sistermans, N.; Smits, L.L.; Pijnenburg, Y.A.; Van Der Flier, W.M.; et al. The Influence of Co-Morbidity and Frailty on the Clinical Manifestation of Patients with Alzheimer's Disease. *J. Alzheimer's Dis.* **2014**, *42*, 501–509. [CrossRef]

20. Marfany, A.; Sierra, C.; Camafort, M.; Domenech, M.; Coca, A. High blood pressure, Alzheimer disease and antihypertensive treatment. *Panminerva Med.* **2018**, *60*, 8–16.

21. Muñoz, C.G.; Navarro, N.G. Manejo de pacientes con enfermedad de Alzheimer: ¿cambio en el paradigma actual? *Revista Científica Sociedad Española Enfermería Neurológica* **2017**, *45*, 30–31. [CrossRef]

22. Kumar, A.; Sidhu, J.; Goyal, A.; Tsao, J.W. Alzheimer Disease–PubMed. Available online: https://pubmed.ncbi.nlm.nih.gov/29763097/ (accessed on 21 April 2020).

23. Attems, J.; Jellinger, K.A. The overlap between vascular disease and Alzheimer's disease–lessons from pathology. *BMC Med.* **2014**, *12*, 206. [CrossRef]

24. Culqui, D.R.; Linares, C.; Ortiz, C.; Carmona, R.; Diaz, J. Association between environmental factors and emergency hospital admissions due to Alzheimer's disease in Madrid. *Sci. Total. Environ.* **2017**, *592*, 451–457. [CrossRef] [PubMed]

25. Dugger, B.N.; Malek-Ahmadi, M.H.; Monsell, S.E.; Kukull, W.A.; Woodruff, B.K.; Reiman, E.M.; Beach, T.G.; Wilson, J. A Cross-Sectional Analysis of Late-Life Cardiovascular Factors and Their Relation to Clinically Defined Neurodegenerative Diseases. *Alzheimer Dis. Assoc. Disord.* **2016**, *30*, 223–229. [CrossRef] [PubMed]

26. Andrew, M.K.; Tierney, M.C. The puzzle of sex, gender and Alzheimer's disease: Why are women more often affected than men? *Women's Health* **2018**, *14*, 174550651881799. [CrossRef]

27. Nucera, A.; Hachinski, V. Cerebrovascular and Alzheimer disease: Fellow travelers or partners in crime? *J. Neurochem.* **2018**, *144*, 513–516. [CrossRef] [PubMed]

28. Ringman, J.M.; Sachs, M.C.; Zhou, Y.; Monsell, S.E.; Saver, J.L.; Vinters, H.V. Clinical predictors of severe cerebral amyloid angiopathy and influence of APOE genotype in persons with pathologically verified Alzheimer disease. *JAMA Neurol.* **2014**, *71*, 878–883. [CrossRef] [PubMed]

29. Campdelacreu, J. Enfermedad de Parkinson y enfermedad de Alzheimer: Factores de riesgo ambientales. *Neurología* **2014**, *29*, 541–549. [CrossRef]

30. Domínguez, R.; Pagano, M.; Marschoff, E.; González, S.; Repetto, M.; Serra, J. Enfermedad de Alzheimer y deterioro cognitivo asociado a la diabetes mellitus de tipo 2: Relaciones e hipótesis. *Neurología* **2014**, *29*, 567–572. [CrossRef]

31. Jefferson, A.L.; Beiser, A.; Himali, J.J.; Seshadri, S.; O'Donnell, C.J.; Manning, W.J.; Wolf, P.A.; Au, R.; Benjamin, E.J. Low cardiac index is associated with incident dementia and Alzheimer disease: The Framingham Heart Study. *Circulation* **2015**, *131*, 1333–1339. [CrossRef]

32. Cunningham, J.B.; McCrum-Gardner, E. Power, effect and sample size using GPower: Practical issues for researchers and members of research ethics committees Joseph. *Evid. Based Midwifery* **2007**, *5*, 132.

33. Alzheimer León Alza su Voz el 21 de Septiembre|Leonoticias. Available online: https://www.leonoticias.com/leon/alzheimer-leon-alza-20180915185052-nt.html (accessed on 21 April 2020).

34. Escala de Downton—Enfermería Creativa. Available online: https://enfermeriacreativa.com/2019/07/08/escala-de-downton/ (accessed on 22 April 2020).

35. Xu, X.; Zou, J.; Geng, W.; Wang, A. Association between glaucoma and the risk of Alzheimer's disease: A systematic review of observational studies. *Acta Ophthalmol.* **2019**, *97*, 665–671. [CrossRef]

36. Ehrenberg, A.J.; Suemoto, C.K.; Resende, E.D.P.F.; Petersen, C.; Leite, R.E.P.; Rodriguez, R.D.; Ferretti-Rebustini, R.E.D.L.; You, M.; Oh, J.; Nitrini, R.; et al. Neuropathologic Correlates of Psychiatric Symptoms in Alzheimer's Disease. *J. Alzheimer's Dis.* **2018**, *66*, 115–126. [CrossRef] [PubMed]

37. Kao, L.; Kang, J.-H.; Lin, H.-C.; Huang, C.-C.; Lee, H.-C.; Chung, S.-D. Rheumatoid Arthritis Was Negatively Associated with Alzheimer's Disease: A Population-Based Case-Control Study. *PLoS ONE* **2016**, *11*, e0168106. [CrossRef] [PubMed]

38. Hachinski, V. The convergence of stroke and dementia TT—A convergência do acidente vascular cerebral e da demência. *Arq. Neuropsiquiatr.* **2018**, *76*, 849–852. [CrossRef] [PubMed]

39. Lu, N.; Dubreuil, M.; Zhang, Y.; Neogi, T.; Rai, S.K.; Ascherio, A.; Hernan, M.; Choi, H.K. Gout and the risk of Alzheimer's disease: A population-based, BMI-matched cohort study. *Ann. Rheum. Dis.* **2015**, *75*, 547–551. [CrossRef] [PubMed]

40. Ihara, M.; Washida, K. Linking Atrial Fibrillation with Alzheimer's Disease: Epidemiological, Pathological, and Mechanistic Evidence. *J. Alzheimer's Dis.* **2018**, *62*, 61–72. [CrossRef]

41. Annweiler, C.; Dursun, E.; Féron, F.; Gezen-Ak, D.; Kalueff, A.V.; Littlejohns, T.; Llewellyn, D.J.; Millet, P.; Scott, T.; Tucker, K.L.; et al. 'Vitamin D and cognition in older adults': Updated international recommendations. *J. Intern. Med.* **2014**, *277*, 45–57. [CrossRef]

42. Lo, R.Y.; Chen, Y.-H. Alzheimer's disease and osteoporosis. *Tzu Chi Med. J.* **2017**, *29*, 138–142. [CrossRef]

43. Lee, H.-Y.; Li, C.-C.; Juan, Y.-S.; Chang, Y.-H.; Yeh, H.-C.; Tsai, C.-C.; Chueh, K.-S.; Wu, W.-J.; Yang, Y.-H. Urinary Incontinence in Alzheimer's Disease. *Am. J. Alzheimer's Dis. Other Dementiasr* **2016**, *32*, 51–55. [CrossRef]

44. Swords, G.; Nguyen, L.; Mudar, R.A.; Llano, D.A. Auditory system dysfunction in Alzheimer disease and its prodromal states: A review. *Ageing Res. Rev.* **2018**, *44*, 49–59. [CrossRef]

45. Rouch, I.; Dorey, J.-M.; Boublay, N.; Henaff, M.-A.; Dibie-Racoupeau, F.; Makaroff, Z.; Harston, S.; Benoit, M.; Barrellon, M.-O.; Fédérico, D.; et al. Personality, Alzheimer's disease and behavioural and cognitive symptoms of dementia: The PACO prospective cohort study protocol. *BMC Geriatr.* **2014**, *14*, 110. [CrossRef]

46. Verbrugge, L.M. Women, men, and osteoarthritis. *Arthritis Rheum.* **1995**, *8*, 212–220. [CrossRef] [PubMed]

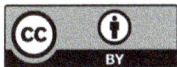

International Journal of
*Environmental Research
and Public Health*

MDPI

Article

Barriers and Facilitators Perceived by Spanish Experts Concerning Nursing Research: A Delphi Study

Alberto González-García [1], Ana Díez-Fernández [1,*], Noelia Martín-Espinosa [2],
Diana P. Pozuelo-Carrascosa [2], Rubén Mirón-González [3] and Montserrat Solera-Martínez [1]

[1] Centro de Estudios Sociosanitarios, Facultad de Enfermería de Cuenca, Universidad de Castilla-La Mancha, 16071 Cuenca, Spain; alberto.gonzalez@uclm.es (A.G.-G.); montserrat.solera@uclm.es (M.S.-M.)
[2] Grupo de Investigación Multidisciplinar en Cuidados (IMCU), Facultad de Fisioterapia y Enfermería de Toledo, Universidad de Castilla-La Mancha, 45071 Toledo, Spain; noelia.martin@uclm.es (N.M.-E.); DianaP.Pozuelo@uclm.es (D.P.P.-C.)
[3] Facultad de Medicina y Ciencias de la Salud, Universidad de Alcalá, Alcalá de Henares, 28805 Madrid, Spain; ruben.miron@uah.es
* Correspondence: ana.diez@uclm.es; Tel.: +34-969-179-100 (ext. 4656); Fax: +34-969-179-178

Received: 6 April 2020; Accepted: 5 May 2020; Published: 6 May 2020

check for updates

Abstract: The identification of research priorities in line with current health needs and nursing competencies is a priority. Nevertheless, barriers and facilitators perceived by nurses to performing nursing research have scarcely been investigated. The main aim of this study was to explore the situation in nursing research in Spain, as perceived by Spanish experts. A Delphi study technique in two phases was applied using an online survey tool. A panel of 20 nursing experts in nursing, teaching and management positions participated. The strengths highlighted were the possibility of reaching the PhD level, the possibility of receiving continuous training in research methodology, and access to scientific knowledge through the Internet. The weaknesses identified were the lack of Spanish nursing journals in which to publish the research results, the lack of funding in nursing care research, and the lack of connection between the healthcare institutions and the university. According to the experts, elements that could enhance leadership in research are the creation of nursing research units in hospitals, the economic recognition of nurses with PhDs, and considering research work as part of their daily tasks in clinical settings. The idea of being subordinated to physicians still remains in nurses' ways of thinking.

Keywords: nurses; nursing research; Delphi method; consensus; Spain

1. Introduction

Over the past two decades, several factors have led to an increase in demand for qualified nursing care: changes in providing health care, economic cutbacks in healthcare organization, and technological developments. Bäck-Pettersson et al. [1] have suggested that nursing research should be geared towards the study of principles for effective and efficient nursing practice and factors affecting perceptions of health and well-being among individuals, families, communities and healthcare services.

The changes which nursing has undergone in Spain in the last two decades, both at an academic and professional level and as to the evolution of the health system, have drawn a favorable framework for the progressive incorporation of nursing professionals in the activities of scientific knowledge generation and communication [2]. Thus, the identification of research priorities in line with current health needs and nursing competencies is a priority in itself.

The Delphi method has been shown to be a widely used and flexible method that is particularly useful in achieving consensus in a given area of uncertainty or lack of empirical evidence [3]. It seeks to gain the most reliable consensus of a group of experts by answering a series of sequential questionnaires or "rounds" intermingled by controlled feedback [4,5]. The Delphi technique has been used in a wide variety of nursing research, such as for determining the priorities of nursing administration research [6] and for the delivery of health care to children [7–9]. With regards to the academic field, the quality of nursing doctoral education and strategic directions for improving quality have been pointed out [10], as well as the identification of characteristics and essential elements of lifelong learning [11,12].

To our knowledge, only one study has tried to identify the barriers and facilitators perceived by nurses to the use of nursing research [13], focused on the Chinese context. The main difficulties identified were lack of authority, lack of time, language difficulties, lack of financial resources and lack of legal protection. The elements in favor were an improvement in management support, the promotion of education to increase the knowledge base and the moderate increase in the time available for implementation. The health center, academic training, and knowledge of the theoretical basis of evidence-based nursing were the factors that influenced these barriers and facilitators' perceptions [13]. Nevertheless, interest in Spain has been focused on establishing research priorities in healthcare [14,15], but not in identifying the weaknesses, threats, strengths and opportunities to research in nursing. In both cases, a list of closed priorities that had been previously agreed upon in a working group was used, but professionals in the field of clinical practice were not included in the group of experts.

It has been recommended to periodically reevaluate the academic programs of the nursing teaching centers to ensure that their approach is adapted to the current challenges, thus improving productivity [16]. In a context in which research excellence is a priority [17], and taking into account that access to external funding sources for the development of research projects requires a high competitive level, it seems logical to examine the current situation to know if it is necessary to make changes. In this sense, the Delphi method itself can provide elements for planning future scenarios [18].

Nurses play a pivotal role in the delivery of effective health care [8]. Considering that nurses and midwives comprise almost 40% of the healthcare workforce, the care that they deliver has a significant impact upon patient outcomes [19]. However, concerns about whether nurses and midwives use the best available evidence to guide their clinical practice have been noticed [20,21]. A lack of research use by nurses and midwives has potentially damaging consequences, with up to 30–40% of patients not receiving appropriate care [22].

For this reason, the main aim of this study was to explore the situation in nursing research in Spain, as perceived by Spanish experts. Secondary aims were to create a consensus on barriers and facilitators to delimit the characteristics of nursing research in Spain at present, and, finally, to identify the difficulties that clinical-care nursing professionals encounter in carrying out this task.

2. Methods

2.1. The Delphi Method

This study was conducted using the Delphi method. This method of study was developed in the 1950s by the RAND Corporation for military use [23]. The Delphi approach is a structured process that utilizes a series of questionnaires or rounds to gather and to provide information without the need for face-to-face meetings. The process continues until group consensus is reached. It is growing in popularity, especially for nurse researchers and for health research in general. It provides a relatively rapid and efficient way to obtain agreement from a wide variety of key informants by presenting a series of questionnaires for ranking. Maintenance of participation levels at 50% to 80% is crucial in reaching the consensus [24].

Google forms™ was used as the vehicle for distribution of the questionnaires. Participants were provided the link to the questionnaires through email correspondence. The study had two rounds.

In addition to sociodemographic and educational characteristics of the panel members, which are regarded as crucial to enable assessment of their credibility, round one was used to generate ideas [25]. Participants were asked two open-ended questions, thus allowing panel members freedom in their responses. These questions were (a) "Comment and describe what are the main strengths, opportunities and elements in favor of nursing in order to carry out your research activity. In other words, what facilitates and/or would facilitate our research work?"; and (b) "Comment and describe what are the main weaknesses, threats and difficulties and elements against nursing in order to carry out your research activity. In other words, what obstructs or would hinder our research work?".

Two researchers read the responses from the open-ended questions in the round one independently, searching for relationships and patterns and classifying them into clusters of similar ideas. The most commonly occurring attributes and concepts were identified and grouped into similar ideas. To validate the concepts that occurred, the individual notes were compared, and a third researcher evaluated the areas that deferred. Two researchers developed then the concepts that most commonly occurred into statements that retained the panelists' collective conceptual meaning. Statements were finally classified into four categories, following the structure of a strengths, weaknesses, opportunities and threats (SWOT) matrix. The number of items generated was 80. After that, two different researchers classified every item into seven main categories created ad hoc: nursing environment, academic level achieved, health administration, support for research from health administration, PhD issues, academic background, and nursing profession.

In round two of the study, participants were asked to rate their agreement with a Likert scale with numerical values attached to the scale range: zero (0) indicated strongly disagree and ten (10) indicated strongly agree. Data were collected between November 2016 and March 2017.

2.2. Sample

Purposive sampling stratified by clusters was used for creating the panel of experts. An expert has been defined as one of a group of informed individuals and specialists in their field or someone who has knowledge about a specific subject [25]. Purposive sampling has been widely supported as an appropriate method of sample selection, especially in qualitative research [26]. The most important requisite of purposeful selection is the identification of experts in disciplines or domains directly and indirectly represented in the research instrument or topic under discussion. In addition to this, purposive sampling within maximum variation sampling is one way to obtain representativeness and rich data by including a wide range of extremes [27]. Maximum variation or heterogeneity sampling is described as a special kind of purposive sampling, which may be used to identify experts or cases (in qualitative research) to provide rich information [27]. This sampling method aims to identify themes or patterns that run through a range of variations.

Taking everything into account, the panel of experts consisted of four clusters: (1) nurses actively working at hospitals or primary health-care centers; (2) nurses working as a lecturer or full-time professor at the university; (3) nurses in a management position at a hospital (managing directors or directors of nursing); and (4) nurses in a management position at the university (dean, vice dean or head of the nursing department). These clusters include the professional fields of a nursing professional in Spain.

Regardless of the group to which they belonged, the research team considered it of great importance that the panelists show active research activity, given the topic of the proposed study. For this reason, active research activity was verified prior to its inclusion in the panel of experts in the form of a minimum of five papers indexed in Web of Science (WOS). There is little agreement about the size of the expert panel. Sample size and heterogeneity depends upon the purpose of the project, design selected and period for data collection. For the conventional Delphi, a heterogeneous sample is used to ensure that the entire spectrum of opinion is determined. Moreover, anonymity provides an equal chance for each panel member to present and react to ideas, unbiased by the identities of other participants. Reactions are given independently, so each opinion carries the same weight and is given equal importance in the analysis [25].

A reference group of twenty nurses representing all the clusters mentioned above was regarded as a convenient group of informed individuals and specialists with the requisite expert knowledge concerning nursing research, thus qualifying them as panel members. The principal investigator emailed them individually, explaining the characteristics of the study and proposing them to be part of the panel of experts. All of them responded positively to the invitation.

2.3. Validity

Content validity was enhanced in some respects. Firstly, open-ended questions from round one and statements from round two were pretested with a representative sample of nurses to ensure that the concepts included in the study were clear. Secondly, the purposive study sample was comprised of a panel of experts who actively participate in nursing profession [28], so that they are representative of the area of knowledge [29]. Thirdly, successive rounds of the questionnaire increase the validity. Finally, the validity of results will be ultimately affected by the response rates [25]. Nevertheless, the findings should be regarded as expert opinions rather than indisputable data, and the validity and credibility of the research depends on the accuracy of conducting and reporting in the study. It is also important to be aware that the results only represent one moment in time [3,24].

2.4. Ethical Considerations

The Ethics Committee of the "Virgen de la Luz" Hospital approved the protocol (registration number 2016/PI0116). Each participant was assigned a code to protect his or her data and affiliation. Informed written consent was required by email. Information was provided on the purpose, risks, benefits and social implications of participation. The right to refuse participation, to decline to answer questions posed or to withdraw at any stage of the process without any penalty or consequence was assured prior to eliciting participation. The ethical principles of the Declaration of Helsinki and the Oviedo Convention of Human Rights and Biomedicine were followed.

2.5. Analysis and Consensus

Rated round two responses were recoded into three levels of agreement: 0–4 (low consensus), 5–7 (medium consensus), and 8–10 (high consensus). Only statements classified as high consensus were analyzed. The percentage of high consensus, mean values and standard deviations were calculated. The high consensus statements, with a percentage of $\geq 65\%$, a mean value of > 8.0 points and a standard deviation of < 2.5 were finally considered as the final conclusion of the Delphi method. Data analysis was performed using the computer package IBM SPSS Statistics version 24 (SPSS, Inc., Chicago, IL, USA).

3. Results

As mentioned above, twenty introductory letters were sent (five from each cluster). Of these, eighteen respondents fully completed both rounds (90%). Demographic and educational characteristics of the panel members who responded to all rounds are presented in Table 1. Ten were female and their ages ranged from 33 to 61 years old (mean = 46.61, SD = 9.84). Experts came from every area of expertise equally: registered nurses ($n = 2$), management nurse positions ($n = 2$), lecturers or professors at the university ($n = 2$) and lecturers or professors in management positions ($n = 2$). Almost all of the participants had reached the PhD level (75%).

Table 1. Characteristics of the study sample (panelists).

Characteristics	Male (*n* = 8)	Female (*n* = 10)	*p* Value
Age (mean ± SD)	41.63 ± 7.58	50.60 ± 9.92	0.051
Degree, n (%)			
Registered nurse (prior to university level)	0 (0.0 %)	1 (100.0 %)	
Registered nurse (prior to EHEA)	6 (45.5 %)	7 (54.5 %)	
Registered nurse (EHEA, bachelor's degree)	2 (50.0 %)	2 (50.0 %)	0.830
Total	8 (44.4 %)	10 (55.6 %)	
Academic level,n (%)			
Bachelor's degree (RN)	1 (100.0 %)	0 (0.0 %)	
Master's degree (MSc)	1 (50.0 %)	1 (50.0 %)	
Doctoral level (PhD)	6 (40.0 %)	9 (60.0 %)	0.498
Total	8 (44.4 %)	10 (55.6 %)	
Work place, n (%)			
Registered nurse	2 (50.0 %)	2 (50.0 %)	
Management nurse position	2 (50.0 %)	2 (50.0 %)	
Lecturer/Professor at the University	2 (50.0 %)	2 (50.0 %)	0.930
Lecturer/Professor at the University, management position	2 (33.3 %)	4 (66.7 %)	
Total	8 (44.4 %)	10 (55.6 %)	

Abbreviations: SD = standard deviation; EHEA = European higher education area; RN = registered nurse; MSc = Master of Science; PhD = doctorate.

High-consensus statements that reached the inclusion criteria are presented in Table 2 following a double classification: on one hand, the structure of a SWOT matrix; on the other hand, the main categories created ad hoc and the items. The items comprise a broad spectrum of nursing research topics, from the nursing environment and profession to support from healthcare providers necessary to develop research in nursing.

The strengths highlighted by the experts revolve around three dimensions or categories: academic level achieved, health administration and support from health administration. The most important ideas were the possibility of reaching the PhD level, the possibility of receiving continuous training in research methodology, and access to scientific knowledge through the Internet. These strengths could be reinforced with the following opportunities: the privileged position of nursing to perform clinical research in all areas of health and care levels, the possibility of economic recognition with the PhD level, the creation of specific clinical research units in nursing in the health services, and giving visibility to nurses as researchers.

The weaknesses identified are related to nursing environment, support for research from health administration and the nursing profession: the lack of Spanish nursing journals in which to publish the research results, the lack of funding in nursing care research, and the lack of connection between healthcare institutions and the university. Threats are also related to health administration and the nursing profession. Firstly, "Care research is considered an extra task that must be performed outside the workday" (Participant 9983H). Secondly, the lack of a research mindset among nursing professionals is explained as "There is no culture of research within the profession" (Participant 9990Q). Thirdly, panelists also point out that "The colleagues themselves make it difficult for professionals with research concerns" (Participants 9990Q, 9989P, 9999Z, 9986L).

Finally, a threat related to the historical identification of nursing as a delegate and subordinate profession to physicians with little leadership capacity is detailed as follows: "Become aware that nursing has its own field of knowledge and that it is not subordinate to other sciences such as medicine" (Participant 9997X), "It is not recognized that the nurse can investigate, and being considered as a profession by organizations" (participant 9998Y), and "The persistence of a delegated, subordinate self-image, along with the low ambition of professionals" (9993T).

The rest of the statements that did not reach the minimum consensus required are included in the Supplementary Table S1, as they can help to provide a full picture of the nursing situation in Spain.

Int. J. Environ. Res. Public Health **2020**, *17*, 3224

Table 2. High-consensus statements after round two.

Strengths	Mean (SD)	% of Agreement
Academic level achieved		
To have achieved direct access to PhD programs	8.78 (1.11)	66.7
To reach academic positions with sufficient power to sustain and represent the voice of nursing	8.39 (1.75)	66.7
Health administration		
Training and permanent updating in research methodology	8.89 (1.41)	77.8
Support from health administration		
Access to scientific knowledge through the Internet	8.67 (1.97)	66.7
Opportunities		
Nursing environment		
There is a wide range of possibilities in clinical research	9.06 (1.06)	77.8
Nursing professionals play an important role in almost all areas and health care levels	8.56 (1.38)	66.7
Health administration		
Economic recognition of nurses with PhD level	8.67 (2.35)	77.8
To create nursing research units in hospitals supported by health management	8.78 (2.21)	72.2
Support from health administration		
Give visibility to nurses as researchers	8.78 (2.05)	77.8
Weaknesses		
Nursing environment		
There are few journals in the area of nursing in Spain, currently any Spanish nursing journal has JCR impact	8.67 (2.14)	66.7
Support for research from health administration		
Nursing care research funding is not a priority policy	8.72 (1.87)	77.8
Nursing profession		
Lack of connection between healthcare institutions and the university	8.61 (1.20)	66.7
Threats		
Health administration		
Care research is considered an extra task that must be performed outside the workday	8.83 (2.30)	83.3
Nursing profession		
There is no research mindset among nursing professionals, or lack of motivation	8.44 (1.91)	66.7
The colleagues themselves make it difficult for professionals with research interests	8.94 (1.11)	66.7
Persistence of nursing self-image as a delegate, subordinate profession with little leadership capacity	8.83 (0.85)	66.7

Abbreviations: SD = standard deviation; PhD = doctorate; JCR = journal citation reports.

4. Discussion

The aim of this study was to explore the situation of nursing research in Spain perceived by Spanish experts. To our knowledge, this study is the first to highlight the barriers and facilitators perceived by nurses concerning nursing research in the Spanish context. When it comes to reaching consensus, sharing knowledge, being able to make reflective statements without being personally confronted, and obtaining responses from colleagues in the panel are described as some of the advantages of the Delphi method. Previous studies have pointed out that the panel members affect each other and may change their point of view during the rounds [24]. Moreover, the number of rounds is variable, and when this number is increased, it becomes more difficult to achieve high participation levels [30]. Therefore, two rounds were performed in our study in order not to bias the panelists' opinions during the process.

When analyzing the international context, some common areas appeared as difficulties for nursing research: lack of time during the workday, language difficulties, and lack of financial resources [13]. Having access to almost all areas and health care levels offers a wide range of possibilities in nursing research, which was previously stated in other contexts [1]. Our study confirmed, as in the Swedish context, that an element in favor of nursing research has been the development of doctoral education programs within nursing science, which was made possible by the increase in the number of registered nurses that have the PhD degree. Certainly, nursing research has increased in both quantity and complexity, according to a recent scoping review that identified four global research priorities: nursing theory development, methodology of nursing research, expertise in advanced nursing and professional nursing practice [17].

While, in a study involving seven countries, it was noted as a concern that research in nursing science may be compromised due to the primary supervision of nursing doctoral students by non-nurse supervisors [10], in our context it does not appear as a threat with a sufficient degree of consensus, although this phenomenon does exist. Nevertheless, it has been recently pointed out that nursing as a discipline is rather young and the theoretical development of nursing knowledge is even more recent [17]. The main difficulty in this field is the lack of connection between the healthcare institutions and the university. Creating nursing research units in healthcare institutions and achieving economic recognition of nurses with the PhD level are considered imperative to increase nursing research.

Previous studies carried out in Spain indicated as main barriers the lack of time during the workday to implement new ideas, that nurses do not perceive as relevant the results of the research for its application in clinical practice and the lack of collaboration of physicians for the implementation of nursing research [31]. Even though they do not coincide exactly with the items that have been proposed in our study, conceptual similarities are found, so that our panelists point out that there is no research mindset among nursing professionals. The lack of collaboration with the medical group was also indicated in round two of our study, but it did not reach a sufficient degree of consensus to be included in the final items. Finally, while, in the first study in Spain, a lack of training in research methodology was pointed out as a weakness [14], our study shows that this difficulty seems to have been overcome because panelists identified it as a strength. In this regard, North American nurses in management positions have recently assured, on the one hand, that they are not prepared with the essential skills to succeed so that training and education are essential. On the other hand, they pointed out that most healthcare institutions have prioritized workflow and productivity over research, which does not favor nursing research [32]. These aspects have been stated in our study.

Our study shows that there is still a self-image as a delegate, subordinate profession with little leadership capacity. This situation is specific to the Spanish context, but it has also been confirmed in other contexts [13,28]. This situation is explained by the historical trajectory of the nursing profession in Spain, given that the profession was conceived as an auxiliary of physicians [33]. Until the transformation from polytechnics to university colleges since 1977, nursing did not become an autonomous profession [34]. Certain factors have previously been stated to enhance nurses' leadership skills: gaining experience in policy development, having role models and incorporating leadership skills in bachelors' curricula [28]. Our study shows that academic positions to represent nursing voices

Int. J. Environ. Res. Public Health **2020**, *17*, 3224

are considered a strength in our country, but nothing is mentioned about achieving management or health policy positions.

Limitations

Our study has several limitations that should be acknowledged. First, this method is not a replacement for rigorous scientific reviews of published reports or for original research. Second, the sample size was small, and this may be considered as a limitation in this study. Nonetheless, it has been stated that a sample of 20–50 experts is recommended for surveys of expert opinions [35]. This type of sampling is particularly useful if the target population from which experts may be drawn is not clearly defined, or if there is great variation in the domain or phenomenon to be studied [36]. In any case, the level of agreement must be set by the researcher prior to implementation; in our case, only high-level consensus and a percentage agreement of > 65% were analyzed. Third, not exploring disagreement or marginalizing dissenting voices may also generate artificial consensus [36]. Fourth, the existence of consensus from a Delphi process does not mean that the correct answer has been found [25], but that a collegiate response has been obtained among the main representatives of the area of knowledge [1], and this response represents an opinion in the instant object of the study; therefore, it may vary over time [24]. Fifth, the sample was selected on purpose, as per the researchers' knowledge of the contribution that the expert panelists could make to the study. This may have resulted in some relevant nurse leaders being excluded.

5. Conclusions

Our study allows us to conclude that the main strengths for nursing research in Spain highlighted by experts were the access and development of PhD programs, as well as the privileged position of nursing in all clinical settings. Elements that could enhance the achievement of leadership in research according to the experts were the creation of nursing research units in hospitals, the economic recognition of nurses with the PhD level, and considering research work as part of the daily tasks of the clinical nurse. Despite the elapsed time, the ideas of being subordinated to physicians and having little leadership capacity apparently remain in nurses' ways of thinking. Experts pointed out that it is necessary to work on the connection between the universities and the healthcare institutions, as well as on raising awareness among professionals in the clinical field about the need for teamwork to achieve leadership in care research. Given that the findings of a Delphi group represent expert opinion rather than indisputable fact, further inquiry to validate the findings and to develop an international panel of experts from different contexts may be important.

Supplementary Materials: The following are available online at http://www.mdpi.com/1660-4601/17/9/3224/s1, Table S1: Rest of the statements after round two (Low and medium-consensus statements).

Author Contributions: Conceptualization, A.G.-G. and A.D.-F.; Data curation, A.G.-G. and M.S.-M.; Formal analysis, A.G.-G., A.D.-F., N.M.-E. and R.M.-G.; Funding acquisition, A.G.-G.; Investigation, A.G.-G., A.D.-F. and M.S.-M.; Methodology, A.G.-G. and A.D.-F.; Project administration, M.S.-M.; Resources, N.M.-E., D.P.P.-C. and R.M.-G.; Software, M.S.-M.; Supervision, A.G.-G.; Validation, N.M.-E., D.P.P.-C. and R.M.-G.; Visualization, A.G.-G. and A.D.-F.; Writing—original draft, A.G.-G., A.D.-F., N.M.-E. and M.S.-M.; Writing—review & editing, A.G.-G., A.D.-F., N.M.-E., D.P.P.-C., R.M.-G. and M.S.-M.. All authors have read and agreed to the published version of the manuscript.

Funding: The Research group "Research in Health and Social Sciences" from the Universidad de Castilla-La Mancha (GI20153025) funded this research.

Acknowledgments: The authors express their gratitude to the panel members who voluntarily participated in the study.

Conflicts of Interest: The authors declare no conflict of interest.

References

1. Bäck-Pettersson, S.; Hermansson, E.; Sernert, N.; Björkelund, C. Research priorities in nursing—A delphi study among swedish nurses. *J. Clin. Nurs.* **2008**, *17*, 2221–2231. [CrossRef] [PubMed]
2. Camaño-Puig, R. The state of information science in Spain. *Rev. Lat. Am. Enferm.* **2002**, *10*, 214–220. [CrossRef] [PubMed]
3. Powell, C. The delphi technique: Myths and realities. *J. Adv. Nurs.* **2003**, *41*, 376–382. [CrossRef] [PubMed]
4. Dalkey, N.; Helmer, O. An experimental application of the delphi method to the use of experts. *Manag. Sci.* **1963**, *9*, 458–467. [CrossRef]
5. Reid, N. *Wards in Chancery*; Royal College of Nursing: London, UK, 1988.
6. Scott, E.; Murphy, L.; Warshawsky, N. Nursing administration research priorities: A national delphi study. *J. Nurs. Adm.* **2016**, *46*, 238–244. [CrossRef] [PubMed]
7. Brenner, M.; Hilliard, C.; Regan, G.; Coughlan, B.; Hayden, S.; Drennan, J.; Kelleher, D. Research priorities for children's nursing in Ireland: A delphi study. *J. Pediatr. Nurs.* **2014**, *29*, 301–308. [CrossRef]
8. Parlour, R.; Slater, P. Developing nursing and midwifery research priorities: A Health Service Executive (HSE) north west study. *Worldviews Evid.-Based Nurs.* **2014**, *11*, 200–208. [CrossRef]
9. Wielenga, J.M.; Tume, L.N.; Latour, J.M.; Van Den Hoogen, A. European neonatal intensive care nursing research priorities: An e-delphi study. *Arch. Dis. Child. Fetal Neonatal Ed.* **2015**, *100*, F66–F71. [CrossRef]
10. Kim, M.J.; Park, C.G.; Mckenna, H.; Ketefian, S.; Park, S.H.; Klopper, H.; Lee, H.; Kunaviktikul, W.; Gregg, M.F.; Daly, J.; et al. Quality of nursing doctoral education in seven countries: Survey of faculty and students/graduates. *J. Adv. Nurs.* **2015**, *71*, 1098–1109. [CrossRef]
11. Davis, L.; Taylor, H.; Reyes, H. Lifelong learning in nursing: A delphi study. *Nurse Educ. Today* **2014**, *34*, 441–445. [CrossRef]
12. Paul, S.A. Assessment of critical thinking: A delphi study. *Nurse Educ. Today* **2014**, *34*, 1357–1360. [CrossRef] [PubMed]
13. Wang, L.P.; Jiang, X.L.; Wang, L.; Wang, G.R.; Bai, Y.J. Barriers to and facilitators of research utilization: A survey of registered nurses in China. *PLoS ONE* **2013**, *8*, e81908. [CrossRef] [PubMed]
14. Moreno-Casbas, T.; Martín-Arribas, C.; Orts-Cortés, I.; Comet-Cortés, P. Identification of priorities for nursing research in Spain: A delphi study. *J. Adv. Nurs.* **2001**, *35*, 857–863. [CrossRef] [PubMed]
15. Comet-Cortés, P.; Escobar-Aguilar, G.; González-Gil, T.; de Ormijana-Sáenz Hernández, A.; Rich-Ruiz, M.; Vidal-Thomas, C.; Córcoles-Jiménez, P.; Izquierdo-Mora, D.; Silvestre-Busto, Y.C. Establecimiento de Prioridades de Investigación En Enfermería En España: Estudio Delphi. *Enferm. Clin.* **2010**, *20*, 88–96. [CrossRef]
16. Kulage, K.M.; Ardizzone, L.; Enlow, W.; Hickey, K.; Jeon, C.; Kearney, J.; Schnall, R.; Larson, E.L. Refocusing research priorities in schools of nursing. *J. Prof. Nurs.* **2013**, *29*, 191–196. [CrossRef]
17. Hopia, H.; Heikkilä, J. Nursing research priorities based on CINAHL database: A scoping review. *Nurs. Open* **2020**, *7*, 483–494. [CrossRef]
18. Rowe, G.; Wright, G. The delphi technique: Past, present, and future prospects—Introduction to the special issue. *Technol. Soc. Chang.* **2011**, *78*, 1487–1490. [CrossRef]
19. Estabrooks, C.A.; Winther, C.; Derksen, L. Mapping the field: A bibliometric analysis of the research utilisation literature in nursing. *Nurs. Res.* **2004**, *9*, 12–21. [CrossRef]
20. Hughes, R. *Patient Safety and Quality: An Evidence-Based Handbook for Nurses*; Agency for Healthcare Research and Quality: Rckville, MD, USA, 2008.
21. Veeramah, V. Utilization of research findings by graduate nurses and midwives. *J. Adv. Nurs.* **2004**, *47*, 183–191. [CrossRef]
22. Squires, J.; Estabrooks, C.A.; Gustavsson, P.; Wallin, L. Individual determinants of reseach utilization by nurses: A systematic review update. *Implement. Sci.* **2011**, *6*, 1. [CrossRef]
23. Dalkey, N. *The Delphi Method: An Experimental Study of Group Opinion*; RAND: Santa Monica, CA, USA, 1969.
24. McKenna, H.P. The delphi technique: A worthwhile research approach for nursing? *J. Adv. Nurs.* **1994**, *19*, 1221–1225. [CrossRef] [PubMed]
25. Keeney, S.; Hasson, F.; McKenna, H.P. A critical review of the delphi technique as a research methodology for nursing. *Int. J. Nurs. Stud.* **2001**, *38*, 195–200. [CrossRef]

26. Burns, N.; Grove, S. *Understanding Nursing Research, Builiding an Evidence-Based Practice*; Saunders Elsevier: St. Louis, MO, USA, 2007.

27. Patton, M. *Qualitative Research and Evaluation Methods*; Sage: Thousand Oaks, CA, USA, 2002.

28. Shariff, N. Factors that act as facilitators and barriers to nurse leaders' participation in health policy development. *BMC Nurs.* **2014**, *13*, 1–13. [CrossRef] [PubMed]

29. Goodman, C.M. The delphi technique: A critique. *J. Adv. Nurs.* **1987**, *12*, 729–734. [CrossRef] [PubMed]

30. Edwards, L.H. Research priorities in school nursing: A delphi process. *J. Sch. Nurs.* **2002**, *18*, 157–162. [CrossRef]

31. Moreno-Casbas, T.; Fuentelsaz-Gallego, C.; González-María, E.; Gil de Miguel, Á. Barreras Para La Utilización de La Investigación. Estudio Descriptivo En Profesionales de Enfermería de La Práctica Clínica y En Investigadores Activos. *Enferm. Clin.* **2010**, *20*, 153–164. [CrossRef]

32. Sun, C.; Prufeta, P. Using a delphi survey to develop clinical nursing research priorities among nursing management. *J. Nurs. Adm.* **2019**, *49*, 156–162. [CrossRef]

33. Siles González, J. *[History of Nursing]*; Difusión Avances de Enfermería: Madrid, Spain, 2011.

34. Warne, T.; Johansson, U.B.; Papastavrou, E.; Tichelaar, E.; Tomietto, M.; den Bossche, K. Van Moreno, M.F.V.; Saarikoski, M. An exploration of the clinical learning experience of nursing students in nine european countries. *Nurse Educ. Today* **2010**, *30*, 809–815. [CrossRef]

35. List, D. *Maximum Variation Sampling for Surveys and Consensus Groups*; Audience Dialogue: Adelaide, Australia, 2004.

36. Bruce, J.C.; Langley, G.C.; Tjale, A.A. The use of experts and their judgments in nursing research: An overview. *Curationis* **2008**, *31*, 57–61.

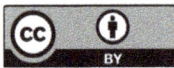

International Journal of
Environmental Research and Public Health

MDPI

Article

Nurse Manager Core Competencies: A Proposal in the Spanish Health System

Alberto González García [1], Arrate Pinto-Carral [2,*], Jesús Sanz Villorejo [3] and Pilar Marqués-Sánchez [4]

1   Department of Nursing and Physiotherapy, Universidad de León, 24401 Ponferrada, Spain; agong@unileon.es
2   SALBIS Research Group, Department of Nursing and Physiotherapy, Universidad de León, 24001 Ponferrada, Spain
3   Director of the University Dental Clinic, European University of Madrid, 28670 Madrid, Spain; jesus.sanz@universidadeuropea.es
4   SALBIS Research Group, Department of Nursing and Physiotherapy, Universidad de León, 24401 Ponferrada, Spain; pilar.marques@unileon.es
*   Correspondence: apinc@unileon.es

Received: 27 March 2020; Accepted: 30 April 2020; Published: 2 May 2020

check for updates

Abstract: Nurses who are capable of developing their competencies appropriately in the field of management are considered fundamental to the sustainability and improvement of health outcomes. These core competencies are the critical competencies to be developed in specific areas. There are different core competencies for nurse managers, but none in the Spanish health system. The objective of this research is to identify the core competencies needed for nurse managers in the Spanish health system. The research was carried out using the Delphi method to reach a consensus on the core competencies and a Principal Component Analysis (PCA) to determine construct validity, reducing the dimensionality of a dataset by finding the causes of variability in the set and organizing them by importance. A panel of 50 experts in management and healthcare engaged in a four-round Delphi study with Likert scored surveys. We identified eight core competencies from an initial list of 51: decision making, relationship management, communication skills, listening, Leadership, conflict management, ethical principles, collaboration and team management skills. PCA indicated the structural validity of the core competencies by saturation into three components (α Cronbach >0.613): communication, leadership and decision making. The research shows that eight competencies must be developed by the nursing managers in the Spanish health system. Nurse managers can use these core competencies as criteria to develop and plan their professional career. These core competencies can serve as a guideline for the design of nurse managers' development programs in Spain.

Keywords: nurse manager; competence; core competencies; governance; leadership

1. Introduction

Economic and social changes have led to an adaptation of healthcare management at all levels and a change in the way in which services are provided [1–6]. The relationship between the economy and sustainability should be causes that make it necessary to develop management competencies with a high level of development, because these competencies are related to higher performance and outcomes [7–10]. To address these changes, nurses need to be part of the core of healthcare [2,4,11,12]. This claim is justified because the nurse is a professional with a high degree of leadership in many healthcare processes [13], because of their closeness to patients, families and the community [14]. Multiple research programs are led by nurses, including oncology, mental health, patient safety, palliative care and childcare, among others, which shows the importance of the nurse in the healthcare system [15–19]. For this reason, the participation of the nurse in the governance of healthcare organizations is recognized as fundamental, both for health outcomes and the sustainability of the health system [20–23].

The American Institute of Medicine, in its report entitled "The future of nursing: leading change in health", already identified nursing in 2010 as a key player in critical decision making and in the transformation of healthcare [24]. In the same way, Weber et al. [25] and McClaringan et al. [20] express themselves by stating that nursing is fundamental to the implementation of shared governance, because their commitment and participation is essential for the sustainability and improvement of health. Panayotou et al. [26] emphasizes nursing within strategic plans, so that their key actions are focused on the creation of a culture of good practice. Brooks-Cleator et al. [27], in his studies on transculturality and governance, focus on the importance of the nurse in establishing a culture of safety. The involvement of nurses in social action committees has achieved a great impact on the everyday problems of people [28], highlighting the importance of their participation in decision making [29]. When the nurse is involved in the different parts of the healthcare process (management and nursing care), better results are achieved [30], communication is enhanced, together with collaboration between the different professional groups, innovation, organizational commitment and retention of staff [23].

Nurse leaders and nurse manager are different roles, although there is a natural overlap of the required competencies [1,10,31]. To develop the role of the nurse in the governance of healthcare organizations, the Global Nursing Leadership Institute (GNLI) in the actions of Nursing Now (2020) has developed a nurse preparation program designed to promote leaders for change, focused on new policies to improve the health of the population [18,32]. Thus, to identify, mentor and train nurse leaders, the management competencies are an essential resource [31]. Furthermore, for the integration of nurses at different levels of organizational management and governance, the nurse should develop management competencies that go beyond the scope of nursing [33–35].

The nurse manager is responsible for planning and managing resources, organizing nursing care, supporting teamwork, evaluating the services provided, and contributing to the achievement of optimal results for the both the organization and the patients [36,37]. Based on the literature review, it is necessary to increase the knowledge of the role of the nurse manager [36,38–41], because the necessary competencies are often not clearly defined [35,42], which would explain this lack of conceptualization of the nurse manager's role. This same absence is evident in the Spanish context since there are no core competencies for carrying out management functions.

Core competencies are the collective learning of the organization, especially with regard to skills related to the generation of a product or service, so that all necessary knowledge and technologies are integrated [43,44]. The core competencies in nursing management are associated with the success of the healthcare organization [45]. Therefore, the core competencies for nurse managers are the set of fundamental competencies needed to ensure their work effectiveness [46]. There are three functional roles within nursing management, the operational nurse manager (performs his or her function at unit level), the logistic nurse manager (performs his or her function at the department level), and the top nurse manager (performs his or her function at the organizational level); all of them should develop the core competencies to help improve the quality of healthcare. [46].

Hence, the main objective of this study is to propose the core competencies to be developed by the nurse manager in the Spanish health system. To achieve this objective, the following specific objectives were set:

- To determine core competencies for each functional level of nursing management by expert consensus;
- To describe the level of development of competencies for each functional level of nursing management by expert consensus;
- To describe the training needed to develop each of the required competencies by expert consensus;
- To evaluate the structural validity of the proposed core competencies.

This paper is laid out as follows: first, the current state of knowledge about the nurse manager is described. The second part explains the research methods. Next, the results are presented and interpreted. Finally, the paper includes a discussion and conclusion.

2. Materials and Methods

2.1. Review Literature

Based on a scoping literature review during 2018-19 to identify existing competencies related to nurse managers, electronic databases were used (Web of Science, Scopus, PubMed and CINAHL) to conduct the search, identifying 56 competencies for nurse managers. Relevant studies were identified, such as that carried out by the American Organization of Nurse Executives (AONE) who established two competency models for nurse managers [47]. In addition, the literature review identified other important research to define competencies—for example, the Chase instrument [48] or the research carried out by Kantanen [42], DeOnna [35] or Pillay [49], among others. The results of this review are the foundation for the execution of the current Delphi study, which assesses the competencies for nurse manager positions.

2.2. Delphi Methodology

The study was carried out through four rounds of the Delphi method. The Delphi method is a method used to obtain a consensus from a group of experts [50], where the overall view will provide more solid information than that offered by a single person on an individual basis, thus reducing the subjectivity [50,51]. The questionnaires were administered through the LimeSurvey online platform. The questionnaires included an instruction form for the expert, the authorization to participate in the research and the instructions. A reminder email was sent every 4 days until a reply was received. After the survey, the researchers selected or excluded the items that received less than 80% agreement among experts.

The objective of the first Delphi round was to reach a consensus among the panel of experts about the core competencies for nurse managers. During the second round, the experts were asked individually if they wished to reconsider their opinions in light of the feedback. In the third round, the experts were asked to provide a consensus about the core competencies at each nurse manager on a functional level. The experts also agreed on the training required for each level of competence (expert, very competent, competent, novice advanced and novice). The fourth round allowed experts to reconsider their opinions in view of the feedback from the third round.

2.2.1. Consensus

In any Delphi study, the definition of consensus should be set a priori. Thus, for this research, we defined the consensus in three ways: (I) if at least 80% of the experts agreed with the competencies, responding "agree" or "complete agreement" in the questionnaires; (II) if at least 80% of the experts agreed with the degree of development of the competencies; (III) if at least 80% of the experts agreed with the type of training required. Where an agreement was not reached, items were deleted for the next Delphi round.

2.2.2. Participants

In this study, we decided to invite experts from two categories and twelve groups: experts in health management (Table 1) and experts in the health environment (Table 1), because experts in these two categories have valuable knowledge on nursing management.

Table 1. Socio-demographic data from the panel of experts.

Demographic Variable			Frequency
Gender			
	Female		32 (64%)
	Male		18 (36%)
Age			
	Mean		49.52
	Standard deviation		11.02
	<40 years		10 (20%)
	41–50 years		15 (30%)
	51–60 years		18 (36%)
	>60 years		7 (14%)
Education			
	Master's degree		34 (68%)
	Ph.D.		14 (28%)
Scope of representation			
Expert group	Group 1	Minister of Health	3 (6.1%)
	Group 2	Head of the Health Department	5 (10%)
	Group 3	General Council of Nurses	3 (6%)
	Group 4	Scientific Association	4 (8%)
	Group 5	Trade Union	3 (6%)
	Group 6	General Manager	5 (10%)
	Group 6	Medical Director	2 (4%)
	Group 6	Nurse Executive	5 (10%)
	Group 6	Management Director	1 (2%)
	Group 7	Middle Nurse manager	2 (4.1%)
	Group 8	Nursing supervisor	3 (6.1%)
	Group 9	Nurse	3 (6.1%)
	Group 9	Doctor	2 (4.1%)
	Group 9	Assistant Nursing Care Technician	2 (4.1%)
	Group 10	Nursing Degree Students	2 (4.1%)
	Group 11	Research/Teaching	4 (8.2%)
	Group 12	Lawyer	1 (2%)

Source: own elaboration.

2.2.3. Variables

The variables of the study were:

- Socio-demographic variables: To define the profile of the experts, information was collected related to age, sex, profession, university education, postgraduate education, professional role, place of study, years of professional practice, years of management experience, management functions performed and international experience;
- Competencies: From the review of the literature emerged the list of competencies to be proposed for the experts.

2.2.4. The Delphi Questionnaires

Two questionnaires were developed ad hoc as measuring instruments.

- Competencies needed for nurse managers (Appendix A): Each participant rated his/her level of agreement or disagreement with each competency according to a one to five Likert scale (1 = complete disagreement, 5 = complete agreement);
- Level of competency development for nurse managers (Appendix B): In order to reach a consensus about the level of development of the competencies at each level of management, the degree of

agreement or disagreement with each competency according to a one to five Likert scale (1 = novice, 5 = expert), and the type of training required to develop the competencies, according to a one to six Likert scale (1 = University Extension Diploma, 2 = Continuing education, 3 = University Expert, 4 = University specialization diploma, 5 = master's degree, 6 = Ph.D.) was recorded.

2.2.5. Level of Development

For this research, the term "level of development" was used to refer to the level of deepening in each competency that the nurse manager should acquire in each of the functional levels, thus the level of development would be:

- Novice: follows the rules and plans;
- Novice advanced: can provide partial solutions to unfamiliar or complex situations;
- Competent: strong demonstration of competency;
- Very competent: significant demonstration of competency;
- Expert: when demonstrating the behavior of the competency model.

2.2.6. Validity and Reliability

The validity and reliability of the questionnaires was carried out with a group of 12 people selected on the basis of the same criteria used for the panel of experts. The reliability of the questionnaires was ensured by carrying out a Cronbach's Alpha Coefficient analysis. The content validity was estimated through expert judgement, which analyzed errors and ambiguities in the formulation of the questions, excess items, proposals for improvement, suggestions for the style of the surveys.

2.3. Principal Component Analysis

The Principal Component Analysis (PCA) is a data transformation technique. The aim of the method is to reduce the dimensionality of multivariate data, while preserving as much of the relevant information as possible [52]. The factor analyses were carried out with respect to the theory of Thurstone [53,54] (3 phases): first, the assessment of the adequacy of the data for factorial analysis, second, the extraction of factors, and finally the rotation and interpretation of factors.

For determining the suitability of the data for factorial analysis, we used the Kaiser–Meyer–Olkin (KMO) test. The next step was the extraction of factors, using Kaiser's criteria, which makes the decision based on an eigenvalue greater than one [55], and a scree plot, which is a graphical representation of the eigenvalues. This graph helps to find the inflexion point and the number of factors above this point that should be retained [56]. Finally, we proceeded with the rotation and interpretation of the factors, through the varimax rotation method and Kaiser standardization, to achieve a structure as simple as possible that was easy to interpret [57].

3. Results

3.1. Demographics of the Expert Panel

A total of 50 experts consented to participate and took part in the Delphi study. Table 1 lists the demographic characteristics of the complete expert panel. The response rate for all of the Delphi rounds was 100%.

3.2. Delphi Study

During the first and second Delphi rounds, 51 competencies were agreed by consensus (more than 80%) from the proposed list. In round 1, the percentage of "total agreement" was 100% ("agreed" or "complete agreement") with the competencies decision making, communication skills, listening and conflict management. In this round, more than 80% of the experts were in "total agreement" with eight competencies (Table·2): decision making, communication skills, listening, leadership, conflict management, ethical principles, collaboration and team management skills.

Experts in round 2 were provided with individual feedback from the round 1 survey. This feedback included the complete expert panel responses. Participants were asked if they agreed or disagreed with the statements that were made in the previous round. From round 2, it appears that the experts showed a "complete agreement" with a percentage equal to 100% in the competencies identified as the core competencies (Table 2). In round 2, the competencies with less than an 80% consensus were eliminated.

Table 2. Core of competencies.

Competency	Total Agreement	
	Round 1	Round 2
Decision making	100%	100%
Relationship management	84%	100%
Communication skills	100%	100%
Listening	100%	100%
Leadership	84%	100%
Conflict Management	100%	100%
Ethical principles	80%	100%
Collaboration and team management skills	88%	100%

Source: own elaboration.

During the third and fourth Delphi rounds, the eight competencies from the core competencies were shown to be necessary for the three levels of nurse manager existing in Spain (operations, logistics and top management), differing in the level of development of the competencies at each level of management ("Expert", "very competent" and "competent"). The panel of experts in round 3 were asked about the level of development of each competency to reach a consensus. The experts in round 4 were again provided with individual feedback from round 3, and asked to indicate their agreement with statements that were made by participants in the previous round. The final consensus is shown in Table 3.

Table 3. Development of core competencies at each level of nurse manager.

Competency	Top Management	Logistics	Operations
Decision making	Expert	Very competent	Very competent
Relationship management	Very competent	Very competent	Very competent
Communication skills	Expert	Very competent	Expert
Listening	Expert	Very competent	Expert
Leadership	Expert	Competent	Expert
Conflict Management	Very competent	Very competent	Very competent
Ethical principles	Expert	Very competent	Expert
Collaboration and team management skills	Expert	Very competent	Expert

Source: own elaboration.

During the third round, the experts were asked to indicate their opinion about the appropriate training to reach the right level of competency. In round 4, experts were again provided with individualized feedback from the previous round. The final consensus is shown in Table 4.

Table 4. Training required by competency level.

Competency Level	Type of Training (Consensus)
Novice	University Extension Diploma (100%)
	Continuing education (98%)
	University Extension Diploma (90%)
Novice advanced	Continuing education (90%)
	University Expert (90%)
	Continuing education (96%)
Competent	University Expert (100%)
	University Specialization Diploma (96%)
	University Expert (96%)
Very competent	University specialization diploma (96%)
	Master's degree (96%)
	Master's degree (96%)
Expert	Ph.D. (96%)

Source: own elaboration.

3.3. Principal Component Analysis

The data were suitable for factoring as the correlation matrix showed a predominance of meaningful results ($p < 0.05$), Bartlett's test was significant ($p < 0.001$) and KMO value was 0.505. The integration of competency listening into the competency communication skills was appropriate for factoring (as shown in Table 5).

Table 5. Principal Component Analysis (PCA) of core competencies.

	CP 1	CP2	CP3
Communication skills	0.851		
Relationship management	0.771		
Conflict Management	0.620		
Leadership		0.877	
Collaboration and team management skills		0.841	
Ethical principles			0.773
Decision making			0.706
Explained variance	28.43%	22.665%	17.576%
Eigenvalue	1.99	1.587	1.230
α Cronbach			0.613

Source: own elaboration. Caption: communication (CP), leadership (CP2), decision making (CP3).

The extraction of factors showed three factors that explained 68.67% of the total accumulated variance. The varimax rotation method yielded a three-factor solution: communication, leadership and decision making (Table 5). The observed convergence between the Kaiser criteria and the scree plot adds certainty to the results. The reliability of the core competencies showed a Cronbach's alpha value of 0.613, indicating a satisfactory result. (Table 5).

4. Discussion

This paper reports on the findings of the core competencies to be developed by the nurse manager in the Spanish health system. Decision making, relationship management, communication skills, listening, leadership, conflict management, ethical principles, collaboration and team management skills were seen as the core competencies for nurse managers. These findings are consistent with the findings from previous studies [47,51,52]. Kantanen et al. [42] emphasizes competency in decision making as a critical competency. McCarthy [58] highlights core competencies that are aligned with our research in communication, relationship management, ethical values and decision making. Our research is also aligned with Pillay [59] and with Gunawan [60], when he described relationship management, conflict management and collaboration and team management as basic competencies.

To emphasize the strength of the core competencies identified in this research, we should say that this were also identified through a scoping review of the literature, with the exception of the listening skills and ethical principles, which were not found among the most frequent results in the review. It should be noted that the frequency of citation in the selected articles was used as a criterion for identifying the core competencies in the literature review.

This study identified that all the core competencies are needed independent of the functional level of nurse managers (executive management, logistics and operational management). Although each functional level requires different levels of competency development to be reached. There was a consensus between the experts in Delphi rounds 3 and 4. These findings are consistent with findings from previous studies (e.g., [47,58]). McCarthy et al. [58] highlighted that core competencies should be common to all three levels of management at different degrees of development. The AONE [61] has shown shared competencies in their different models ("Nurse Manager Competency", "Nurse Executive Competencies" and "Nurse Executive Competencies: CNE system"), and in the Nurse Executive Competency Assessment Tool, which differentiates the degree of development of each competency. In another sense, the AONE also defined non-shared competencies in their models.

With regard to the development of competencies, an agreement was reached in Delphi rounds 3 and 4. The experts agreed that competencies should be developed at "competent" (this was considered to have been reached when there is a strong demonstration of competency), "very competent" (level reached when there is a significant demonstration of competency) and "expert" level (level reached when it demonstrates the behavior of the competency model). This proposal is in agreement with AONE, who use the levels competent, proficient and expert for the development of competencies, emphasizing how these levels are reached through master's degree studies or a Ph.D. [62,63]. In contrast, in other studies such as "Nurse manager competencies", the focus is on the degree to which the competencies contribute to the nurse manager's work (minimally, moderately, significantly and essentially) [48]. Furthermore, the results of the current study emphasize the need for a high level of competence development, in the same way that Crawford et al. [64] demonstrated by indicating how executive practice would require a high degree of specialization and a specific development of competencies.

During Delphi rounds 3 and 4, the expert panel achieved a consensus about the training to be developed by the nurse manager on the three competency levels ("expert", "very competent" and "competent"). The "competent" level is reached through continuing education, University Expert and University specialization diploma. With regard to the "very competent" level, the consensus was reached with University expert, University specialization diploma or master's degree. Finally, the "expert" level is reached through master's and Ph.D. studies. We should keep in mind how work experience and education significantly influence the development of competencies of nurse managers [65]. However, experience as a nurse manager does not prepare them for the wide range of skills needed, requiring specialized training and work experience in concrete situations [33,66]. Learning experientially as a nurse manager should be accompanied by prior planning and close mentoring [67]. Previous studies show that the quality and level of training are responsible for orienting nurse managers towards good governance and the acquisition of the global vision of the organization [33,68,69]. Furthermore, the results of the current study emphasize how it is possible to appreciate differences between nurse managers who have completed advanced management programs with respect to others who have not participated in this type of training program, adding evidence to previous studies [68,70]. We share the recommendations given by the Joint Commission for Accreditation of Healthcare Organizations regarding the development of different career levels for nurses according to their level of education, training and experience [71]. In addition, and just like Fralic [72] affirmed, our results suggest that the training received by nurse managers would be one of the key aspects, because they are responsible for managing the area with the largest number of people, to make decisions about resource management and other areas such as quality of care, patient safety, research, training, expenditure or investment. The present study, along with other previous studies such as the research carried out by Herrin et al. [73], support that the master's degree training allows the nurse manager to be able to carry out adequate decision making, as well as for the effective management of health processes. In the same way, Rizani et al. [74] point out that the average competence of nurses is higher when they have developed advanced studies (master's degree or Ph.D.), increasing with time their level of competency to a higher degree than those nurses who have not developed advanced training.

The PCA verified the core competencies by defining three principal components named communication (communication skills, relationship management, conflict management), leadership (leadership and team management skills) and decision making (decision making and ethical principles), which would therefore constitute the competency factors to develop the role of a nurse manager in Spain (Table 6). The strength of the eigenvalue confirms the importance of the relationship between decision making and ethical principles [75], the need for strong leadership in working groups [76] and communication as a fundamental element in conflict resolution [77]. By comparing the core competencies emerging from our research with the most relevant international studies into core competencies for nurse managers, we would find a shared factor with communication, which should indeed be presented as a shared factor [25,78,79].

Table 6. Comparison of core competencies.

Core Competencies	Leach et al. [79]	Weber [25]	Aone [47]
Communication	Organizational Management	Influence	Leadership
Leadership	Interpersonal effectiveness	Emotional Intelligence	Professionalism
Decision making	Systemic thinking	Result orientation	Communication
	Creative thinking	Change Management	Leadership
	Technical skills	Communication	Knowledge of the health environment
	Ability to adapt	Management vision	
	Customer Service		
	Personal domain		

Source: own elaboration.

The communication ability that would be expected from the nurse manager should include the ability to convey critical thinking and generate reflection in nurse teams prior to action [36]. In the same way, it should, for example, facilitate conflict resolution and shared decision making, as well as creation, participation and team management [80]. The differences that would arise between all the core competencies could be related to the different health contexts in which management practice takes place [58].

The purpose of this study was to determine the core competencies for each functional level of nursing management by expert consensus. Our research contributes strong and important evidence to the nursing management field. Firstly, we provide a baseline of competencies for nurses who intend to carry out functions as nurse managers. Secondly, our study is also useful as a tool for evaluating and detecting areas for improvement for nurse managers. Finally, the core competencies should be useful for planning the professional development of nurse managers.

With regard to the limitations of this research, we should mention the different healthcare contexts from which the body of research knowledge is derived. Nursing management has specific characteristics for each of these contexts.

5. Conclusions

This study found core competencies for nurse managers in Spain. The successful nurse manager should develop all these competencies (as relevant to their practice) in today's rapidly evolving healthcare system. In conclusion, this study yielded a consensus on eight core competencies for nurse managers in Spain: decision making, relationship management, communication skills, listening, leadership, conflict management, ethical principles, collaboration and team management skills, oriented towards leadership and good governance of health organizations, and on the basis of the social responsibility of health professionals. The nurse manager is responsible for the largest area of a healthcare organization, managing large budgets and large numbers of nurses. Therefore, a nurse should not be promoted to the role of a nurse manager without advanced management training.

Our research shows the precise level of development of each competency for the different functional levels of nurse manager. The nurse manager at any functional level should develop these core competencies before being promoted to other roles as a nurse manager.

Any nurse who wishes to develop his or her professional career as a nurse manager should first develop the core competencies shown here.

Moreover, our research shows the necessary education required to acquire the competency development necessary for each different nursing management role. Both nurses who want to be promoted to nurse managers and current nurse managers should follow the educational programs shown in order to adapt their knowledge to the requirements of the role.

These core competencies may have implications for practice, organizational policy, and education related to nursing management. The proposed core competencies may contribute to nurse manager role design, selection processes, and nurse manager curriculum design for traditional academic institutions and organizational continued professional development programs. Further understanding of core competencies is likely to inform interventions, which may improve nurses' work environment, patient care, patient safety and organizational outcomes.

The following research should develop the characteristics corresponding to each of these competencies and training situations.

Author Contributions: Conceptualization, A.G.G.; A.P.-C.; P.M.-S.; and J.S.V.; methodology, A.P.-C.; A.G.G.; validation, M.P.-S.; formal analysis, M.P.-S.; A.P.-C.; investigation, A.G.G. and P.M.-S.; resources, J.S.V.; and writing—original draft preparation, A.G.G. and P.M.-S.; writing—review and editing, A.G.G.; A.P.-C.; P.M.-S.; J.S.V. All authors have read and agreed to the published version of the manuscript.

Funding: This research received no external funding.

Appendix A. Competencies Needed for Nurse Managers

Please select the appropriate answer for each concept:

Table A1. List of competencies.

Level of Agreement Competency	1	2	3	4	5
Financial skills					
Analytical Thinking					
Decision-making					
Innovation					
Strategic Management					
Human Resources Management					
Legal aspects					
Marketing					
Organizational Management					
Relationship Management					
Communication skills					

Table A1. *Cont.*

Level of Agreement Competency	1	2	3	4	5
Feedback					
Evaluation of information and its sources					
Listening					
Information systems and computers					
Technology					
Leadership					
Career planning					
Influence					
Change Management					
Delegate					
Conflict Management					
Ethical principles					
Power and Empowerment					
Critical thinking					
Collaboration and team management skills					
Interpersonal Relations					
Multi-professional management					
Team Building Strategies					
Result orientation					
Care Management Systems					
User care skills					
Health policy					
Identification and responsibility with the organization					
Knowledge of the health environment					
Quality and Safety					
Quality and improvement processes					
Clinical skills					
Infection control practices					
Standard Nursing Practice					
Nurse Research					
Nursing Theories					
Care Planning					
Nursing training planning					
Professionalism					
Integrity					
Awareness of Personal Strengths and Weaknesses					
Strategic Vision					
Personal and professional balance					
Compassionate					
Diversity					
Emotional Intelligence					
Serve as a model					
Basic Oral English					
English medium level of writing					
English medium reading level					

Caption: 1 = Complete disagreement; 2 = Disagreement; 3 = No disagreement/No agreement; 4 = Agreement 5 = Complete agreement.

Appendix B. Level of Competency Development for Nurse Managers

In this section, you should mark which functional level(s) each competency corresponds to, taking into account that the competency may be necessary for all three levels.

You should also indicate the level of development of this competence.

Table A2. Development of competencies

Competency		Novice	Novice Advancing	Competent	Very Competent	Expert
Decision-making	Operations Logistics Top managment					
Relationship Management	Operations Logistics Top managment					
Communication skills	Operations Logistics Top managment					
Listening	Operations Logistics Top managment					
Leadership	Operations Logistics Top managment					
Conflict Management	Operations Logistics Top managment					
Ethical principles	Operations Logistics Top managment					
Collaboration and team management skills	Operations Logistics Top managment					

Indicate to which degree of training each competence level should be developed:

Table A3. Type of training required

	U. Ext D	C. Edu.	U. Exp	U. Spec. D.	Master	Ph.D.
Novice						
Novice advanced						
Competent						
Very competent						
Expert						

Caption: University Extension Diploma (U. Ext D); Continuing education (C. Edu); University Expert (U. Exp); University specialization diploma (U. Spec. D.); Master's degree (Master); Ph.D (Ph.D.).

References

1. Kantanen, K.; Kaunonen, M.; Helminen, M.; Suominen, T. Leadership and management competencies of head nurses and directors of nursing in Finnish social and health care. *J. Res. Nurs.* **2017**, *22*, 228–244. [CrossRef]
2. Nursing Now. Vision Nursing Now. 2019. Available online: https://www.nursingnow.org/vision/?doing_wp_cron=1577348723.0888390541076660156250 (accessed on 26 December 2019).
3. Cathcart, E.B.; Greenspan, M. A new window into nurse manager development. *J. Nurs. Adm.* **2012**, *42*, 557–561. [CrossRef] [PubMed]
4. Cummings, G.; MacGregor, T.; Davey, M.; Lee, H.; Wong, C.A.; Lo, E.; Muise, M.; Stafford, E. Leadership styles and outcome patterns for the nursing workforce and work environment: A systematic review. *Int. J. Nurs. Stud.* **2010**, *47*, 363–385. [CrossRef] [PubMed]
5. Fennimore, L.; Wolf, G. Nurse Manager Leadership Development: Leveraging the Evidence and System-Level Support. *J. Nurs. Adm.* **2011**, *41*, 204–210. [CrossRef] [PubMed]
6. Ding, B.; Liu, W.; Tsai, S.B.; Gu, D.; Bian, F.; Shao, X. Effect of patient participation on nurse and patient outcomes in inpatient healthcare. *Int. J. Environ. Res. Public Health* **2019**, *16*, 1344. [CrossRef]
7. Boyatzis, R.E. *The Competent Manager: A Model for Effective Performance*; John Wiley & Sons: Toronto, CA, Canada, 1982; ISBN 0-471-09031-X.
8. Groves, K. Talent management best practices: How exemplary health care organizations create value in a down economy. *Health Care Manag. Rev.* **2011**, *3*, 227–240. [CrossRef]
9. Kerfoot, K.M.; Luquire, R. Alignment of the system's chief nursing officer: Staff or direct line structure? *Nurs. Adm. Q.* **2012**, *36*, 325–331. [CrossRef]

10. MacMillan-Finlayson, S. Competency development for nurse executives: Meeting the challenge. *J. Nurs. Adm.* **2010**, *40*, 254–257. [CrossRef]

11. Thorne, S. Nursing now or never. *Nurs. Inq.* **2019**, *26*, e12326. [CrossRef]

12. Aiken, L.H.; Cimiotti, J.P.; Sloane, D.M.; Smith, H.L.; Flynn, L.; Neff, D.F. Effects of nurse staffing and nurse education on patient deaths in hospitals with different nurse work environments. *Med. Care* **2011**, *49*, 1047–1053. [CrossRef]

13. Savage, C.; Kub, J. Public health and nursing: A natural partnership. *Int. J. Environ. Res. Public Health* **2009**, *6*, 2843–2848. [CrossRef] [PubMed]

14. McHugh, G.A.; Horne, M.; Chalmers, K.I.; Luker, K.A. Specialist community nurses: A critical analysis of their role in the management of long-term conditions. *Int. J. Environ. Res. Public Health* **2009**, *6*, 2550–2567. [CrossRef] [PubMed]

15. McPherson, C.; Ndumbe-Eyoh, S.; Betker, C.; Oickle, D.; Peroff-Johnston, N. Swimming against the tide: A Canadian qualitative study examining the implementation of a province-wide public health initiative to address health equity. *Int. J. Equity Health* **2016**, *15*, 0419–0424. [CrossRef] [PubMed]

16. Cummings, G.; Lee, S.D.; Tate, K.C. The evolution of oncology nursing: Leading the path to change. *Can. Oncol. Nurs. J.* **2018**, *28*, 314–317.

17. Lasater, K.; Sloane, D.; McHugh, M.; Aiken, L. *End of Life Care Quality Remains a Problem–Nurses May be a Solution*; University of Pennsylvania School of Nursing: Philadelphia, PA, USA, 2019; Available online: https://www.nursing.upenn.edu/live/news/1276-end-of-life-care-quality-remains-a-problem-nurses (accessed on 27 December 2019).

18. Campbell, L. Leadership-Patients: Empowering professionalism and celebrating the future. Patient Blood Management: Challenges of Providing a State-wide Service. In Proceedings of the Nursing &Midwifery Leadership Conference, Perth, Australia, 28–29 November 2019.

19. Rogers, J.; Middleton, S.; Wilson, P.H.; Johnstone, S.J. Predicting functional outcomes after stroke: An observational study of acute single-channel EEG. *Top. Stroke Rehabil.* **2019**, *9*, 1–12. [CrossRef]

20. McClarigan, L.; Mader, D.; Skiff, C. Yes, We Can and Did: Engaging and Empowering Nurses through Shared Governance in a Rural Health Care Setting. *Nurse Lead.* **2019**, *17*, 65–70. [CrossRef]

21. Kerfoot, K. Four measures that are key to retaining nurses. *Hosp Health Netw.* 2015. Available online: https://www.hhnmag.com/articles/3253-four-measures-that-are-key-to-retaining-nurses (accessed on 27 December 2019).

22. Press Ganey. *Nursing Special Report: The Influence of Nurse Manager Leadership on Patient and Nurse Outcomes and the Mediating Effects of the Nurse Work Environment Nurse*; Press Ganey: South Bend, IN, USA, 2017; Volume 26, pp. 3–23.

23. Ho, E.; Principi, E.; Cordon, C.P.; Amenudzie, Y.; Kotwa, K.; Holt, S.; Macphee, M. The Synergy Tool: Making Important Quality Gains within One Healthcare Organization. *Adm. Sci.* **2017**, *7*, 32. [CrossRef]

24. Institute of Medicine of the National Academies. *The Future of Nursing: Leading Change, Advancing Health*; Institute of Medicine of the National Academies: Washington, DC, USA, 2010; Volume 40, pp. 1–4.

25. Weber, E.; Ward, J.; Walsh, T. Nurse leader competencies: A toolkit for success. *Nurs. Manag.* **2015**, *46*, 47–50. [CrossRef]

26. Panayotou, M.S.; Cefaratti, D.; Hanscom, H.; Petto, P.N.; Turner, R.R.; Talley, L. Shared governance strategic plan creation and implementation. *Nurs. Manag.* **2019**, *50*, 9–12. [CrossRef]

27. Brooks-Cleator, L.; Phillipps, B.; Giles, A. Culturally Safe Health Initiatives for Indigenous Peoples in Canada: A Scoping Review. *Can. J. Nurs. Res.* **2018**, *50*, 202–213. [CrossRef]

28. Kanninen, T.H.; Häggman-Laitila, A.; Tervo-Heikkinen, T.; Kvist, T. Nursing shared governance at hospitals–it's Finnish future? *Leadersh. Health Serv. (Bradf. Engl.)* **2019**, *32*, 558–568. [CrossRef]

29. Clavelle, J.; Porter O'Grady, T.; Drenkard, K. Structural empowerment and the nursing practice environment in magnet organizations. *J. Nurs. Adm.* **2013**, *43*, 566–573. [CrossRef]

30. Whitt, M.; Baird, B.; Wilbanks, P.; Esmail, P. Tracking decisions with shared governance. *Nurse Lead.* **2011**, *9*, 53–55. [CrossRef]

31. Meadows, M.T.; Dwyer, C. AONE continues to guide leadership expertise with post-acute competencies. *Nurse Lead.* **2015**, *13*, 21–25. [CrossRef]

32. Catton, H. International Council of Nurses: Putting nurses at the centre of the world's policymaking has benefits for us all. *Int. Nurs. Rev.* **2019**, *66*, 299–301. [CrossRef] [PubMed]

33. Baxter, C.; Warshawsky, N. Exploring the acquisition of nurse manager competence. *Nurse Lead.* **2014**, *12*, 46–59. [CrossRef]
34. Chase, L.K. Are you confidently competent? *Nurs. Manag.* **2012**, *43*, 50–53. [CrossRef] [PubMed]
35. DeOnna, J. Developing and Validating an Instrument to Measure the Perceived Job Competencies Linked to Performance and Staff Retention of First-Line Nurse Managers Employed in a Hospital Setting. Ph.D. Thesis, The Pennsylvania State University, College of Education, State College, PA, USA, 2006.
36. Scoble, K.B.; Russell, G. Vision 2020, part I: Profile of the future nurse leader. *J. Nurs. Adm.* **2003**, *33*, 324–330. [CrossRef]
37. AONE. AONE Nurse Executive Competencies. Available online: http://www.aone.org/resources/nurse-leader-competencies.shtml (accessed on 12 November 2019).
38. Meadows, M.T. New Competencies for System Chief Nurse Executives. *J. Nurs. Adm.* **2016**, *46*, 235–237.
39. Pihlainen, V.; Kivinen, T.; Lammintakanen, J. Management and leadership competence in hospitals: A systematic literature review. *Leadersh. Health Serv.* **2016**, *29*, 95–110. [CrossRef]
40. Shirey, M.R. Stress and coping in nurse managers: Two decades of research. *Nurs. Econ.* **2006**, *24*, 193–203. [PubMed]
41. Vance, M. Scotland the brave: Statutory supervision transformed. *Pract. Midwife* **2009**, *12*, 16–77. [PubMed]
42. Kantanen, K.; Kent, B.; Kaunonen, M.; Helminen, M.; Suominen, T. The development and pilot of an instrument for measuring nurse managers' leadership and management competencies. *J. Res. Nurs.* **2015**, *20*, 667–677. [CrossRef]
43. Tampoe, M. Exploiting the core competences of your organization. *Long Range Plan.* **1994**, *27*, 66–77. [CrossRef]
44. Higgins, J.M. Innovation: The core competence. *Plan Rev.* **1995**, *23*, 32–36. [CrossRef]
45. Garman, A.N.; Johnson, M.P. Leadership Competencies: An Introduction. *J. Healthc. Manag.* **2006**, *51*, 13–17. [CrossRef] [PubMed]
46. Prahalad, C.K.; Hamel, G. The Core Competence of the Corporation. *Harv. Bus. Rev.* **1990**, *68*, 1–15.
47. AONE. AONE Nurse Executive Competencies. *Nurse Lead.* **2015**, *3*, 15–22.
48. Chase, L. Nurse Manager Competencies. Ph.D. Thesis, University of Iowa, Iowa City, IA, USA, 2010.
49. Pillay, R. Towards a competency-based framework for nursing management education. *Int. J. Nurs. Pract.* **2010**, *16*, 545–554. [CrossRef]
50. Linstone, H.A.; Turoff, M.; Helmer, O. *The Delphi Method*; Addison-Wesley: Redeading, MA, USA, 1975; ISBN 0-201-04294-0.
51. Varela-Ruiz, M.; Díaz-Bravo, L.; García-Durán, R. Descripción y usos del método Delphi en investigaciones del área de la salud. *Investig. Educ. Méd.* **2012**, *1*, 90–95.
52. Sewell, M. *Principal Component Analysis*; University College London: London, UK, 2008.
53. Thurstone, L.L. Multiple factor analysis. *Psychol. Rev.* **1931**, *38*, 406–427. [CrossRef]
54. Thurstone, L.L. *Multiple Factor Analysis*, 5th ed.; University of Chicago Press: Chicago, IL, USA, 1957.
55. Kaiser, H.F. The Application of Electronic Computers to Factor Analysis. *Educ. Psychol. Meas.* **1960**, *20*, 141–151. [CrossRef]
56. Cattell, R.B. The scree test for the number of factors. *Multivar. Behav. Res.* **1966**, *1*, 245–276. [CrossRef] [PubMed]
57. Carroll, J.B. An analytical solution for approximating simple structure in factor analysis. *Psychometrika* **1953**, *18*, 23–38. [CrossRef]
58. McCarthy, G.; Fitzpatrick, J.J. Development of a Competency Framework for Nurse Managers in Ireland. *J. Contin. Educ. Nurs.* **2009**, *40*, 346–350. [CrossRef]
59. Pillay, R. The skills gap in nursing management in South Africa: A sectoral analysis: A research paper. *J. Nurs. Manag.* **2010**, *18*, 134–144. [CrossRef]
60. Gunawan, J.; Aungsuroch, Y.; Fisher, M.L. Factors contributing to managerial competence of first-line nurse managers: A systematic review. *Int. J. Nurs. Pract.* **2018**, *24*, 1–12. [CrossRef]
61. AONE. Competencies Assessment. Available online: http://www.aone.org/resources/online-assessments.shtml (accessed on 18 August 2019).
62. Waxman, K.T.; Roussel, L.; Herrin-Griffith, D.; D'Alfonso, J. The AONE Nurse Executive Competencies: 12 Years Later. *Nurse Lead.* **2017**, *15*, 120–126. [CrossRef]

63. Crawford, C.L.; Omery, A.; Spicer, J. An Integrative Review of 21st-Century Roles, Responsibilities, Characteristics, and Competencies of Chief Nurse Executives: A Blueprint for the Next Generation. *Nurs. Adm. Q.* **2017**, *41*, 297–309. [CrossRef]

64. Sandehang, P.M.; Hariyati, R.T.; Rachmawati, I.N. Nurse career mapping: A qualitative case study of a new hospital. *BMC Nurs.* **2019**, *18*, 1–9. [CrossRef]

65. Kuraoka, Y. Effect of an experiential learning-based programme to foster competence among nurse managers. *J. Nurs. Manag.* **2018**, *26*, 1–9. [CrossRef] [PubMed]

66. Warshawsky, N.; Cramer, E. Describing Nurse Manager Role Preparation and Competency: Findings from a National Study. *J. Nurs. Adm.* **2019**, *49*, 249–255. [CrossRef] [PubMed]

67. Kleinman, C.S. Leadership Roles, Competencies, and Education: How Prepared Are Our Nurse Managers? *J. Nurs. Adm.* **2003**, *33*, 451–455. [CrossRef] [PubMed]

68. ANA. *Nursing Administration: Scope and Standards of Practice*, 2nd ed.; Nursesbooks.org; ANA: Washington, DC, USA, 2018; ISBN 9781558106444.

69. West, M. Evaluation of a nurse leadership development programme. *Nurs. Manag.* **2016**, *22*, 26–31. [CrossRef] [PubMed]

70. Rees, S.; Glynn, M.; Moore, R.; Rankin, R.; Stevens, L. Supporting nurse manager certification. *J. Nurs. Adm.* **2014**, *44*, 368–371. [CrossRef] [PubMed]

71. Joint Comission on Accreditation of Healthcare Organizations. Health Care at the Crossroads: Strategies for Addressing the Evolving Nursing Crisis. Available online: Shorturl.at/mCDTV (accessed on 24 August 2019).

72. Fralic, M.F. Patterns of preparation. The nurse executive. *J. Nurs. Adm.* **1987**, *17*, 35–38. [CrossRef]

73. Herrin, D.; Hathaway, D.; Jacob, S.; McKeon, L.; Norris, T.; Spears, P.; Stegbauer, C. A model academic-practice partnership. *J. Nurs. Adm.* **2006**, *36*, 547–550. [CrossRef]

74. Rizany, I.; Hariyati, R.T.; Handayani, H. Factors that affect the development of nurses' competencies: A systematic review. *Enferm. Clin.* **2018**, *28*, 154–157. [CrossRef]

75. Loreggia, A.; Mattei, N.; Rossi, F.; Venable, K.B. Preferences and Ethical Principles in Decision Making. In Proceedings of the 2018 AAAI/ACM Conference on AI, Ethics and Society-AIES '18, New York, NY, USA, 2–3 February 2018.

76. Berrios Martos, P.; Lopez Zafra, E.; Aguilar Luzon, M.C.; Auguste, J.M. Relationship between leadership style and attitude toward working groups. *Int. J. Psychol.* **2008**, *43*, 444.

77. Codier, E.; Codier, D.D. Could Emotional Intelligence Make Patients Safer? Specific skills might help nurses to improve communication, conflict resolution, and individual and team performance. *Am. J. Nurs.* **2017**, *117*, 58–62. [CrossRef]

78. Carlson, E.E.; Kline, M.M.; Zangerle, C.M. AONE Competencies: Preparing Nurse Executives to Lead Population Health. *Nurse Lead.* **2016**, *14*, 108–112. [CrossRef]

79. Leach, L.S.; McFarland, P. Assessing the professional development needs of experienced nurse executive leaders. *J. Nurs. Adm.* **2014**, *44*, 51–62. [CrossRef] [PubMed]

80. Garman, A.N.; Fitz, K.D.; Fraser, M.M. Communication and relations management. *J. Healthc. Manag.* **2006**, *51*, 291–294. [PubMed]

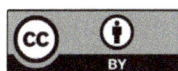

International Journal of
Environmental Research and Public Health

MDPI

Article

Analyzing the Job Demands-Control-Support Model in Work-Life Balance: A Study among Nurses in the European Context

Virginia Navajas-Romero [1,*], Antonio Ariza-Montes [2] and Felipe Hernández-Perlines [3]

1   Department of Statistics, Management and Applied Economy. Universidad de Córdoba, 14014 Córdoba, Spain
2   Management Departament, Universidad Loyola Andalucía, 14014 Córdoba, Spain; ariza@uloyola.es
3   Departament of Business Administration; Universidad de Castilla La Mancha, 13071 Ciudad Real, Spain; felipe.HPerlines@uclm.es
*   Correspondence: vnavajas@uco.es

Received: 1 April 2020; Accepted: 18 April 2020; Published: 21 April 2020

check for
updates

Abstract: The balance of personal life with professional life is a topical issue that is increasingly worrisome due to globalization, the rapid introduction of new technologies into all areas of human life, the overlap between time between work and family, new organizational systems, and changes in the nature of work. This problem is accentuated by professions subjected to intense labor demands, as is the case of nurses. Adopting the Job Demand–Control–Support model, the main purpose of this research is to analyze how these factors lead to a greater or lesser degree of work–life balance. The research proposes a logistic regression model, which was constructed with a sample of 991 nursing professionals from the V European Working Conditions Survey. The results obtained confirm, on the one hand, that there is a significant effect of physical demands (but not psychological demands) on work–life balance. On the other hand, the moderating effects of job control are partially confirmed for psychological demands, and those of supervisor support (but not co-worker support) are partially confirmed for physical demands. In conclusion, the present research shows that effective management of nurses' work context can decisively contribute to finding the difficult balance between personal and professional time.

Keywords: job demands; job control; social support; work–life balance; nurses

1. Introduction

The balance of personal life with professional life is a topical issue that is increasingly worrisome due to globalization, the intrusion of new technologies into personal life, the overlap between work time and family time, new organizational systems, and changes in the nature of work [1]. This problem is accentuated in professions with intense working hours or schedules [2]. Nursing professionals are without a doubt in this situation. The role of a nurse is very demanding, as quick and effective responses are required to deal with the health needs of the community. Furthermore, it is an industry with an intensive work environment, which operates 24 h a day, 365 days a year, and sometimes requires exceeding the standard 40 h week of full-time employment for the production of services [3].

Work–life balance (WLB) is understood as several individual and structural constraints of their way of harmonizing work time and personal time according to an individual system of values, goals, and aspirations [4]. Although much research on the WLB has focused its analysis on the challenge of caring for children and the elderly [5–7], this is a topic of great importance in current academic research [8] because achieving an optimal WLB is critical to personal well-being [9,10]. Despite this, given the intense interconnectedness of work and personal time, many workers have

297

serious difficulties defining the boundaries between them and often cross those boundaries, which has harmful consequences to their health and well-being [11]. Due to the changing nature of the current workforce, the WLB has a broader and higher perspective on the EU political agenda, encompassing aspects such as business organizational culture in terms of gender equality and social protection. In fact, at the Social Summit for Fair Employment and Growth held in Gothenburg in November 2017, the WLB was proclaimed as a European pillar of social rights [12]. Despite this, the peculiarities of the work environment that surrounds the nursing profession makes it difficult to reconcile work and family life, preventing a high level of work satisfaction from being achieved [13,14].

The job demand–control–support model (JDCS) [15–18] constitutes a very useful theoretical approach for understanding the characteristics of work and its consequences for the occupational health of employees [19]. In fact, this model has been used in many professions with the aim of studying a wide range of reactions that provoke tension in workers [20–27]. In particular, the JDC model establishes that factors such as the level of labor demands and the control the workers have over their work will affect the development of WLB. In subsequent model improvements, the level of perceived support at work was included as another relevant factor (the JDCS model).

Following this idea, the present study analyzes the effects caused by certain factors related to the context of work in nursing personnel (demands, control, and social support) and how they influence the WLB of these professionals. According to the JDCS model approach, the worst situation of WLB for workers would be manifested in those occupations characterized by high job demands, low control, and little social support. Previous studies with this model support the association between poor work results (for example, exhaustion, stress, poor well-being, etc.) with high levels of demands or work load (for example, [28–30]), low control over work, or the degree of autonomy in the application of labor decisions (for example, [31–33]). In addition, the low level of support perceived by colleagues or supervisors also influences (for example, [27,34]). The literature in general terms suggests that a low family–work balance is related to lower job satisfaction, higher turnover intentions, exhaustion, and deterioration of health [35,36], and a high family–work balance is related to higher levels of professional commitment and lower intentions to leave the profession [28,37,38]. However, although there are some studies that have tested the JDCS model with nursing personnel [28,39,40], the investigations that have related the model with the WLB are practically nonexistent.

Undoubtedly, nursing professionals carry out work of special interest to society, given the leading role of the health system in the welfare of any nation. Despite this, the work of nurses is characterized by high job demands: direct contact with patients, exhausting workdays, night shifts [41], and limited job control over the tasks they perform. This last circumstance is a result of the numerous regulations and operating protocols that regulate and limit the activity of these professionals, regulations that tend to be more rigorous when written by personnel outside the health care profession [42]. The other pillar on which the JDCS model is built is social support. Nursing requires much collaboration and teamwork. In this context, perceived social support is of great importance because, as Schwarzer and Knoll (2007) note, conflicts in work teams multiply when employees perceive little support from their supervisors and/or co-workers [43–45].

The consequences of the scenario described above are multifaceted: stress, alienation, low organizational commitment, and burnout. One of the least researched outcomes in academia from the perspective of the JDCS model is the problem that nurses have with balancing work time with personal time. Studies in other occupations suggest that the combination of high job demands and a great deal of autonomy can help reduce work–life conflict [46]. In contrast, individuals in professions that face many job demands within a context of low autonomy will have more difficulty achieving an adequate WLB [44]. Additionally, various studies suggest that supervisor and/or co-worker support contributes decisively to improving WLB [47].

Unlike other professionals, nurses offer an intangible service that is inextricably linked with the professional who performs it. Good management of work–family conflicts will improve the WLB of these professionals, which will translate into positive effects for the worker and the organization [48].

The purpose of this study is to contribute on the idiosyncrasies of the profession and the value the profession provides for citizens and the welfare state. The majority of studies on WLB adopt an approach based on worker health [49]. However, in the European context, there is little empirical research that analyzes both the main effects of the JDCS model and the multiplicative model in their relationship with WLB, which means that the impacts of job demands, job control, and social support have not received the attention they deserve in a profession so relevant in the European context [50]. Taking into account everything raised so far, this research seeks to (i) analyze job demands, job control, and social support in nursing staff, as well as assess whether these factors lead to a greater or lesser degree of WLB in European hospitals; and (ii) explore whether these models differ from those identified in the previous literature. The following research question is derived from these objectives: Does this organizational model allow its workers to have a high WLB according to the JDCS model that relates labor demands, labor control, and social support?

2. Managing Demands, Control and Support in an Organizational Context in Nursing

Health is one of the fundamental pillars of a welfare society. The World Health Organization estimates that the health care sector workforce in 2013 included 20.7 million nurses out of a total of 43.5 million health workers worldwide [51,52]. The well-being of workers is essential for the health of society [49]. Balancing work and family life in the nursing sector to achieve a high degree of well-being is crucial for the development of the service [53], since well-being impacts the quality of patient care [54], with poor well-being increasing the risk of negligence and/or abuse [55].

The sector is characterized by high job demands, both physical and psychological. The situation with respect the physical demands of nurse workers reflects the need to work with limited resources, both in terms of personnel and equipment [56], which causes a level of emotional strain that approaches exhaustion [52,53]. The nursing sector is the sector with the highest rate of nonfatal occupational diseases and injuries, which causes an increase in sick leave [57]. Factors such as stress, poor health, and depression negatively affect WLB [58,59]. Regarding the psychological demands, nurses must make urgent and critical decisions that involve a vital risk for the patient [60]; thus, nursing professionals are continuously exposed to traumatic events [61]. Health care services are needed 24 h a day, seven days a week. This need may contribute to greater job stability in health care than in other sectors [62], but it also implies an internal organization based on exhausting workloads and 12 h continuous work shifts, which hinder the conciliation of work with personal and family life [63].

From the perspective of job control, it deepens knowledge of the skill discretion and the decision authority of this sector, and nursing work requires multiple skills [64]. According to Ulrich, Barden, Cassidy, and Varn-Davis, there are different skills that workers in this sector have to have, such as communication, collaboration, and resource management and leadership skills [65]. At the same time, nursing professionals usually have little autonomy in carrying out their work activities [66], which greatly limits their decision-making capacity [67]. However, nurses who have higher levels of work autonomy tend to be high-performing, satisfied, and committed workers [68]. With respect to social support in health, Olmedo (2009) reports the presence of a complex web of interpersonal relationships with conflicting power dynamics between physicians (who are mostly male) and nurses, whose profession is still highly feminized [69,70]. Work pressures, limited control, and the complex social system trigger deterioration of the work environment [71], resulting in absenteeism, high turnover, depression, and even suicide [72]. Nurses who consider these conditions unsustainable eventually abandon the profession in search of jobs with fewer demands and better working conditions that will improve their personal quality of life, including the balance between work and family time [73].

Although some previous studies have applied the JDCS model in the nursing sector, they have generally done so from analytical approaches and perspectives that differ from those presented in this article. From the perspective of job demands, Heijden et al. (2018) confirm that job demands are positively correlated with job turnover, while the availability of resources and the experience of nurses are inversely related to turnover [74]. At the end of the last century, De Jonge et al. (1999) claimed that the combination of job demands and job control can predict the health of employees [75,76]. From the perspective of job control, the work of Yamaguchi et al. (2016) confirms that the absence of job control increases the likelihood that nursing personnel will abandon nursing as a career [77]. More recently, Mark and Smith (2012) have added that rewards, decision-making skills, and skill discretion decrease depression and anxiety among these professionals, which is often motivated by a lack of resources and a lack of time to attend to patients [78,79]. Finally, from social support perspective, Sigurdardottir et al. (2015) show that training programs improve nursing professionals' perceptions of social support (from both supervisors and co-workers) [80,81]. Stress is another topic of interest analyzed with this model. Thus, Nabirye et al. (2011) note that the role conflict and ambiguity that characterize the work of more experienced nurses lead to increased stress [82,83].

The effects that such a demanding profession exerts on health and well-being have also been the subject of analysis in academia [84]. The study of Xanthopoulou et al. (2009) provides key evidence of pathways leading to the well-being of nursing personnel in general hospitals [85]. Another study using the JDCS model in Uganda concluded that younger nurses are more satisfied than older nurses [82]. These authors suggest that with age, family responsibilities increase, and consequently, the likelihood of conflicts between personal and professional life increases. Other authors focus on analyzing the most important antecedents of the psychosocial well-being of nurses, highlighting the importance of social support to improve job satisfaction and stress [86]. Following this idea, two studies carried out in Sweden show the positive effect that empowerment [87] and social support [88] exert against burnout in nursing personnel.

3. Research Hypotheses

The three previously described job strain variables should have an interactive effect on the WLB of nurses. Additionally, the interaction among these variables can reduce the relationship between job demands and employees' WLB. Against the reference framework described in the previous paragraphs and based on the literature review, the following research hypotheses are proposed:

Hypothesis 1. *The high job demands faced by nursing professionals will be negatively associated with work–life balance.*

Hypothesis 2. *Job control will reduce the effects of job demands on work–life balance.*

Hypothesis 3. *Supervisors/co-workers will reduce the effects of job demands on work–life balance.*

The following Figure 1 summarizes the theoretical model and research hypotheses.

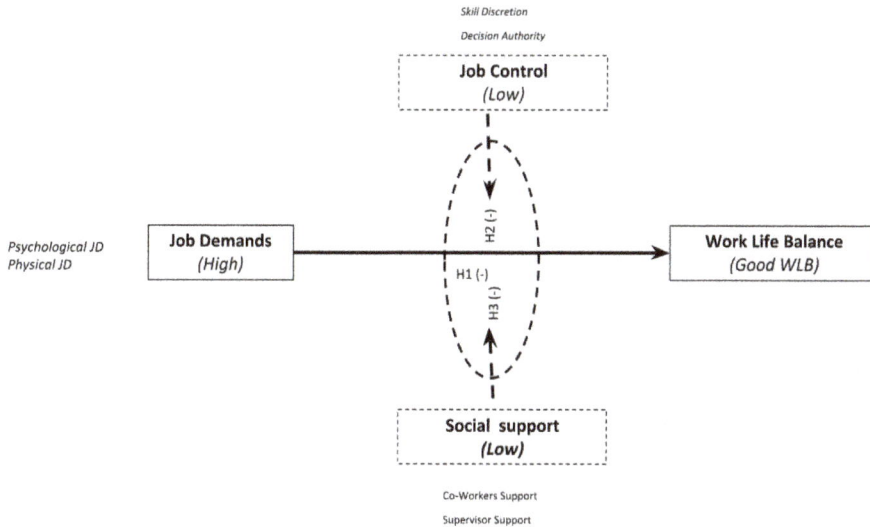

Figure 1. Research model. Source: Prepared by the authors.

4. Methodology

4.1. Data Collection and Sampling

For the development of this research, information collected by the European Foundation for the Improvement of Living and Working Conditions regarding the work environment and working conditions in 35 European countries was used (EU28, Norway, Switzerland, Albania, the former Yugoslav Republic of Macedonia, Montenegro, Serbia, and Turkey during the period from February to September 2015. The European Working Conditions Survey (EWCS) (The complete questionnaire can be found in the European Foundation for the Improvement of Living and Working Conditions (2019). See the following link: https://www.eurofound.europa.eu/sites/default/files/page/field_ef_documents/6th_ewcs_2015_final_source_master_questionnaire.pdf) is conducted every five years based on a questionnaire-based interview. A subsample of 991 nursing professionals (ISCO Code 222) (Classification structure of the International Labor Organization (ILO) that organizes jobs according to tasks and functions. Specifically, group 222 includes "Nursing and midwifery professionals") was extracted to achieve the objectives of this study. The majority of the respondents were women (89.1% of the total), with an average age of 42.8 years (SD = 11.0).

4.2. Measures and Methodology: The Binary Logistic Regression Model

The dependent variable of this study was WLB, measured by an indicator composed of four items that ask the following: (a) How are your working time arrangements set? (b) How do your working hours fit in with your family or social commitments outside work? (c) How often have you worked during your free time to meet work demands? (d) Would you say that arranging to take an hour or two off during working hours to take care of personal or family matters is easy or not? The Cronbach's α of the four-item scale was 0.898. Subjects with good WLB were coded as 1, while those with a lower level of WLB were coded as 0.

As indicated by Rugulies et al. (2010), the Copenhagen Psychosocial Questionnaire is considered a very effective tool for assessing the psychosocial work environment [89]. Different authors, such as Widerszal-Bazyl (2017), have demonstrated the psychometric properties of this questionnaire [90]. The extensive information provided by the European Working Conditions Survey permits the rigorous reproduction of the different scales included in the Copenhagen Psychosocial Questionnaire [9]. To meet the objectives of the present study, five indexes related to job demands, work organization, relationships, leadership, etc. were calculated. Twenty-three items from the EWCS were used to generate five indexes: (1) Psychological Job Demands (Cronbach's $\alpha = 0.736$); (2) Skill Discretion (Cronbach's $\alpha = 0.695$); (3) Decision Authority (Cronbach's $\alpha = 0.770$); (4) Co-worker Support (only one item); and (5) Supervisor Support (Cronbach's $\alpha = 0.905$).

Finally, physical job demands were measured with the Job Content Questionnaire (JCQ). This scale evaluates the social and psychological characteristics of a particular job. Some examples of the 13 items used to measure the risk of physical job demands are the following: "Are you exposed at work to high temperatures that make you perspire even when you are not working?", "Do you handle or have skin contact with chemical products or substances?" or "Does your main job involve lifting or moving people?" Cronbach's Alpha for this scale was 0.772.

The statistical analysis applied in this study was the binary logistic regression model. This method is one of the most frequently applied statistical approaches for developing social prediction models with binary results [91,92]. Logistic regression has been used with the Karasek model for example [93–95] and specifically in the field of nursing (for example, [96–98]). This method allows the determination of the probability that a certain event—good balance between personal and professional life—will occur compared with the probability that the opposite event will occur. In this study, the Hosmer–Lemeshow goodness of fit test was used as a measure of overall validity, and the Wald test was used for the analysis of individual variables.

5. Results

In the initial estimate of the central variable of this study, the general sample of the nursing professionals appears to present some problems balancing their personal time and work time, with an average score of only 0.5071 on a scale of 0 (poor WLB) to 1 (good WLB). In addition, this problem seems slightly more pressing among women (0.5067) than among men (0.5102).

In relation to the demands to which nursing professionals are subjected, it must be emphasized that the weight of psychological demands (0.3513) is, in all cases, greater than that of physical demands (0.2384). Additionally, women perceive more demands than men, both physical (0.2387 vs. 0.2364) and psychological (0.3524 vs. 0.3421).

Nursing professionals have greater skill discretion (0.6607) than decision authority (0.5698). This general trend does not differ by gender, although male nurses have greater skill discretion than female nurses (0.6667 vs. 0.6600), while female nurses have greater decision authority than male nurses (0.5714 vs. 0.5563).

Finally, the perceived supervisor support (0.2564) is much higher than the perceived support from co-workers (0.1893), a circumstance that should be the subject of analysis and deep debate within the profession. In addition, male nurses have more social support mechanisms than female nurses in regard to support from both supervisors (0.2617 vs. 0.2558) and co-workers (0.1952 vs. 0.1886).

5.1. Job Demand–Control–Support Factors and Work-Life Balance

The individual relationships between the different factors of the JDCS model and WLB are presented in Table 1. First, it should be noted that the fundamental principles of the JDCS model are confirmed. The high job demands, the low job control, and the low social support are negatively correlated with the outcome variable, i.e., the WLB indicator. However, these results must be taken with caution because the only variables that are statistically significant are those related to the physical ($\beta = -0.613$, $p = 0.000$) and psychological demands ($\beta = -0.520$, $p = 0.001$) on the nursing professionals. In fact, these two scales have the strongest relationship with the outcomes variable, followed by the two scales of social support and, finally, the measures of job control.

An examination of each of the individual components shows that physical demands are more important than psychological demands for predicting WLB among nursing and professionals.

In addition, the association between "low decision authority" ($\beta = -0.188$, $p = 0.250$) and WLB is more intense than the association between "low skill discretion" ($\beta = -0.087$, $p = 0.555$) and WLB. Likewise, the influence of supervisor support on WLB balance ($\beta = -0.412$, $p = 0.178$) is greater than the association between support from co-workers and WLB ($\beta = -0.257$, $p = 0.260$).

Table 1. Logistic regression: factors that determine work–life balance (high/low score).

Variables in the Model					Odds Ratios		
						95% C.I. for OR	
Variables	B	Standard	Wald	*p*	OR	Lower	Upper
Job Demands							
Psychological JD (high)	−0.520	0.151	11.863	0.001	0.594	0.442	0.799
Physical JD (high)	−0.613	0.15	16.711	0.000	0.542	0.404	0.727
Job Control							
Skill discretion (low)	−0.087	0.148	0.348	0.555	0.917	0.686	1.224
Decision authority (low)	−0.188	0.163	1.324	0.250	0.829	0.602	1.141
Social Support							
Co-worker support (low)	−0.257	0.228	1.271	0.260	0.773	0.494	1.209
Supervisor support (low)	0.412	0.306	1.811	0.178	0.662	0.364	1.207

5.2. Strain Model

The original proposal of the Karasek model (1979) is presented in Table 2, which shows the analysis of the association between WLB and job demands (physical and psychological) and job control (skill discretion and decision authority) and the interaction between both dimensions [16].

Table 2. Adjusted association between job demands, decision latitude, their interaction, and work–life balance index (Strain Model).

Variables in the Model					Odds Ratios		
						95% C.I. for OR	
Variables	B	Standard	Wald	*p*	OR	Lower	Upper
Job Demands							
Psychological JD (high)	0.025	0.321	0.006	0.937	1.026	0.546	1.926
Physical JD (high)	−0.397	0.193	4.223	0.040	0.672	0.460	0.982
Job Control							
Skill discretion (low)	0.320	0.248	1.673	0.196	1.377	0.848	2.237
Decision authority (low)	−0.095	0.216	0.192	0.661	0.917	0.596	1.389
Moderator effect of JC							
PhyJD x JC (Skill)	−0.257	0.329	0.541	0.462	0.785	0.412	1.495
PhyJD x JC (Dauth)	0.007	0.320	0.000	0.983	1.007	0.538	1.886
PsyJD x JC (Skill)	−0.533	0.195	7.467	0.006	0.587	0.400	0.860
PsyJD x JC (Skill)	−0.302	0.313	0.929	0.335	0.739	0.400	1.366

The results show a direct negative relationship between physical job demands and WLB ($\beta = -0.397$, $p < 0.05$). These results partially confirm Hypothesis 1.

Additionally, to test for interaction effects, interaction terms were introduced in the logistic regression model. Table 2 shows that the effect of psychological job demands on WLB is moderated when skill discretion is involved ($\beta = -0.533$, $p < 0.01$). This means that control over work (discretion to solve problems on your own and performing varied activities for which it is necessary to learn new skills) enriches nurses' work and possibly their personal life, cushioning the negative effect that the psychological demands of the profession exert on WLB. In other words, in the presence of low job control, the negative effect of psychological demands on WLB is more intense ($\beta = -0.533$, Sig. 0.006) than when greater job control is present ($\beta = -0.520$, Sig. 0.001). These results partially support Hypothesis 2 because the moderating effect of decision authority in the job demands–WLB relationship does not obtain statistically significant results for physical demands ($\beta = 0.007$, Sig. 0.983) or for psychological demands ($\beta = -0.302$, Sig. 0.335).

5.3. Iso-Strain Model

Subsequently, variables related to social support were incorporated into the model to contrast the hypotheses of the iso-strain model. Table 3 shows the adjusted association between WLB and job demands (physical and psychological), job control (skill discretion and decision authority), and social support (co-workers and supervisors) and their respective interactions.

Table 3. Adjusted association between job demands, decision latitude, social support, and their interaction and work–life balance index (iso-strain model).

Variables in the Model					Odds Ratios		
						95% C.I. for OR	
Variables	B	Standard	Wald	p	OR	Lower	Upper
Job Demands							
Psychological JD (high)	−0.122	0.466	0.069	0.793	0.885	0.355	2.206
Physical JD (high)	−0.397	0.193	4.223	0.040	0.672	0.460	0.982
Job Control							
Skill discretion (low)	−0.041	0.351	0.014	0.906	0.960	0.483	1.908
Decision authority (low)	−0.175	0.301	0.337	0.562	0.840	0.466	1.515
Moderator effect of JC							
PhyJD x JC (Skill)	0.259	0.485	0.285	0.594	1.295	0.500	3.354
PhyJD x JC (Dauth)	−0.341	0.461	0.548	0.459	0.711	0.288	1.754
PsyJD x JC (Skill)	−0.348	0.487	0.511	0.475	0.706	0.272	1.834
PsyJD x JC (Skill)	−0.621	0.264	5.543	0.019	0.538	0.321	0.901
Social Support							
Co-worker support (low)	0.029	0.466	0.004	0.950	1.03	0.413	2.566
Supervisor support (low)	−0.215	0.485	0.196	0.658	0.807	0.312	2.087
Moderator effect of Social Support							
PhyJD x JC (Skill)	0.769	0.521	2.178	0.140	2.157	0.777	5.989
PhyJD x JC (Dauth)	−0.749	0.267	7.848	0.005	0.473	0.280	0.799
PsyJD x JC (Skill)	−0.814	0.519	2.457	1.117	0.443	0.160	1.226
PsyJD x JC (Skill)	0.522	0.492	1.126	0.289	1.686	0.642	4.423

The new model presents some novelties regarding the formulated hypotheses. The most notable results are as follows. First, the direct relationship of job demands with WLB disappears from the overall model. The association of physical and psychological demands with WLB occurs in interaction with variables related to job control and social support. Thus, Table 3 shows that the strain-by-control interaction term at the 0.05 level only manifests when decision authority is present. This variable exerts a moderating effect on the psychological job demands–WLB relationship ($\beta = -0.621$, $p < 0.05$). This result partially confirms research hypothesis 2 as it indicates that decision authority, but not skill discretion, has a modulating effect.

Finally, the strain-by-support interaction term at the 0.05 level was analyzed. Table 3 shows that supervisor support moderates the effect of physical demands on WLB ($\beta = -0.749$, $p < 0.01$). This result partially confirms research hypothesis 3 as it indicates that supervisor support, but not co-worker support, has a moderating effect.

6. Discussion

The main objective of the present study was to test the efficacy of the JDCS model for predicting WLB among nursing professionals. Nursing presents its own particularities and is critical for maintaining the welfare state in Europe; however, nursing care takes place in one of the most stressful work environments that exists [96]. As noted by Karatepe and Uludag (2007), the health care sector is unique due to its high level of stress and its intense physical, psychological, and emotional demands [99].

Some studies, such as that of Ghislieri et al. (2017) performed with a sample of 500 nurses working in an Italian hospital, confirm that nurses have difficulties balancing work time and personal time [100]. To examine this issue among nursing professionals, the current study adopts the JDCS model as a reference framework, developing several logistic regression models that attempt to explain the direct and interactive effects of three fundamental variables: job demands, job control, and social support. The results obtained from a large sample of 991 European nursing professionals partially confirm both the strain hypothesis and the iso-strain hypothesis of the Johnson and Hall (1988) and Karasek (1979) models [16,17].

First, with respect to Hypothesis 1, a significant effect of physical (but not psychological) demands on WLB is confirmed. The physical demands that most affect nurses are, in the following order, handling or being in direct contact with materials that can be infectious, such as waste, bodily fluids, laboratory materials, etc.; lifting or moving people; having to maintain tiring or painful positions; performing repetitive hand or arm movement; handling or being in skin contact with chemical products or substances; and carrying or moving heavy loads. Being subjected to such physical demands causes nurses to feel that their work does not fit well with family or social commitments. The high physical demands cause a decrease in the well-being of workers linked to the work–family conflict because it includes aspects of physical fatigue, pain, and insecurity in the work environment [101], reducing the physical resources that a worker has to their WLB [47]. According to the World Health Organization, poor well-being in the workplace is one of the most important causes of absenteeism, turnover, and poor performance in the workplace [51]. This result is consistent with the study by Hussain et al. (2012), who highlight the high job demands that nurses face as well as the very poor working conditions, which translate into serious difficulties reconciling work and family time [102]. These authors warn of the risk that nurses will abandon the profession in search of less demanding and stressful options. The physical and psychological demands that nursing professionals face are well known and are overwhelmingly related to their close interactions with patients [103,104]. The results of our study indicate that nurses experience greater strain from physical demands than from psychological demands, perhaps because, as Qureshi (2018) warns, direct contact with patients requires high physical effort to lift or move people or heavy objects, maintain tiring or uncomfortable positions, and perform repetitive tasks or movements with one's hands or arms [105]. Similarly, Greenglass et al. (2001) and Garrett and McDaniel (2001) suggest that high physical demands may originate from the excessive workload and atypical schedules that include shift work, weekends, and nights [106–109]. These factors cause an imbalance between professional and personal demands, which manifests as lower organizational commitment, exhaustion, work stress, dissatisfaction, and, directly related to the object of this research, a worse personal–professional life balance [110].

Hypothesis 2 of this research was examined in a second phase intended to demonstrate the modulating effect of job control on WLB. The results of this study confirm this moderating effect in the case of psychological demands, which suggests that increasing the decision-making capacity of nursing professionals will improve their mood, vitality, and general interest, thus cushioning the direct effect that the demanding work exerts on stress, overwork, and personal life–professional life conflict [111]. Therefore, this research empirically confirms that being able choose the order in which one will perform tasks, being able to work at one's own pace and using one's own methods, being consulted about objectives that affect one's work, being able to influence the decisions that are important, or having the opportunity to apply one's own ideas at work, among other discretionary acts, cushions the negative effect that the psychological pressure of nursing work exerts on WLB. These results are in line with the study by Pisarski et al. (2006), who show that increased control in the workplace generates better WLB, especially when the individual is able to control his or her work hours and/or experiences an increase in schedule flexibility [112–115]. For many health professionals, their commitment to their work and professional career is a priority that takes them away from family and social relationships and causes them to dedicate less time than they would like to family responsibilities [116]. This extreme and rigid dedication causes a high level of exhaustion and a sensation of lethargy and depersonalization [117]. The debate on the effects of this professional dedication on WLB as one's health care career advances has a long history, but the issue seems far from a closed topic [118]. Decades ago, Hirschman (1970) reported the need to introduce changes in hospital work practices to correct this problem [119]. More recently, Mushfiqur et al. (2018) emphasize the moral obligation to change matters related to the management of health institutions, including work hours and locations, the relationship with the environment, and, of course, better balance between personal life and professional life [120]. Increasing the flexibility of work schedules is one of the most common strategies to mitigate this problem. Thus, the Medical Women's Federation (MWF) (2018) and Adisa et al. (2017) promote part-time work as a way to effectively improve WLB and create a positive impact on both Social Security and the lives of workers [118–121].

Finally, Hypothesis 3 of this research aimed to verify the moderating effect of social support in the job demand–WLB relationship. This moderating effect is partially confirmed for physical demands in the presence of supervisor support; that is, the negative effect of physical demands on WLB is mitigated when supervisor support is available. In conclusion, the physical demands (handling potentially infectious materials, moving patients, maintaining painful positions) that nursing professionals face generate problems with WLB, but these problems are reduced if nurses have the support of their immediate supervisors. A similar conclusion was reached by Abdul-Rashid et al. (2017), who applied a structural equations model in a sample of nurses from public hospitals in Malaysia [122]. Social support is decisive in an occupation in which teamwork, specifically cooperative work, occupies a leading role [123,124]. The creation of a work environment based on open communication and social support from co-workers and supervisors necessarily increases WLB [125]. Professionals in nursing units face complex problems that require very specific skills, support, and a great capacity for adaptation [126]. In this sense, support from both co-workers and supervisors can moderate the harmful effects of nursing demands on WLB. The studies of Tucker et al. (2018), Somers et al. (2018), and Jennings (2007) confirm that positive interpersonal relationships with supervisors improve safety, mutual respect, and positive feelings, which translate to greater WLB [127–129]. The results of our research support the cushioning effect of social support (at least in terms of supervisor support) in the job demands–WLB relationship, thus supporting Hypothesis 3.

7. Conclusions and Limitations

This study yields important theoretical and practical implications for the nursing profession in Europe. At the theoretical level, understanding how the JDCS model works in a sector such as nursing, where complex and dynamic tasks are performed, can decisively contribute to improving the WLB of professionals subjected to intense work demands. From a practical perspective, the findings of this study corroborate the idea that job demands are not the only variables that affect WLB, particularly when employees perceive job control and/or social support from their organizations. Consequently, the industry must analyze the workplace factors that affect WLB. Human resource managers should explore new tools to provide employees with control over their daily activities, especially in an occupation such as nursing, which involves direct contact with patients and in which the quality of the services provided is conditioned by the workers' decision-making capacity and freedom of actions. All progress in this regard (for example, modifying action protocols) will lead to greater autonomy, which should translate into better WLB. In addition, managers should promote a cooperative work environment based on an organizational culture of support, and teamwork should be encouraged. Investing in the training of work teams will improve aspects such as the organizational climate and social support, which will translate into improvements within the organization (for example, in the organization of work shifts) and in the attitude towards patient service. These strategies should reduce job stress and, as a result, increase the WLB of workers.

As is often the case in empirical research conducted in the field of social sciences, the results obtained should be interpreted with caution. First, a causal relationship between variables cannot be established since this is a cross-sectional study. Second, the study of the JDCS model is based on self-assessed measures and is therefore susceptible to bias; however, Pelfrene et al. (2002) corroborated that studies based on self-assessed measures support the strain hypothesis of the model to a greater extent than studies that use more objective evaluations [130]. Third, the research was developed in a specific socio-geographic scenario (Europe) where very different health systems and labor codes coexist that condition the fundamental variables of the JDCS model. Fourth, no control variables have been introduced, despite being a highly feminized profession. Therefore, it would not be prudent to generalize these assumptions and ideas to other work environments. Future studies should investigate other groups in the health industry (for example, doctors or hospital managers) and analyze the influence of different geographic areas to allow comparisons among different cultural environments.

Author Contributions: "Conceptualization, V.N-R and A.A.-M.; Methodology, A.A.-M. and F.H-P.; Software, F.H.-P. Validation, V.N-R and A.A.-M.; Formal Analysis, V.N.-R. and A.A.-M; Investigation, V.N-R. and A.A.-M.; Resources, F.H.-P. and A.A.-M.; Data Curation, A.A.-M. Writing—Original Draft Preparation, V.N.-R. and F.H.-P.; Writing—Review & Editing, A.A.-M. and V.N.-R.; Visualization, F.H.-P. and A.A.-M.; Supervision, A.A.-M. and F.H.-P.; Project Administration, V.N.-R. All authors have read and agreed to the published version of the manuscript.

Funding: This research received no external funding.

Acknowledgments: We thank Eurofound for providing the data set for this research. Reference [9], European Working Conditions Survey Integrated Data File, 1991–2015, [data collection], UK Data Service. SN: 7363, https://doi.org/10.5255/UKDA-SN-7363-4.

Conflicts of Interest: The authors declare no conflict of interest.

References

1. Babatunde, A.; Mordi, C.; Simpson, R.; Adisa, T.; Oruh, E. Time Biases: Exploring the Work-Life Balance of Single Nigeria Managers and Professionals. *J. Manag. Psychol.* **2019**, *35*, 35–70. [CrossRef]
2. Lee, D.J.; Sirgy, M.J. Work-Life Balance in the Digital Workplace: The Impact of Schedule Flexibility and Telecommuting on Work-Life Balance and Overall Life Satisfaction. *Thriving Digit. Work.* **2019**, 355–384. [CrossRef]
3. Kowitlawkul, Y.; Yap, S.F.; Makabe, S.; Chan, S.; Takagai, J.; Tam, W.W.S.; Nurumal, M.S. Investigating nurses' quality of life and work-life balance statuses in Singapore. *Int. Nurs. Rev.* **2019**, *66*, 61–69. [CrossRef] [PubMed]
4. Casper, W.J.; Vaziri, H.; Wayne, J.H.; DeHauw, S.; Greenhaus, J. The jingle-jangle of work–nonwork balance: A comprehensive and meta-analytic review of its meaning and measurement. *J. Appl. Psychol.* **2018**, *103*, 182. [CrossRef] [PubMed]
5. Duxbury, L.E.; Higgins, C.A. Gender differences in work-family conflict. *J. Appl. Psychol.* **1991**, *76*, 60. [CrossRef]
6. Williams, L.J.; Bozdogan, H.; Aiman-Smith, L. Inference problems with equivalent models. In *Advanced Structural Equation Modeling: Issues and Techniques*; Erlbaum: Mahwah, NJ, USA, 1996; pp. 279–314.
7. Ozer, E.M. The impact of childcare responsibility and self-efficacy on the psychological health of professional working mothers. *Psychol. Women Q.* **1995**, *19*, 315–355. [CrossRef]
8. Crompton, R.; Lyonette, C. Work-life 'balance' in Europe. *Acta Sociol.* **2006**, *49*, 379–393. [CrossRef]
9. Parent-Thirion, A.; Fernandez Macias, E.; Hurley, J.; Vermeylen, G. *Fourth European Working Conditions Survey*; European Foundation for the Improvement of Living and Working Conditions: Dublin, Ireland, 2007.
10. Lee, J.M.; Choi, H.G. Influence of organizational culture supporting work-life balance on well-being and depression mediated by work-life balance. *Korean J. Ind. Organ. Psychol.* **2019**, *32*, 1–27. [CrossRef]
11. Niessen, C.; Müller, T.; Hommelhoff, S.; Westman, M. The impact of preventive coping on business travelers' work and private life. *J. Organ. Behav.* **2018**, *39*, 113–127. [CrossRef]
12. Rodríguez González, S. Desigualdad por causa de género en la Seguridad Social: Carreras de cotización y prestaciones. *Lan Harremanak. Rev. Relac. Laborales* **2017**, *38*, 93–125.

13. Cramer, E.; Hunter, B. Relationships between working conditions and emotional wellbeing in midwives. *Women Birth.* **2019**, *32*, 521–532. [CrossRef] [PubMed]

14. Hayes, B.; Prihodova, L.; Walsh, G.; Doyle, F.; Doherty, S. Doctors don't Do-little: A national cross-sectional study of workplace well-being of hospital doctors in Ireland. *BMJ Open* **2019**, *9*, e025433. [CrossRef] [PubMed]

15. Nielsen, M.B.; Einarsen, S.V. What we know, what we do not know, and what we should and could have known about workplace bullying: An overview of the literature and agenda for future research. *Aggress. Violent Behav.* **2018**, *42*, 71–83. [CrossRef]

16. Karasek, R. Job demands, job decision latitude, and mental strain: Implications for job redesign. *Adm. Sci. Q.* **1979**, *24*, 285–308. [CrossRef]

17. Karasek, R. *Healthy Work: Stress, Productivity, and the Reconstruction of Working Life*; Basic Books: New York, NY, USA, 1990.

18. Johnson, V.J.; Hall, E.M. Job strain, work place social support, and cardiovascular disease: A cross-sectional study of a random sample of the Swedish working population. *Am. J. Public Heal.* **1988**, *78*, 1336–1342. [CrossRef]

19. Salin, D. Risk factors of workplace bullying for men and women: The role of the psychosocial and physical work environment. *Scand. J. Psychol.* **2015**, *56*, 69–77. [CrossRef]

20. Ariza-Montes, A.; Arjona-Fuentes, J.M.; Han, H.; Law, R. Work environment and well-being of different occupational groups in hospitality: Job Demand–Control–Support model. *Int. J. Hosp. Manag.* **2018**, *73*, 1–11. [CrossRef]

21. Asif, F.; Javed, U.; Janjua, S.Y. The job demand-control-support model and employee wellbeing: A meta-analysis of previous research. *Pak. J. Psychol. Res.* **2018**, *33*, 1.

22. Mivšek, P.; Äimälä, A.M.; Žvanut, B.; Tuomi, J. Midwifery students' well-being among undegradutes in Slovenia: A pilot study. *Midwifery* **2018**, *61*, 63–65. [CrossRef]

23. Rong, Y.; Guo, K.R.; Yin, H.F.; Wu, Y.F.; Li, S.; Sun, D.Y. Evaluating the level of occupational stress and its influence factors among traffic police in a district in Shanghai. *Chin. J. Ind. Hyg. Occup. Dis.* **2019**, *37*, 352–356. [CrossRef]

24. Schernhammer, E.S.; Feskanich, D.; Liang, G.; Scott, A.J.; Singh, R.B.; Anjum, B.; Takahashi, M. Stress and Burnout in Doctors. *Camb. Handb. Psychol. Health Med.* **2019**, *27*, 361.

25. Schilling, R.; Colledge, F.; Ludyga, S.; Pühse, U.; Brand, S.; Gerber, M. Does cardiorespiratory fitness moderate the association between occupational stress, cardiovascular risk, and mental health in police officers? *Int. J. Environ. Res. Public Health* **2019**, *16*, 2349. [CrossRef] [PubMed]

26. Chambel, M.J.; Carvalho, V.S.; Cesário, F.; Lopes, S. *The Work-to-Life Conflict Mediation between Job Characteristics and Well-Being at Work, Career Development International*; Emerald Publishing Limited: Bingley, UK, 2017.

27. Ibrahim, R.Z.A.R.; Saputra, J.; Bakar, A.A.; Dagang, M.M.; Nazilah, S.; Ali, M.; Yasin, M.A.S.M. Role of Supply Chain Management on the Job Control and Social Support for Relationship between Work-Family Conflict and Job Satisfaction. *Int. J. Sup. Chain* **2019**, *8*, 907.

28. Goller, M.; Harteis, C.; Gijbels, D.; Donche, V. Engineering students' learning during internships: Exploring the explanatory power of the job demands-control-support model. *J. Eng. Educ.* **2020**, 1–18. [CrossRef]

29. Ogunyemi, A.O.; Babalola, S.O.; Akanbi, S.O. Job Demands and Mental Strain Relationship: The Moderating Effect of Perceived Organizational Support on the Mediating Role of Job Decision Latitude among Nigerian Immigration Officers. *KIU J. Soc. Sci.* **2019**, *5*, 141–150.

30. Rana, F.A.; Javed, U. Psychosocial job characteristics, employee well-being, and quit intentions in Pakistan's insurance sector. *Glob. Bus. Organ. Excel.* **2019**, *38*, 38–45. [CrossRef]

31. Vassos, M.; Nankervis, K.; Skerry, T.; Lante, K. Can the job demand-control-(support) model predict disability support worker burnout and work engagement? *J. Intellect. Dev. Disabil.* **2019**, *44*, 139–149. [CrossRef]

32. Park, H.; Oh, H.; Boo, S. The Role of Occupational Stress in the Association between Emotional Labor and Mental Health: A Moderated Mediation Model. *Sustainability* **2019**, *11*, 1886. [CrossRef]

33. Schmitt, H. Job Demands, Job Control, and Social Support on Burnout: Why Type Matters. Ph.D. Thesis, Alliant International University, Alhambra, CA, USA, 2019.

34. Ding, G.; Liu, H.; Huang, Q.J. Enterprise social networking usage as a moderator of the relationship between work stressors and employee creativity: A multilevel study. *Inf. Manag.* **2019**, *56*, 103165. [CrossRef]

35. Grzywacz, J.G.; Frone, M.J.; Brewer, C.S.; Kovner, C.T. Quantifying work–family conflict among registered nurses. *Res. Nurs. Heal.* **2006**, *29*, 414–426. [CrossRef]

36. Cortese, C.G.; Ghislieri, C.; Colombo, L. Determinants of nurses' job satisfaction: The role of work–family conflict, job demand, emotional charge and social support. *J. Nurs. Manag.* **2010**, *18*, 35–43. [CrossRef] [PubMed]

37. Russo, M.; Buonocore, F. The relationship between work–family enrichment and nurse turnover. *J. Manag. Psychol.* **2012**, *27*, 216–236. [CrossRef]

38. Tummers, L.G.; Den Dulk, L. The effects of work alienation on organisational commitment, work effort and work-to-family enrichment. *J. Nurs. Manag.* **2013**, *21*, 850–859. [CrossRef]

39. Lecca, L.I.; Finstad, G.L.; Traversini, V.; Lulli, L.G.; Gualco, B.; Taddei, G. The Role of Job Support as a Target for the Management of Work-Related Stress: The State of Art. *Qual. Access Success* **2020**, *21*, 174.

40. Liu, Y.; Zhang, J.; Hennessy, D.A.; Zhao, S.; Ji, H. Psychological strains, depressive symptoms, and suicidal ideation among medical and non-medical staff in urban china. *J. Affect. Disord.* **2019**, *245*, 22–27. [CrossRef] [PubMed]

41. Henson, J.S. The Effectiveness of a Robotic Seal on Compassion Satisfaction in Acute Care Nurses: A Mixed Methods Approach. Ph.D. Thesis, The University of Texas at Tyler, Tyler, TX, USA, 2019.

42. Papastavrou, E.; Andreou, P.; Tsangari, H.; Schubert, M.; De Geest, S. Rationing of nursing care within professional environmental constraints: A correlational study. *Clin. Nurs. Res.* **2014**, *23*, 314–335. [CrossRef] [PubMed]

43. Schwarzer, R.; Knoll, N. Functional roles of social support within the stress and coping process: A theoretical and empirical overview. *Clin. Nurs. Res.* **2007**, *42*, 243–252. [CrossRef]

44. McGinnity, F.; Russell, H.; Watson, D.; Kingston, G.; Kelly, E. *Winners and Losers? The Equality Impact of the Great Recession in Ireland*; Economic and Social Research Institute (ESRI): Redlands, CA, USA, 2014; ISBN 978-1-908275-67-7.

45. Lahana, E.; Tsaras, K.; Kalaitzidou, A.; Galanis, P.; Kaitelidou, D.; Sarafis, P. Conflicts management in public sector nursing. *Int. J. Health Manag.* **2019**, *12*, 33–39. [CrossRef]

46. Russo, M.; Shteigman, A.; Carmeli, A. Workplace and family support and work–life balance: Implications for individual psychological availability and energy at work. *J. Posit. Psychol.* **2016**, *11*, 173–188. [CrossRef]

47. Haar, J.M.A.; Sune, A.; Russo, M.; Ollier-Malaterre, A. A cross-national study on the antecedents of work–life balance from the fit and balance perspective. *Soc. Indic. Res.* **2019**, *142*, 261–282. [CrossRef]

48. Cheng, S.Y.; Lin, P.C.; Chang, Y.K.; Lin, Y.K.; Lee, P.H.; Chen, S.R. Sleep quality mediates the relationship between work–family conflicts and the self-perceived health status among hospital nurses. *J. Nurs. Manag.* **2019**, *27*, 381–387. [CrossRef] [PubMed]

49. Neeson, J. Nurses are human beings too. *Nurs. Stand.* **2017**, *31*, 32. [CrossRef] [PubMed]

50. Lu, H.; Zhao, Y.; While, A. Job satisfaction among hospital nurses: A literature review. *Int. J. Nurs. Stud.* **2019**, *94*, 21–31. [CrossRef] [PubMed]

51. World Health Organization. *World Health Statistics: Monitoring Health for the SDGs Sustainable Development Goals*; World Health Organization: Geneva, Switzerland, 2018.

52. Lemieux-Cumberlege, A.; Taylor, E.P. An exploratory study on the factors affecting the mental health and well-being of frontline workers in homeless services. *Health Soc. Care Community* **2019**, *27*, e367–e378. [CrossRef]

53. Maslach, C.; Schaufeli, W.B.; Leiter, M.P. Job burnout. *Annu. Rev. Psychol.* **2001**, *52*, 397–422. [CrossRef]

54. Barnett, M.D.; Martin, K.J.; Garza, C.J. Satisfaction with work–family balance mediates the relationship between workplace social support and depression among hospice nurses. *J. Nurs. Sch.* **2019**, *51*, 187–194. [CrossRef]

55. Griffith, R. The elements of negligence liability in nursing. *Br. J. Nurs.* **2020**, *29*, 176–177. [CrossRef]

56. Harrod, M.; Petersen, L.; Weston, L.E.; Gregory, L.; Mayer, J.; Samore, M.H.; Drews, A.; Krein, S.L. Understanding workflow and personal protective equipment challenges across different healthcare personnel roles. *Clin. Infect. Dis.* **2019**, *69*, 185–191. [CrossRef]

57. Bureau of Labor Statistics Nonfatal Occupational Injuries and Illnesses Requiring Days Away From Work. *Industry Injury and Illness Data–2015*; Bureau of Labor Statistics, US Department of Labor: Washington, DC, USA, 2015; pp. 1–28.

58. Khan, S.A.; Waqas, M.; Siddiqui, M.; Ujjan, B.U.; Khan, M.; Bari, M.E.; Azeem, M.A. Work-life balance amongst residents in surgical and non-surgical specialties in a tertiary care hospital in Karachi. JPMA. *J. Pak. Med. Assoc.* **2020**, *70*, 252. [CrossRef]

59. Daxini, S.; Mehta, N. A Study on Impact of Work Stress on Work-Life balance Among Full Time Women Faculties in Self Financing Courses in Mumbai Suburban. *Adv. Innov. Res.* **2019**, *29*, 130–139.

60. Lin, Y.L.; Tomasi, J.; Guerguerian, A.M.; Trbovich, P. Technology-mediated macrocognition: Investigating how physicians, nurses, and respiratory therapists make critical decisions. *J. Crit. Care* **2019**, *53*, 132–141. [CrossRef] [PubMed]

61. Fukumori, T.; Miyazaki, A.; Takaba, C.; Taniguchi, S.; Asai, M. Traumatic Events Among Cancer Patients That Lead to Compassion Fatigue in Nurses: A Qualitative Study. *J. Pain Symptom Manag.* **2020**, *59*, 254–260. [CrossRef] [PubMed]

62. Hysong, S.J.; Amspoker, A.B.; Hughes, A.M.; Woodard, L.; Oswald, F.L.; Petersen, L.A.; Lester, H.F. Impact of team configuration and team stability on primary care quality. *Implement. Sci.* **2019**, *14*, 22. [CrossRef] [PubMed]

63. Hussain, I.R.; Mujtaba, B.G. The relationship between work-life conflict and employee performance: A study of national database and registration authority workers in Pakistan. *J. Knowl. Manag. Econ. Inf. Technol.* **2012**, *2*, 1–11.

64. Dobber, J.; Latour, C.; Snaterse, M.; van Meijel, B.; terRiet, G.; Scholte op Reimer, W.; Peters, R. Developing nurses' skills in motivational interviewing to promote a healthy lifestyle in patients with coronary artery disease. *Eur. J. Cardiovasc. Nurs.* **2019**, *18*, 28–37. [CrossRef]

65. Ulrich, B.; Barden, C.; Cassidy, L.; Varn-Davis, N. Frontline nurse manager and chief nurse executive skills: Perceptions of direct care nurses. *Nurse Leader* **2019**, *17*, 109–112. [CrossRef]

66. Dello Russo, S.; Mascia, D.; &Morandi, F. Individual perceptions of HR practices, HRM strength and appropriateness of care: A meso, multilevel approach. *Int. J. Hum. Resour. Manag.* **2018**, *29*, 286–310. [CrossRef]

67. Ronquillo, C.; Boschma, G.; Wong, S.T.; Quiney, L. Beyond greener pastures: Exploring contexts surrounding Filipino nurse migration in Canada through oral history. *Nurs. Inq.* **2011**, *18*, 262–275. [CrossRef]

68. Labrague, L.J.; McEnroe-Petitte, D.M.; Tsaras, K. Predictors and outcomes of nurse professional autonomy: A cross-sectional study. *Int. J. Nurs. Pr.* **2019**, *25*, e12711. [CrossRef]

69. Olmedo, G.R. Medicalización, psiquiatrización … ¿despsiquiatrización? *Con-Cienc. Soc. Anu. Didáctica Geogr. Hist. Cienc. Soc.* **2009**, *13*, 17–40.

70. Azizi, S.; Jafari, S.; Ebrahimian, A. Shortage of Men Nurses in the Hospitals in Iran and the World: A Narrative Review. *Sci. J. Nurs. Midwifery Paramed. Fac.* **2019**, *5*, 6–23.

71. White, E.M.; Aiken, L.H.; Sloane, D.M.; McHugh, M.D. Nursing home work environment, care quality, registered nurse burnout and job dissatisfaction. *Geriatr. Nurs.* **2019**, *52*. [CrossRef] [PubMed]

72. McGilton, K.S.; Tourangeau, A.; Kavcic, C.; Wodchis, W.P. Determinants of regulated nurses' intention to stay in long-term care homes. *J. Nurs. Manag.* **2013**, *21*, 771–781. [CrossRef] [PubMed]

73. Ropponen, A.; Koskinen, A.; Puttonen, S.; Härmä, M. Exposure to working-hour characteristics and short sickness absence in hospital workers: A case-crossover study using objective data. *Int. J. Nurs. Stud.* **2019**, *91*, 14–21. [CrossRef]

74. Van Der Heijden, B.I.; Peeters, M.C.; Le Blanc, P.M.; Van Breukelen, J.W.M. Job characteristics and experience as predictors of occupational turnover intention and occupational turnover in the European nursing sector. *J. Vocat. Behav.* **2018**, *108*, 108–120. [CrossRef]

75. De Jonge, J.; Mulder, M.J.; Nijhuis, F.J. The incorporation of different demand concepts in the job demand-control model: Effects on health care professionals. *Soc. Sci. Med.* **1999**, *48*, 1149–1160. [CrossRef]

76. Scanlan, J.N.; Still, M. Relationships between burnout, turnover intention, job satisfaction, job demands and job resources for mental health personnel in an Australian mental health service. *BMC Health Serv. Res.* **2019**, *19*, 62. [CrossRef]

77. Yamaguchi, Y.; Inoue, T.; Harada, H.; Oike, M. Job control, work-family balance and nurses' intention to leave their profession and organization: A comparative cross-sectional survey. *Int. J. Nurs. Stud.* **2016**, *64*, 52–62. [CrossRef]

78. Mark, G.; Smith, A.P. Occupational stress, job characteristics, coping, and the mental health of nurses. *Br. J. Health Psychol.* **2012**, *17*, 505–521. [CrossRef]

79. Smith, J.H.; Sweet, L. Becoming a nurse preceptor, the challenges and rewards of novice registered nurses in high acuity hospital environments. *Nurse Educ. Pr.* **2019**, *36*, 101–107. [CrossRef]

80. Sigurdardottir, A.O.; Svavarsdottir, E.K.; Juliusdottir, S. Family nursing hospital training and the outcome on job demands, control and support. *Nurse Educ. Today* **2015**, *35*, 854–858. [CrossRef] [PubMed]

81. Chiu, Y.L.; Tsai, C.C.; Chiang, C.Y.F. The relationships among nurses' job characteristics and attitudes toward web-based continuing learning. *Nurse Educ. Today* **2013**, *33*, 327–333. [CrossRef] [PubMed]

82. Nabirye, R.C.; Brown, K.C.; Pryor, E.R.; Maples, E.H. Occupational stress, job satisfaction and job performance among hospital nurses in Kampala, Uganda. *J. Nurs. Manag.* **2011**, *19*, 760–768. [CrossRef] [PubMed]

83. Sheridan, P.; Carragher, L.; Carragher, N.; Treacy, J. Development and validation of an instrument to measure stress among older adult nursing students: The Student Nurse Stressor-15 (SNS-15) Scale. *J. Clin. Nurs.* **2019**, *28*, 1336–1345. [CrossRef]

84. Kelly, L.A.; Lefton, C.; Fischer, S.A. Nurse Leader Burnout, Satisfaction, and Work-Life Balance. *JONA: J. Nurs. Adm.* **2019**, *49*, 404–410. [CrossRef]

85. Xanthopoulou, D.; Bakker, A.B.; Demerouti, E.; Schaufeli, W.B. Work engagement and financial returns: A diary study on the role of job and personal resources. *J. Occup. Organ. Psychol.* **2009**, *82*, 183–200. [CrossRef]

86. McVicar, A. Scoping the common antecedents of job stress and job satisfaction for nurses (2000–2013) using the job demands–resources model of stress. *J. Nurs. Manag.* **2016**, *24*, E112–E136. [CrossRef]

87. Hochwälder, J. The psychosocial work environment and burnout among Swedish registered and assistant nurses: The main, mediating, and moderating role of empowerment. *Nurs. Health Sci.* **2007**, *9*, 205–211. [CrossRef]

88. Sundin, L.; Hochwälder, J.; Bildt, C.; Lisspers, J. The relationship between different work-related sources of social support and burnout among registered and assistant nurses in Sweden: A questionnaire survey. *Int. J. Nurs. Stud.* **2007**, *44*, 758–769. [CrossRef]

89. Rugulies, R.; Aust, B.; &Pejtersen, J.H. Do psychosocial work environment factors measured with scales from the Copenhagen Psychosocial Questionnaire predict register-based sickness absence of 3 weeks or more in Denmark? *Scand. J. Public Health* **2010**, *38*, 42–50. [CrossRef]

90. Widerszal-Bazyl, M. Copenhagen psychosocial questionnaire (copsoq). *Medycynapracy* **2017**, *68*, 329–349.

91. Van Smeden, M.; Moons, K.G.; de Groot, J.A.; Collins, G.S.; Altman, D.G.; Eijkemans, M.J.; Reitsma, J.B. Sample size for binary logistic prediction models: Beyond events per variable criteria. *Stat. Methods Med Res.* **2019**, *28*, 2455–2474. [CrossRef] [PubMed]

92. Debray, T.P.; Damen, J.A.; Riley, R.D.; Snell, K.; Reitsma, J.B.; Hooft, L.; Collins, G.; Moons, K.G. A framework for meta-analysis of prediction model studies with binary and time-to-event outcomes. *Stat. Methods Med Res.* **2019**, *28*, 2768–2786. [CrossRef] [PubMed]

93. Birolim, M.M.; Mesas, A.E.; González, A.D.; Santos, H.G.D.; Haddad, M.D.C.F.L.; Andrade, S.M.D. Job strain among teachers: Associations with occupational factors according to social support. *Cienc. Saudecoletiva* **2019**, *24*, 1255–1264. [CrossRef]

94. Tam, J.Z.; Mohamed, Z.; Puteh, S.E.W.; Ismail, N.H. A systematic review on identifying associated factors in deciding work-relatedness of chronic back pain among employee. *Malays. J. Public Health Med.* **2019**, *19*, 1–14.

95. Nguyen Ngoc, A.; Le ThiThanh, X.; Le Thi, H.; Vu Tuan, A.; Nguyen Van, T. Occupational Stress Among Health Worker in a National Dermatology Hospital in Vietnam, 2018. *Frontiers in Psychiatry.* **2020**, *10*, 950. [CrossRef]

96. Wesołowska, K.; Elovainio, M.; Gluschkoff, K.; Hietapakka, L.; Kaihlanen, A.M.; Lehtoaro, S.; Heponiemi, T. Psychosocial work environment and cross-cultural competence among native and foreign-born registered nurses. *Res. Nurs. Health* **2019**, *42*, 349–357. [CrossRef]

97. BagheriHosseinabadi, M.; Ebrahimi, M.H.; Khanjani, N.; Biganeh, J.; Mohammadi, S.; Abdolahfard, M. The effects of amplitude and stability of circadian rhythm and occupational stress on burnout syndrome and job dissatisfaction among irregular shift working nurses. *J. Clin. Nurs.* **2019**, *28*, 1868–1878. [CrossRef]

98. Arnetz, J.; Sudan, S.; Goetz, C.; Counts, S.; Arnetz, B. Nurse work environment and stress biomarkers: Possible implications for patient outcomes. *J. Occup. Environ. Med.* **2019**, *61*, 676–681. [CrossRef]

99. Karatepe, O.M.; Uludag, O. Conflict, exhaustion, and motivation: A study of frontline employees in Northern Cyprus hotels. *Int. J. Hosp. Manag.* **2007**, *26*, 645–665. [CrossRef]

100. Ghislieri, C.; Gatti, P.; Molino, M.; Cortese, C.G. Work–family conflict and enrichment in nurses: Between job demands, perceived organisational support and work–family backlash. *J. Nurs. Manag.* **2017**, *25*, 65–75. [CrossRef] [PubMed]

101. Voydanoff, P. The effects of work demands and resources on work-to-family conflict and facilitation. *J. Nurs. Manag.* **2004**, *66*, 398–412. [CrossRef]

102. Hussain, A.; Rivers, P.A.; Glover, S.H.; Fottler, M.D. Strategies for dealing with future shortages in the nursing workforce: A review. *Health Serv. Manag. Res.* **2012**, *25*, 41–47. [CrossRef] [PubMed]

103. Mc Carthy, V.J.; Wills, T.; Crowley, S. Nurses, age, job demands and physical activity at work and at leisure: A cross-sectional study. *Appl. Nurs. Res.* **2018**, *40*, 116–121. [CrossRef]

104. Nam, S.; Lee, S.J. Occupational factors associated with obesity and leisure-time physical activity among nurses: A cross sectional study. *Int. J. Nurs. Stud.* **2016**, *57*, 60–69. [CrossRef]

105. Qureshi, M.A.; Ab Hamid, K.B.; Jeihoony, P.; Ali, R.; Brohi, N.A.; Magsi, R.; Shah, S.M.M. Is Supervisor Support Matter in Job Satisfaction? A Moderating Role of Fairness Perception among Nurses in Pakistan. *Acad. Strateg. Manag. J.* **2018**, *17*, 1–10.

106. Greenglass, E.R.; Burke, R.J.; Fiksenbaum, L. Workload and burnout in nurses. *J. Community Appl. Soc. Psychol.* **2001**, *11*, 211–215. [CrossRef]

107. Garrett, D.K.; McDaniel, A.M. A new look at nurse burnout: The effects of environmental uncertainty and social climate. *JONA J. Nurs. Adm.* **2001**, *31*, 91–96. [CrossRef]

108. Haluza, D.; Schmidt, V.M.; Blasche, G. Time course of recovery after two successive night shifts: A diary study among Austrian nurses. *J. Nurs. Manag.* **2019**, *27*, 190–196. [CrossRef]

109. Vedaa, Ø.; Harris, A.; Erevik, E.K.; Waage, S.; Bjorvatn, B.; Sivertsen, B.; Moen, B.E.; Pallesen, S. Short rest between shifts (quick returns) and night work is associated with work-related accidents. *Int. Arch. Occup. Environ. Health* **2019**, *92*, 829–835. [CrossRef]

110. Mahendran, A.V.; Panatik, S.A.; Rajab, A.; Nordin, N. The Influence of Work-life Balance on Burnout among Nurses. *Indian, J. Public Health Res. Dev.* **2019**, *10*, 3338. [CrossRef]

111. Bae, J.; Jennings-McGarity, P.; Hardeman, C.P.; Kim, E.; Lee, M.; Littleton, T.; Saasa, S. Compassion Satisfaction Among Social Work Practitioners: The Role of Work–Life Balance. *J. Soc. Serv. Res.* **2019**, 1–11. [CrossRef]

112. Pisarski, A.; Brook, C.; Bohle, P.; Gallois, C.; Watson, B.; Winch, S. Extending a model of shift-work tolerance. *Chronobiol. Int.* **2006**, *23*, 1363–1377. [CrossRef] [PubMed]

113. Chunta, K.S. New Nurse Leaders: Creating a Work-Life Balance and Finding Joy in Work. *J. Radiol. Nurs.* **2020**. [CrossRef]

114. Dousin, O.; Collins, N.; Kaur Kler, B. Work-Life Balance, Employee Job Performance and Satisfaction Among Doctors and Nurses in Malaysia. *Int. J. Hum. Resour. Stud.* **2019**, *9*, 306–319. [CrossRef]

115. Fuentes, R. Implementing a Self-Scheduling Model to Decrease Nurse Turnover in Medical-Surgical Nursing. Ph.D. Thesis, Walden University, Minneapolis, MI, USA, 2019.

116. Ahmed, J.; Saleem, N.; Fatima, K. Factors Influencing Work Life Balance of Women Entrepreneurs: A Case of Quetta (Pakistan). *Dialogue* **2019**, *14*, 93.

117. Zaghini, F.; Fiorini, J.; Piredda, M.; Fida, R.; Sili, A. The relationship between nurse managers' leadership style and patients' perception of the quality of the care provided by nurses: Cross sectional survey. *Int. J. Nurs. Stud.* **2020**, *101*, 103446. [CrossRef]

118. De Souza, B.; Ramsay, R. Medical Women's Federation celebrates its long history. *BMJ* **2019**, *336*, 90. [CrossRef]

119. Hirschman, A.O. *Exit, Voice, and Loyalty: Responses to decline in Firms, Organizations, and States*; Harvard University Press: Cambridge, MA, USA, 1970; Volume 25.

120. Mushfiqur, R.; Mordi, C.; Oruh, E.S.; Nwagbara, U.; Mordi, T.; Turner, I.M. The impacts of work-life-balance (WLB) challenges on social sustainability: The experience of Nigerian female medical doctors. *Empl. Relat.* **2018**, *40*, 868–888. [CrossRef]

121. Adisa, T.A.; Gbadamosi, G.; Osabutey, E.L. What happened to the border? The role of mobile information technology devices on employees' work-life balance. *Pers. Rev.* **2017**, *46*, 1651–1671. [CrossRef]

122. Abdul-Rashid, S.H.; Sakundarini, N.; Raja Ghazilla, R.A.; Thurasamy, R. The impact of sustainable manufacturing practices on sustainability performance: Empirical evidence from Malaysia. *Int. J. Oper. Prod. Manag.* **2017**, *37*, 182–204. [CrossRef]

123. Kim, J.H.; Kim, M.Y. Factors affecting organizational commitment of general hospital nurses in small and medium sized cities. *J. Korean Acad. Nurs. Adm.* **2019**, *25*, 14–24. [CrossRef]

124. Tabriz, A.A.; Birken, S.A.; Shea, C.M.; Fried, B.J.; Viccellio, P. What is full capacity protocol, and how is it implemented successfully? *Implement. Sci.* **2019**, *14*, 73. [CrossRef]

125. Wallace, A.S.; Pierce, N.L.; Davisson, E.; Manges, K.; Tripp-Reimer, T. Social resource assessment: Application of a novel communication tool during hospital discharge. *Patient Educ. Couns.* **2019**, *102*, 542–549. [CrossRef] [PubMed]
126. Baris, V.K.; Seren Intepeler, S. Cross-cultural adaptation and psychometric evaluation of the Turkish version of the Self-Efficacy for Preventing Falls-Nurse. *J. Nurs. Manag.* **2019**, *27*, 1791–1800. [CrossRef] [PubMed]
127. Tucker, M.K.; Jimmieson, N.L.; Bordia, P. Supervisor support as a double-edged sword: Supervisor emotion management accounts for the buffering and reverse-buffering effects of supervisor support. *Int. J. Stress Manag.* **2018**, *25*, 14. [CrossRef]
128. Somers, M.J.; Birnbaum, D.; Casal, J. Supervisor support, control over work methods and employee well-being: New insights into nonlinearity from artificial neural networks. *Int. J. Hum. Resour. Manag.* **2018**, 1–23. [CrossRef]
129. Jennings, K.N. In the balance: Work/life balance of senior development professionals within higher education. Ph.D. Thesis, Iowa State University, Ames, IA, USA, 2007.
130. Pelfrene, E.; Vlerick, P.; Kittel, F.; Mak, R.P.; Kornitzer, M.; Backer, G.D. Psychosocial work environment and psychological well-being: Assessment of the buffering effects in the job demand–control (–support) model in BELSTRESS. *Stress Health* **2002**, *18*, 43–56. [CrossRef]

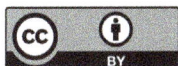

International Journal of
Environmental Research and Public Health

MDPI

Article

Workplace Violence and Its Effects on Burnout and Secondary Traumatic Stress among Mental Healthcare Nurses in Japan

Yudai Kobayashi, Misari Oe *, Tetsuya Ishida, Michiko Matsuoka, Hiromi Chiba and Naohisa Uchimura

Department of Neuropsychiatry, Kurume University School of Medicine, Asahi-machi 67,
Kurume 830-0011, Japan
* Correspondence: oe_misari@kurume-u.ac.jp

Received: 17 March 2020; Accepted: 14 April 2020; Published: 16 April 2020

check for
updates

Abstract: Workplace violence (WPV) in healthcare settings has drawn attention for over 20 years, yet few studies have investigated the association between WPV and psychological consequences. Here, we used a cross-sectional design to investigate (1) the 12-month prevalence of workplace violence (WPV), (2) the characteristics of WPV, and (3) the relationship between WPV and burnout/secondary traumatic stress among 599 mental healthcare nurses (including assistant nurses) from eight hospitals. Over 40% of the respondents had experienced WPV within the past 12 months. A multivariate logistic regression analysis indicated that occupation and burnout were each significantly related to WPV. Secondary traumatic stress was not related to WPV. Our results suggest that WPV may be a long-lasting and/or cumulative stressor rather than a brief, extreme horror experience and may reflect specific characteristics of psychological effects in psychiatric wards. A longitudinal study measuring the severity and frequency of WPV, work- and non-work-related stressors, risk factors, and protective factors is needed, as is the development of a program that helps reduce the psychological burden of mental healthcare nurses due to WPV.

Keywords: workplace violence; mental healthcare nurses; secondary traumatic stress; burnout; nursing license

1. Introduction

Workplace violence (WPV) is defined as any incident in which a person is abused, threatened, or assaulted in circumstances related to their work; this can include verbal abuse and threats as well as physical attacks [1,2]. The International Labor Organization reported that the magnitude of exposure to violence at work depends not only on a person's occupation but also upon the circumstances named "situations at risk," including those associated with working alone (e.g., small shops); working with the public (e.g., railway workers); working with valuables (e.g., financial institutions); working with people in distress (e.g., healthcare workers); working in an environment that is increasingly open to violence (e.g., school teachers); working in conditions of special vulnerability (e.g., immigrant workers); working in military and paramilitary organizations; and working in zones of conflict [3].

Workplace violence (WPV) in healthcare settings has been drawing attention for over 20 years [2,4–8] and has been reported in many places, including Europe [9], Asia [10–12], the U.S. [13], and the Middle East [14]. According to a recent review, the prevalence of WPV against healthcare workers was higher in Asian and North American countries than that in other countries [15]. Female nurses were reported to be the victims of verbal abuse more often than male nurses, and male nurses were reported to be more commonly the victims of physical abuse [7]. Most of the WPV in healthcare settings occurs in psychiatric departments, emergency services, polyclinics/waiting rooms, and geriatric units [8].

According to a review of WPV in psychiatric wards over the past 20 years, studies of WPV have examined mainly its occurrence rate, risk assessment, and risk management; fewer investigations have assessed the physical and psychological consequences of WPV [2]. WPV may cause not only physical injuries but also psychological impacts, resulting in higher rates of fear or anxiety, anger, insecurity, depression, emotional exhaustion, suicidal thoughts, post-traumatic stress symptoms, guilt, self-blame, and shame [2,8]. The consequences of WPV include decreased job satisfaction, increased intent to leave the organization, and lowered health-related quality of life [2].

WPV and its consequences among nurses in Japan have been described [10,16–20]. Of respondents to previous surveys, 33–47% of the nurses had experienced WPV during the prior 12 months [16–18]. The proportion of nurses who experienced physical aggression and verbal abuse was significantly high in psychiatric wards [16]. Another study showed that nurses who had encountered verbal abuse or violence by patients in psychiatry departments had experienced severe psychological impacts such as secondary traumatic stress and low satisfaction with family support [10]. The characteristics of WPV itself in Japan have been evaluated, but few studies have examined the psychological effects of WPV in detail.

Burnout is defined as a syndrome conceptualized as resulting from chronic workplace stress that has not been successfully managed [21]. It is characterized by three dimensions: feelings of energy depletion or exhaustion; increased mental distance from one's job or feelings of negativism or cynicism related to one's job; and reduced professional efficacy [21]. In the International Classification of Diseases, 11th revision (ICD-11), the definition is more detailed: "burnout refers specifically to phenomena in the occupational context and should not be applied experiences in other areas of life" [22]. Among healthcare workers, nurses are known to struggle with burnout symptoms the most, and this poses serious consequences for patients, other healthcare professionals, and healthcare organizations [23]. A meta-analysis on burnout in mental healthcare nurses showed that variables such as work overload, work-related stress, professional seniority, male gender, being single, and aggression at work contributed to burnout development [24]. Burnout is regarded as one of the relevant consequences of WPV [2,25]. Associations between WPV and burnout, turnover intention [26,27], and intention to leave [28] have been described.

Secondary traumatic stress (STS) is a syndrome including intrusion, avoidance, and arousal resulting from indirect traumatic exposure in a professional context [29]. A study conducted in Israel showed that psychiatric nurses reported higher levels of STS symptoms compared to community nurses [30]. Another study revealed a high correlation between work-related post-traumatic stress disorder (PTSD) symptoms (due to traumatic stressors such as WPV), STS, and burnout in psychiatric nurses [31].

We conducted the present study to investigate the prevalence of WPV and its effects on burnout and STS among mental healthcare nurses in Japan. We focused on mental healthcare nurses because there have been few investigations of the association between WPV and psychological consequences. We conducted a large-scale, multicenter study to clarify the psychological impact of WPV by using questionnaires about the respondents' well-being, psychological distress, alcohol use disorder, and anger related to harmful experiences, as well as compassion satisfaction, burnout and STS. We tested our hypothesis that mental healthcare nurses who have experienced WPV have a higher rate of burnout and higher secondary traumatic stress.

2. Participants and Methods

2.1. Study Design

This is a questionnaire-based cross-sectional study.

2.2. Participants and Procedures

Mental health nurses and mental health assistant nurses working at the mental health ward of a university hospital or one of seven mental health hospitals (i.e., psychiatric inpatient, outpatient, and day-treatment centers) on the island of Kyushu in Japan were recruited using the convenience (i.e., not randomized) sampling method. The inclusion criterion was age 20–79 years old. Candidates who could not understand the questionnaires in Japanese were excluded.

The researcher in charge (Y.K.) explained the purpose and methods of the research to the head nurse of the psychiatric neurology ward of A University Hospital (pseudonym) and the head of each hospital both in a letter of request and orally. After obtaining the hospital's consent to participate in the research in a letter of consent, the researcher in charge distributed a set of questionnaires to the person in charge of the target hospital (the person in charge of the facility at the head of each ward or the secretary-level depending on the hospital). The researcher in charge verbally explained the freedom of research participation, significance, the purpose of use, method of use, questionnaire items, the protection of personal information, the questionnaire handling after collection, and contact information, etc. to the person in charge at the facility. That person then verbally explained the study to the research subjects, i.e., nurses. Participants were encouraged to fill out the questionnaires when they were alone outside of work hours. The questionnaires were hand-delivered by a person in charge at each hospital, and the enclosed envelopes were sealed up to 2 weeks after distribution. The completed questionnaires were dropped into collection boxes placed temporarily at each hospital. The researcher in charge retrieved the questionnaires.

The respondents' data were collected from October 18 to November 30, 2019. The questionnaires were administered and completed anonymously. We collected sociodemographic data such as sex, age, marital status, occupation, years of experience as a registered nurse or as an assistant nurse, the type of present workplace (acute ward or others). Of 650 eligible nurses, 599 nurses and assistant nurses participated in the study (response rate, 92.2%). We did not obtain the sociodemographic information of the non-respondents.

2.3. Measures

2.3.1. Well-Being

The World Health Organization-Five Well-Being Index (WHO-5) is a five-item self-report questionnaire developed by the WHO; it measures the respondent's current mental well-being [32]. The total raw score, ranging from 0 to 25, is multiplied by 4 to give the final score, with 0 representing the worst imaginable well-being and 100 representing the best imaginable well-being. The Japanese version of the WHO-5 was validated by Awata et al. [33,34] and showed sufficient reliability and validity in community-dwelling elderly persons and in diabetic patients. A cutoff score of the Japanese WHO-5 version at 11/12 or 12/13 of the raw total score for detecting depression was recommended by Awata et al. for the Japanese version [33]. In the present study, we used 12/13 as the cutoff score for low well-being according to Awata's recommendation. Cronbach's alpha of the present study was 0.89.

2.3.2. Psychological Distress

The Kessler six-item scale (K6) is a self-report questionnaire measuring psychological distress; it consists of six brief questions [35]. The total score (ranging from 0 to 24) has been used as an indicator of serious mental illness or mood and anxiety disorders in the general population. The Japanese version of the K6 showed screening performance that was essentially equivalent to that of the original English version [36,37]. We adopted the 12/13 cut-off according to Kessler's recommendation [35]. The Cronbach's alpha of the present study was 0.88.

2.3.3. Alcohol Use Disorder

The Alcohol Use Disorder Identification Test (AUDIT), which was developed by the WHO for the screening of excessive drinking, is a 10-item self-report questionnaire [38]. The Japanese version of the AUDIT was validated by Kawada et al. [39] and showed satisfactory internal reliability. The score ranges from 0 to 40. In Japan, a total score ≥11 is considered indicative of alcohol abuse [40]. The Cronbach's alpha of the present study was 0.79.

2.3.4. Anger Related to Harmful Experience

The Dimensions of Anger Reaction-5 (DAR-5) is a five-item self-report questionnaire regarding the respondent's anger reaction after a harmful experience such as violence. The DAR-5 was developed and validated by Forbes et al. [41,42]. The score ranges from 5 to 25. Because the Japanese version of the DAR-5 has not been developed, we used a back-translated version provided by a principal researcher in this study. According to Forbes et al., the cutoff point of 12 was used for high risk. The Cronbach's alpha of the present study was 0.80.

2.3.5. Workplace Violence

For assessing WPV, we asked eight questions that were used in a prior study's questionnaire regarding WPV [43]; that questionnaire was derived from the "WPV in the Health Sector Country Case Studies Research Instruments Survey Questionnaires" [44] as set out by an International Labor Office/International Council of Nurses/WHO/Public Services International (ILO/ICN/WHO/PSI) project. Because there was no Japanese version for these questions, we used a back-translated version provided by a principal researcher. Among the eight questions, four were qualitative yes/no questions (the existence of violence within the past 12 months, the existence of physical injury, whether the respondent thinks that this violence was avoidable, and the presence of help-seeking behavior); one was a quantitative question (psychological influence), and the remaining three questions were qualitative multiple-choice questions (characteristics of violence, perpetrator, type of coping behaviors).

2.3.6. Burnout, Secondary Traumatic Stress, and Compassion Satisfaction

We used the ProQOL (Professional Quality of Life) scale to measure burnout and secondary traumatic stress simultaneously. As a 30-item self-report questionnaire developed by Stamm [45], the ProQOL consists of three subscales: compassion satisfaction, burnout, and secondary traumatic stress. "Compassion satisfaction" is about the pleasure that a person derives from being able to do his/her work well. Burnout and secondary traumatic stress are negative aspects of one's professional quality of life. In the ProQOL scale, burnout is indicated by exhaustion, frustration, anger, and depressive symptoms. An example of the scale's burnout subscale questions is "I feel connected to others." Secondary traumatic stress is about work-related secondary exposure to people who have experienced extremely or traumatically stressful events. The negative effects of secondary traumatic stress can include fear, sleep difficulties, intrusive images, and avoiding reminders of the person's traumatic experiences. An example of the ProQOL scale's secondary traumatic stress question is "I jump or am startled by unexpected sounds."

The Japanese version of the ProQOL was validated by Fukumori et al. [46]. According to those authors, a high risk of compassion satisfaction is indicated by a score of ≤26 points, a high risk of burnout by a score of ≥33 points, and a high risk of secondary traumatic stress by ≥28 points [46]. The Cronbach's alpha of the present study was 0.78. We considered the fact that burnout and secondary traumatic stress were clearly separated as subscales to be an advantage in the present study.

2.4. Statistical Analyses

All statistical analyses were conducted using JMP Pro for Windows, ver. 14 (SAS Institute, Cary, NC, USA). The chi-square (χ^2) test was used for testing relationships between categorical variables.

The Shapiro–Wilk test was used to check normal distributions of the continuous variables. Only the compassion satisfaction subscale of the ProQOL showed a normal distribution. In light of these results, we decided to use non-parametric analyses. The Mann–Whitney U test was used for comparisons of two independent groups. We performed a multivariate logistic regression analysis to test the association between a categorical dependent variable and a set of independent variables. All tests were two-sided and based on a 0.05 level of significance. Pairwise deletion was conducted for missing data.

2.5. Ethical Considerations

All subjects gave their informed consent for inclusion before they participated in the study. The study was conducted in accord with the Declaration of Helsinki, and the protocol was approved by the Ethical Committee of Kurume University, Japan (approval no. 19100, approved on 9 September 2019).

3. Results

3.1. Sociodemographic Characteristics of the Participants

The sociodemographic characteristics of the study participants are summarized in Table 1. Females accounted for 65.4% of the participants, and the mean age was 47.1 years. Regarding the specific nursing occupations, 66.4% of the participants were certified nurses, and 32.6% had an assistant nurse certification. Concerning marital status, 353 (58.9%) of the participants were married, 122 (20.4%) participants were single, 87 (14.5%) participants were divorced, and 30 (5.0%) participants were widowed (missing data; $n = 7$). There were 258 (43.6%) participants working at acute wards, and the others were working at chronic wards or at an outpatient division.

Table 1. Sociodemographics and comparison of the groups with and without workplace violence within the past 12 months ($n = 599$).

Variables	Total ($n = 599$)	With WPV ($n = 265$)	Without WPV ($n = 328$)	Test	Probability
	n	n (%)	n (%)	x^2	p
Sex					
Female	390	169 (43.7)	218 (56.3)		
Male	206	95 (46.3)	110 (53.7)	0.4	0.5
Missing	3				
Occupation					
Nurse	398	197 (49.5)	201 (50.5)		
Assistant nurse	195	64 (33.5)	127 (66.5)	13.6 *	<0.01
Missing	6				
Ward					
Acute ward	258	129 (50.2)	128 (49.8)		
Others	334	134 (40.5)	197 (59.5)	5.5 *	0.02
Missing	7				
	Mean (SD)	**Mean (SD)**	**Mean (SD)**	**|z|**	**p**
Age, years	47.1 (13.2)	45.7 (11.9)	48.4 (14.0)	2.5 *	0.01
Duration as nurse, years	19.8 (13.4)	19.0 (11.9)	20.5 (14.5)	0.8	0.4
WHO-5 final score	48.2 (19.0)	45.5 (18.7)	50.3 (19.0)	2.8 *	<0.01
K6	5.4 (4.5)	6.2 (4.9)	4.7 (4.1)	3.8*	<0.01
AUDIT	3.9 (4.7)	3.9 (4.8)	3.8 (4.6)	0.4	0.7
DAR-5	7.3 (2.6)	7.9 (3.0)	6.8 (2.2)	5.2 *	<0.01
Compassion satisfaction	24.4 (8.7)	23.5 (9.0)	25.2 (8.4)	2.3*	0.02
Burnout	25.4 (6.4)	26.5 (5.8)	24.4 (6.8)	3.3*	<0.01
Secondary traumatic stress	12.0 (6.8)	13.6 (7.1)	10.6 (6.2)	5.4*	<0.01

WPV: workplace violence; WHO-5: World Health Organization-Five Well-Being Index; K6: Kessler Six-Item Scale; AUDIT: Alcohol Use Disorder Identification Test; DAR-5: Dimensions of Anger Reaction-5. * $p < 0.05$.

3.2. Prevalence of WPV within the Past 12 Months and the Characteristics of the WPV

Among these 599 mental health nurses (including assistant nurses), 265 participants (44.7%) answered that they had experienced WPV within the past 12 months. Regarding the types of violence (multiple choices were available), verbal violence was reported by 165 participants (62.3% of 265 victims); physical violence was reported by 160 participants (60.4%); and sexual violence was reported by seven participants (2.6%). Sex did not affect the percentages of the types of violence. The mean age among the nurses who experienced physical violence was significantly lower than that of the nurses who had not had this experience: (mean ± SD) 44.7 ± 12.0 vs. 48.2 ± 13.4, $|z| = 2.9$, $p < 0.01$). The percentages of verbal violence and sex violence were not significantly different among the types of working wards, but the percentage of physical violence in the participants working at acute wards (33.3%) was significantly higher than that of the participants working at other places (22.0%, $\chi^2 = 9.4$, $p < 0.01$). The percentage of sexual violence did not differ by occupation, but there was a significantly higher percentage of verbal violence among the nurses (31.1%) than among the assistant nurses (21.4%, $\chi^2 = 6.1$, $p = 0.01$), and a significantly higher percentage of physical violence among the nurses (30.8%) than among the assistant nurses (18.2%, $\chi^2 = 10.5$, $p < 0.01$).

The perpetrators of WPV were the subject of a multiple-choice question: 223 participants (84.2% of 265 victims) reported that the perpetrator was a patient, 11 participants (4.2%) described a patient's family member, 35 participants (13.2%) reported a work colleague, and 33 participants (12.5%) responded that their boss or supervisor was the perpetrator of WPV.

3.3. Mental Health Status of Nurses Who Experience WPV

The mean values and standard deviations of the mental health status results are summarized in Table 1. The number of participants who attained a low value of well-being as the WHO-5 raw score was 310 (52.6%) participants. The number of participants with high psychological distress on the K6 was 42 (7.1%). Fifty-six (10.1%) participants reported problem drinking, and 41 (7.2%) participants were at high risk of anger related to harmful experiences. The number of participants at high risk of compassion satisfaction was 332 (59.4%); that of burnout was 62 (10.9%); and that of secondary traumatic stress was 18 (3.2%).

3.4. Comparisons of the Groups with and without Workplace Violence

The results of our comparisons of mental health status between the participants with ($n = 265$) and without ($n = 328$) WPV (missing data; $n = 6$) are provided in Table 1. The χ^2 analyses revealed that there were significant differences between these two groups in occupation and type of workplace (wards). The nurses had experienced WPV more than the assistant nurses had, and the nurses who were working at acute wards had experienced WPV more compared to the nurses who worked at other wards. There was no significant difference in the experience of WPV based on marital status. The Mann–Whitney U-tests showed that there were significant differences in age, the well-being score, psychological distress, anger, and three subscales of professional quality of life. The participants who experienced WPV were younger and showed lower well-being, higher psychological distress, higher anger, lower compassion satisfaction, higher burnout, and higher secondary traumatic stress.

3.5. Risk Factors of Workplace Violence

To investigate the risk factors of WPV, we conducted a multivariate logistic regression analysis using sociodemographic characteristic variables (sex, age, years of experience, occupation, and ward type) and symptom measures (well-being, psychological distress, alcohol use, anger, (low) compassion satisfaction, burnout, and secondary traumatic stress) as listed in Table 2. Among them, occupation and burnout were each identified as a significant factor related to WPV. The odds ratio of nurses experiencing WPV compared to the assistant nurses was 2.03.

Table 2. Multivariate logistic regression analysis for workplace violence within the past 12 months.

Independent Variable	Beta	Wald	*p*	OR	95% CI
Sex, 1: male, 0: female	−0.08	0.57	0.45	0.85	0.55–1.31
Age	−0.01	0.70	0.40	0.99	0.96–1.01
Years of experience	−0.005	0.16	0.69	1.00	0.97–1.01
Occupation, 1: Nurse, 0: Assistant nurse	0.35	9.96	<0.01	2.03	1.31–3.15
Ward, 1: Acute ward, 0: other	0.09	0.72	0.39	1.19	0.80–1.78
WHO-5, 1: raw score ≤12, 0: others	0.04	0.17	0.68	1.09	0.72–1.67
K6, 1: ≥13, 0: others	0.28	1.70	0.19	1.75	0.75–4.06
AUDIT, 1: ≥11, 0: others	0.13	0.53	0.47	1.29	0.65–2.55
DAR-5, 1: ≥12, 0: others	0.29	2.09	0.15	1.78	0.81–3.90
Compassion satisfaction, 1: ≤26, 0: others	0.05	0.24	0.62	1.11	0.73–1.70
Burnout, 1: ≥33, 0: others	0.34	4.33	0.04	1.99	1.04–3.81
Secondary traumatic stress, 1: ≥28, 0: others	0.22	0.46	0.50	1.55	0.44–5.50

4. Discussion

4.1. Main Findings

The respondents' questionnaire results demonstrated that >40% of the respondents had experienced WPV within the prior 12 months. Compared to the nurses who did not experience WPV, the respondents who experienced WPV were younger and showed lower well-being scores, higher psychological distress, higher anger, lower compassion satisfaction, higher burnout, and higher secondary traumatic stress. These results revealed that WPV affects the mental health status of staff. The high prevalence of WPV observed in this study population is consistent with those of studies conducted in Japan [16] and other countries [43,47]. The effects of WPV on the present nurses' mental health status are also in line with those of previous investigations [2,8].

However, our present findings do not support our hypothesis that WPV is associated with higher burnout and higher secondary traumatic stress. In the multivariate regression analysis, only burnout was associated with WPV; secondary traumatic stress was not. The association we observed between WPV and burnout is in agreement with previous studies [25,48,49]. A cross-sectional study conducted in the Netherlands revealed that physical aggression was positively associated with the staff's burnout symptoms [48], and this association remained in the same study sample over a two-year longitudinal study [49]. The advantage of the present investigation is that we examined burnout and secondary traumatic stress using the ProQOL scale, which can avoid overlapping of symptoms. Our finding that WPV was not associated with secondary traumatic stress suggests that the psychological burden of mental healthcare nurses that is due to WPV may be recognized as a long-lasting and/or cumulative stressor rather than as a brief, extreme horror experience, and it may reflect specific characteristics of psychological effects in psychiatric wards.

Researchers in Israel investigating mental healthcare nurses reported that the association between WPV and burnout/secondary traumatic stress was observed only indirectly via general work stress in the prior month [50]. Those authors explained that mental healthcare nurses may feel that WPV is an integral component of their job, and low burnout/secondary traumatic stress may be an adjusted reaction to their work environment [50,51]. Our present data showing a direct association between WPV and burnout may call this idea into question, and it may suggest that mental healthcare nurses with WPV feel a psychological overload as maladaptation to their work environment.

Interestingly, we also observed that the type of nursing license was a risk factor for WPV; the questionnaire results demonstrated that the nurses experienced more WPV than the assistant nurses. This is not consistent with a recent Japanese study investigating job-related stress [52]. In that study, assistant nurses who were working at psychiatry hospitals experienced more irritability and somatic symptoms than the nurses working there. The authors of that study speculated that stronger stress reactions of assistant nurses were observed because of their lesser education period compared to the certified nurses. In our study, we asked about the existence of WPV, which is categorized into an objective variable. The reason for the higher frequency of WPV among nurses may be because nurses tend to play a more responsible role; for example, persuading a patient to accept medication or a medical treatment or conducting forced treatment. A U.S. study investigating work-related violence based on the type of nursing license (between registered nurses and licensed practical nurses) showed that the risk of physical assault was increased for the licensed practical nurses working with neonatal/pediatric patients, whereas the registered nurses' risk was decreased; the registered nurses' risk of physical violence increased while providing patient care, whereas the licensed practical nurses' risk increased while supervising patient care [53].

Although we did not find an association in multivariate analysis, our present study revealed that psychiatric nurses working at acute wards had encountered more physical violence compared to that in other workplaces for nurses. This is consistent with a study that showed that patients with mental illness (affected by dementia, mental retardation, drug and substance abuse, or other psychiatric disorders) were the most frequent perpetrators of physical violence in a general hospital [54]. It is also of note that verbal violence was observed equally in acute wards and in other places including chronic wards in the present study.

4.2. Recommendations for Further Research

We raise four major challenges for further research. First, because we did not measure the severity and frequency of WPV, a study measuring them may play a role. Second, we detected an association between WPV and burnout, but we did not ask the participants about their stressors other than WPV. Moreover, our study was cross-sectional. It is thus necessary to conduct a large-scale longitudinal cohort study to assess the impacts of WPV, work-related stressors, and non-work-related stressors. It has been reported that both WPV and burnout were positively associated with turnover intention [26]. Third, not only risk factors but also factors that protect against negative psychological impacts after WPV should be examined. A study in Canada investigated the role of relational occupational coping self-efficacy against workplace incivility and burnout and revealed that self-coping is a protective factor [55]. Fourth, a program that helps reduce the psychological burden of mental healthcare nurses due to WPV should be developed. A study demonstrated that the life satisfaction of mental healthcare nurses was affected more by staff resilience, post-traumatic growth, and job stress than by WPV [56]. A program with strategies for increasing occupational coping self-efficacy, resilience, and post-traumatic growth may be effective.

4.3. Study Limitations

There are several limitations to be considered in this study. (1) The study's design was cross-sectional, and we cannot discuss causality. (2) We did not include a comparison group such as nurses working in an internal medicine ward. (3) We did not use validated versions of the evaluations for anger and WPV. (4) We did not obtain the sociodemographic information of the non-respondents; this may have caused selection bias.

5. Conclusions

The results of our study demonstrated that mental healthcare nurses who experienced WPV showed a poorer mental health status, and WPV was associated with burnout among mental healthcare nurses in Japan. Further research is merited, including longitudinal studies, investigations assessing

Int. J. Environ. Res. Public Health **2020**, *17*, 2747

risk and protective factors, and the development of an intervention program for the psychological burden experienced after WPV. An expansion of the existing call to action by the implementation of policy changes is also important to mitigate workplace violence in healthcare settings.

Author Contributions: Conceptualization, Y.K., M.O., M.M., and T.I.; methodology, M.O.; writing—original draft preparation, Y.K. and M.O.; writing—review and editing, M.M., T.I., H.C., and N.U.; project administration, M.O.; funding acquisition, H.C. and M.O. All authors have read and agreed to the published version of the manuscript.

Funding: This work was supported by JSPS KAKENHI Grant Number JP19K17121. The article processing charge was funded by JSPS KAKENHI Grant Number JP19K17121.

Conflicts of Interest: The authors declare no conflict of interest.

References

1. Health and Safety Executive. Work-related Violence. Available online: http://www.hse.gov.uk/violence/index.htm. (accessed on 1 April 2020).
2. d'Ettorre, G.; Pellicani, V. Workplace Violence Toward Mental Healthcare Workers Employed in Psychiatric Wards. *Saf. Health Work* **2017**, *8*, 337–342. [CrossRef]
3. Chappell, D.; Di Martino, V. *Violence at Work*, 3rd ed.; International Labour Office: Geneva, Switzerland, 2006.
4. Schnieden, V. Violence against doctors. *Br. J. Hosp. Med.* **1993**, *50*, 9.
5. Martinez, A.J. Managing Workplace Violence with Evidence-Based Interventions: A Literature Review. *J. Psychosoc. Nurs. Ment. Health Serv.* **2016**, *54*, 31–36. [CrossRef]
6. D'Ettorre, G.; Pellicani, V.; Mazzotta, M.; Vullo, A. Preventing and managing workplace violence against healthcare workers in Emergency Departments. *Acta Biomed.* **2018**, *89*, 28–36. [CrossRef] [PubMed]
7. Edward, K.L.; Stephenson, J.; Ousey, K.; Lui, S.; Warelow, P.; Giandinoto, J.A. A systematic review and meta-analysis of factors that relate to aggression perpetrated against nurses by patients/relatives or staff. *J. Clin. Nurs.* **2016**, *25*, 289–299. [CrossRef] [PubMed]
8. Mento, C.; Silvestri, M.C.; Bruno, A.; Muscatello, M.R.A.; Cedro, C.; Pandolfo, G.; Zoccali, R.A. Workplace violence against healthcare professionals: A systematic review. *Aggress. Violence Behav.* **2020**, *51*, 101381. [CrossRef]
9. Firenze, A.; Santangelo, O.E.; Gianfredi, V.; Alagna, E.; Cedrone, F.; Provenzano, S.; La Torre, G. Violence on doctors. An observational study in Northern Italy. *Med. Lav.* **2020**, *111*, 46–53. [CrossRef] [PubMed]
10. Inoue, M.; Tsukano, K.; Muraoka, M.; Kaneko, F.; Okamura, H. Psychological impact of verbal abuse and violence by patients on nurses working in psychiatric departments. *Psychiatry Clin. Neurosci.* **2006**, *60*, 29–36. [CrossRef] [PubMed]
11. Shi, L.; Li, G.; Hao, J.; Wang, W.; Chen, W.; Liu, S.; Yu, Z.; Shi, Y.; Ma, Y.; Fan, L.; et al. Psychological depletion in physicians and nurses exposed to workplace violence: A cross-sectional study using propensity score analysis. *Int. J. Nurs. Stud.* **2020**, *103*, 103493. [CrossRef]
12. Lee, H.L.; Han, C.Y.; Redley, B.; Lin, C.C.; Lee, M.Y.; Chang, W. Workplace Violence Against Emergency Nurses in Taiwan: A Cross-Sectional Study. *J. Emerg. Nurs.* **2020**, *46*, 66–71.e64. [CrossRef]
13. Phillips, J.P. Workplace Violence against Health Care Workers in the United States. *N. Engl. J. Med.* **2016**, *375*, e14. [CrossRef] [PubMed]
14. Alshehry, A.S.; Alquwez, N.; Almazan, J.; Namis, I.M.; Cruz, J.P. Influence of workplace incivility on the quality of nursing care. *J. Clin. Nurs.* **2019**, *28*, 4582–4594. [CrossRef] [PubMed]
15. Liu, J.; Gan, Y.; Jiang, H.; Li, L.; Dwyer, R.; Lu, K.; Yan, S.; Sampson, O.; Xu, H.; Wang, C.; et al. Prevalence of workplace violence against healthcare workers: A systematic review and meta-analysis. *Occup. Environ. Med.* **2019**, *76*, 927–937. [CrossRef] [PubMed]
16. Fujita, S.; Ito, S.; Seto, K.; Kitazawa, T.; Matsumoto, K.; Hasegawa, T. Risk factors of workplace violence at hospitals in Japan. *J. Hosp. Med.* **2012**, *7*, 79–84. [CrossRef] [PubMed]
17. Fujimoto, H.; Greiner, C.; Hirota, M.; Yamaguchi, Y.; Ryuno, H.; Hashimoto, T. Experiences of Violence and Preventive Measures Among Nurses in Psychiatric and Non-Psychiatric Home Visit Nursing Services in Japan. *J. Psychosoc. Nurs. Ment. Health Serv.* **2019**, *57*, 40–48. [CrossRef]
18. Sato, K.; Wakabayashi, T.; Kiyoshi-Teo, H.; Fukahori, H. Factors associated with nurses' reporting of patients' aggressive behavior: A cross-sectional survey. *Int. J. Nurs. Stud.* **2013**, *50*, 1368–1376. [CrossRef]

19. Saeki, K.; Okamoto, N.; Tomioka, K.; Obayashi, K.; Nishioka, H.; Ohara, K.; Kurumatani, N. Work-related aggression and violence committed by patients and its psychological influence on doctors. *J. Occup. Health* **2011**, *53*, 356–364. [CrossRef]

20. Kimura, Y.; Inoue, M. Factors Associated with the Level of Psychological Impact of Patients' Offensive Language/Violence on Psychiatric Nurses Varying in Years of Experience. *Jpn. J. Occup. Med. Traumatol.* **2017**, *65*, 137–142.

21. World Health Organization. International Classification of Diseases 11th Revision. Available online: https://icd.who.int/ (accessed on 1 November 2019).

22. The World Health Organization. Burn-Out an "Occupational Phenomenon": International Classification of Diseases. Available online: https://www.who.int/mental_health/evidence/burn-out/en/ (accessed on 5 April 2020).

23. Woo, T.; Ho, R.; Tang, A.; Tam, W. Global prevalence of burnout symptoms among nurses: A systematic review and meta-analysis. *J. Psychiatr. Res.* **2020**, *123*, 9–20. [CrossRef]

24. López-López, I.M.; Gómez-Urquiza, J.L.; Cañadas, G.R.; De la Fuente, E.I.; Albendín-García, L.; Cañadas-De la Fuente, G.A. Prevalence of burnout in mental health nurses and related factors: A systematic review and meta-analysis. *Int. J. Ment. Health Nurs.* **2019**, *28*, 1032–1041. [CrossRef]

25. Gascon, S.; Leiter, M.P.; Andrés, E.; Santed, M.A.; Pereira, J.P.; Cunha, M.J.; Albesa, A.; Montero-Marín, J.; García-Campayo, J.; Martínez-Jarreta, B. The role of aggressions suffered by healthcare workers as predictors of burnout. *J. Clin. Nurs.* **2013**, *22*, 3120–3129. [CrossRef] [PubMed]

26. Liu, W.; Zhao, S.; Shi, L.; Zhang, Z.; Liu, X.; Li, L.; Duan, X.; Li, G.; Lou, F.; Jia, X.; et al. Workplace violence, job satisfaction, burnout, perceived organisational support and their effects on turnover intention among Chinese nurses in tertiary hospitals: A cross-sectional study. *BMJ Open* **2018**, *8*, e019525. [CrossRef] [PubMed]

27. Choi, S.H.; Lee, H. Workplace violence against nurses in Korea and its impact on professional quality of life and turnover intention. *J. Nurs. Manag.* **2017**, *25*, 508–518. [CrossRef] [PubMed]

28. Wu, Y.; Wang, J.; Liu, J.; Zheng, J.; Liu, K.; Baggs, J.G.; Liu, X.; You, L. The impact of work environment on workplace violence, burnout and work attitudes for hospital nurses: A structural equation modelling analysis. *J. Nurs. Manag.* **2019**. [CrossRef]

29. Figley, C.R.; Carbonell, J.L.; Boscarino, J.A.; Chang, J. A clinical demonstration model for assessing the effectiveness of therapeutic interventions: An expanded clinical trials methodology. *Int. J. Emerg. Ment. Health* **1999**, *1*, 155–164.

30. Zerach, G.; Shalev, T.B. The relations between violence exposure, posttraumatic stress symptoms, secondary traumatization, vicarious post traumatic growth and illness attribution among psychiatric nurses. *Arch. Psychiatr. Nurs.* **2015**, *29*, 135–142. [CrossRef]

31. Tirgari, B.; Azizzadeh Forouzi, M.; Ebrahimpour, M. Relationship Between Posttraumatic Stress Disorder and Compassion Satisfaction, Compassion Fatigue, and Burnout in Iranian Psychiatric Nurses. *J. Psychosoc. Nurs. Ment. Health Serv.* **2019**, *57*, 39–47. [CrossRef]

32. Topp, C.W.; Østergaard, S.D.; Søndergaard, S.; Bech, P. The WHO-5 Well-Being Index: A systematic review of the literature. *Psychother. Psychosom.* **2015**, *84*, 167–176. [CrossRef]

33. Awata, S.; Bech, P.; Yoshida, S.; Hirai, M.; Suzuki, S.; Yamashita, M.; Ohara, A.; Hinokio, Y.; Matsuoka, H.; Oka, Y. Reliability and validity of the Japanese version of the World Health Organization-Five Well-Being Index in the context of detecting depression in diabetic patients. *Psychiatry Clin. Neurosci.* **2007**, *61*, 112–119. [CrossRef]

34. Awata, S.; Bech, P.; Koizumi, Y.; Seki, T.; Kuriyama, S.; Hozawa, A.; Ohmori, K.; Nakaya, N.; Matsuoka, H.; Tsuji, I. Validity and utility of the Japanese version of the WHO-Five Well-Being Index in the context of detecting suicidal ideation in elderly community residents. *Int. Psychogeriatr.* **2007**, *19*, 77–88. [CrossRef]

35. Kessler, R.C.; Barker, P.R.; Colpe, L.J.; Epstein, J.F.; Gfroerer, J.C.; Hiripi, E.; Howes, M.J.; Normand, S.L.; Manderscheid, R.W.; Walters, E.E.; et al. Screening for serious mental illness in the general population. *Arch. Gen. Psychiatry* **2003**, *60*, 184–189. [CrossRef]

36. Furukawa, T.A.; Kawakami, N.; Saitoh, M.; Ono, Y.; Nakane, Y.; Nakamura, Y.; Tachimori, H.; Iwata, N.; Uda, H.; Nakane, H.; et al. The performance of the Japanese version of the K6 and K10 in the World Mental Health Survey Japan. *Int. J. Methods Psychiatr. Res.* **2008**, *17*, 152–158. [CrossRef] [PubMed]

37. Sakurai, K.; Nishi, A.; Kondo, K.; Yanagida, K.; Kawakami, N. Screening performance of K6/K10 and other screening instruments for mood and anxiety disorders in Japan. *Psychiatry Clin. Neurosci.* **2011**, *65*, 434–441. [CrossRef] [PubMed]

38. Reinert, D.F.; Allen, J.P. The alcohol use disorders identification test: An update of research findings. *Alcohol. Clin. Exp. Res.* **2007**, *31*, 185–199. [CrossRef] [PubMed]

39. Kawada, T.; Inagaki, H.; Kuratomi, Y. The alcohol use disorders identification test: Reliability study of the Japanese version. *Alcohol* **2011**, *45*, 205–207. [CrossRef]

40. Hiro, H.; Shima, S. Availability of the Alcohol Use Disorders Identification Test (AUDIT) for a complete health examination in Japan. *Jpn. J. Alcohol Stud. Drug Depend.* **1996**, *31*, 437–450.

41. Forbes, D.; Alkemade, N.; Hopcraft, D.; Hawthorne, G.; O'Halloran, P.; Elhai, J.D.; McHugh, T.; Bates, G.; Novaco, R.W.; Bryant, R.; et al. Evaluation of the dimensions of anger reactions-5 (DAR-5) scale in combat veterans with posttraumatic stress disorder. *J. Anxiety Disord.* **2014**, *28*, 830–835. [CrossRef]

42. Forbes, D.; Alkemade, N.; Mitchell, D.; Elhai, J.D.; McHugh, T.; Bates, G.; Novaco, R.W.; Bryant, R.; Lewis, V. Utility of the Dimensions of Anger Reactions-5 (DAR-5) scale as a brief anger measure. *Depress. Anxiety* **2014**, *31*, 166–173. [CrossRef]

43. Cheung, T.; Yip, P.S. Workplace violence towards nurses in Hong Kong: Prevalence and correlates. *BMC Public Health* **2017**, *17*, 196. [CrossRef]

44. International Labour Office; International Council of Nurses; World Health Organisation; Public Services International. Workplace Violence in the Health Sector Country Case Studies Research Instruments Survey Questionnaires. Available online: https://www.who.int/violence_injury_prevention/violence/interpersonal/en/WVfocusgroupdiscussion.pdf (accessed on 1 April 2020).

45. Stamm, B.H. *The Concise ProQOL Manual*, 2nd ed. Pocatello, ID ProQOL.org. 2010. Available online: https://proqol.org/uploads/ProQOLManual.pdf (accessed on 15 April 2020).

46. Fukumori, T.; Goto, T.; Sato, H. Development, reliability, and validity of a Japanese version of the Professional Quality of Life Scale for Nurses. *Jpn. J. Psychol.* **2018**, *89*, 150–159. [CrossRef]

47. Chen, W.C.; Hwu, H.G.; Kung, S.M.; Chiu, H.J.; Wang, J.D. Prevalence and determinants of workplace violence of health care workers in a psychiatric hospital in Taiwan. *J. Occup. Health* **2008**, *50*, 288–293. [CrossRef] [PubMed]

48. de Looff, P.; Nijman, H.; Didden, R.; Embregts, P. Burnout symptoms in forensic psychiatric nurses and their associations with personality, emotional intelligence and client aggression: A cross-sectional study. *J. Psychiatr. Ment. Health Nurs.* **2018**, *25*, 506–516. [CrossRef] [PubMed]

49. de Looff, P.; Didden, R.; Embregts, P.; Nijman, H. Burnout symptoms in forensic mental health nurses: Results from a longitudinal study. *Int. J. Ment. Health Nurs.* **2019**, *28*, 306–317. [CrossRef] [PubMed]

50. Itzhaki, M.; Bluvstein, I.; Peles Bortz, A.; Kostistky, H.; Bar Noy, D.; Filshtinsky, V.; Theilla, M. Mental Health Nurse's Exposure to Workplace Violence Leads to Job Stress, Which Leads to Reduced Professional Quality of Life. *Front. Psychiatry* **2018**, *9*, 59. [CrossRef]

51. Baby, M.; Glue, P.; Carlyle, D. 'Violence is not part of our job': A thematic analysis of psychiatric mental health nurses' experiences of patient assaults from a New Zealand perspective. *Issues Ment. Health Nurs.* **2014**, *35*, 647–655. [CrossRef]

52. Yada, H.; Abe, H.; Omori, H.; Ishida, Y.; Katoh, T. Job-related stress in psychiatric assistant nurses. *Nurs. Open* **2018**, *5*, 15–20. [CrossRef]

53. Nachreiner, N.M.; Hansen, H.E.; Okano, A.; Gerberich, S.G.; Ryan, A.D.; McGovern, P.M.; Church, T.R.; Watt, G.D. Difference in work-related violence by nurse license type. *J. Prof. Nurs.* **2007**, *23*, 290–300. [CrossRef]

54. Ferri, P.; Silvestri, M.; Artoni, C.; Di Lorenzo, R. Workplace violence in different settings and among various health professionals in an Italian general hospital: A cross-sectional study. *Psychol. Res. Behav. Manag.* **2016**, *9*, 263–275. [CrossRef]

55. Fida, R.; Laschinger, H.K.S.; Leiter, M.P. The protective role of self-efficacy against workplace incivility and burnout in nursing: A time-lagged study. *Health Care Manag. Rev.* **2018**, *43*, 21–29. [CrossRef]

56. Itzhaki, M.; Peles-Bortz, A.; Kostistky, H.; Barnoy, D.; Filshtinsky, V.; Bluvstein, I. Exposure of mental health nurses to violence associated with job stress, life satisfaction, staff resilience, and post-traumatic growth. *Int. J. Ment. Health Nurs.* **2015**, *24*, 403–412. [CrossRef]

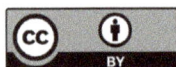

International Journal of
*Environmental Research
and Public Health*

MDPI

Article

Satisfaction with Social Support Received from Social Relationships in Cases of Chronic Pain: The Influence of Personal Network Characteristics in Terms of Structure, Composition and Functional Content

Rosario Fernández-Peña [1,*], José Luis Molina [2] and Oliver Valero [3]

[1] Department of Nursing, University of Cantabria (Spain), SALBIS Research Group, Nursing Research Group IDIVAL, 39008 Santander, Spain

[2] Department of Social and Cultural Anthropology, GRAFO, Universitat Autònoma de Barcelona, 08193 Barcelona, Spain; joseluis.molina@uab.cat

[3] Servei d'Estadística Aplicada, Universitat Autònoma de Barcelona, 08193 Barcelona, Spain; oliver.valero@uab.cat

* Correspondence: roser.fernandez@unican.es; Tel.: +34-942-202-241

Received: 4 February 2020; Accepted: 10 April 2020; Published: 15 April 2020

check for updates

Abstract: The worldwide burden of chronic illnesses, constitutes a major public health concern and a serious challenge for health systems. In addition to the strategies of self-management support developed by nursing and health organizations, an individual's personal network represents a major resource of social support in the long-term. Adopting a cross-sectional design based on personal network analysis methods, the main aim of this study is to explore the relationship between satisfaction with the social support received by individuals suffering chronic pain and the structure, composition, and functional content in social support of their personal networks. We collected personal and support network data from 30 people with chronic pain (20 person's contacts (alters) for each individual (ego), 600 relationships in total). Additionally, we examined the level of satisfaction with social support in each of the 600 relationships. Bivariate and multivariate tests were performed to analyze the satisfaction with the social support received. Using cluster analysis, we established a typology of the 600 relationships under study. Results showed that higher satisfaction was associated with a balance between degree centrality and betweenness (i.e., measures of network cohesion and network modularity, respectively). Finally, new lines of research are proposed in order to broaden our understanding of this subject.

Keywords: social support; patient satisfaction; chronic disease; chronic pain

---

1. Introduction

Chronic illness constitutes a critical public health challenge that affects both social and economic development worldwide. Chronic illness also represents a major challenge for health services. Data from the WHO reveals that noncommunicable diseases (NCDs) cause 41 million deaths annually, equivalent to 71% of all deaths globally [1].

The steady increase in the prevalence of chronic illnesses is due, in part, to the progressive aging of the population, together with an increased life expectancy. Thus, people with several illnesses or chronic conditions live longer than in the past [2]. Faced with this scenario, health services are undergoing a reorganizational shift from a model centered on illness and treatment, to one centered on the individual and their particular chronic conditions. Both institutional and personal environments are also very important to chronic illness patients, comprising sources of support outside the more formal health and/or social systems.

A key element of the models developed to face chronicity is self-management. This concept emphasizes the patient's role in managing health and has been defined as an 'individual's ability to manage the symptoms, treatment, physical, and psychosocial consequences and lifestyle changes inherent in living with a chronic condition' [3]. This is a changing construct, which reflects the different types of support needed throughout the progression of the illness, mediated by such factors as the stage of the illness, its stability over time, the symptoms, and the physical limitations, among others [4]. However, as proposed by Morris et al. [5], the notion of self-management is questionable, as an individual construct, namely because many practices concerning the management of illnesses involve the support and/or negotiation of roles within the framework of relationships. Therefore, in essence, chronic illnesses are not restricted to the individual, rather they are 'embedded in family, community, and societal conditions that shape and influence—and may constrain—the choices people make, or can make' [6]. Based on this change in paradigm, the Innovate Care for Chronic Conditions (ICCC) of the WHO, propose a framework for health systems to improve the management of chronic conditions. This framework proposes the following micro, meso, and macro levels of health care systems: The level of interaction with the patient (micro), the organization of healthcare at the community level (meso), and the level of politics (macro). Each level dynamically interacts and influences the other two over time, via feedback loops [7]. According to the ICCC framework, optimal outcomes are achieved when a partnership exists between health care teams, community partners, and patients and their families [8], i.e., when individual self-management is embedded in the social systems of support that make it possible. Furthermore, certain aspects of the community are highly relevant, such as associations for patients and their families, making caregivers increasingly influential [9].

Along these lines, different dedicated programs and interventions have been developed by health organizations to improve self-management, including assessments based on the perspectives of both patients and health professionals [10–12]. Likewise, other programs have used a community approach, focusing on supporting the self-management of chronic illness on behalf of the individual's social networks [5,13–17]. However, these latter approaches do not provide tie-level measures of the social environments in which self-management may be developed. In addition, they use the terms 'social support' and 'social networks' interchangeably, conflating two related but unidentical social phenomena. Social support has been defined as 'support accessible to an individual through social ties to other individuals, groups, and the larger community' [18]. Instead, social networks have been described as 'the direct and indirect ties linking a group of individuals over certain definable criteria, such as kinship, friendship, and acquaintances.' Therefore, social networks provide a structural framework in which support may, or may not, be accessible to the individual [19]. We aim to contribute to the research in this field by providing detailed social tie-level information about the social environment of individuals in situations of chronic pain on one hand, and information about the content of the relationship on the other without prejudging the existence of social support.

Furthermore, in the study of social support, three differentiated aspects of social ties are distinguished: (1) the existence or number of relationships as a reflection of social integration, (2) the formal structure of the same or social networks, and the functional content, in this case, social support (3) and the influence of the structure of social relationships on functional content in social support [20,21].

Social network analysis (SNA) is a research method that examines the interactions between individuals, groups, and organizations, which has been applied in a variety of research areas. In the context of health, this approach has led to academic literature which has significantly increased in recent decades, prioritizing the role of social structure, including the areas of community and primary health, care and nursing research [22–26], identifying new challenges and providing opportunities for innovative research.

Social support has been studied in several contexts, one of which is informal caregiving [27,28]. Compared to other approaches in social support research, personal network analysis (PNA), also labeled as egocentric network analysis in the literature [29], is based on the ensemble of relationships that surround an individual (ego) across social settings (i.e., family, work colleagues, neighbors, ...), as well as the relationships between the person's contacts (alters) [30,31]. This enables the simultaneous study of micro phenomena (interactions) and meso phenomena (the social networks and institutions that the individual belongs to on a community level) [32]. Previous research has noted the effects of personal networks on individual outcomes based on theoretical frameworks, such as the social capital and the social influence through diffusion and social support, with the latter being one of the most studied areas based both on this approach and on different disciplines [33]. From this perspective, a PNA, constitutes an excellent approach to the study of social support in the context of informal care in chronic illness, since this can be used to measure the structure and composition of personal networks and the functional content of social support. This enables the possibility of differentiating the personal network from the support network (comprising both support providers and non-providers), as well as relating these personal network characteristics, including the structural variables, with other variables of interest. Whereas, in general, social support studies evaluate the quality, or the quantity, of a person's social ties, studies based on PNA regard these ties as being potentially of interest [34]. This is based on the importance of the relationships between the interacting units [30]. Therefore, the structural variables of these relationships are commonly included in the analysis.

In the study of social support, one dimension of interest is the quality or sense of satisfaction. This dimension reflects the discrepancy among the interactions between real and desired (or necessary) support. The relevance of this distinction is that satisfaction with social support provides a better explanation of the quality of life and health outcomes when compared with the mere provision or number of support providers [35,36]. Regarding the assessment of satisfaction, although it has been used in some instruments intended to evaluate social support [37], there is a gap in the literature regarding the role of the personal networks' characteristics in the quality or satisfaction with social support. Thus, this study focuses on the quality of social support received from personal networks in the context of chronic pain. This dimension has seldom been researched [36,38] despite being a highly relevant health problem due to its prevalence, complexity, and the consequences for both the individual and the social environment in which it is embedded [39,40]. Our approach provides a rich set of measures at the tie level that allows us to measure with detail personal networks' structure, composition, and functional content of social support along with its perceived quality. Just having this type of detailed information, it is possible to suggest ways to improve the effective self-management of individuals in chronic pain situations.

2. Materials and Methods

This research is part of a larger study aimed at examining social support and quality of life in the context of chronic pain [41]. In a prior publication, the descriptive results of this larger study were presented using a mixed approach [42], showing that different types of personal networks were associated with self-reported quality of life, which scored below the populational mean in all dimensions considered.

2.1. Design

A descriptive, cross-sectional study using personal network analysis.

2.2. Sample Description

The inclusion criteria of participants were people over the age of 18 diagnosed with chronic pain, and receiving care at Marques de Valdecilla University Hospital Pain Unit of Santander (Spain), without mental or cognitive decline and who agreed to participate voluntarily in the study. Convenience sampling was used to select participants: An equal number of men and women (15 in each case) that met the inclusion criteria and were recommended by professionals working at the pain management unit among their patients. All voluntary participants were briefed about the goals and methods of the research and signed an informed consent form (see Section 2.6 below). All of them agreed to be interviewed several times if necessary, either at the hospital or participants' homes, according to their health status and personal preferences. Nobody requested to quit the research, probably because of the positive assessment of both the attention and feedback about their personal networks they received during the interviews. Fieldwork and data analysis were conducted between July 2014 and July 2015. The personal networks of the 30 cases amounted to a total of 600 personal relationships (20 relationships per ego).

2.3. Variables

The data collection included participant variables (ego), their contacts (alter) and details regarding their personal network (see [41,42] for further information regarding the variables):

(a) Sociodemographic data (ego characteristics): sex, age, civil status, level of studies, and work situation.
(b) Variables regarding the composition of the personal network (alter characteristics): Age, sex, type of tie with ego, place of residence, and proximity.
(c) Social support (function): type (emotional, instrumental, informational, and combinations of the same), satisfaction, reciprocity, variation over time, frequency, and channel of transmission.
(d) Variables regarding the structure of the personal network: density, degree centrality (two measures; mean of the alter-alter matrix and at node level), betweenness centrality (two measures; mean of a personal network and at node level), number of components and number of isolates.

2.4. Data Collection Instruments

Personal network: EgoNet open-source software (https://sourceforge.net/projects/egonet/), was used to collect and analyze each ego's personal network data. Additionally, UCInet software [43] was used to calculate degree, and betweenness centrality for each of the 600 alters studied. Sociodemographic, pain variables, and personal network data were collected based on an ad hoc questionnaire designed in accordance with the study objectives.

2.5. Data Analysis

Bivariate linear mixed models were used to analyze the satisfaction with the social support received. These were converted into the following numerical values: very unsatisfactory = 0, quite unsatisfactory = 1, satisfactory = 2, quite satisfactory = 3, and very satisfactory = 4. Ego characteristics and structure, composition, and functional content in social support of their personal network were considered as explanatory variables. The ego was included as a random effect for the analysis of the structure and composition of alter variables. Variables with a p-value of 0.2 were included in a multivariate logistic regression model to identify which factors were related to satisfactory or very satisfactory support.

Additionally, a multiple correspondence analysis (MCA) combined with classification methods were used in order to establish typologies for the 600 relationships examined in terms of the quality of the social support received from the ego's point of view. MCA is a descriptive, exploratory technique designed to analyze multi-way contingency tables with cases as rows and categories of variables as columns [44]. Components obtained from the MCA were submitted to a cluster analysis applying Ward's hierarchical clustering method [45,46]. Results were represented in a tree dendrogram using R-squared distance. Bivariate tests were conducted between each of the explanatory variables and the profiles, using chi-square tests to describe the obtained profiles.

The statistical analysis was performed using SAS v9.4 software (SAS Institute Inc., Cary, NC, USA), and the significance level was set at $p < 0.05$.

2.6. Ethical Considerations

The Clinical Research Ethics Committee of Cantabria (Spain) provided ethical approval for this study (internal code 2014.32). All study participants received verbal and written information concerning the study objectives and procedure. Participation was voluntary, and all participants provided their signed informed consent. Furthermore, this study adhered to national and international ethical guidelines (Code of Ethics and Declaration of Helsinki) and fulfilled data confidentiality legislation (Spanish organic law 15/1999 of 13 December on the protection of personal data).

3. Results

3.1. Sociodemographic Variables

In total, 30 people participated in the study (15 women and 15 men). The mean age of participants was 54.57 years (SD 11.64, range 30–73 years). Their marital status was married or with a partner ($n = 27$); divorced ($n = 1$); and widowed ($n = 2$). Their educational level was primary education ($n = 16$), vocational education ($n = 8$), secondary education ($n = 4$), and higher education ($n = 2$). Their employment status at the time of the interview was: retired ($n = 10$), active ($n = 9$), on sick leave due to pain ($n = 6$), and homemaker ($n = 5$). The mean length of time since the onset of chronic pain was 12.2 years (SD 9.18, range 1–35 years) in men and 16.6 years (SD 12.39, range 1–39) in women.

3.2. Bivariate Analysis

The satisfaction with the social support received in the 600 personal relationships studied was distributed as follows: very satisfactory 12.3%, quite satisfactory 22%, satisfactory 26%, quite unsatisfactory 6.5%. The very unsatisfactory category was present in 33.2%, corresponding to relationships where no support was provided (see also [27] for descriptive analysis of other variables related to social support function).

3.2.1. Ego Variables

From the bivariate analysis, no statistically significant relationships were observed (p-value > 0.05) between satisfaction with social support received and the following ego variables: Age, gender, level of studies, work situation, civil status, level of pain, pain duration, and the number of cohabitants. However, the results obtained, when comparing the means of age and duration of pain variables for the ego, are notable. The quality of social support received decreased as the ego's age increased, and as the time with chronic pain increased.

Age of ego (p-value 0.174): for the categorical variable age, as age increased, satisfaction decreased (for every 10 years, satisfaction values decreased by 0.16 units):

- Participants aged between 30 and 51 years; mean satisfaction 2.01 (SD 0.19).
- Participants aged between 52 and 63 years; mean satisfaction 1.72 (SD 0.17).
- Participants aged between 65 and 73 years; mean satisfaction 1.51 (SD 0.18).

Duration of pain (p-value 0.096): using the categorical variable model and recoding the duration of pain variable, we observed that, as the duration of pain increased, satisfaction decreased:

- Duration of pain between 1 and 8 years; mean satisfaction 2.04 (SD 0.18).
- Duration of pain between 9 and 19 years; mean satisfaction 1.67 (SD 0.18).
- Duration of pain between 20 and 39 years; mean satisfaction 1.5 (SD 0.18).

3.2.2. Composition Variables

Regarding the composition variables (Table 1), the most satisfactory support was defined by an adult female alter, with whom the ego had a strong tie, who was a close family member (partner, parents, and children) and who lived geographically close.

Table 1. Satisfaction and composition variables of the personal network.

Variable	Category	Mean (SD)
Age of the alter *	≤30 years	1.36 (0.17)
	31–50 years	1.95 (0.13)
	51–60 years	1.67 (0.16)
	>60 years	1.69 (0.14)
Sex of the alter *	Women	1.91 (0.12)
	Men	1.56 (0.12)
Tie with the ego *	Partner	3.22 (0.26)
	Parents	3.03 (0.33)
	Brothers	1.75 (0.18)
	Children	2.77 (0.19)
	Other family members	1.32 (0.13)
	Friends	1.61 (0.14)
	Other ties	1.41 (0.18)
Strength of the tie *	Very close	2.83 (0.13)
	Quite close	2.19 (0.12)
	Close	1.50 (0.12)
	Not very close	0.74 (0.13)
	Not at all close	0.21 (0.20)
Place of residence of the alter compared to the ego	Same locality	1.89 (0.13)
	Same province	1.66 (0.13)
	Other province/country	1.53 (0.18)

* *p*-value < 0.05.

3.2.3. Structural Variables

Regarding the structural variables of the personal network (Table 2), the quality of the social support received increased as the density of the network increased. In contrast, the quality of support decreased as the number of isolates and components increased. Regarding the node, as the degree centrality of the alter increased (a measure related to the density of the network), satisfaction increased. Likewise, satisfaction increased as the betweenness centrality of the alter increased.

Table 2. Satisfaction and structure variables of the personal network and alters.

Variable	Range/Category	Mean (SD)
Density *	<40%	1.57 (0.15)
	41–60%	1.64 (0.16)
	>60%	2.28 (0.22)
Degree centrality (alter) *	0–5	1.35 (0.14)
	6–11	1.60 (0.13)
	12–19	2.35 (0.15)
Betweeness Centrality (alter) *	0	1.44 (0.13)
	0.1–1.2	1.69 (0.15)
	1.2–114.3	2.12 (0.14)
Components	1	2 (0.16)
	2	1.54 (0.20)
	3–11	1.58 (0.18)
Isolates	0	1.89 (0.14)
	1	1.63 (0.23)
	2–9	1.46 (0.22)

* *p*-value < 0.05.

3.2.4. Functional Social Support

Regarding the social support characteristics, of the 600 relationships examined, 401 support-providing relationships were identified (66.83%) and 199 relationships in which support was not provided (33.17%). Thus, the mean number of providers and non-providers was 13 and 7, respectively, for each ego. The functional variables concerning social support (Table 3), reveal that the personal relationships offering greater quality support from the ego's perspective were characterized by offering various types of support (multiplexity). This was provided face-to-face or combined with daily telephone calls, which could become more frequent over time and occurred in reciprocal support relationships.

Table 3. Satisfaction and social support variables.

Variable	Category	Mean (SE)
Social support variables in provider relationships (*n* = 401)		
Type *	Emotional	2.37 (0.07)
	Emotional and instrumental	3.18 (0.10)
	Emotional, instrumental and informational	3.62 (0.18)
	Other types of support	2.55 (0.14)
Frequency *	Daily	3.26 (0.09)
	Weekly	2.57 (0.08)
	Biweekly	2.42 (0.12)
	Monthly	1.94 (0.11)
	>2 months	1.83 (0.15)
Transmission channel *	Face-to-face	2.70 (0.09)
	By telephone	2.22 (0.13)
	Face-to-face and by telephone	2.74 (0.10)
	Internet/Telephone + internet	2.16 (0.28)
Variation of support *	Increases	3.22 (0.18)
	No variation	1.47 (0.12)
	Decreases	1.73 (0.19)
Reciprocity *	Yes	1.97 (0.10)
	No	0.99 (0.14)

SE = Standard Error.* *p*-value < 0.05.

3.3. Multivariate Logistic Regression Model

From the multivariate logistic regression model, we obtained that the variables which were related to the satisfactory or very satisfactory support were: Age of the ego (the level of satisfaction with the social support received decreased as the age of the ego increased), sex of the alter (women offered more satisfactory support compared to men), tie with the ego (close family members, friends, and neighbors provide more satisfactory support), reciprocal relationships in the support and relationships in which the ego has a very strong tie.

3.4. Cluster Analysis

In order to explore the 600 relationships examined in terms of the quality of the social support received a multiple correspondence analysis was performed. Variables included in the analysis were the sex of the alter, tie with the ego, type of support, satisfaction, frequency, transmission channel, reciprocity, and proximity. We obtained 11 factors that accounted for 75% of the total variability. Applying a classification algorithm to these factors, three clusters were obtained, which comprise the totality of the 600 studied relationships. The satisfaction profiles presented the following distribution: Profile 1 (237 relationships), represented by a majority of satisfactory relations with the social support received; Profile 2 (164 relationships), represented by a majority of very and quite satisfactory relationships considering the social support received, and Profile 3 (199 relationships), represented in its totality by very unsatisfactory relationships, and corresponding to the non-providers of social support present in the personal networks studied.

Table 4 displays the distribution of egos among the three profiles according to age. In consonance with the results of the bivariate analysis presented above and which revealed a decrease of satisfaction as the age of the ego increases, the relationships containing cluster 3 and valued as being very unsatisfactory with the social support received corresponded with egos over the age of 65 in almost 50% of cases.

Table 4. Age of ego and relationships according to the three profiles (%).

Category	Profile 1	Profile 2	Profile 3
30–49 years	38.4	31.1	19.1
50–64 years	35.9	37.2	37.2
65 and over	25.7	31.7	43.7
Total	100	100	100

Graphically, these relations are grouped, forming three profiles, as shown in the following dendrogram (Figure 1). The horizontal axis represents individuals that are grouped by horizontal lines at a height that represent the distance between the two linked clusters.

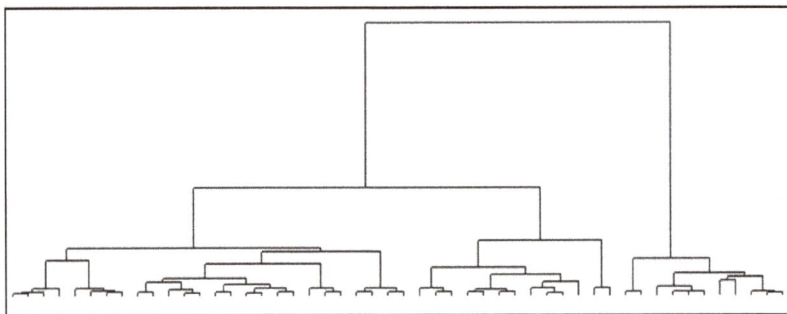

Figure 1. Dendrogram of the hierarchical cluster analysis.

3.4.1. Composition Variables

Table 5 presents the distribution of the personal network composition variables across the three profiles (bivariate tests between the explanatory variables and the profiles). The social support that was deemed more satisfactory was provided by (a) women, (b) close family members (followed by the friends), (c) middle-aged people, (d) those with whom the ego has a strong tie, (e) reciprocal support relationships, and (f) people living geographically close to the ego. Although to a lesser degree, there was a presence of more unsatisfactory relations with non-providers in the case of close adult family members.

For the analysis of the family roles, we have considered: (a) close family members: partner, parents, siblings, and children; (b) family members: Aunts/uncles, grandchildren, cousins, grandparents, nephews/nieces, and brothers/sisters-in-law, and (c) other family members: family roles not included in (a) and (b). The variable 'proximity' was examined based on five categories, which were recoded into two categories: A = strong tie: very close, quite close, and close, and (b) weak tie: not very close and not close at all.

Table 5. Composition variables of the personal network according to the three profiles (%).

Variable	Category	Profile 1	Profile 2	Profile 3
Age of the alter *	<20	2.1	7.3	15.1
	20–39	21.5	24.4	19.6
	40–59	45.6	45.2	32.7
	>60	30.8	23.1	32.6
Sex of the alter *	Male	45.1	41.5	57.8
	Female	54.9	58.5	42.2
Relationship with ego *	Close family members	17.3	59.8	14.1
	Family members	24.9	7.9	24.1
	Other family member	4.2	9.1	17.6
	Friends	35.9	17.1	32.2
	Neighbors	8.4	3	6.5
	Work and professional colleagues	9.3	3	5.5
Strength of the tie *	Strong tie	77.2	100	49.2
	Weak tie	22.8	0	50.8
Place of residence of the alter compared to the ego *	Same location	35	58	43.2
	Same province	43	32.9	40.2
	Other province	17.4	8.5	12.6
	Other province/country	4.6	0.6	4

* p-value < 0.05.

3.4.2. Structural Variables

Table 6 presents the multivariate analysis findings considering the importance that structural measures have on the personal network for the quality of the support, in consonance with the results of the bivariate analysis presented above. In this manner, the personal network providing the most highly-valued level of satisfaction combined both a degree centrality and high density with a high betweenness centrality, both of which were above the overall mean. Likewise, the findings reveal a tendency for satisfaction levels to decrease in networks that were more fragmented, with less cohesion or with a greater number of isolates and components.

Table 6. Structural variables of the personal network. Profile and global means.

Variable	Profile 1	Profile 2	Profile 3	Global Mean
Density	0.44	0.53	0.41	0.45
Degree Centrality [a]	7.08	12.44	7.25	8.60
Betweeness Centrality [a]	2.41	8.53	2.10	3.98
Components	2.41	2.11	3.03	2.53
Isolates	0.91	0.74	1.62	1.10

[a] Alters' centrality measures

3.4.3. Functional Social Support

Regarding the specific characteristics of the social support provided (Table 7), the greatest quality was associated with the combination of different types of support, especially emotional and instrumental support. Likewise, the frequency of the provision of support and face-to-face contact or combined with the provision of telephone support represents the most satisfactory support relationships.

Below, we display the graphs of two study participants with different levels of satisfaction with the social support received. The most satisfactory support network (Figure 2) corresponds to a woman aged 40 years who had chronic pain for 14 years, whereas the graph that illustrates the least satisfactory support network (Figure 3) is that of a man aged 66 years who had experienced chronic pain for 35 years. Table 8 shows the legend of graphs, and Table 9 displays the quantitative results of the differences in these three personal network dimensions examined, as well as the quality of social support.

Table 7. Social support variables in the three profiles (%).

Variable	Category	Profile 1	Profile 2	Profile 3
	Emotional	83.5	34.8	0
	Instrumental	5.1	2.4	0
	Informative	2.1	0	0
	All three types of support	0.4	12.8	0
Type *	Emotional and instrumental	3.4	46.3	0
	Emotional and informative	3.4	3.7	0
	Instrumental and informative	0.4	0	0
	Professional	1.7	0	0
	None	0	0	100
	Daily	7.6	63.4	0.5
	Weekly	39.2	31.7	0.5
Frequency *	Biweekly	17.3	3.7	0
	Monthly	23.6	0.6	0
	Every 2 or 3 months	6.3	0.6	0
	Every 3 months or more	5.9	0	99
	Face-to-face	43.5	54.3	0
	By telephone	24.1	3.7	0
Channel of	Internet	3	0.6	0
transmission *	Face-to-face and by telephone	27.8	41.5	0
	Telephone and internet	1.7	0	0
	No support	0	0	100
	Has not varied	70.5	61	92
Variation *	More support	13.1	31.1	0
	Less support	16.5	7.9	8
Reciprocity *	Yes	78.9	93.3	59.3

* *p*-value < 0.05.

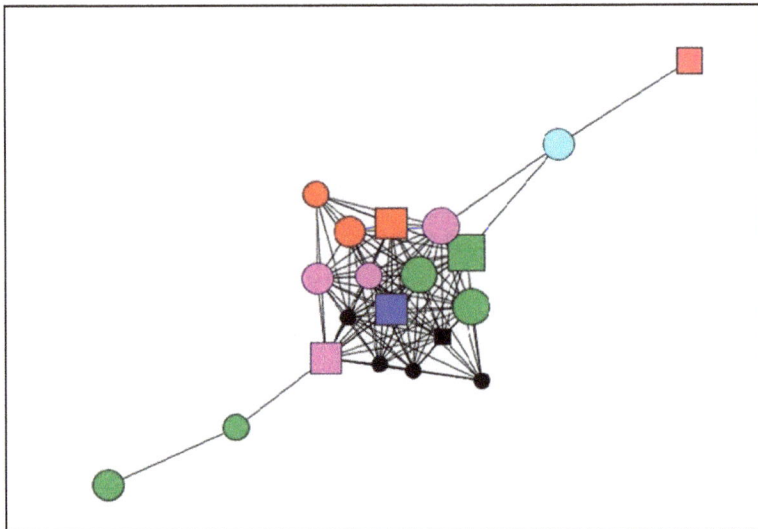

Figure 2. Graph Case 1. Woman (40 years old), living with chronic pain for 14 years.

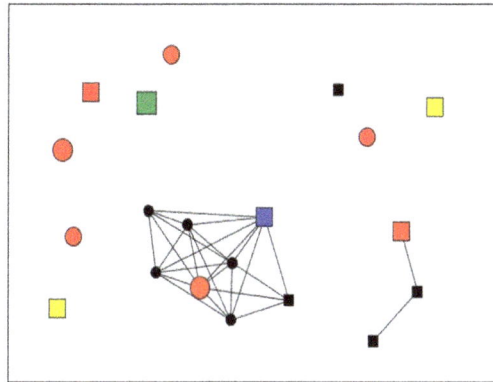

Figure 3. Graph Case 28. Man (66 years old), living with chronic pain for 35 years.

Table 8. Legend of graphs.

Node Shape: Sex	Node Size: Satisfaction	Node Colour: Type of Social Support
Circle: Women Square: Men	Large: More satisfaction Small: Less satisfaction	Red: Emotional Dark blue: Instrumental Pink: Emotional and instrumental Yellow: Informational Green: All types Black: Non-providers Light blue: Emotional and informational Orange: Professional

Table 9. Descriptive analysis of social support at the ego level.

		Case 01	Case 28
Satisfaction (%)	Very satisfactory	20	0
	Quite satisfactory	35	15
	Satisfactory	20	40
	Quite unsatisfactory	0	0
	Very unsatisfactory	25	45
Structure	Density	0.605	0.137
	Degree Centrality (mean)	11.5	2.6
	Betweenness Centrality (mean)	5.7	0.25
	Components	1	11
	Isolates	0	9
Composition (%)	Sex of the alters Women (vs. men)	70	50
	Strength of the tie Strong tie (vs. weak)	80	90
	Place of residence of alters Same locality as ego	80	15
	Reciprocity Yes	45	90
Social support (%)	Type of support All three types	25	5
	Emotional and instrumental	20	0
	Non-providers	25	45
	Variation of support Increases	55	15
	Frequency of support Daily	25	5
	2 or 3 times per week	10	0
	Transmission channel Face-to-face	65	45
	Face-to-face and telephone	10	10

In addition to the differences of age and time since onset of pain in each of the two cases presented, the comparison of these two networks reveals differences affecting the structure, composition, and content of the social support as well as the satisfaction with the social support received by each of the two participants.

4. Discussion

This study aimed to examine the structure, composition, and functional content of social support in the context of personal networks, in relation to satisfaction from the ego perspective. It is important to consider these conditions in order to assess social support as a relational element that is contained and transmitted within social relations [20].

4.1. Composition Variables

The most highly-valued social support was provided by middle-aged female alters, with whom the ego maintained a close relationship and who lived geographically close to the ego. These characteristics highlight the importance of the age of the alter on the ability to offer support (children and older people as non-providers) or the geographical proximity of the alter, which is considered key, especially for the provision of instrumental or tangible support [47–49]. Regarding the type of tie with the ego, our results add to the existing literature, which underlines the significant role of the family and friends in the provision of social support [50]. Nonetheless, it is necessary to consider that, although family roles represent 76.8% of the most satisfactory relationships, they also represent 55.8% of the total number of relationships in the profile identified as the most unsatisfied with the social support received. Therefore, when considering social support in the framework of social relationships, it should be appreciated that not all aspects of so-called close relationships are positive [20,51]. Negative interactions, together with social loss and loneliness, constitute adverse aspects of social interactions [52], which can be detrimental to a person's health by influencing the sense of wellbeing, life stress, less supportive networks, and psychological distress [53–55]. Likewise, specifically in cases of chronic pain, it is also necessary to consider the impact of pain and the resultant effects on a person's social and family relationships [39,40,56], including effects on their partners [57–60]. Therefore, these findings suggest the need for contextual and longitudinal assessments of support in long-term conditions, as these factors affect both the receiver, as well as the provider of support and the relationship dynamics.

4.2. Structural Variables

Our results have shown that quality in the provision of social support is related to certain levels of density as well as with a relatively high betweenness centrality. Nonetheless, none of these explain separately the maximum level of satisfaction. Therefore, the results suggest that the ideal support network should strive for a certain balance between a dense center and a periphery that may act as a bridge with other more diverse relationships.

From a sociological point of view, social structures affect and are affected by human behavior [61]. In the field of health, several studies have underlined the role that the network structure plays in different health outcomes, such as the effect of the same on health-related behaviors [62–64] in the transmission of sexually transmitted diseases [65,66] in mental health [67] or the relation between network structure and health status [68]. Likewise, some studies have found certain benefits derived from having a network with different social domains and with a diverse typology of alters, as these can act as facilitators of other resources offering different types of support [69,70]. Therefore, an alter with a high betweenness, as shown by our results, represents a quality support resource for ego, which can benefit from these indirect relationships. Conversely, some studies have found that density is not automatically related to social support [71,72] and that networks with low density are more adaptive and offer greater support according to determined contexts [73]. We contend that this idea of *balance* among density and intermediation in the structure of the personal network is important when evaluating social support. For the case of chronic pain, a dense network may guarantee the availability of emotional support in which strong ties mainly are represented by kin and close relationships. However, the same relationships over time may lead to a redundancy of the already-known support resources, and alters with a high betweenness might enable access to new support resources (information, contacts, etc.) of great value for ego. Although certain levels of density are necessary for achieving a feeling of safety, something necessary in a healthy personal context, the effectiveness of the network in relation to social support is based on ties that allow access to diverse resources with alternative ways of thinking and acting [74,75], and that the person may use as 'social capital' assets [76]. Therefore, in certain contexts, density and intermediation offer different advantages and may, in fact, be complementary [77].

4.3. Functional Social Support

Concerning the types of support provided, emotional support was most highly-valued, followed by the combination of emotional and instrumental support, reinforcing the importance of a multiplexity or diversity of resources [34]. Thus, in the context of chronic pain, emotional support may guarantee a feeling of accompaniment, understanding, and empathy for the other person's situation, as well as constituting a coping resource, enhancing the ability to adapt to the situation and acting as a facilitator of self-management. Furthermore, in the case of chronic pain, having the instrumental support of others is necessary because of the impairments associated with the performance of basic activities of daily living such as, for example, mobilization, hygiene, or personal grooming. Our findings support previous research [78–80] showing that relationships characterized by reciprocal support are those that are most highly-valued, highlighting the importance of this characteristic in relationships involving health aspects. In addition, increasing and frequent face-to-face support is a characteristic of the most highly-valued support relationships. It is important to note that these findings may be related to caregiver burden as a consequence of caring for people with chronic illnesses in the long term [81–83].

According to previous studies [84], and highlighting the importance of the dynamic nature of personal relationships throughout the life cycle, our findings reveal that satisfaction with the social support received decreases as the age of the ego increases and as the time since the onset of pain increases. This aspect is highly relevant in chronic illness and, more specifically, in the case of chronic pain, mainly because of: (a) the increased prevalence of this disorder in aging populations [39,56], (b) the changes in personal networks at the ego-alter level, i.e., the alters that are lost and are added to the personal network over time, and (c) changes in the characteristics of the relationships as a consequence of life events (e.g., marriage, divorce, chronic illness, retirement, etc.) that may affect the content in social support [85–87].

Personal contexts, namely the characteristics of relationships and personal networks, are key elements that help us understand the complexity of satisfaction with social support for self-management in chronic illnesses.

Future research with a longitudinal design is recommended, focused on the study of variations in social support over time in individuals with chronic pain. Lastly, comparative studies involving personal network research may reveal possible differences in structure, composition, and content in the social support of personal networks according to the age of the ego, as well as providing further information on the support networks of older people.

5. Conclusions

The satisfaction with the informal care received by people with chronic pain, via their personal network resources, is different according to personal characteristics, such as age, pain, the amount of time since the onset of chronic pain, as well as characteristics related to their personal network. Person-centered care implies considering the different social and relational contexts in which people live their lives. Support for self-management in situations of chronic illness includes the support provided by primary care nursing professionals and health organizations via different strategies, as well as the support from the social and personal environment surrounding the person and, therefore, both can be considered as being complementary. From the point of view of the support provided by the personal network, we have shown that a balance between degree centrality and betweenness (an indicator of the existence of various social circles connected through the ego) is needed in order to achieve higher satisfaction with the support received. This finding may help to enhance the self-management capabilities of this type of patient by introducing small adjustments to their personal network structures. In this vein, cases in which insufficient or inappropriate social support are detected in an individual's personal environment could benefit from the implementation of strategies, based on specially designed network interventions, with the aim of guaranteeing the continuity and appropriateness of care and support over time.

Author Contributions: R.F.-P. and J.L.M. conceived of the study and designed the research. O.V. analyzed the data. R.F.-P. and J.L.M. wrote the initial manuscript. All authors have read and agreed to the published version of the manuscript.

Funding: This research received no external funding.

Acknowledgments: We thank all the people who agreed to take part in the study for their availability and kindness even in times of illness. We also thank the health professionals at the Marqués de Valdecilla University Hospital Pain Unit for their valuable assistance during field work.

Conflicts of Interest: The authors declare no conflict of interest.

References

1. WHO Noncommunicable Diseases. Available online: https://www.who.int/news-room/fact-sheets/detail/noncommunicable-diseases (accessed on 2 April 2020).
2. Wagner, E.H.; Austin, B.T.; Davis, C.; Hindmarsh, M.; Schaefer, J.; Bonomi, A. Improving chronic illness care: Translating evidence into action. *Health Aff.* **2001**, *20*, 64–78. [CrossRef] [PubMed]
3. Barlow, J.; Wright, C.; Sheasby, J.; Turner, A.; Hainsworth, J. Self-management approaches for people with chronic conditions: A review. *Patient Educ. Couns.* **2002**, *48*, 177–187. [CrossRef]
4. Van Houtum, L.; Rijken, M.; Heijmans, M.; Groenewegen, P. Self-management support needs of patients with chronic illness: Do needs for support differ according to the course of illness? *Patient Educ. Couns.* **2013**, *93*, 626–632. [CrossRef] [PubMed]
5. Morris, R.L.; Kennedy, A.; Sanders, C. Evolving 'self'-management: Exploring the role of social network typologies on individual long-term condition management. *Heal. Expect.* **2015**, *19*, 1044–1061. [CrossRef]
6. Kendall, P.R.W. *Investing in Prevention:Improving Health and Creating Sustainability*; Bristish Columbia: Vancouver, Canada, 2010.
7. World Health Organization. *Innovative Care for Chronic Conditions: Building Blocks for Action*; WHO: Geneva, Switzerland, 2002.
8. Epping-Jordan, J.E. Integrated approaches to prevention and control of chronic conditions. *Kidney Int.* **2005**, *68*, 86–88. [CrossRef]
9. Nuño, R.; Coleman, K.; Bengoa, R.; Sauto, R. Integrated care for chronic conditions: The contribution of the ICCC Framework. *Health Policy* **2012**, *105*, 55–64. [CrossRef]
10. Barlow, J.H.; Brancroft, G.V.; Turner, A.P. Self-management training for people with chronic disease: A shared learning experience. *J. Health Psychol.* **2005**, *10*, 863–872. [CrossRef]
11. Davies, F.; Wood, F.; Bullock, A.; Wallace, C.; Edwards, A. Interventions to improve the self-management support health professionals provide for people with progressive neurological conditions: Protocol for a realist synthesis. *BMJ Open* **2017**, *7*, e014575. [CrossRef]
12. Nøst, T.H.; Steinsbekk, A.; Bratås, O.; Grønning, K. Expectations, effect and experiences of an easily accessible self-management intervention for people with chronic pain: Study protocol for a randomised controlled trial with embedded qualitative study. *Trials* **2016**, *17*, 325.
13. Crotty, M.M.; Henderson, J.; Ward, P.R.; Fuller, J.; Rogers, A.; Kralik, D.; Gregory, S. Analysis of social networks supporting the self-management of type 2 diabetes for people with mental illness. *BMC Health Serv. Res.* **2015**, *15*, 257. [CrossRef]
14. Gallant, M.P. The influence of social support on chronic illness self-management: A review and directions for research. *Heal. Educ. Behav.* **2003**, *30*, 170–195. [CrossRef] [PubMed]

15. Vassilev, I.; Rogers, A.; Blickem, C.; Brooks, H.; Kapadia, D.; Kennedy, A.; Sanders, C.; Kirk, S.; Reeves, D. Social networks, the "Work" and work force of chronic illness self-management: A survey analysis of personal communities. *PLoS ONE* **2013**, *8*, e59723. [CrossRef] [PubMed]

16. Koetsenruijter, J.; Van Lieshout, J.; Vassilev, I.; Portillo, M.C.; Serrano, M.; Knutsen, I.; Roukova, P.; Lionis, C.; Todorova, E.; Foss, C.; et al. Social support systems as determinants of self-management and quality of life of people with diabetes across Europe: Study protocol for an observational study. *Health Qual. Life Outcomes* **2014**, *12*, 29. [CrossRef] [PubMed]

17. Reeves, D.; Blickem, C.; Vassilev, I.; Brooks, H.; Kennedy, A.; Richardson, G.; Rogers, A. The contribution of social networks to the health and self-management of patients with long-term conditions: A longitudinal study. *PLoS ONE* **2014**, *9*, e98340. [CrossRef] [PubMed]

18. Lin, N.; Ensel, W.; Simeone, R.; Kuo, W. Social support, stressful life events, and illness: A model and an empirical test. *J. Heal. Soc. Behav.* **1979**, *20*, 108–119. [CrossRef]

19. Lin, N.; Dean, A.; Ensel, W.M. Social support scales: A methodological note. *Schizophr. Bull.* **1981**, *7*, 73–89. [CrossRef]

20. House, J.S. Social support and social structure. *Sociol. Forum* **1987**, *2*, 135–146. [CrossRef]

21. House, J.S.; Landis, K.R.; Umberson, D. Social relationships and health. *Science* **1988**, *241*, 540–545. [CrossRef]

22. Rn, D.C.B.; Rn, F.P.; Benton, D.C.; Pérez-Raya, F.; Fernández-Fernández, M.P.; González-Jurado, M.A. A systematic review of nurse-related social network analysis studies. *Int. Nurs. Rev.* **2014**, *62*, 321–339.

23. Bae, S.H.; Nikolaev, A.N.; Seo, J.; Castner, J. Health care provider social network analysis: A systematic review. *Nurs. Outlook* **2015**, *63*, 566–584. [CrossRef]

24. Scherlowski, H.; Guimaraes de Araújo, M.; Andrade, J.; Feijó, T.; Souza, V.; dos Santos, R. Social network analysis in primary health care: An integrative review. *Integr. Rev.* **2018**, *31*, 108–115.

25. Hawe, P.; Webster, C.; Shiell, A. A glossary of terms for navigating the field of social network analysis. *J. Epidemiol. Community Health* **2004**, *58*, 971–975. [CrossRef] [PubMed]

26. Parnell, J.M.; Robinson, J.C. Social network analysis: Presenting an underutilised method for nursing research. *J. Adv. Nurs.* **2018**, *74*, 1310–1318. [CrossRef] [PubMed]

27. Del-Pino-Casado, R.; Frías-Osuna, A.; Palomino-Moral, P.; Ruzafa-Martínez, M.; Ramos-Morcillo, A. Social support and subjective burden in caregivers of adults and older adults: A meta-analysis. *PLoS ONE* **2018**, *13*, e0189874. [CrossRef] [PubMed]

28. Rodríguez-Madrid, M.N.; del Río-Lozano, M.; Fernandez-Peña, R.; Jiménez-Pernett, J.; García-Mochón, L.; Lupiañez-Castillo, A.; García-Calvente, M.M. Gender differences in social support received by informal caregivers: A personal network analysis approach. *Int. J. Environ. Res. Public Health* **2019**, *16*, 91. [CrossRef] [PubMed]

29. Perry, B.; Pescosolido, B.; Borgatti, S. *Egocentric Network Analysis: Foundations, Methods, and Models*; Cambridge University Press: Cambridge, UK, 2018.

30. McCarty, C. Structure in personal networks. *J. Soc. Struct.* **2002**, *3*, 20.

31. Hâncean, M.; Molina, J.L.; Lubbers, M.J. Recent advancements, developments and applications of personal network analysis. *Int. Rev. Soc. Res.* **2016**, *6*, 137–145. [CrossRef]

32. Molina, J.L. El estudio de las redes personales: Contribuciones, métodos y perspectiva. *Empiria Rev. Metodol. Cienc. Soc.* **2005**, *10*, 71–105.

33. McCarty, C.; Lubbers, M.J.; Vacca, R.; Molina, J.L. How personal networks have been used so far. In *Conducting Personal Network Research. A Practical Guide*; The Guilford Press: New York, NY, USA, 2019; p. 270.

34. Smith, K.; Christakis, N. Social networks and health. *Annu. Rev. Sociol.* **2008**, *34*, 405–418. [CrossRef]

35. Doeglas, D.; Suurmeijer, T.; Briançon, S.; Moum, T.; Krol, B.; Bjelle, A.; Sanderman, R.; Van der Heuvel, W. An international study on measuring social support: Interactions and satisfaction. *Soc. Sci. Med.* **1996**, *43*, 1389–1397. [CrossRef]

36. Franks, H.M.; Cronan, T.A.; Oliver, K. Social support in women with fibromyalgia: Is quality more important than quantity? *J. Community Psychol.* **2004**, *32*, 425–438. [CrossRef]

37. Tardy, C. Social support measurement. *Am. J. Community Psychol.* **1985**, *13*, 187–202. [CrossRef]

38. Bernardes, S.F.; Forgeron, P.; Fournier, K.; Reszel, J. Beyond solicitousness: A comprehensive review on informal pain-related social support. *Pain* **2017**, *158*, 2066–2076. [CrossRef] [PubMed]

39. Breivik, H.; Collett, B.; Ventafridda, V.; Cohen, R.; Gallacher, D. Survey of chronic pain in Europe: Prevalence, impact on daily life, and treatment. *Eur. J. Pain* **2006**, *10*, 287–333. [CrossRef]

40. Dueñas, M.; Ojeda, B.; Salazar, A.; Mico, J.A.; Failde, I. A review of chronic pain impact on patients, their social environment and the health care system. *J. Pain Res.* **2016**, *9*, 457–467. [CrossRef]

41. Fernández Peña, R. El Estudio del Apoyo Social y la Calidad de Vida Desde las Redes Personales: El Caso del Dolor Crónico. Ph.D. Thesis, Universidad Autónoma de Barcelona, Barcelona, Spain, 2015.

42. Fernández-Peña, R.; Molina, J.L.; Valero, O. Personal network analysis in the study of social support: The case of chronic pain. *Int. J. Environ. Res. Public Health* **2018**, *15*, 2695.

43. Borgatti, S.P.; Everett, M.G. *Analyzing Social Networks*; Sage Publications: London, UK, 2013.

44. Greenacre, M. *Correspondence Analysis in Practice*, 2nd ed.; Chapman & Hall: London, UK, 2007.

45. Ward, J.H., Jr. Hierarchical grouping to optimize an objective function. *J. Am. Stat. Assoc.* **1963**, *58*, 236–244. [CrossRef]

46. Hartigan, J.A. *Clustering Algorithms*; Wiley & Sons: New York, NY, USA, 1975.

47. Weiner, A.S.B.; Hannum, J.W. Differences in the quantity of social support between geographically close and long-distance friendships. *J. Soc. Pers. Relat.* **2012**, *30*, 662–672. [CrossRef]

48. Fernández, M. Social support networks in Spain: The factors that determine models of choice. *Int. Sociol.* **2012**, *27*, 384–402.

49. Mok, D.; Wellman, B. Did distance matter before the Internet? Interpersonal contact and support in the 1970s. *Soc. Netw.* **2007**, *29*, 430–461. [CrossRef]

50. Tomini, F.; Tomini, S.M.; Groot, W. Understanding the value of social networks in life satisfaction of elderly people: A comparative study of 16 European countries using SHARE data. *BMC Geriatr.* **2016**, *16*, 203. [CrossRef] [PubMed]

51. Antonucci, T.C.; Akiyama, H.; Lansford, J.E. Negative effects of close social relations. *Fam. Relat.* **1998**, *47*, 379–384. [CrossRef]

52. Cohen, S.; Janicki-Deverts, D. Can we improve our physical health by altering our social networks? *Perspect. Psychol. Sci.* **2009**, *4*, 375–378. [CrossRef] [PubMed]

53. Rook, K.S. The negative side of social interaction: Impact on psychological well-being. *J. Pers. Soc. Psychol.* **1984**, *46*, 1097–1108. [CrossRef] [PubMed]

54. Rook, K.S. Exposure and reactivity to negative social exchanges: A preliminary investigation using daily diary data. *J. Gerontol.* **2003**, *58*, 100–111. [CrossRef] [PubMed]

55. Newsom, J.T.; Rook, K.S.; Nishishiba, M.; Sorkin, D.H.; Mahan, T.L. Understanding the relative importance of positive and negative social exchanges: Examining specific domains and appraisals. *J. Gerontol.* **2005**, *60*, 304–312. [CrossRef]

56. Català, E.; Reig, E.; Artés, M.; Aliaga, L.; López, J.S.; Segú, J.L. Prevalence of pain in the Spanish population: Telephone survey in 5000 homes. *Eur. J. Pain* **2002**, *6*, 133–140. [CrossRef]

57. Geisser, M.E.; Cano, A.; Leonard, M. Factors associated with marital satisfaction and mood among spouses of persons with chronic back pain. *J. Pain* **2005**, *6*, 518–525. [CrossRef]

58. Leonard, M.T.; Cano, A.; Johansen, A.B. Chronic pain in a couples context: A review and integration of theoretical models and empirical evidence. *J. Pain* **2006**, *7*, 377–390. [CrossRef]

59. Cano, A.; Leonard, M. Integrative behavioral couple therapy for chronic pain: Promoting behavior change and emotional acceptance. *J. Clin. Psychol.* **2006**, *62*, 1409–1418. [CrossRef]

60. Roy, R. What happens to spouses? In *Social Relations and Chronic Pain*; Kluwer Academic Publishers: New York, NY, USA, 2002; pp. 57–70. ISBN 0306471973.

61. Entwisle, B.; Faust, K.; Rindfuss, R.R.R.; Kaneda, T. Networks and contexts: Variation in the structure of social ties. *Am. J. Sociol.* **2007**, *112*, 1495–1533. [CrossRef]

62. Jolly, A.; Muth, S.; Wylie, J.; Potterat, J. Sexual networks and sexually transmitted infections: A tale of two cities. *J. Urban Heal.* **2001**, *78*, 433–446. [CrossRef] [PubMed]

63. Smith, A.M.A.; Grierson, J.; Wain, D.; Pitts, M.; Pattison, P. Associations between the sexual behaviour of men who have sex with men and the structure and composition of their social networks. *Sex. Transm. Infect.* **2004**, *80*, 455–458. [CrossRef] [PubMed]

64. Birkett, M.; Kuhns, L.; Latkin, C.; Muth, S.; Mustanski, B. The sexual networks of racially diverse young men who have sex with men. *Arch. Sex. Behav.* **2015**, *44*, 1787–1797. [CrossRef] [PubMed]

65. Morris, M. Sexual networks and HIV in four african populations: The use of standardized behavioral surveys with biological markers. In *Network Epidemiology: A Handbook for Survey Design and Data Collection*; Oxford University Press on Demand: Oxford, UK, 2004; pp. 58–84. ISBN 9780199269013.

66. Bearman, P.S.; Moody, J.; Stovel, K. Chains of affection: The structure of adolescent romantic and sexual networks. *Am. J. Sociol.* **2004**, *110*, 44–91. [CrossRef]

67. Hansen, L.R.; Pedersen, S.B.; Overgaard, C.; Torp-Pedersen, C.; Ullits, L.R. Associations between the structural and functional aspects of social relations and poor mental health: A cross-sectional register study. *BMC Public Health* **2017**, *17*, 860. [CrossRef]

68. Haas, S.A.; Schaefer, D.R.; Kornienko, O. Health and the structure of adolescent social networks. *J. Health Soc. Behav.* **2010**, *51*, 424–439. [CrossRef]

69. Agneessens, F.; Waege, H.; Lievens, J. Diversity in social support by role relations: A typology. *Soc. Netw.* **2006**, *28*, 427–441. [CrossRef]

70. Platt, J.; Keyes, K.M.; Koenen, K.C. Size of the social network versus quality of social support: Which is more protective against PTSD? *Soc. Psychiatry Psychiatr. Epidemiol.* **2014**, *49*, 1279–1286. [CrossRef]

71. Stokes, J.P. Predicting satisfaction with social support form social network structure. *Am. J. Community Psychol.* **1983**, *11*, 141–152. [CrossRef]

72. Ashida, S.; Heaney, C.A. Differential associations of social support and social connectedness with structural features of social networks and the health status of older adults. *J. Aging Health* **2008**, *20*, 872–893. [CrossRef] [PubMed]

73. Hirsch, B.J. Natural support systems and coping with major life changes. *Am. J. Community Psychol.* **1980**, *8*, 159–172. [CrossRef]

74. Burt, R.S. Structural holes and good ideas. *Am. J. Sociol.* **2004**, *110*, 349–399. [CrossRef]

75. Wellman, B.; Wortley, S. Different strokes from different folks: Community ties and social support. *Am. J. Sociol.* **1990**, *96*, 558–588. [CrossRef]

76. Coleman, J.S. Social capital in the creation of human capital. *Am. J. Sociol.* **1988**, *94*, S95–S120. [CrossRef]

77. Putnam, R.D. Bowling alone: America's declining social capital. In *Culture and Politics*; Palgrave Macmillan: New York, NY, USA, 2000; pp. 223–234.

78. Chandola, T.; Marmot, M.; Siegrist, J. Failed reciprocity in close social relationships and health: Findings from the Whitehall II study. *J. Psychosom. Res.* **2007**, *63*, 403–411. [CrossRef]

79. Knowlton, A.R.; Yang, C.; Bohnert, A.; Wissow, L.; Chander, G.; Arnsten, J.A. Informal care and reciprocity of support are associated with HAART adherence among men in baltimore. *AIDS Behav.* **2011**, *15*, 1429–1436. [CrossRef]

80. Mercken, L.; Candel, M.; Willems, P.; De Vries, H. Disentangling social selection and social influence effects on adolescent smoking: The importance of reciprocity in friendships. *Addiction* **2007**, *102*, 1483–1492. [CrossRef]

81. Adelman, R.D.; Tmanova, L.; Delgado, D.; Dion, S.; Lachs, M.S. Caregiver burden: A clinical review. *J. Am. Med. Assoc.* **2014**, *311*, 1052–1059. [CrossRef]

82. Jones, S.L.; Hadjistavropoulos, H.D.; Janzen, J.A.; Hadjistavropoulos, T. The relation of pain and caregiver burden in informal order adult caregivers. *Pain Med.* **2011**, *12*, 51–58. [CrossRef]

83. Rodakowski, J.; Skidmore, E.R.; Rogers, J.C.; Schulz, R. Role of social support in predicting caregiver burden. *Arch. Phys. Med. Rehabil.* **2012**, *93*, 2229–2236. [CrossRef] [PubMed]

84. Shaw, B.A.; Krause, N.; Liang, J.; Bennett, J. Tracking changes in social relations throughout late life. *J. Gerontol.* **2007**, *62*, 90–99. [CrossRef] [PubMed]

85. Feld, S.L.L.; Suitor, J.J.J.; Gartner, J.G.; Hoegh, J.G.; Gartner, J.G. Describing changes in personal networks over time. *Field Methods* **2007**, *19*, 218–236. [CrossRef]

86. Mollenhorst, G.; Volker, B.; Flap, H. Changes in personal relationships: How social contexts affect the emergence and discontinuation of relationships. *Soc. Netw.* **2014**, *37*, 65–80. [CrossRef]

87. Fischer, C.S.; Beresford, L. Changes in support networks in late middle age: The extension of gender and educational differences. *J. Gerontol. Ser. B Psychol. Sci. Soc. Sci.* **2015**, *70*, 123–131. [CrossRef] [PubMed]

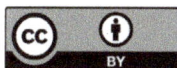

International Journal of
Environmental Research and Public Health

MDPI

Review

Experiences of Homeless Families in Parenthood: A Systematic Review and Synthesis of Qualitative Evidence

Filipa Maria Reinhardt Andrade [1,*], Amélia Simões Figueiredo [2], Manuel Luís Capelas [2], Zaida Charepe [2] and Sérgio Deodato [2]

[1] Institute of Health Sciences, Doctorate Student of the Doctorate Degree in Nursing, Universidade Católica Portuguesa, 1649-023 Lisbon, Portugal
[2] Institute of Health Sciences, Centre for Interdisciplinary Research in Health (CIIS), Universidade Católica Portuguesa, 1649-023 Lisbon, Portugal; simoesfigueiredo@ics.lisboa.ucp.pt (A.S.F.); luis.capelas@ics.lisboa.ucp.pt (M.L.C.); Zaidacharepe@ics.lisboa.ucp.pt (Z.C.); sdeodato@ics.lisboa.ucp.pt (S.D.)
* Correspondence: fandrade@ics.lisboa.ucp.pt

Received: 6 March 2020; Accepted: 7 April 2020; Published: 15 April 2020

check for
updates

Abstract: The objective of this systematic review was to identify the available qualitative data and to develop a framework to address the life experiences of homeless families in parenthood. The research was performed in the PubMed and CINAHL Complete databases, for works published in Portuguese, English, French and Spanish. Studies that included qualitative data, or both qualitative and quantitative data, were considered for this research. A total of 358 articles were obtained, of which 37 were assessed for eligibility, and 26 were rejected. In the end, 11 studies were selected. The Joanna Briggs Institute Critical Appraisal Checklist for Qualitative Research was used. These studies were conducted mostly in the United States, in temporary/transitional shelters for nuclear or single-parent families (led by women) in a homeless situation. In this context, the area which arose as the more relevant one was mental health, followed by the social studies. Two types of dimensions emerged from the results: mediating dimensions (which include the categories "Insecurity", "Lack of Privacy", "Isolation", "Stigma" and "Disempowerment") that are responsible for difficulties related to education, and behavioural changes in both the parents and the children; and supporting dimensions (which include the categories "Context as a Facilitator", "Relationship with Others" and "Parents' and children's Self") that lead to motivation, as well as the acquisition of strategies by the parents, to resolve parenting issues. This research helps expand nursing knowledge and presents a synthesis of the life experiences of homeless families in parenthood. Nursing can respond to the vulnerable population, due to its predominant role in promoting their health.

Keywords: family; homeless; nursing; parenting; parents; vulnerable population

1. Introduction

Parenthood is considered "the recognition of a mother's/father's responsibilities, the assumption of behaviours that promote the children's growth and development, as well as the internalisation of expectations expressed by individuals, families, friends and society, regarding the parental role's appropriate or inappropriate behaviours"(own translation, from: Ordem dos Enfermeiros) [1] (p. 66). Parenthood is understood as a transition [2–4]. Life transitions correspond to periods of greater vulnerability and increased health risk, which is why they have been increasingly considered a central concept for nursing [2,5]. Nurses are aware of the needs and changes brought upon by transitions, and they prepare the patient/family to better cope with such events, through learning and acquiring new skills [2].

The transition experience requires, as outcome indicators: the incorporation of new knowledge; the change of behaviours; the redefinition of the meanings associated with the occurred events; and, consequently, the redefinition of oneself within the social context [5]. Concerning possible constraints to the transition process, the author refers that, although community resources are able to create conditions which facilitate transition (family support, relevant information, referral, decision-making support), they may also create transition-inhibiting conditions (inappropriate counselling, insufficient information, etc.). The author points out that the society's development stage has a similar dual effect on transition—it may either facilitate the process, through the creation of laws and regulations, or inhibit it, through stigma, stereotypes, and marginalization [3].

In this regard, parenthood is considered to be an important, complex, challenging and highly responsible task for the human being, since it concerns the preparation of another human being for the challenges of development, namely physical, economical and psycho-social adversities [6]. While being an activity that usually involves the children, the parents and other family members in an interaction throughout life, it is not exclusive for these players and may involve other people, such as nurses, teachers, friends, partners, and even strangers [7]. In this sense, any person that participates in the care and development of a child is part of the parenthood process [8]. This concept emphasises that, in order to acquire the sense of being a father, or a mother, and to meet all the relevant requirements, it is not enough to just become a parent. It is necessary to go through a complex, conscious—and sometimes unconscious—process of role appropriation. Although parenthood is a subjective concept, because it is influenced by cultural beliefs, the dimensions and structural tasks of the parent-child relationship tend to remain similar, thus allowing its assessment (i.e., the evaluation of parental skills and competences) and producing data adequate for research purposes [6]. In this sense, Cruz considers five assessable parental functions: (1) Satisfaction of the basic survival and health needs—Where he emphasizes that the inability to assume this function may be related to socio-economic constraints, natural disasters, drug addiction, or parents' disease; (2) Providing of an organized and predictable physical world for the child—Which includes safety-promoting routines (severely dysfunctional families reveal a great difficulty in performing this function); (3) Responding to the needs of cognitive understanding with respect to extra-family realities—Stresses the difficulty of families that are more isolated or less permeable in ensuring this function; (4) Satisfaction of the needs of affection, trust and safety—This function is associated with the construction of attachment, which has proved to be a fundamental predictor of personal adaptation throughout life; (5) Satisfaction of the child's social interaction needs—The family should perform this function because, as the original nucleus of the child's socialization, it influences the future integration of the child in broader social contexts [9].

Furthermore, Figueiredo uses the life cycle stages ("Family with young children", "Family with children at school", and "Family with adolescent children") to define several assessment categories with respect to the parental role's competence. The aforesaid categories differ in terms of knowledge dimension, as well as adhesion behaviour. This author relates the knowledge of the role with the available information and the ability to learn skills, in order to identify the need to acquire new knowledge conducive to behavioural changes. She also relates the adhesion behaviour dimension to those aspects which highlight the parents' actions that reflect the full incorporation of parenthood through the identity of the role. That incorporation is evidenced by trust and competence in the role's performance. The evaluative categories of knowledge and adhesion behaviour are related to: physical care (which includes nourishment, elimination, personal hygiene and physical exercise); leisure activities; health surveillance; safety and prevention of accidents; attachment; cognitive, psychosexual, emotional and social development; structuring rules; a positive interaction with the child; adaptation to school; and the parents' involvement in education [10].

When we observe the different conditions that should be involved in the parental process/activity, the complexity associated with the process of educating a child becomes evident. In this sense, family plays a key role: it constitutes the most immediate space for the child's care, affections, dependence and socialization; it defines habits, health care routines, education, and the contexts to which the child is exposed (friends, school, neighbourhood, etc.); and it influences the present, the future and the development of the child. However, the family is not always able to provide a homogeneous environment and can have a negative impact on the child's well-being [11].

Within the family, there may be risk factors (internal or external), which represent a deficit in the children's development potential. On the other hand, the existence of protective factors (internal or external) that encourage the full development of the child can also occur. The internal protection factors relate to the quality of the interactions between family members. or to the involvement in stimulant activities. The external protective factors are associated with socioeconomic patterns, such as the family's structure, the parents' adequate working conditions, or the social support provided by public policies. As for external risk factors, they are related to demographic variables (e.g., having a single/adolescent mother, father's absence, separations and divorces) and to socioeconomic patterns (e.g., poverty, inequalities, mother's lack of education, violence, lack of social support, and restricted access to public policies regarding health and education). In contrast, the internal risk factors are associated with parental practices and parent-child interaction styles (e.g., abuse, neglect, negative communication, inconsistent discipline) [11]. In homeless families, many of those internal and external risk factors are simultaneously present, which accounts for their greater vulnerability [12]. From a nursing care perspective, vulnerability has always been considered a priority. As such, these families are a focus of interest for the nursing practice, often being the target of the aforementioned care [13].

A homeless person is an individual who, "regardless of his/her nationality, racial or ethnic origin, religion, age, sex, sexual orientation, socio-economic status, and physical and mental health status, is: homeless, living in a public space, in an emergency shelter, or in a precarious location; or homeless, living in a temporary accommodation destined for that purpose" (own translation, from: Ministério do Trabalho, Solidariedade e Segurança Social) [14] (p. 3925).

The reasons for the families' homelessness are different from those that lead to homelessness in adults. Most families are left homeless by: domestic violence [15–17]; repeated episodes of trauma and violence throughout life; child abuse; relationship breakups [15,16]; neighbourhood harassment; mental health problems involving parents and/or children [15,16,18]; special educational needs [15,16]; lack of family and social support networks; lack of access to statutory services [15–17,19]; social and emotional problems [17,20]; chronic instability; compromised health [19]; family head with a physical disability, with chronic health problems or with mental health problems [17]; poor financial situations and/or low income streams [21]; precarious housing situations; financial problems due to underemployment or unemployment; past mistakes (e.g., high school or college dropouts); and premature responsibilities, such as assuming a parental role at a young age [19]. The characteristics of these homeless families are heterogeneous. The most common are single-parent families led by (single) women [16,17,22]; with two children, generally under 11 years of age [16].

The lack of housing brings high social costs [23] and in families, has profound consequences, including the risk of health deterioration in family members [24,25]; the disruption of family dynamics, and the separation of parents and children [25]. Homeless families present multiple problems and needs that are interrelated (e.g., social, educational and health care) [15]. Homelessness is rarely an isolated event. Children from homeless families are prone to have a history of: low birth weight; anaemia; tooth decay; delayed immunizations; growth deficits; increased accident frequency, mainly injuries and burns [16]; developmental deficits; mental health problems [16,24,26,27]; behaviour disorders (e.g., sleep disorders, eating disorders, aggression and hyperactivity in young children); anxiety and post-traumatic stress [16]. A combination of multiple adverse childhood experiences may weaken their resilience [28] and they may become homeless as adults [28,29].

The protective factors for children belonging to homeless families include: school, due to its social stability, its routines and the parents' sense of achievement when they are capable of maintaining their child in the same school [16]; and the positive relationships between parents and children, which can mitigate the negative effects of homelessness in childhood, by helping the children to better manage their emotions, by promoting self-regulation, by forming positive relationships and by improving the children's functioning [30].

Homeless families face unique conditions that can affect the health and well-being of both the parents and the children. They may also affect parental practices, a better understanding of the homeless parents' life experiences being necessary in order to increasingly meet the real needs of this population. The Canadian Homeless Press Observatory argues that the support given to families, through the strengthening of relationships, is essential to avoid situations of homeless youth [29].

The European Federation of National Organisations Working with the Homeless (*Fédération Européenned' Associations Nationales Travaillant avec les Sans-Abri*—FEANTSA) suggests future research, highlighting the importance of studies in the following areas: homeless families, in order to further unveil the existing challenges and the strategies to be implemented, concerning the relationship with these families; parenting, in order to identify the constraints and strategies that homeless women (and men) face in their parental roles, as well as in the construction of their parental identities [31].

A preliminary search in the PubMed and CINAHL databases revealed the inexistence of systematic reviews on this topic and that none is currently in progress. Hence the necessity of aggregating knowledge to better comprehend the parental experiences of homeless individuals, and to identify useful factors for the monitoring of these vulnerable families. This will contribute to the understanding of how professionals can support families in managing their situation.

It is important to highlight the importance of this work for the scientific area of nursing, since nurses are considered the health professionals closest to the population, playing a fundamental role in health promotion and disease prevention, especially among the vulnerable population, as is the case of homeless families. This work is part of the Special Issue of the International Journal of Environmental Research and Public Health, since it emphasizes the importance of nursing for society as promoters of the population's health.

In this sense, we decided to conduct this systematic review, in order to better recognize the main research lines that have been explored up to this date, and to respond to the challenge proposed by the FEANTSA. For that purpose, we employed a scientific methodology which follows the Joanna Briggs Institute (JBI) protocol for systematic reviews of qualitative evidence [32].

The objective of this systematic review was to identify available qualitative evidence and to develop a framework to address the life experiences of homeless families in parenthood. We intended to answer the following research question, formulated according to the PICo acronym, [32] (Population, phenomenon of Interest and Context): What are the parenthood (I) experiences of the homeless (C) family (P)?

2. Methods

This systematic review adopts the method suggested by Moher, Liberati, Tetzlaff, Altman and the PRISMA group [33].

2.1. Inclusion Criteria

Population—This review considered all the studies that focus on homeless families constituted by adult parents (over 18 years of age) and their children (under 18 years of age). The parents and/or family correspond to the individuals who are responsible for providing care to the child/adolescent [32]. The following types of family were included: nuclear family (a man and a woman, who may or may not be legally married, with one or more biological/adopted children); reconstructed family (a couple in which at least one of the elements had a previous marital relationship and has a child who resulted from that relationship); single-parent family (a single parent and one or more children, being identified the gender of the person who represents the parental figure); extended family (a nuclear family, plus other relatives, or people who share with them bonds other than kinship) [10].

Phenomenon of interest—This review considered all the studies that address the parenthood experiences of homeless families, with parenthood being based on the evaluative categories of the parental role proposed by Figueiredo [10], and also the five parental functions of Cruz [9].

Context—This review considered studies conducted with homeless families. To that end, we employed the definition of "Homeless" recommended by the ENIPSSA [14].

Type of studies—Primary studies, of mixed or qualitative nature, published in Portuguese, French, English and Spanish, without a previously defined time span.

2.2. Exclusion Criteria

We excluded text (review) articles, opinion articles, letters to the editor, response letters, dissertations and reports, since priority was given to the numerous original research articles.

2.3. Search Strategy

The research strategy that was used aimed to find published studies indexed in certain databases. It comprised three stages. The first stage included an initial search in the PubMed and CINAHL databases, to analyse the keywords; it also encompassed the analysis of the MeSH Health Sciences descriptors in the respective query platform, as well as in CINAHL. The MeSH terms were then used in the PubMed database, while the corresponding MeSH headings were used in the CINAHL database. After selecting the relevant Boolean operators, descriptors, and indexed terms used to describe them, a second search was conducted in all the included databases—PubMed and CINAHL Complete (through EBSCOhost). The keywords which were used corresponded to the ones defined according to the PICo acronym (Population, phenomenon of Interest and Context). The research strategy was sensitive to the specific characteristics of each selected database (Table 1).

Table 1. Search strategy.

Database	Search Strategy
PubMed	(((((((((((((((parenting) OR parenting styles) OR parenting practices) OR parent education) OR childrearing) OR family practice) OR parenting education) OR parenting education) OR parental behaviour) OR parent* behaviour) OR parent* education) OR parent* attitudes) OR altered parenting) OR parent* roll) OR parenthood)) AND ((((homeless persons) OR homeless people) OR homelessness) OR vulnerable populations)) AND ((((((((((((parent* OR biological parents) OR child of impaired parents) OR marriage) OR spouses) OR mothers) OR fathers) OR parents) OR only child) OR nuclear family) OR single parent) OR single parent family) OR family)
CINAHL	(parent* OR biological parents OR child of impaired parents OR marriage OR spouses OR mothers OR fathers OR parents OR only child OR nuclear family OR single parent OR single parent family OR family) AND (homeless persons OR homeless people OR homelessness OR vulnerable populations) AND ((MH "Parenting") OR (MH "Altered Parenting (NANDA)") OR (MH "Parenting (Iowa NOC)") OR (MH "Parenting Alteration (Saba CCC)") OR (MH "Parenting Education") OR (MH "Risk for Altered Parenting (NANDA)" OR parenting styles OR parenting practices OR child-rearing OR family practice OR parental behaviour OR parent* behaviour OR parent* education OR parent* attitudes OR parent* role OR parenthood)

The searches were carried out between January 9th and January 30th, 2019. Duplicates were removed and, subsequently, two independent reviewers performed an analysis of the terms and descriptors found in the titles and abstracts of the articles. Studies that did not meet the inclusion criteria were excluded. Afterwards, the selected articles were read in full. Those that did not satisfy the inclusion criteria, or corresponded to the exclusion criteria, were eliminated. Finally, in a third stage, the selected articles' bibliographic references were analysed, in order to identify additional relevant studies. This review was not recorded in any systematic review database.

Before their integration in the final sample, all the selected articles were subjected to a methodological quality assessment.

2.4. Evaluation of the Methodological Quality

The methodological quality evaluation was conducted by two independent reviewers, using the JBI Critical Appraisal Checklist for Qualitative Research [32]. Disagreements between the reviewers were resolved through debating. The evaluation's purpose was to analyse the strengths and weaknesses of each selected work. The reviewers critically appraised the articles, which were accepted for inclusion if there was congruence between the research methodology, the research's objectives, and the methods used for data collection, representation and analysis.

2.5. Data Extraction

Data was extracted from all the works included in the review, using the JBI-QARI standardized data extraction tool [32]. The extracted data encompassed specific details about each research's objectives, scientific area, type of study (design and data collection method), population, context, phenomena of interest, and significant findings for our research question and objective.

2.6. Data Synthesis

The qualitative research's results were grouped and categorized based on the similarity of meaning, with at least two findings per category, using the JBI-QARI tool [32]. The different categories were created through a process of consensus between the reviewers. Data was then aggregated and subjected to synthesis, resulting in a single comprehensive set of findings that can provide a basis for evidence-based practice. The findings were classified as "credible" or "unquestionable" (according to their credibility level), using the JBI-QARI tool.

3. Results

We obtained a preliminary total of 358 articles through the database search. After duplicate removal, 349 works were subjected to relevance assessment based on their title and abstract. Of these, 248 were excluded after title evaluation and 64 were excluded after abstract evaluation, because they did not meet the established inclusion criteria. The remaining 37 studies were subjected to an eligibility assessment, and 26 were rejected, since they did not meet the inclusion criteria. Thus, a total of 11 articles were subjected to critical evaluation, with none being excluded. Figure 1 shows a PRISMA flowchart of the studies' identification and selection process for inclusion in the review.

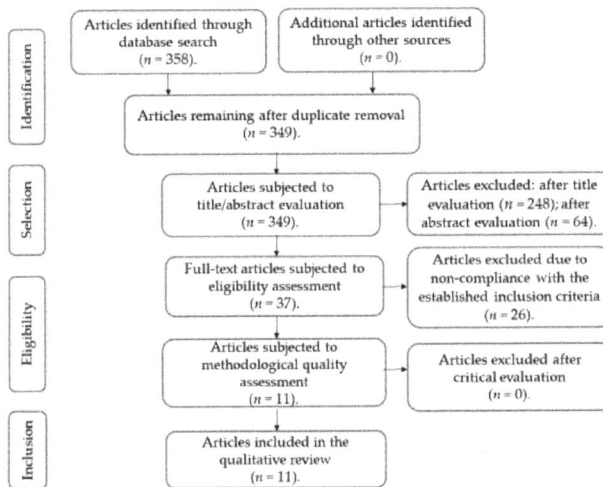

Figure 1. PRISMA flowchart detailing the search's results and the studies' selection/inclusion process (based on the method suggested by Moher, Liberati, Tetzlaff, Altman and the PRISMA group) [33].

3.1. Methodological Quality

All the 11 selected works were included in the analysis. These studies met the inclusion criteria and were considered methodologically rigorous, regarding the evaluation criteria. They offered useful descriptions of the daily life of homeless families. They also showed congruence between the research methodology, the research's objectives, the methods used for data collection, representation and analysis, and the methods employed to interpret the results. Most of the data represented the participants' opinions adequately. Despite the high quality of the selected articles, there was a lack of information in some of them. For instance, only 18% presented a statement contextualising the researchers' cultural and/or theoretical background. Furthermore, only 54.55% of the reported conclusions were derived from data interpretation. Prior to the critical evaluation, the reviewers decided that these shortcomings were not essential criteria that needed to be met for the article's inclusion. Table 2 presents the final assessment of the included works, specifying the research design's accuracy, as well as the quality of the resulting reports.

Table 2. Final evaluation of the included studies (according to the method used by Lockwood) [32].

Quote	Q1	Q2	Q3	Q4	Q5	Q6	Q7	Q8	Q9	Q10
Anderson et al. 2006 [15]	Y	Y	Y	Y	Y	N	Y	Y	N	Y
Anthony et al., 2017 [34]	Y	Y	Y	Y	Y	N	Y	Y	Y	Y
Cosgrove and Flynn, 2005 [35]	N	Y	Y	NC	Y	N	Y	Y	N	NC
Haskett et al., 2018 [36]	Y	Y	Y	Y	Y	Y	Y	Y	Y	Y
Holtrop et al., 2015 [37]	Y	Y	Y	Y	Y	N	Y	Y	Y	NC
Lindsey, 1997 [38]	Y	Y	Y	Y	Y	N	N	Y	N	NC
Morris and Butt, 2003 [39]	N	Y	Y	Y	Y	N	Y	Y	Y	Y
Roche et al., 2018 [40]	Y	Y	Y	Y	Y	N	Y	Y	Y	Y
Sylvestre et al., 2018 [25]	Y	Y	Y	Y	Y	Y	Y	Y	Y	Y
Tischler et al., 2004 [41]	Y	Y	Y	NC	Y	N	Y	NC	Y	N
Vanleit et al., 2006 [42]	Y	Y	Y	Y	Y	N	Y	Y	Y	N
% Yes	81.82	100	100	81.82	100	18.18	90.91	90.91	72.73	54.55

N: No; NC: Not Conclusive; Y: Yes.

Q1. Is there congruence between the declared philosophical perspective and the research methodology? Q2. Is there consistency between the research methodology and the research's question(s)/objective(s)? Q3. Is there consistency between the research methodology and the data collection methods? Q4. Is there congruence between the research methodology and the data's representation and analysis? Q5. Is there congruence between the research methodology and the results' interpretation? Q6. Is there a statement that contextualises the researcher from a cultural or theoretical point of view? Q7. Are the researcher's influence in the research and the inverse phenomenon addressed? Q8. Are the participants and their opinions adequately represented? Q9. Is the research considered ethical, according to the current criteria, or, for recent studies, is there evidence of ethical approval by an appropriate committee? Q10. Do the conclusions drawn in the research report derive from the data's analysis/interpretation? Note: Q1, Q2, Q3, etc., refer to the questions included in the JBI Critical Appraisal Checklist for Qualitative Research [32].

Regarding the CONQual results, most of the selected studies obtained a moderate score [37–40,42], four reached a high score [15,25,34,36], one obtained a low score [35], and one achieved a very low score [41]. Despite their low classification, these last two articles were not eliminated, because their findings were unique and contributed to the knowledge of the phenomenon. Additional details can be seen in Tables S1 and S2, which are available in electronic format.

3.2. Results of the Extracted Data

Concerning the research design, the studies are mostly qualitative in nature [15,25,34,35,38–40,42]. Only three works present a mixed nature, with qualitative and quantitative approaches [36,37,41].

Two of the articles are grounded in theory [38,39], while the remaining did not declare any specific methodology, merely stating that they used a qualitative approach. The methods applied in the 11 articles were diverse, namely: qualitative individual interviews, family interviews, focus groups with parents, participant observation, diaries and reflection activities.

The works are scattered over time (from 1997 to 2018). After the first article, which appears in 1997, there is a large gap, whilst the remaining articles were published between the time period 2003 to 2018. The first article that appears after this gap is the nursing study. They were mainly conducted in the United States, except for two studies that were performed in the United Kingdom [15,41] and one study that was carried out in Australia [40]. The context of the studies corresponded to temporary/transitional shelters for nuclear families [15,25,34,36,37,41] or single-parent families led by homeless women [35,38,42]. Only one study was conducted in multiple contexts (shelters, motels and transition houses) for homeless nuclear families [39]. Another research was carried out with single-parent families led by homeless men, who were recruited for the study by agencies that provide support to the homeless [40].

As for the number of families interviewed, the majority were single-parent families led by women, with a total of 506 families, and in two studies the number of interviews was not mentioned [35,38]. Next, the largest number of records were single-parent families led by men with a total of 51 interviews, 40 of whom were part of the same study [40]. Finally, there were 22 nuclear families (couple with children) in two of the studies [15,41], and five interviews that were represented by relatives in one of the studies [39].The most frequent research field was mental health [15,25,35–37,41], followed by social sciences [34,38,40], occupational therapy [42], education (in one of the psychology studies) [35], and nursing [39]. Further details about the included studies are presented in Table S3 that will be available in electronic form.

3.3. Synthesis of the Qualitative Research's Results

Taking into account the objective of the study, which sought to develop a structure to address the experiences of homeless families in parenthood, we extracted a total of 74 results from the 11 studies. Those findings were combined to form 12 categories based on similarity of meaning. The categories were grouped into two dimensions: "Parenthood Mediating Dimensions" and "Parenthood Supporting Dimensions". As mediating dimensions, we considered situations of transition to a higher parenthood stage, where the transition's inhibiting factors are highlighted. As supporting dimensions, we considered situations which reveal the transition process, emphasising the facilitating resources for that transition. The mediating dimensions include the categories "1—Insecurity", "2—Lack of Privacy", "3—Isolation", "4—Stigma", and "5—Disempowerment", which support the categories "6—Education Difficulties", "7—Changes in Parents' Behaviour", and "8—Changes in Children's Behaviour". On the other hand, the supporting dimensions include the categories "9—Context as a Facilitator", "10—Relationship with Others", and "11—Parents' and Children's Self", which lead to the additional category "12—Parenting Motivation and Strategies" that addresses parenting issues.

Next, we will present the synthesis of our findings, in the form of a narrative text, followed by an overview of the obtained results associated with the aforesaid findings and the established categories.

3.4. Synthesis of the Findings

3.4.1. Parenthood Mediating Dimensions

This synthesis derives from 53 findings and the following eight categories: "Insecurity", "Lack of Privacy", "Isolation", "Stigma", "Disempowerment", "Education Difficulties", "Changes in Parents' Behaviour", and "Changes in Children's Behaviour".

The mediating dimension of the "Insecurity" category is sustained by the following findings: lack of security; lack of hygiene; racism; intimidation; attacks from shelter residents; and negative influences from others. In the "Lack of Privacy" category, it is supported by: space limitations;

restrictive environment; and the need for privacy to play. In the "Isolation" category, it is sustained by: shelters located far from family, school and city centre; separation from friends and family; distancing from children; and the existence of loneliness feelings. In the "Stigma" category, it is supported by: feelings of stigmatization, humiliation, disrespect, and judgment. The "Disempowerment" category is divided into 3 subcategories: "Routine Change", sustained by the changes in the shelter's routines, the difficulty in maintaining routines, and the involvement of other adults; "**Rule Enforcement**", supported by shelter rules not consistent with previous parenthood options, as well as by the imposition of external rules; and "Parents' Needs", sustained by the need for practical, material and financial help, employment, education, transport, housing assistance, mental health promotion, pregnancy support, and time for oneself and one's children, as well as by the inability to play the role of provider and guide. The "Changes in Children's Behaviour" category includes: mental health problems; disobedience; mood swings; disrespect for authority; aggression; feelings of anguish, boredom and confusion; eating disorders; development regressions; concerns; and hiding the reality of living in shelters. The "Changes in Parents' Behaviour" category encompasses the lack of availability and conditions to meet the child's needs, as well as the dependence on the shelter's resources. Finally, the "Education Difficulties" category includes: difficulty in establishing discipline; the need for help when dealing with school; difficulty in integrating the school's community; difficulty in identifying school absenteeism as a problem; inability to help the child with school tasks, to maintain the child in a single school system throughout the year, and to identify academic problems; abdication of the responsibilities concerning school; absence of regular school attendance; and education barriers related to communication.

3.4.2. Parenthood Supporting Dimensions

This synthesis derived from 21 findings and 4 categories: "Context as a Facilitator", "Relationship with Others", "Parents' and Children's Self", and "Parenting Motivation and Strategies". It demonstrates that the homeless situation experienced in temporary/transitional shelters seems to enhance parenthood issues in some families, since they lead to motivation and acquisition of strategies by the parents, in order to deal with those issues. Some parents perceive this "Context as a Facilitator", because: it gives them access to services and resources; it is a safe place; it strengthens family practices and cohesion; and it is a stabilising experience that highlights the parental role. Additionally, they consider that it promotes the "Relationship with Others", defending that: it is a social opportunity; it provides a sense of community and of collective parenting; it provides supportive relationships, positive encounters with community service providers, and social support from family and friends. In addition, it seems to encourage the "Children's Self", since a young person demonstrated having resilience and perseverance, despite being homeless. It also seems to promote the "Parents' Self", since they reveal: the ability to help their children to deal with emotions; the ability to identify academic problems; optimism; hope for the future; perseverance; self-efficacy; resilience; resistance; the ability to set goals; and that they can do without help. Despite the homelessness situation, in some families parenthood seems to be enhanced, and it is even verified that the children function as a source of "Motivation", leading parents to seek improvement regarding their life situation and employment status, as well as to seek help to promote their mental health and maintain their morale. Parenthood also appears to feed the desire to move forward, in order to provide a better life for the respective children. Furthermore, to cope with the various challenges, the parents seek "Strategies", such as: reading; writing a diary; keeping focus; attending church; and talking to the respective support team, friends and family.

Figure 2 shows the relationship between the categories and the synthesised findings, to illustrate the general synthesis process.

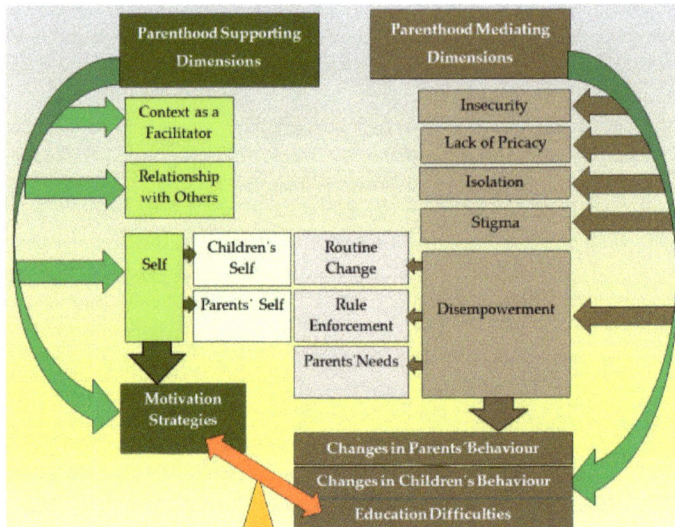

Figure 2. Overview of the synthesised findings.

4. Discussion

This systematic review sought to gather the best available evidence on the parenthood experiences of homeless families. As stated previously, the aggregation of 11 qualitative research articles resulted in the finding of two types of parenthood dimensions. On the one hand, we found "Parenthood Mediating Dimensions" (corresponding to transitional states), which include: "Insecurity", "Lack of Privacy", "Isolation", "Stigma", and "Disempowerment" (the latter pertaining to routine changes, rule enforcement and the multiple needs of the parents). On the other hand, we found "Parenthood Supporting Dimensions", which encompass: "Context as a Facilitator" (of access to services and resources, by acting as a stabilising experience for the family, and by highlighting the parental role), "Relationship with Others", and finally the "Parents' and Children's Self". In their turn, these categories led to relevant findings. The "Parenthood Mediating Dimensions" sustain changes in the parents' and children's behaviour, but, above all, they are associated with difficulties in education. Conversely, the "Parenthood Supporting Dimensions" lead to motivation and to the acquisition of strategies by the parents, with respect to parenting issues.

We found that some of the considered dimensions fit into the concept of parenthood recommended by the International Council of Nurses [1], as well as into the one suggested by Figueiredo [10]. Nevertheless, most of the dimensions corresponded to experiences, or feelings, reported by the parents. Some reflected difficulties in exercising the parental role, while others revealed protective factors related to the homelessness situation. This was one of the limitations we encountered in this study. In the "Parenthood Supporting Dimensions", the transition process is revealed through: the need of establishing relationships with others, as sources of support and information; the interaction with others; and the use of resources and coping strategies, to deal with the situation. This is in line with the findings presented by Meleis [3].

We encountered another limitation in this study, related to the context of the included works (all were conducted in temporary or transitional shelters). The research should be extended to other contexts of homelessness, such as: the street/public spaces, precarious locations, pensions, and rooms paid for by the social services.

We also found that the families identified in the study fit the characteristics of the different types of homeless families, such as single-parent families led by (single) women [16,17]. Additionally, we identified multiple problems and needs in the studied families, which is in accordance with the results obtained by Anderson et al. [15], as well as multiple risk/protection factors (both internal and external), in line with the findings of Macana and Comim [11].

Regarding the limitations of this review, we stress that only articles published in English, Portuguese, French and Spanish were included, and there might have been relevant findings in works published in other languages. Another limitation relates to the use of a small number of databases, since its extension would have led to a broader research, and to the possibility of including other significant contributions. Another possible limitation concerns the priority given to the search for articles, thus excluding other kinds of text, such as opinion documents, dissertations and reports. Since the literature available for inclusion was limited to published original research articles, there is always the risk that relevant studies may not have been identified.

Despite the effort to find all relevant articles, some significant research works may have been overlooked. There is the possibility that both reviewers may have neglected important studies, during the screening process of the 358 articles initially obtained. On the other hand, the bibliographic search allowed the identification of articles produced in various professional fields, such as psychiatry, psychology, social sciences, occupational therapy, and nursing. This provided a broader picture of the homeless parents' experiences.

Some of the obtained articles corresponded to secondary findings related to the parenthood experiences of homeless families, being thus included in the review. For instance, the purpose of one of the selected articles was to identify the parents' and the employees' perceptions, regarding their experience with the family support team, and also to recognise ways of improving this service in the future [15]. Although the focus was on the experience with the family support team, some of this study's findings were considered relevant to the objective of the present systematic review, being, therefore, included in it. This would not have been possible using a more restrictive bibliographic search strategy.

When we critically evaluated the 11 included articles, they revealed a variety of strengths and limitations. All works showed coherence between the research methodology and the research's question(s)/objective(s), the data collection methods and the results' interpretation. Nonetheless, two of the studies did not present congruence between the stated philosophical perspective and the research methodology [35,39], and there were two articles that did not present congruence between the research methodology and the data's representation and analysis [35,41].

The absence of an appropriate statement enhanced the complexity of evaluating the congruence between the philosophical perspective and the research methodology. Additionally, the inexistence of congruence, regarding the data's presentation and analysis, increased the difficulty of the data's evaluation. Although the reviewers did not consider these phenomena a reason for exclusion, the congruence between the philosophical perspective and the research methodology, as well as between the research methodology and the data's representation and analysis, would have been preferable, to strengthen the studies' credibility.

Data were collected through participant observation, individual interviews, written diaries, reflection activities, and group interviews/focus groups. The fathers' perspectives were under-represented, because most of the interviewees belonged to single-parent families led by women, thus highlighting the perspective of homeless mothers. However, in one of the studies, it was possible to analyse exclusively the male perspective, since it encompassed single-parent families led by men [40]. This unequal representation might be considered a limitation, because homeless fathers may have different experiences from homeless mothers. Even so, it may provide a realistic picture of homeless families.

Most of the studies were conducted in the United States, except for two which were carried out in the United Kingdom [15,41], and one that was performed in Australia [39]. This geographical distribution can result in limitations related to cultural differences, concerning the way homeless parenthood is viewed. It is important to note that these results can also refer to refugee families, which are becoming more important today. Such divergences may be relevant, since they can have implications

Int. J. Environ. Res. Public Health **2020**, *17*, 2712

for the practice in various settings and cultures. Nonetheless, we consider the studies' heterogeneity a strength, because it represents the complexity and diversity of the parenthood experiences in homelessness situations.

5. Conclusions

This review's findings contributed to the scientific knowledge about the complexities of homeless families/fathers/mothers and the challenges faced by them. Homeless parents living in temporary or transitional shelters are confronted with the intricacy of parental experiences influenced by insecurity, lack of privacy, isolation, stigma and disempowerment. On the other hand, to some families, the homelessness experience lived in temporary or transitional shelters seems to enhance parenthood, since they regard that context as a facilitator of the parental role, which promotes family cohesion, the relationships within the family and with others, as well as the parents' and the children's self. During the complicated journey of homeless parenthood, the parents use coping strategies and see their children as a great source of motivation, where they find strength to fight against the multiple difficulties they experience.

This review adds scientific knowledge on the experiences of homeless families, by revealing several parenthood mediating and parenthood supporting dimensions. However, the specific knowledge about parental experiences is still limited. The concept of homeless parenthood is scarcely researched; there exists a need for further studies in other homeless contexts, and in the field of Nursing, in order to adapt nursing responses to those families. While conducting this review, we found a reduced number of articles about the studied topic, which justifies the presented need and encourages additional research in the area of homeless parenthood. We stress the need for further research on paediatric nursing care, in the above-mentioned area. Regarding our methodological approach, we conclude that it was appropriate, since it allowed answering the research question.

Supplementary Materials: The following are available online at http://www.mdpi.com/1660-4601/17/8/2712/s1, Table S1. Final evaluation of the included studies (according to the method used by Lockwood), Table S2 Summary of the conclusions reached through the CONQual tool (adapted from the one proposed in the Joanna Briggs Institute's Methodological Manual), Table S3. Characterization of the included studies.

Author Contributions: Conceptualization, F.M.R.A. and A.S.F.; methodology, F.M.R.A., A.S.F., M.L.C. and Z.C.; software, F.M.R.A., A.S.F. and M.L.C.; validation, F.M.R.A., A.S.F.; formal analysis, F.M.R.A., A.S.F.; investigation, F.M.R.A., A.S.F., M.L.C., Z.C. and S.D.; resources F.M.R.A., A.S.F., M.L.C., Z.C. and S.D.; data curation, F.M.R.A., A.S.F., M.L.C. and Z.C.; writing—original draft preparation, F.M.R.A. and A.S.F.; writing—review and editing, F.M.R.A. and A.S.F.; visualization, F.M.R.A., A.S.F., M.L.C., Z.C. and S.D.; supervision, F.M.R.A., A.S.F., M.L.C., Z.C. and S.D.; project administration, F.M.R.A. and A.S.F.; funding acquisition, S.D. All authors have read and agreed to the published version of the manuscript.

Funding: This research was funded by Universidade Católica Portuguesa—Centre for Interdisciplinary Research in Health (CIIS).

Conflicts of Interest: The authors declare the absence of any conflicts of interest.

References

1. Ordem dos Enfermeiros. *CIPE®Versão2—Classificação Internacional Para a Prática de Enfermagem*; Ordem Dos Enfermeiros: Lisboa, Portugal, 2011.
2. Meleis, A.I.; Sawyer, L.M.; Im, E.O.; Messias, D.K.H.; Schumacher, K. Experiencing transitions: An emerging middle-range theory. *Adv. Nurs. Sci.* **2000**, *23*, 2–28. [CrossRef] [PubMed]
3. Meleis, A.I. *Transitions Theory: Middle Range and Situation Specific Theories in Nursing Research and Practice*; Springer Publishing Company: New York, NY, USA, 2010.
4. Meleis, A.I. *Theoretical Nursing: Development and Progress*, 5th ed.; Wolters Kluwer Health/Lippincott Williams & Wilkins: Philadelphia, PA, USA, 2012.
5. Meleis, A.I. *Theoretical Nursing: Development and Progress*, 4th ed.; Lippincott Williams & Wilkins: Philadelphia, PA, USA, 2007.

6. Barroso, R.G.; Machado, C. Definições, dimensões e determinantes da parentalidade. *Psychologica* **2010**, *52*, 211–229. [CrossRef]
7. Hoghughi, M. Parenting: An introduction. In *Handbook of Parenting: Theory and Research for Practice*; Hoghughi, M., Long, N., Eds.; SAGE Publications Ltd.: London, UK, 2004.
8. Ordem dos Enfermeiros. *Guia Orientador de Boa Prática: Adaptação à Parentalidade Durante a Hospitalização*; Ordem dos Enfermeiros: Lisboa, Portugal, 2015.
9. Cruz, O. *Parentalidade*; LivPsic: Porto, Portugal, 2005.
10. Figueiredo, M.H. *Modelo Dinâmico de Avaliação e Intervenção Familiar: Uma Abordagem Colaborativa em Enfermagem de Família*, 1st ed.; Lusociência—Edições Técnicas e Científicas, Lda: Loures, Portugal, 2012.
11. Macana, E.C.; Comim, F. O papel das práticas e estilos parentais no desenvolvimento da primeira infância. In *Fundamentos da Família Como Promotora do Desenvolvimento Infantil: Parentalidade em Foco*; Pluciennik, G.A., Lazzari, M.C., Chicaro, M.F., Eds.; Fundação Maria Cecilia Souto Vidigal: São Paulo, Brasil, 2015.
12. Nichiata, L.Y.I.; Bertolozzi, M.R.; Takahashi, R.F.; Fracolli, L.A. The use of the "Vulnerability" concept in the nursing area. *Rev Latino Am. Enferm.* **2008**, *16*, 923–928. [CrossRef] [PubMed]
13. Meleis, A.I. *Theoretical Nursing: Development and Progress*, 6th ed.; Wolters Kluwer: Philadelphia, PA, USA, 2018.
14. Ministério do Trabalho, Solidariedade e Segurança Social. Estratégia Nacional para a Integração das Pessoas em Situação de Sem-Abrigo (ENIPSSA) 2017-2023. In Presidência do Conselho de Ministros, Resolução do Conselho de Ministros n.º 107/2017, Diário da República n.º 142/2017—Série, I. Available online: https://data.dre.pt/eli/resolconsmin/107/2017/07/25/p/dre/pt/html (accessed on 5 January 2019).
15. Anderson, L.; Stuttaford, M.; Vostanis, P. A family support service for homeless children and parents: User and staff perspectives. *Child Fam. Soc. Work* **2006**, *11*, 119–127. [CrossRef]
16. Vostanis, P. Mental health of homeless children and their families. *Adv. Psychiatr. Treat* **2002**, *8*, 463–469. [CrossRef]
17. Kim, K.; Garcia, I. Why Do Homeless Families Exit and Return the Homeless Shelter? Factors Affecting the Risk of Family Homelessness in Salt Lake County (Utah, USA) As a Case Study. *Int. J. Environ. Res. Public Health* **2019**, *16*, 4328. [CrossRef]
18. Simões Figueiredo, A.; Seabra, P.; Sarreira-Santos, A.; Vollrath, A.; Medeiros Garcia, L.; Vidal, T.; Neves Amado, J. Nursing consultation in a public bathhouse: A community resource for the vulnerable population in a European capital. *Issues Ment. Health Nurs.* **2019**, *40*, 28–32. [CrossRef]
19. Gultekin, L.; Brush, B.L. In their own words: Exploring family pathways to housing instability. *J. Fam. Nurs.* **2017**, *23*, 90–115. [CrossRef]
20. Simões Figueiredo, A.; Vidal, T.; Sarreira-Santos, A.; Medeiros-Garcia, L.; García-Padilla, F.; Seabra, P. Nursing consultation in public showers: What lies beyond the results? *Issues Ment. Health Nurs.* **2019**, *40*, 535–536. [CrossRef]
21. Grant, R.; Gracy, D.; Goldsmith, G. Twenty-five years of child and family homelessness: Where are we now? *Am. J. Public Health* **2013**, *103*, e1–e10. [CrossRef]
22. Pleace, N. Family Homelessness in Europe. In *Homeless in Europe. Family Homelessness in Europe*; Feantsa: Brussels, Belgium, 2019; Available online: https://www.feantsa.org/public/user/Resources/magazine/2019/Autumn/Homeless_in_Europe_Magazine_Autumn2019_final.pdf (accessed on 18 November 2019).
23. Baptista, I.; Marlier, E. *Fighting Homelessnes Sand Housing Exclusion in Europe: A Study of National Policies*; European Commission: Brussels, Belgium, 2019.
24. Martin-Fernandez, J.; Lioret, S.; Vuillermoz, C.; Chauvin, P.; Vandentorren, S. Food Insecurity in Homeless Families in the Paris Region (France): Results from the ENFAMS Survey. *Int. J. Environ. Res. Public Health* **2018**, *15*, 420. [CrossRef]
25. Sylvestre, J.; Kerman, N.; Polillo, A.; Lee, C.M.; Aubry, T.; Czechowski, K. A qualitative study of the pathways into and impacts of family homelessness. *J. Fam. Issues* **2018**, *39*, 2265–2285. [CrossRef]
26. Bassuk, E.L.; Richard, M.K.; Tsertsvadze, A. The prevalence of mental illness in homeless children: A systematic review and meta-analysis. *J. Am. Acad. Child Adoles. Psychiatr.* **2015**, *54*, 86–96. [CrossRef] [PubMed]
27. Haskett, M.E.; Armstrong, J.M.; Tisdale, J. Developmental status and social-emotional functioning of young children experiencing homelessness. *Early Child. Educ. J.* **2015**, *44*, 19–125. [CrossRef]

28. Mzwandile, A.; Mabhala, M.A.; Yohannes, A. Being at the Bottom Rung of the Ladder in an Unequal Society: A Qualitative Analysis of Stories of People without a Home. *Int. J. Environ. Res. Public Health* **2019**, *16*, 4620. [CrossRef]

29. Gaetz, S.; O'grady, B.; Kidd, S.; Schwan, K. Without a Home: The National Youth Homelessness Survey. Available online: https://homelesshub.ca/sites/default/files/WithoutAHome-final.pdf (accessed on 21 January 2019).

30. Perlman, S.; Sheller, S.; Hudson, K.M.; Wilson, C.L. Parenting in the face of homelessness. In *Supporting Families Experiencing Homelessness. Current Practices and Future Directions*; Haskett, M., Perlman, S., Cowan, B.A., Eds.; Springer: New York, NY, USA, 2014.

31. Baptista, I. Women and homelessness. In *Homelessness Research in Europe: Festschrift for Bill Edgar and Joe Doherty*; O'Sullivan, E., Busch-Geertsema, V., Quilgars, D., Pleace, N., Eds.; Feantsa: Brussels, Belgium, 2010.

32. Lockwood, C.; Porrit, K.; Munn, Z.; Rittenmeyer, L.; Salmond, S.; Bjerrum, M.; Loveday, H.; Carrier, J.; Stannard, D. Chapter 2: Systematic reviews of qualitative evidence. In *Joanna Briggs Institute Reviewer's Manual*; Aromataris, E., Munn, Z., Eds.; The Joanna Briggs Institute: Adelaide, Australia, 2017; Available online: https://reviewersmanual.joannabriggs.org/ (accessed on 30 January 2019).

33. Moher, D.; Liberati, A.; Tetzlaff, J.; Altman, D.G. The PRISMA Group. Preferred Reporting Items for Systematic Reviews and Meta-Analyses: The PRISMA Statement. *PLoS Med.* **2009**, *6*, e1000097. [CrossRef]

34. Anthony, E.R.; Vincent, A.; Shin, Y. Parenting and child experiences in shelter: A qualitative study exploring the effect of homelessness on the parent-child relationship. *Child. Fam. Soc. Work* **2017**, *23*, 8–15. [CrossRef]

35. Cosgrove, L.; Flynn, C. Marginalized mothers: Parenting without a home. *Anal. Soc. Issues Public Policy* **2005**, *5*, 127–143. [CrossRef]

36. Haskett, M.E.; Armstrong, J.; Neal, S.C.; Aldianto, K. Perceptions of triple P-positive parenting program seminars among parents experiencing homelessness. *J. Child Fam. Stud.* **2018**, *27*, 1957–1967. [CrossRef]

37. Holtrop, K.; McNeil, S.; McWey, L.M. It's a struggle but I can do it. I'm doing it for me and my kids: The psychosocial characteristics and life experiences of at-risk homeless parents in transitional housing. *J. Marital Fam. Ther.* **2015**, *41*, 177–191. [CrossRef]

38. Lindsey, E.W. The process of restabilization for mother-headed homeless families: How social workers can help. *J. Fam. Soc. Work* **1997**, *2*, 49–72. [CrossRef]

39. Morris, R.I.; Butt, R.A. Parents' perspectives on homelessness and its effects on the educational development of their children. *J. Sch. Nurs.* **2003**, *19*, 43–50. [CrossRef] [PubMed]

40. Roche, S.; Barker, J.; McArthur, M. 'Performing' fathering while homeless: Utilising a critical social work perspective. *Br. J. Soc. Work* **2018**, *48*, 283–301. [CrossRef]

41. Tischler, V.; Karim, K.; Rustall, S.; Gregory, P.; Vostanis, P. A family support service for homeless children and parents: Users' perspectives and characteristics. *Health Soc. Care Community* **2004**, *12*, 327–335. [CrossRef] [PubMed]

42. Vanleit, B.; Starrett, R.; Crowe, T.K. Occupational concerns of women who are homeless and have children: An occupational justice critique. *Occup. Ther. Heal. Care* **2006**, *20*, 47–62. [CrossRef] [PubMed]

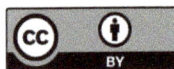

International Journal of
*Environmental Research
and Public Health*

MDPI

Article

I Am a Nursing Student but Hate Nursing: The East Asian Perspectives between Social Expectation and Social Context

Luis Miguel Dos Santos

Woosong Language Institute, Woosong University, Daejeon 34514, Korea; luisdossantos@woosong.org

Received: 12 March 2020; Accepted: 7 April 2020; Published: 10 April 2020

check for
updates

Abstract: From the East Asian social and cultural perspectives and contexts, this study aimed to understand the relationships and behaviors between nursing students' sense of filial piety and their decision-making behind selecting nursing education as their major. Forty-two traditional-age nursing students (i.e., six men and 36 women) at their final year of a bachelor's degree program in nursing were invited. The findings indicated that many nursing students disliked their university major and the potential career pathway as a nursing professional, as none of them selected the major based on their choice and interest. The environmental context and family's recommendations were the major impacts to influence the decision-making process of the participants. The result also indicated that filial piety, parents' recommendations, and elderly people's suggestions were the key factors to influence the selections and decisions of university major and career development pathways. The study provided a blueprint for related staff and professionals to create and design career counselling and services for East Asian youths to enable life investment and development.

Keywords: career development; counselling; cultural perspective; decision-making process; East Asian perspective; filial piety; nursing education; nursing shortage; nursing student; turnover

---

1. Introduction

Nursing education and training are popular university majors for secondary school graduates, university students, and even adult returning students wishing to pursue life-long personal investment and development [1]. Every year, a large number of secondary school graduates and returning students decide to study nursing as their university major and to develop their careers. Although many individuals start their university education directly after completing secondary school, there are also a large number of adult returning students deciding to start their college and university study during mid-adulthood [2]. The selection of one's university major and career development path are decisions that impact the rest of one's life [3]. However, individuals' social, family, personal, educational, and economic patterns influence their decision-making processes, particularly for East Asian people, who have a strong sense of collectivism [4]. The expression of decision-making for career development is more likely employed when describing that process, which can happen at different stages of life [5].

Although nursing education is a very famous and popular university major, an inappropriate matching and mismatching of career development continues to happen in this profession. One study [6] collected information from 648 questionnaires at three hospitals in Taiwan about nurses' job satisfaction and intention to quit their position. The results indicated that a large number of nurses planned to leave their positions due to significant levels of stress and burnout at their workplace. Although they understand their job natures and responsibilities before entering the profession, many nurses decide to switch their career profession due to ideas of balancing work and family [7].

One study [8] employed the Ward Organizational Features Scales (WOFS) to measure the relationship between job satisfaction and work responsibilities of 834 acute ward nurses in the United Kingdom. The relationship between nurses and other medical staff was one of the most critical elements for their career decision. Additionally, many nurses indicated that the workload of their positions always negatively impacted their job satisfaction due to unbalanced responsibilities. It is worth noting that the negative measurement affected the career decisions of these nurses, who worked in a stressful environment [9].

A recent study [10] about the relationship between disappointment and nursing student retention collected data from 17 nursing students during the third year of their nursing program at university level. The report indicated that many nursing students decided to join the nursing profession because of the desire to provide a caring service, a personal background with the healthcare profession, modelling from peers, and potential career advancement. One study [11] indicated that a number of nursing students explained that negative experiences regarding their training, teaching staff, placement experience, and teammates always affected their career decisions. For example, some participants indicated that the excessive responsibilities and expectations from their supervisors could influence their career decisions due to negative placement experiences. Based on the results, it is not hard to predict that many nursing students or fresh graduate nurses may leave the nursing profession within the first few years of their career [11].

Another study indicated that nursing programs always have a high dropout rate due to the unique nature of the profession [12]. Unlike doctors who can provide individualized medical treatments to patients, nurses tend to assist other medical professionals. In other words, nurses cannot offer individual services without the supervision of other medical professionals. Therefore, once nursing students understand the nature of the profession, many decide to drop out [13].

Expectation is another element of dropout [14]. Providing a caring service is meaningful for many individuals who want to join social care and health services. However, the responsibilities of nurses are unique. Unlike social workers and counsellors who provide counselling and mental health services to individuals with problems, nurses need to provide both psychological and physical labor services from cleaning to operation room assistance. Therefore, the responsibilities are more comprehensive than for many professions in the field of social care and healthcare. As a result, after students understand the relationship between the duties and their expectations, they may drop out or leave the profession [15].

However, many individuals decide to enter the nursing profession due to stable job advancement and salary, particularly in developing countries [16]. Nursing, teaching, and social work are three demanding professions in society internationally. Many enter these fields due to financial, family, and personal considerations. Although these professions always welcome learners and second-career professionals, inappropriate matching is not uncommon. However, for various reasons, some mismatched individuals never leave their positions. In such cases, low-level performance, motivation, and morale prevail in the workplace [17].

One study [18] indicted that East Asian students are more likely to select a university major based on the interests and expectations of their parents, while most European students tend to select their major based on their own interests. Jin [19] indicated that East Asians' major selection tends to be influenced by filial piety toward parents. The researcher employed the Career-Related Filial Piety Scale (C-FPS) to investigate the relationship between parents' decisions and students' choices. The results indicated that students usually tend to study at universities their parents like and enter professional fields according to their parents' preferences. More recently, a study [20] conducted in Hong Kong reflected this as well. The study collected information from 522 undergraduate students about their reciprocal and authoritarian behaviors and senses about the relationship between students' filial piety and career decisions. The results indicated that although many students select their career pathways based on their interests, most respect their parents' wishes according to the traditional East Asian perspective [21]. Perhaps the social and cultural environment in Hong Kong influences young adults' career decisions due to the westernized nature of that society; most Chinese students and participants tend to listen to their parents in order to avoid arguments and misunderstanding [22].

Purpose of the Study

The researcher has conducted research in the fields of social care, human resource management, school administration, and organizational psychology. The personnel shortage in the areas of social caring and nursing has been an issue for decades. Although many human resource professionals, policymakers, school administrators, leaders of social care departments, and researchers always establish plans to encourage potential medical professionals to work in the field. However, the results of these plans were not always effective. Due to the social and cultural expectations, the researcher wants to understand how the East Asian perspective influenced these issues. Currently, studies with a focus on nursing education and nurses' career development tend to explore participants' elements from a westernized perspective [7,11,13,16], in which individualism is the primary social norm and practice [4]. Therefore, this study aimed to understand the relationship between East Asian nursing students' sense of filial piety and their decision-making behind selecting nursing education as their major [23–34].

There are two purposes of this study. First, every year, a significant number of students decide to enroll in nursing education programs for initial training. Based on the literature review, various reasons for this have been found among these students [7]. However, many of them drop out of the programs or leave the nursing profession within the first few years of their career development [14]. Therefore, this study sought to study a group of traditional-age nursing students enrolled in a nursing education program but who will not enter the nursing profession after graduation. Second, the study sought to understand the factors that contribute to the relationship between East Asian university students' filial piety [20,35–37] and their decision-making behind selecting their university major and career development pathway in nursing [38]. The elements studied included outcome expectations, interests, and goals [38].

As a result, little empirical evidence exists for East Asia regarding the relationships between expectations, social-economic backgrounds, social environmental factors, and personal interests of young individuals and their selection of university subjects and career paths [8–11]. It is worthwhile to note that, unlike in Western cultures, Asian young people tend to highly respect their parents' suggestions, as well as the recommendations of their elders, such as parents, grandparents, teachers, and elder siblings, due to traditions of filial piety [8]. In short, this study serves as one of the first attempts to understand the relationship between filial piety and the decision-making of East Asian university students regarding their major selection and career development [23–34]. Unlike with Westerners, the values of filial piety, collectivism, and sense of family union are essential elements for East Asian people [39]. Therefore, this study will help provide opportunities for readers, university administrators, international school staff, educators, and international student service professionals to establish effective counselling services to assist this particular group of students.

2. Materials and Methods

The employment of qualitative research methods [40] would be appropriate. Unlike quantitative research, qualitative research method allows the researcher to collect rich and in-depth data information from the participants. The researcher could access the information and lived stories which could not be answered by statistics and numbers [41]. Although the researcher had aimed to collect information from one single university counselling centre for a case study, the researcher believed the data information from one single source might not be able to express the holistic pictures of the current problem. Therefore, the researcher decided to employ the general qualitative approach [40,42–44], which may better apply to this study. Thomas [44] indicated that the general qualitative approach is an inductive approach that may meet most of the requirements for qualitative researchers. Moreover, without additional requirements, qualitative researchers could freely collect data information from the targeted groups. As the current study might not fit other qualitative methods, such as case study, the general qualitative approach would be the selection [41,44].

2.1. Participants

Fort-two traditional-age nursing students (i.e., six men and 36 women) at their final year of a bachelor's degree program in nursing were invited. All agreed to participate in this study. All the participants were local Taiwanese students. Five out of the 42 were indigenous Taiwanese. All were born and raised in Taiwanese families with the traditional East Asian conceptions. The age range was 18-22 years. The researchers invited these participants with the snowball sampling strategy [40,42,43]. In other words, the researcher invited participants based on the networking from other participants. Participants were enrolled at five different universities in Taiwan. The participants needed to meet the following criteria, which were:

1. he/she is currently enrolled at a nursing education program in Taiwan;
2. he/she is currently enrolled in the final year of the program;
3. he/she was born and raised in Taiwan;
4. he/she needed to meet the age requirement.

2.2. Data Collection

Two types of tools were employed, including individual and focus group activities [40,43,45]. The individual interviews were conducted to explore their understanding, life experience, and family issues under a private sharing environment [46–48]. The focus group activities were conducted to explore some similar background, social and family expectations, social bias, and interests. Both research tools were particularly useful in regard to listening to the voices by engaging them individually and collectively.

All participants have voluntarily participated in this study. The general inductive approach [44] was employed for qualitative data collection and analysis. The researcher was the collector of the data information. In order to seek meaningful data information, first, the semi-structured interview sessions were created. According to Seidman [49], individuals are less likely to share lived stories and personal background to others without any prior relationships. Therefore, in order to overcome this issue, the researcher decided to conduct two sessions of semi-structured, one-on-one, and private interviews in a private room at a community centre for each participant. Each interview lasted up to 40 min. One of the directions of this study was to explore the direct effect of filial piety on a career decision. Therefore, the protocol interview questions for both individual interview sessions tended to focus on the relationship between an East Asian perspective and the social context and issues. Appendix A shows the protocol interview questions for both interview sessions.

Second, after each participant completed the individual interview sections, all participants were invited into six focus group activities, each with seven participants. As the schedule of each participant was different, the focus group activity hosted seven members regardless of their university enrolments. The focus group activities were hosted at the same community centre. Appendix B shows the protocol interview questions for the focus group activities.

As it might be difficult for participants to share their understanding and experience in English language and a language other than their mother tongue, all the sections were conducted in Chinese Mandarin and translated into English. All the interview and focus group activities were audio-recorded and transcribed into written documents for data analysis. Member checking was done after the data analysis procedure. In order to protect the personal rights of each participant, all participants were given a pseudonym.

2.3. Data Analysis

After the data collection procedure, 543 pages of written transcripts were created based on the semi-structured interviews and focus group activities. Qualitative researchers [40,43,45] advocated that large-size data information should be narrowed down to meaningful themes and patterns. Therefore, the researcher followed the general inductive approach (GIA) [44] for data analysis. First, the researcher used the open-coding procedure for the initial themes. After the initial themes were formed, the axial-coding procedure was employed for the second-level themes. As a result, two themes and seven subthemes were merged.

2.4. Human Subject Protection

All the signed and unsigned agreements, personal contact, audio recording, written transcripts, computer, and related materials were locked in a password-protected cabinet. Only the researcher had the means to open it. After the study was completed, the researcher immediately destroyed and deleted all related materials for personal privacy.

Due to the agreement, the university information and place of origin was masked due to privacy. Most of the students were concerned that their university information would be disclosed. Due to the small population and closed professional networks, the researcher needed to protect the information of the participants. However, the participants allowed the researcher to show their gender for this study. Therefore, the following part will outline their gender with their discussion. It is worth noting that a small number of participants agreed to disclose their place of origin. The researcher reported this information with the discussion of the findings.

All subjects gave their informed consent for inclusion before they participated in the study. The study was conducted in accordance with the Declaration of Helsinki, and the protocol was approved by the Ethics Committee of The Youth Caring Association (2018/2019/SummerFall).

3. Findings and Discussion

During each interview and focus group activity section, the participants answered the same general semi-structured questions that asked for their opinions and feedback. Although all participants had a similar family and social background in the same country, having come from one of the Taiwanese areas, their personal sharing, lived stories, and life experiences were not the same. Unlike in other studies, which have focused on westernized cultural perspectives, all participants reported that their major selection (i.e., nursing) was influenced by their family members, parents, and social expectations. In order to help answer the research questions, the findings were categorized into two superordinate themes and seven subthemes. It is surprising to note that all 42 participants were studying a university major that was not their own selection or interest. In other words, upon graduation, they would receive a degree, initial license, and potentially develop their long-term career pathways in a direction in which they have no strong interests. More importantly, many expressed that they will leave the nursing profession after graduation. Table 1 outlines the themes and subthemes of this study.

Table 1. A list of themes and subthemes for this study.

		Themes and Subthemes
3.1.		**Influences from the Participants' Contextual Environment**
	3.1.1.	The East Asian Perspective on Occupational and Role Expectations
	3.1.2.	Academic Results
	3.1.3.	Financial Influence
3.2.		**Influences from the Participants' Family and Elders**
	3.2.1.	Parental Recommendations
	3.2.2.	Teachers' Recommendations
	3.2.3.	Pressures from Family Members
	3.2.4.	Comparison with Other Relatives

3.1. Influences from the Participants' Contextual Environment

Before the session began, the researcher needed to indicate that the statements about I hate nursing. I dislike the medical career had been recorded 356 times. It was very surprising that the mismatching of major and human resources (i.e., students) was significant in the current Taiwanese university environment, particularly in the faculty of nursing. Although the current study could not represent the overall situation in Taiwan and the East Asian region, the significant results from this study may explore and contribute to an understanding of how these extreme situations [14] happen in the East Asian region [31].

By listening to the stories and life experiences of the participants, the researcher identified several elements that impacted their major decisions. The findings of this study discovered that all did not follow their personal goals and interests when selecting their major (i.e., nursing). The results reflected that the participants' behaviors also tended not to follow their own interests in choosing a career, which goes against a large number of previous findings [7,15,16]. It is worth noting that in most cases in East Asia, university students are not allowed to switch their major once they have been accepted. In other words, students are required to complete the major and degree that they submitted as their choice with their application. Therefore, the contextual and environmental factors that prevailed during their secondary school period highly influenced their life-long developments and career decisions [50]. A group of participants expressed that nursing was a choice of their parents during the application period, saying, "I can apply up to six universities and majors ... But once I admitted with a school and major ... I cannot switch ... but the major application was written by my mother without my agreement ... " (P#5, Male, Interview).

The results of this study supported the idea that youth have their own ways of thinking about career developments [7,51,52]. However, because the university's constraints on their university decisions and their overall contextual factors limited their opportunities, most were unable to exercise the career pathways that they might have decided on their own [14]. A discussion of the influences on the career decisions of the participants follows.

3.1.1. The East Asian Perspective on Occupational and Role Expectations

All 42 participants expressed that the East Asian perspectives about occupational and role expectations influenced their decisions about the major they were studying, their university enrollment, and their career decisions [53]. In the traditional East Asian perspective, medical practitioners are considered to be upper-class citizens with a high level of social status [54]. Although more than half of the participants expressed their desire to become an artist, reporter, chef, journalist, or photographer, none of them selected the majors associated with those occupations. One participant expressed that almost all artists and performers in the fine arts could not become famous until their death, saying, "Although I want to be an artist, I may become a nurse and do some part-time art activities ... But I am not sure will I become a nurse become I hate this occupation now ... " (P#2, Male, Focus Group). Another participant (P#4, Female, Interview) believed her hobbies in dancing could not be a long-term occupation, sharing,

> I chose nursing was because I think medical professionals are very smart in our society ... I really enjoy the perspective of medical professionals ... Although I want to become an artist with my wish and interests ... both athlet[e]s and dancers can only work in their occupation until the early 30s. After that, the lucky one[s] can work as [a] coach. The others are living under the poverty line .... .but now, I don't know ... should I become a nurse? I hate this career .... . (P#4, Female, Interview)

It is worth noting that not only these two participants, but all 42 participants also expressed the ideas *I hate nursing and I dislike medical professions* in this category. Many expressed interests in other fields but had no chances and opportunities. Although the participants tried to escape from the major (i.e., nursing) they were not interested, they still needed to complete the degree and training due to the East Asian perspective and expectation from the society.

The lack of long-term career development in Taiwan always prohibited youths from joining their dream professions [55], particularly in the humanities and fine art occupations. A participant (P#24, Male, Focus Group) shared an idea:

> *I like[d] botany and plant biology from [a] young age. I wish[ed] I c[ould] become a botanist from 8 years ago . . . [but] the long-term development of [a] botanist is unclear. No one can guarantee jobs after graduation, as there are more than 3,000 graduates in this field yearly. Also, Taiwanese people don't really consider Botanist as a professional. So if I can, I [will] select nursing instead. At least the general public will consider doctors as upper professionals . . . . (P#24, Male, Focus Group)*

It was not surprising to hear that in East Asia, university subject selections were not based on the students' own interests and desires for career development [23–34]. For example, the above participants wished to join botanical biology during her secondary school period. But due to the social context and social expectation [39], she needed to select the alternative (i.e., nursing) as her sixth choice on her application. One participant (P#36, Female, Interview) shared about enrolling in a nursing school instead of an electronic engineering program based on the gender-oriented bias and social expectation of gender-oriented occupations, saying,

> *. . . my parents and the society . . . in East Asian countries believe engineers, doctors, pharmacists, and emergency medical technicians must be males. I love science and engineering . . . I want to become a medical engineer in the future . . . but I mother told me that in many Taiwanese universities, there are only a few female students in any of the engineering programmes . . . it is ugly to be the only girl . . . . (P#36, Female, Interview)*

Most described their selection of their university major as having been significantly influenced by the East Asian perspective, social context, and social expectations [23–34]. More importantly, the sense of collectivism [4] was highly represented in these groups of individuals. For example, several of the female participants refused to study one of the STEM subjects because of the social norms and social expectations of men in these areas. Female individuals, however, were expected to study and join the workforce in lesser industries, such as nursing, administration, elementary school education, and social work [56]. Due to the strong East Asian perspective, social context, and social expectation on selecting an academic major and career, it is worth noting that some young adults might give up on following their own interests merely on the basis of the enrollment of students of the opposite gender in a program for which they had prepared for more than four years [19].

3.1.2. Academic Results

Standardized exams and university admission placement tests are widely used in many countries [57]. In Taiwan, a widely used standardized exam is the General Scholastics Ability Test (GSAT). Although there are alternative pathways for enrollment, the GSAT is the most common admission exam for local Taiwanese students. Nearly 30 of the student respondents expressed that their low GSAT scores prohibited their enrollment in the university of their choice and also their selection of university subjects. Unlike in the American educational system, with the community college options, students are allowed to select an undecided major pathway. But Taiwanese students have to select their university enrollment and major during their final semester of 12th grade in secondary school. One participant (P#38, Female, Focus Group) expressed,

> *I wish I c[ould] follow my will to become a medical doctor. But my low score . . . I can only apply for the nursing program . . . However, I cannot enrol at a community college or vocational college because there are no ways to build-up to the medical doctor's programme in the future . . . If I want to study but not re-take the exam for one more year, the only selection would be nursing . . . But again, I hate nursing . . . because it is not the same . . . . (P#38, Female, Focus Group)*

It is less likely for students to switch their university major once enrolled in many East Asian contexts due to unbalanced admission requirements and university policies. Unlike universities in the United States, students started their general education requirement during the first two-year of university education. Except for in special circumstances, students can switch and re-design their university major after the first or the second year of university education. The following participant (P#10, Male, Interview) shared his negative stories about the switching issue in Taiwan, saying,

> *Once I studied nursing during my first year at university, I discovered that I don't like this subject. However, in order to change my university subject, I have to be [among] the top-rated students for the purpose of switching. Otherwise, I have to re-apply for the entire GSAT steps again ... I hate nursing, I hate it so much ... But I cannot switch it due to the administrative requirement ... Also, the social expectation of my nursing career ... What can I do ... . (P#10, Male, Interview)*

In addition to their university enrollment and their selection of a major, the participants' academic results also limited their selection of university location. Some reported that they were forced by their parents and teachers to go to an urban university due to their high score of GSAT. One participant (P#11, Female, Interview) reported,

> *I was partially willing to study nursing actually if I could stay in my hometown ... In the southern part of Taiwan, there is a very good university and the nursing department. The enrolment of this university is my goal. But I received a high score in my GSAT. Therefore, my mother and school principal forced me to come to the capital city with a university that I dislike. I don't like the university, the social expectation of the university, and how people believed this university should create good nurses ... So I hate nursing because of the social expectation ... . (P#11, Female, Interview)*

It is worth noting that this participant (P#11, Female, Interview) was willing to study nursing if she could stay in her hometown. However, the East Asian perspective, social context, and social expectation [23–34] about her testing score, university, major, and potential career development destroyed her career perspective and beliefs. Although she wanted to become a nurse, she will now suffer due to the stresses and pressures from all different directions of her life.

Almost all described their GSAT scores, regardless of the level, as being a factor in their university enrollment, the decision about their academic major, and career development. Because the GSAT score was the most significant element, the decision about university subjects, the location of the university, and even the ability to switch university subjects after enrollment were not controlled by the participants. However, more importantly, a large number of participants expressed that based on their academic results, their parents, teachers, and even school leaders [35] expected them to enroll at top-tier universities and in a specific academic major. Almost all participants were forced to study in an academic major based on the recommendations from their parents and school staff. For example, a participant (P#32, Female, Focus Group) said, "I cannot cho[ose] which school and which location [where] can I study, I have to listen to my parents and teachers".

3.1.3. Financial Influence

Everyone experienced the stress of financial factors. Due to the East Asian traditions and cultural perspectives [34], children are responsible for taking care of their parents and even grandparents after their university graduation. Although the Taiwanese government does not regulate any policies about birth control, many contemporary Taiwanese families have fewer than two children.

Nearly two-thirds of the participants expressed that they would be the one who would take care of their parents and even grandparents after graduation, so they needed to select a career pathway that would allow them to make a significant amount of money. In fact, such East Asian perspectives on family engagements and responsibilities highly influenced the decision-making processes of these participants [31]. One participant (P#33, Male, Focus Group) told the researcher that being a nurse was almost the only way to take care of his parents and four grandparents after his graduation. In the same focus-group activity section, another participant (P#35, Female, Focus Group) echoed that situation with her own, saying,

In many families, taking care of parents [is] expected. My parents expected me to take care of their late [years] ... although I wanted to study music ... I must study nursing, [in] which [I] can make money ... But this must not be my wills ... I really hate nursing ... I don't want to become a nurse after university ... I want my life back as an adult after university ... I did not tell my mother about this yet ... But I am sure I will not become a nurse ... I dislike nursing not matter what .... (P#35, Female, Interview)

Another Participant (P#25, Male, Focus Group) grew up in a rural community in central Taiwan. He also identified this family expectation and financial difficulties as a villager in the countryside. As mentioned above, many East Asian elderly were expected to be cared for by their children. Therefore, as a male child, the participant felt a need to send financial resources to his parents after university graduation. Consequently, this participant considered nursing as one of the occupations that could provide financial security, saying,

... my parents sent me to university due to financial stress. I wish I c[ould] work in my family-run farm. But my parents want me to work in an upper social occupation ... I need to listen ... Moreover, my mother is a disabled person ... I need to take care of her after I finished my university ... But I want to continue my study in physical therapy in the future ... I like the medical profession, but I surely dislike nursing as my life-long career development ... I will explore a master's degree or another qualification soon .... (P#25, Male, Focus Group)

It is worth noting that this participant has a very strong sense in the field of the medical profession. Although he took nursing as his alternative during his university application period, he will continue his career development in physical therapy due to these personal goals and financial considerations.

In addition to their concerns about post-graduation financial stress, participants also experienced pre-graduation financial stress due to their lower-income status. One participant (P#9, Female, Focus Group) used to plan to study in a culinary arts and bakery programs based on her goals and interests. However, most of the culinary arts and bakery program required higher tuition fees and supplemental fees. Because her family could not afford the extra fees, she had to give up her own goals and enroll in the nursing program. Another participant (P#8, Female, Focus Group) also shared similar stories, saying,

I was planning to apply for the film major. But the department required [me] to have several expensive cameras and lenses, a high-quality computer, as well as the extra tuition fees for fine art lectures. I don't want to spend all the saving[s] of my family ... I have to select a university major ... which I hate ... that can make money .... (P#8, Female, Focus Group)

In short, the East Asian perspective, social context, and social expectation about the nursing and medical professions always limited their opportunities and career choices [6,25]. Unlike many studies conducted in the westernized societies and communities, many Taiwanese nursing students decided to enroll into one of the nursing programs based the social and cultural expectations [21]. Although university major and career development should be a selection of individuals, such preferences are not widely available in eastern societies. Furthermore, securing financial resources for their parents and elderly always forced them to enter the medical profession due to the stable salary and other financial considerations [29]. Although registered nurses may earn a reasonable salary for their family, it is unfair for both registered nurses and patients in this case in Taiwan. Although career mismatching always happens due to various reasons, this study discovered some significant findings which may gradually be detrimental to the medical and social health care system [11].

3.2. Influences from the Participants' Contextual Environment

3.2.1. Parental Recommendations

"I do this degree for my parents" (P#13, Female, Interview). It is worth noting that the perspective of "I have to do this degree for my parents" was shared 320 times based on the transcripts.

Young adults and recent secondary school graduates usually do not have significant work and life experience from which to select a major that may, in turn, be an investment in their long-term career plans. One potential way to obtain recommendations is from their parents. Due to the ideas of collectivism, many East Asian people tended to conduct activities and behaviors based on the benefits of the groups and communities. Without the permissions from family members and group members, East Asian people usually conduct nothing further because of the ideas of respectfulness.

All advocated the ideas of collectivism with the traditional East Asian perspective [4] due to their respectfulness towards family members and elders in their cohort [25]. In fact, they consulted with their parents and even grandparents about university selection, academic major, and career development before they submitted their university application. One participant (P#20, Female, Interview) recalled a story about marking her major selections, saying,

> My mother asked me to study nursing as both of my parents are medical professionals in the national-level hospital. Perhaps I am not a good medical profession as I do not have any passion for my patients. But I have to listen to my parents as they are the one who took care of my life. I have to be respectful to them as a good child … This is traditional of us … Although I hate nursing … you don't know how much I hate nursing and the career development of a registered nurse … But I have to do this degree for my parents … . (P#20, Female, Interview)

Another participant (P#28, Female, Interview) also shared a similar situation at the same focus group activity section, saying,

> My father is a doctor, and my mother is a nurse … they expected my sister and I [to] become medical practitioners … so, my sister was asked to enrol in a nursing school and so am I … my interest and career goal is to become a news reporter. But what can I do? Can I not listen to my parents? They spent almost half of their life for two of us … I cannot just say no to them … I hate nursing … But I am doing this degree for them … but for my own interests and goals … . (P#28, Female, Interview)

From the above sharing, many participants selected their major and career development based on their parents' desires and recommendations instead of their own [29]. A study indicated that East Asian people tended to listen to their parents and cohort members as recommendations for their decision. Unlike people in the westernized society, East Asian people advocate the notion of respectfulness towards their parents, elders, and community members. Therefore, this study also reflected the practices of the current participants.

In addition to parental recommendations being an extension of the parents' original occupations, a large number of participants advocated that they were asked to study a major that their parents had not been able to achieve during their own youth. In fact, these expectations from parents are not uncommon in the East Asian perspective [27]. During the last century, most of the East Asian countries and regions were developing as third-world countries. Therefore, youth and students at that time did not have chances for university education. Therefore, parents of this generation and even the society have a higher-level of expectations in the current social context. One participant (P14, Female, Focus Group) was one of many with this case, saying,

> My mother was raised in a low-income family and wished to become a nurse during her childhood … but she couldn't … now, she asked me to complete her dream. But she did not ask me if I want to do so. As a daughter, I hope I can complete her dream for the purpose of respectfulness … however, I can tell you that I hate nursing … I studied this nursing degree for my mother … I will not join the nursing profession afterwards … absolutely no … . (P14, Female, Focus Group)

Similarly, another participant (P#17, Female, Focus Group) also shared a case of a comparable situation, saying,

> My parents did not go to university during their young age … [so they] forced me to go to university … during my early teenage [years], they asked me to [study] medical biology. I have no interest …

but my mother liked this ... I [studied]. Now, my parents want me to study nursing ... I enrolled at my nursing programme now ... because I want to be a good girl ... but I am sure that I hate this nursing subject and I studies this degree for them obviously ... I will not join this nursing profession afterwards ... But I have to study this for my parents ... . (P#17, Female, Focus Group)

After P#17 shared her experience in a focus-group activity section, another participant (P#18, Female, Focus Group) echoed her similar case, saying,

I am sure a lot of students selected their major based on some expectations of the East Asian perspectives ... I am sure more than half of us [classmates]' majors were selected by parents or someone at home ... at least four women in my dorm room were ... I am so surprised that four girls [roommates] in our room were forced to study nursing because of our parents' decision ... We won't join the nursing profession afterwards as we all studied that for our parents ... We all understood that we hate nursing so much ... . (P#18, Female, Focus Group)

When the researcher asked questions about the interrelationships of financial responsibility, academic major, and career decision and development, one participant (P#42, Female, Interview) exclaimed that due to pressure and expectations from her parents,

I absolutely want to become an early childhood teacher ... but my mother just wanted me to study nursing in the capital city ... if I cannot complete the degree, who is going to take care of her late [in] life? I am just a machine to take care of the elderly. But I have to take care of her, due to the filial piety ... this makes me hate nursing so much ... . (P#42, Female, Interview)

One participant (P#25, Female, Interview) expressed that she had to listen to her parents' suggestion to attend medical school instead of the school of agriculture, due to financial considerations. Based on her life stories, the participant showed a solid awareness of her interests and career goals in the farming industry. However, her sense of filial piety limited her arguments because her parents' suggestions were a higher consideration than her own interests and career goals [31].

In short, all participants advocated that their major selections and career developments were chosen by their parents due to the East Asian perspective, social context, and social expectation, particularly parental recommendations and respectfulness [23–34]. The finding from this section was hardly found in much of the current literature with a westernized perspective. It is worth noting that all participants always respected their parents instead of their own interests and goals. Although respectfulness is encouraged, such mismatching may damage the health and social care system.

3.2.2. Teachers' Recommendations

In addition to the recommendations from parents, teachers also controlled the participants' decisions about their university enrollment, academic major, and career development. Nearly all participants revealed that their secondary school principal and homeroom teacher[s] had forced them to go to a nursing program because their enrollment would increase the reputation of the secondary school. One participant (P#23, Female, Interview) shared,

My secondary school is located in a rural community ... I am the first graduate who receive[d] a first-rated GSAT score ... [my] school principal asked me to go to the capital city and stud[y] a bachelor's degree in nursing science, so the secondary school can promote my name and achievement in the city hall. I have asked my parents, family member[s], teachers, counsellors, and social workers about this. All of them advocated the relocation to the capital city and nursing school ... It seems like I have no choice ... but I want to study ocean studies ... . (P#23, Female, Interview)

Teachers' recommendations did not influence just a single student's decision, but a large number of participants. Questions about teachers' recommendations were asked during both the individual and focus-group activity sections, and nearly two-thirds of the participants shared their opinions on how teachers' recommendation influenced their decision. Several significant opinions are listed below. For example, a participant (P#39, Female, Interview) shared negative experience, saying,

> *... my 12th grade homeroom teacher told me that the shortage of medical doctor[s] would be terminated within a decade. So I listened and obeyed her opinion and switch[ed] to nursing. This is the worst recommendation so far in my life ... I want to be a doctor ... not a nurse ... I hate nursing, I like to be a medical doctor as my career development ... It looks like I am studying for my teacher ... I am so angry and upset ... . (P#39, Female, Interview)*

Another participant (P#22, Female, Interview) also told her lived stories between her teachers and herself to the focus group participants, saying,

> *... my teacher asked us to fill up the application form in front of her. She assigned us with the particular subject[s]. If we [did] not listen to her, I think that would be a little bit irresponsible? So I just listened to her. But this is certainly not my own will ... So like, I am studying this degree for my teacher or what? (P#22, Female, Interview)*

In short, nearly all participants exhibited filial piety and respectfulness to their teachers and other school professionals [23–34]. Although some of them argued that their university enrollment and academic major, and their career decisions, were not their first choice, they felt that as good students they had to show the required filial piety and respectfulness.

3.2.3. Pressures from Family Members

Besides family and teachers who had daily interactions with the participants, other family members, such as cousins, uncles, and aunts, also revealed expectations about the participants' decisions regarding their university enrollment, academic major, and career pathway. Almost all participants expressed experience in this subtheme. One participant (P#3, Female, Focus Group) shared that her decisions were forced by her uncle, saying,

> *... my uncle told my mother that he used to work in a hospital and believed the nurses can make a lot of money. So, he highly recommended [to] my mother ... [that] I select this direction. My mother and my uncle sent me the nursing brainwashing messages everyday ... respectfulness, listening, orders from the parents ... I am sure I hate nursing now ... but I am studying this degree exclusively for these two people ... . (P#3, Female, Focus Group)*

Another participant (P#1, Female, Focus Group) also added to this theme and said,

> *... my uncle is [in] upper leadership in chained clinics in the capital city. He always convinced my mother, and I worked for him. So, he called my mother every day and asked me to study nursing ... nursing is a subject that I hated ... But the pressure from my uncle and mother ... I have to follow this pathway ... for them ... . (P#1, Female, Focus Group)*

During the same focus group activity section, Participant (P#29, Focus Group) shared a negative experience, saying,

> *I was the only one who was forced by other family members ... in the Taiwanese society, many people believe being a doctor or medical practitioner is an excellent occupation. I agreed. But this is not something that I want to do for my whole life. I always thought I was tricked by my family as well as the society ... . (P#29, Focus Group)*

In short, many participants expressed negative opinions and experiences about the influence of family [23–34]. Because East Asian people tend to respect their elders' recommendations [29], nearly all participants followed the wills of their family members instead of their own personal interests. It is worth noting that not only parents but also related family members, had the authority to order the participant to choose a particular direction for study and career choice.

3.2.4. Comparison with Other Relatives

Many participants seemed to have had common experiences about how their parents compared their (i.e., the participants') university enrollment, major, and even GSAT scores with those of other children with similar backgrounds. When one of the participants (P#19, Female) was asked how she had decided to start her undergraduate study in nursing, she said that her parents compared her GSAT score and university application form with those of other children who were living in the same neighbourhood. The following remarks made by some of the participants seem to show similar situations of negative experiences. For example, a participant (P#16, Female, Interview) shared,

> *My mother asked [about] other people's academic major selections in the community centre. Afterwards, she came back and asked me to study that nursing ... I was very surprised that my career and major are decided and selected by a group of aunts in the community centre ... I hate nursing for sure ... But as a Taiwanese girl ... I needed to listen to our cohort and members of my family ... If I don't, I cannot show the respectfulness to the community ... . (P#16, Female, Interview)*

Another participant (P#1, Male, Interview) also shared that his mother brought his application form to the community centre and asked opinions from other children. Besides sending their information and report cards to the community centre, some participants told the researcher their parents had even brought all their family members and relatives to their home for discussion. One participant (P#23, Female) shared her experience, saying,

> *During the application period, my parents called everyone to my home for suggestions and discussions. My elder cousins provided more than 20 suggestions. My parents always compare[d] my scores, university enrolment, and major intentions to everyone ... they compared my scores and major ... my score was not excellent. Some of them even laughed ... after they laughed, I still had to follow my mother's decision ... . (P#1, Male, Interview)*

Another participant (P#26, Female, Interview) shared a similar situation, saying,

> *My GSAT score was high enough to apply [for] most of the appropriate majors. I would like to go to a university in the southern part of Taiwan, as I wanted to escape from my family ... but my parents wanted me to study near them. So I stayed ... my parents wanted me to study medicine. Even if I want to study nursing, I have to follow their wills ... because they are my parents ... . (P#26, Female, Interview)*

Last but not least, the cohort and community-based collectivism always influenced how East Asian people behave. In this case, although the participants have their own goals and interests for major and career development, they did not have many choices due to the perspective of collectivism and respectfulness from their elders, family members, and members in their community. The results of this study outlined the relationship between the East Asian perspective, social context, and social expectation. The researcher used nursing students as a sample to explore and discover how this relationship exists in contemporary society. Without a doubt, many behaviors, ideas and perspectives were influenced by this relationship [23–34].

Attention should be paid to the directives given by the parents and family members. Although filial piety is a traditional aspect of the East Asian culture that may not change in the short term in Taiwan, the opinions and expressions of youth should be respected [36]. It is important to note that individuals' academic and career interests and goals significantly influence their career pathways and career development [58,59]. Parents and family members should avoid ordering their children to base their decisions about university enrollment and university subject selections on the desires of their elders. One participant (P#41, Female, Interview) indicated that playing a musical instrument as an academic major was her desire because that hobby was developed based on the decisions of her parents. However, she had no choices due to her parents' decision and application. Therefore, parents should also learn that they need to release more authority to their children and that the children should be taught career development navigation, such as vocational skills training [60].

4. Conclusions

To the best of the knowledge, this is one of the very first nursing studies that is based on the approach of the relationship between an East Asian perspective, social context, and social expectation for East Asian university students' decision-making about their major selections and career developments. In some other countries, in which individuals do not have the significant sense of filial piety and obedience toward their parents and elders that East Asians do, individuals may follow their own interests and career goals for university enrollment and selection of their academic major, particularly in the field of nursing education [1,7,16].

In addition to the East Asian educational systems and structures that exist at the macro-level, at the micro-level filial piety and family negotiation continue to play a vital role for young adults in their decision-making about university enrollment, academic majors, and career progression, and that role could influence their long-term career investment and development [23–34]. Based on the data and experiences shared by this study's 42 participants, all students indicated that their decisions and intentions were solid but were made unwillingly. However, due to their sense of filial piety, almost all of them had tended to listen to and obey suggestions or orders from their parents, teachers, and elders [35].

Some readers may argue that parents accept opinions from the youth in contemporary society. However, because this study was conducted recently in Taiwan with several dozen young adults, it seems clear that their sense of filial piety in the decision-making process is not likely to change in the short run. In general, secondary school graduates are usually under the age of 18 years old. Therefore, their university applications and related forms must be signed by parents or guardians. Although their sense of filial piety would not change even if the students had reached the age of 18 years old, young university students in their early adulthood should have greater authority to decide their own career pathways. The study's findings indicate that some young adults choose to avoid the dictates of filial piety and instead pursue their own interests and career goals. For those interviewed here, the pursuit of their own interests and career goals combined with those directed by filial piety sometimes occurred [20,35–37]. For example, they may have pursued a double university subject major and minor study, to also satisfy their own desires.

4.1. Limitations

Every research study has its limitations. Two limitations have been found in this study. First, this study was a qualitative research study with 42 traditional-age nursing students. However, as mentioned before, nursing education and career development are famous career selections for many university students and second-career changers. Therefore, future research may expand the population to non-traditional age students, second-career changers, returning students, and adult students.

4.2. Implementations

In recent decades, some vocational higher education institutions have created vocation-oriented undergraduate degree programs for students who want to develop hands-on skills for their career pathways [61]. In addition to vocational undergraduate degree programs, some educational systems also allow individuals to take their first and second year of university education with a university subject as undecided. Both of those educational elements are significant blueprints for reforming Taiwanese and even all East Asian higher education institutions and universities, with the goal of expanding the current curriculum and policies for students with non-traditional backgrounds.

Instead of changing the sense of filial piety, the universities, departments of education, and related agencies could reform specific policies in order to avoid putting limitations on young adults. As discussed above, some participants expressed that the university policy did not allow them to switch their university subject. However, recent graduates of secondary school and young adults usually do not have enough life experience to choose appropriate career pathways during their late teenage years. Thousands of university graduates do not participate in the industry or subject area in which they received their undergraduate degree. As a result, if universities would allow enrolled students to switch their academic major after their registration and enrollment, that potentially could increase the graduation rate and interest levels of students and contribute to their learning and enjoyment. It is also worth noting that the relevant agencies should discuss creating an undecided academic major for students who encounter difficulty deciding on a specific major.

Parents also can learn skills and techniques for sharing short-term, middle-term, and long-term career goals and academic interests with their children, while providing the children with the appropriate rewards, appreciation, encouragement, support, and involvement. In addition, parents can learn the significance of helping their children explore and discover their own academic interests and career goals, by bringing them on field trips to university campuses and organizations, introducing them to various cultural backgrounds and diversities, and increasing their understanding of particular subject matters. By conducting these parenting steps, the parents can help their children to exercise filial piety by a show of respectfulness toward their parents, while at the same time making their own decisions about university enrollment, university subject selection, and career development.

Funding: This research was funded by Woosong University Academic Research Funding 2020.

Conflicts of Interest: The authors declare no conflict of interest.

Appendix A

Interview Protocol Questions: The First Interview

(1) Why do you want to study nursing as your bachelor's degree major? Please tell me more.
(2) Do you enjoy your major? Why or why not?
(3) How did you select your university major during secondary school?
(4) If you can select it again, would you select nursing as your major?
(5) How would you think filial piety for your university major selection and other related behaviors?
(6) Further questions will be asked as follow-up questions.

Appendix B

Interview Protocol Questions: The Second Interview

(1) Let's think about the biggest reasons why would you select nursing as your major?
(2) Without this reason, would you select nursing again?
(3) Who select this major (i.e., nursing)? Yourself, families, friends, peers influence, parents etc.?
(4) Would other people influence your major selection/career development/university choice etc.?
(5) Would you think filial piety take some positions in the selection process?
(6) Further questions will be asked as follow-up questions.

References

1.   Foronda, C.L.; Alfes, C.M.; Dev, P.; Kleinheksel, A.J.; Nelson, D.A.; O'Donnell, J.M.; Samosky, J.T. Virtually Nursing. *Nurse Educ.* **2017**, *42*, 14–17. [CrossRef] [PubMed]
2.   Dos Santos, L.M. The motivation and experience of distance learning engineering programmes students: A study of non-traditional, returning, evening, and adult students. *Int. J. Educ. Pract.* **2020**, *8*, 134–148. [CrossRef]
3.   Ginzberg, E. Career development. In *Career Choice and Development: Applying Contemporary Theories to Practice*; Brown, D., Brooks, L., Eds.; Jossey-Bass: San Francisco, CA, USA, 1984; pp. 172–190.
4.   Han, C.M. Individualism, collectivism, and consumer animosity in emerging Asia: Evidence from Korea. *J. Consum. Mark.* **2017**, *34*, 359–370. [CrossRef]

5. Super, D. A Life-span, life-space approach to career development. In *The Jossey-Bass Management Series and the Jossey-Bass Social and Behavioral Science Series. Career Choice and Development: Applying Contemporary Theories to Practice*; Brown, D., Brooks, L., Eds.; Jossey-Bass: San Francisco, CA, USA, 1990; pp. 197–261.
6. Tzeng, H.-M. The influence of nurses' working motivation and job satisfaction on intention to quit: An empirical investigation in Taiwan. *Int. J. Nurs. Stud.* **2002**, *39*, 867–878. [CrossRef]
7. Mohamed, L.K. First-career and second-career nurses' experiences of stress, presenteeism and burn-out during transition to practice. *Evid. Based Nurs.* **2019**, *22*, 85. [CrossRef]
8. Adams, A.; Bond, S. Hospital nurses' job satisfaction, individual and organizational characteristics. *J. Adv. Nurs.* **2000**, *32*, 536–543. [CrossRef]
9. Nantsupawat, A.; Kunaviktikul, W.; Nantsupawat, R.; Wichaikhum, O.; Thienthong, H.; Poghosyan, L. Effects of nurse work environment on job dissatisfaction, burnout, intention to leave. *Int. Nurs. Rev.* **2017**, *64*, 91–98. [CrossRef]
10. Ten Hoeve, Y.; Castelein, S.; Jansen, G.; Roodbol, P. Dreams and disappointments regarding nursing: Student nurses' reasons for attrition and retention. A qualitative study design. *Nurse Educ. Today* **2017**, *54*, 28–36. [CrossRef]
11. Connors, C.A.; Dukhanin, V.; March, A.L.; Parks, J.A.; Norvell, M.; Wu, A.W. Peer support for nurses as second victims: Resilience, burnout, and job satisfaction. *J. Patient Saf. Risk Manag.* **2020**, *25*, 22–28. [CrossRef]
12. Jones, M. Career Commitment of Nurse Faculty. *Res. Theory Nurs. Pract.* **2017**, *31*, 364–378. [CrossRef]
13. Bakker, E.J.M.; Verhaegh, K.J.; Kox, J.H.A.M.; van der Beek, A.J.; Boot, C.R.L.; Roelofs, P.D.D.M.; Francke, A.L. Late dropout from nursing education: An interview study of nursing students' experiences and reasons. *Nurse Educ. Pract.* **2019**, *39*, 17–25. [CrossRef]
14. Salmi, E.; Vehkakoski, T.; Aunola, K.; Määttä, S.; Kairaluoma, L.; Pirttimaa, R. Motivational sources of practical nursing students at risk of dropping out from vocational education and training. *Nord. J. Vocat. Educ. Train.* **2019**, *9*, 112–131. [CrossRef]
15. Jacob, E.R.; McKenna, L.; D'Amore, A. Educators' expectations of roles, employability and career pathways of registered and enrolled nurses in Australia. *Nurse Educ. Pract.* **2016**, *16*, 170–175. [CrossRef]
16. Rainbow, J.G.; Steege, L.M. Transition to practice experiences of first- and second-career nurses: A mixed-methods study. *J. Clin. Nurs.* **2019**, *28*, 1193–1204. [CrossRef] [PubMed]
17. Hama, T.; Takai, Y.; Noguchi-Watanabe, M.; Yamahana, R.; Igarashi, A.; Yamamoto-Mitani, N. Clinical practice and work-related burden among second career nurses: A cross-sectional survey. *J. Clin. Nurs.* **2019**, *28*, 1–11. [CrossRef] [PubMed]
18. Tang, M.A. Comparison of Asian American, Caucasian American, and Chinese College Students: An Initial Report. *J. Multicult. Couns. Devel.* **2002**, *30*, 124–134. [CrossRef]
19. Jin, L. *The Role of Personality and Filial Piety in the Career Commitment Process among Chinese University Students*; The University of Hong Kong: Hong Kong, China, 2009.
20. Hui, T.; Yuen, M.; Chen, G. Career-related filial piety and career adaptability in Hong Kong university students. *Career Dev. Q.* **2018**, *66*, 358–370. [CrossRef]
21. Vuong, Q.-H.; Bui, Q.-K.; La, V.-P.; Vuong, T.-T.; Nguyen, V.-H.T.; Ho, M.-T.; Nguyen, H.-K.T.; Ho, M.-T. Cultural additivity: Behavioural insights from the interaction of Confucianism, Buddhism and Taoism in folktales. *Palgrave Commun.* **2018**, *4*, 143. [CrossRef]
22. Cubillo, M.; Sanchez, J.; Cervino, J. International students' decision-making process. *Int. J. Educ. Manag.* **2006**, *20*, 101–115. [CrossRef]
23. Cooper, C.E.; McLanahan, S.S.; Meadows, S.O.; Brooks-Gunn, J. Family structure transitions and maternal parenting stress. *J. Marriage Fam.* **2009**, *71*, 558–574. [CrossRef]
24. Sung, K. Filial Piety in Modern Times: Timely Adaptation and Practice Patterns. *Australas. J. Ageing* **1998**, *17*, 88–92. [CrossRef]
25. Li, H.; Lin, Y.; Lee, I. The impact of traditional filial piety between older people and their children in Taiwan. *J. Compr. Nurs. Res. Care* **2016**, *1*, 103.
26. Hwang, K.K. Filial piety and loyalty: Two types of social identification in Confucianism. *Asian J. Soc. Psychol.* **1999**, *2*, 163–183. [CrossRef]
27. Cheung, C.K.; Kwan, A. The erosion of filial piety by modernisation in Chinese cities. *Ageing Soc.* **2009**, *29*, 179–198. [CrossRef]

28. Sung, K.-T. A New Look at Filial Piety: Ideals and Practices of Family-Centered Parent Care in Korea. *Gerontologist* **1990**, *30*, 610–617. [CrossRef]

29. Canda, E.R. Filial Piety and Care for Elders: A Contested Confucian Virtue Reexamined. *J. Ethn. Cult. Divers. Soc. Work* **2013**, *22*, 213–234. [CrossRef]

30. Sung, K. Elder respect: Exploration of ideals and forms in East Asia. *J. Aging Stud.* **2001**, *15*, 13–26. [CrossRef]

31. Croll, E. The Intergenerational Contract in the Changing Asian Family. *Oxford Dev. Stud.* **2006**, *34*, 473–491. [CrossRef]

32. Chong, A.M.L.; Liu, S. Receive or give? Contemporary views among middle-aged and older Chinese adults on filial piety and well-being in Hong Kong. *Asia Pac. J. Soc. Work Dev.* **2016**, *26*, 2–14. [CrossRef]

33. Sun, Y. Among a Hundred Good Virtues, Filial Piety is the First: Contemporary Moral Discourses on Filial Piety in Urban China. *Anthropol. Q.* **2017**, *90*, 771–799. [CrossRef]

34. Zhang, M.; Lin, T.; Wang, D.; Jiao, W. Filial piety dilemma solutions in Chinese adult children: The role of contextual theme, filial piety beliefs, and generation. *Asian J. Soc. Psychol.* **2019**. [CrossRef]

35. Kwan, K. Counseling Chinese peoples: Perspectives of filial piety. *Asian J. Couns.* **2000**, *7*, 23–41.

36. Chen, W.-W. The relations between filial piety, goal orientations and academic achievement in Hong Kong. *Educ. Psychol.* **2016**, *36*, 898–915. [CrossRef]

37. Sun, P.; Liu, B.; Jiang, H.; Qian, F. Filial piety and life satisfaction among Chinese students: Relationship harmony as mediator. *Soc. Behav. Personal. Int. J.* **2016**, *44*, 1927–1936. [CrossRef]

38. Lent, R.W.; Brown, S.D.; Hackett, G. Toward a unifying social cognitive theory of career and academic interest, choice, and performance. *J. Vocat. Behav.* **1994**, *45*, 79–122. [CrossRef]

39. Nguyen, V.; Nguyen, N.; Khuat, T.; Nguyen, P.; Do, T.; Vu, X.; Tran, K.; Ho, M.; Nguyen, H.; Vuong, T.; et al. Righting the Misperceptions of Men Having Sex with Men: A Pre-Requisite for Protecting and Understanding Gender Incongruence in Vietnam. *J. Clin. Med.* **2019**, *8*, 105. [CrossRef]

40. Merriam, S.B. *Qualitative Research: A Guide to Design and Implementation*; Jossey Bass: San Francisco, CA, USA, 2009.

41. Sharan, B.; Merriam, E.J.T. *Qualitative Research: A Guide to Design and Implementation*, 4th ed.; Jossey-Bass: San Francisco, CA, USA, 2015.

42. Creswell, J. *Qualitative Inquiry and Research Design: Choosing Among Five Approaches*; SAGE Publications: Thousand Oaks, CA, USA, 2007.

43. Creswell, J. *Qualitative Inquiry and Research Design: Choosing Among Five Approaches*; Sage: Thousand Oaks, CA, USA, 2012.

44. Thomas, D.R. A general inductive approach for analyzing qualitative evaluation data. *Am. J. Eval.* **2006**, *27*, 237–246. [CrossRef]

45. Tang, K.H.; Dos Santos, L.M. A brief discussion and application of interpretative phenomenological analysis in the field of health science and public health. *Int. J. Learn. Dev.* **2017**, *7*, 123–132. [CrossRef]

46. Dos Santos, L.M. Experiences and expectations of international students at historically black colleges and universities: An interpretative phenomenological analysis. *Educ. Sci.* **2019**, *9*, 189. [CrossRef]

47. Dos Santos, L.M. Rural Public Health Workforce Training and Development: The Performance of an Undergraduate Internship Programme in a Rural Hospital and Healthcare Centre. *Int. J. Environ. Res. Public Health* **2019**, *16*, 1259. [CrossRef]

48. Dos Santos, L.M. Promoting safer sexual behaviours by employing social cognitive theory among gay university students: A pilot study of a peer modelling programme. *Int. J. Environ. Res. Public Health* **2020**, *17*, 1804. [CrossRef] [PubMed]

49. Seidman, I. *Interviewing as Qualitative Research: A Guide for Researchers in Education and the Social Sciences*, 4th ed.; Teachers College Press: New York, NY, USA, 2013.

50. Dos Santos, L.M. Mid-life career changing to teaching profession: A study of secondary school teachers in a rural community. *J. Educ. Teach.* **2019**, *45*, 225–227. [CrossRef]

51. Kim, M.S.; Seo, Y.S. Social cognitive predictors of academic interests and goals in South Korean engineering students. *J. Career Dev.* **2014**, *41*, 526–546. [CrossRef]

52. Evans, V.; Salcido, K. *Career Paths: Nursing*; Express Publishing: Newbury, UK, 2019.

53. Yu, M.; Lee, M. Managers' career development recognition in Taiwanese companies. *Asia Pac. Manag. Rev.* **2015**, *20*, 11–17. [CrossRef]

54. Chen, L.; Reich, M. *Medical Education in East Asia: Past and Future*; Indiana University Press: Bloomington, IN, USA, 2017.
55. Remmert, D. *Young Adults in Urban China and Taiwan: Aspirations, Expectations, and Life Choices*; Routledge: London, UK, 2016.
56. Milliken, E. Feminist theory and social work practice. In *Social Work Treatment: Interlocking Theoretical Approaches*; Turner, F.J., Ed.; Oxford University Press: Oxford, UK, 2017; pp. 191–208.
57. Gökdağ Baltaoğlu, M.; Güven, M. Relationship between self-efficacy, learning strategies, and learning styles of teacher candidates (Anadolu University example). *S. Afr. J. Educ.* **2019**, *39*, 1–11. [CrossRef]
58. Dickinson, J.; Abrams, M.D.; Tokar, D.M. An examination of the applicability of social cognitive career theory for African American college students. *J. Career Assess.* **2017**, *25*, 75–92. [CrossRef]
59. Carrico, C.; Matusovich, H.M.; Paretti, M.C. A qualitative analysis of career choice pathways of college-oriented rural central appalachian high school students. *J. Career Dev.* **2019**, *46*, 94–111. [CrossRef]
60. Bodycott, P.; Lai, A. The role of Chinese parents in decisions about overseas study. In *Understanding Higher Education Internationalization. Global Perspectives on Higher Education*; Mihut, G., Altbach, P., Wit, H., Eds.; Sense Publishers: Rotterdam, The Netherlands, 2017; pp. 197–201.
61. Lapan, R.; Shaughnessy, P.; Boggs, K. Efficacy expectations and vocational interests as mediators between sex and choice of math/science college majors: A longitudinal study. *J. Vocat. Behav.* **1996**, *49*, 277–291. [CrossRef]

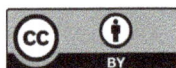

International Journal of
Environmental Research and Public Health

MDPI

Article

Effectiveness of Blended Learning in Nursing Education

María Consuelo Sáiz Manzanares [1,*] , María del Camino Escolar Llamazares [1] and Álvar Arnaiz González [2]

1   Departamento de Ciencias de la Salud, Facultad de Ciencias de la Salud, Universidad de Burgos, C/ Comendadores s/n, 09001 Burgos, Spain; cescolar@ubu.es
2   Departamento de Ingeniería Informática, Escuela Politécnica Superior, Universidad de Burgos, Avda. Cantabria s/n, 09006 Burgos, Spain; alvarag@ubu.es
*   Correspondence: mcsmanzanares@ubu.es; Tel.:+34-673192734

Received: 15 January 2020; Accepted: 26 February 2020; Published: 1 March 2020

check for updates

Abstract: Currently, teaching in higher education is being heavily developed by learning management systems that record the learning behaviour of both students and teachers. The use of learning management systems that include project-based learning and hypermedia resources increases safer learning, and it is proven to be effective in degrees such as nursing. In this study, we worked with 120 students in the third year of nursing degree. Two types of blended learning were applied (more interaction in learning management systems with hypermedia resources vs. none). Supervised learning techniques were applied: linear regression and K-means clustering. The results indicated that the type of blended learning in use predicted 40.4% of student learning outcomes. It also predicted 71.19% of the effective learning behaviors of students in learning management systems. It therefore appears that blended learning applied in Learning Management System (LMS) with hypermedia resources favors greater achievement of effective learning. Likewise, with this type of Blended Learning (BL) a larger number of students were found to belong to the intermediate cluster, suggesting that this environment strengthens better results in a larger number of students. Blended learning with hypermedia resources and project-based learning increase students´ learning outcomes and interaction in learning management systems. Future research will be aimed at verifying these results in other nursing degree courses.

Keywords: learning management system; higher education; nursing; data mining

---

1. Introduction

In approximately the last decade there has been a marked interest in investigating ways of teaching other than traditional face-to-face. The incorporation of technological resources such as virtual platforms and hypermedia resources, combined with other innovative, methodological techniques such as project-based or problem-based learning, have revolutionized the teaching–learning process. The aim is to teach in the most efficient way possible and to make the most of resources while ensuring sustainability. These technological and methodological resources have been applied to different disciplines, especially in the field of health sciences (medicine, pharmacy, psychology, veterinary, etc.). However, in recent years these resources have been incorporated into nursing studies. Next, an approach will be made for the most relevant concepts of teaching in a virtual platform, which has been called blended teaching, as well as the implementation of methodological resources for project-based learning. Likewise, special importance will be given to its application for the formation of future nursing programs by analyzing the pros and cons of this form of teaching and learning in the society of the 21st century. For this reason, the most relevant concepts of these new forms of teaching and their specific application to the nursing degree will be dealt with below. The final objective of this work is to study the effectiveness of different blended learning environments in the teaching of future nurses.

Twenty-first century society requires students and graduates to develop a series of skills related to two important leitmotifs: collaborative work and operation of information and communications technology (ICT). It is increasingly necessary to possess effective and rapid problem-solving skills and to develop digital competences [1]. The use of learning management systems (LMS) is, therefore, a reference in instructional practice, especially in higher education, as is the implementation of collaborative work in these methodological settings for the resolution of tasks and problems. A good example might be the use of project-based learning (PBL) methodology [2]. Recent investigations have confirmed that if such a methodology is accompanied by the use of hypermedia resources (e.g., flipped learning experiences, quizzes, use of wikis, on-line glossaries, etc.), then acquisition of deep learning is strengthened in students [3]. Deep learning is a concept developed in the framework of the taxonomy of Bloom [4]. It corresponds to the highest level of learning competences (comprehending, analyzing, summarizing, and evaluating their own learning). One of the currents of thought in LMS learning environments suggests that learning in these environments implies deeper learning from the point of view of cognitive and metacognitive complexity, as these facilitate self-regulated learning (SRL) and meaningful learning [5].

Likewise, LMS permit a more precise analysis of interactions which are logged in records (or logs). The logs represent units of information and registration that stores precise data on the frequency of user interactions and their duration [6]. LMS also facilitates the inclusion of hypermedia resources [7]. The use of these resources is especially relevant in health science degrees (nursing, medicine, pharmacy, etc.) since it implements practical assumptions in the work, which has been proven to reduce errors in the workplace [8].

There are various stages in this instruction process that will facilitate or inhibit the efficiency and depth of the learning process. One of them is the design of learning tasks in LMS [9,10]. Another essential element is that the teacher plans for process-oriented feedback [11].

1.1. Teaching through Learning Management Systems

The teacher has to reflect, among other points, on the following points: (1) the aims of the subject module, (2) to whom it is addressed, (3) what previous knowledge is required for a successful approach to the subject matter, (4) the type of learning tasks that facilitate content acquisition, (5) the metacognitive skills of the students prior to the instruction, (6) the cognitive and the metacognitive skills in each task needed for its effective solution, and (7) when and where the teaching–learning process will be developed. Likewise, the teacher has to plan follow-up with both the individual student and the group behavior on the platform. As has been argued, solving problems in a collaborative way is one of the most demanding skills in 21st century society. These types of competences are key references in educational and technological areas and for entry into employment. Collaborative work facilitates the construction of deep and effective learning in the students [10]. A scheme for the preparation of pedagogic design in the LMS may be seen in Table 1.

Table 1. Preliminary elements to take into account for the design of learning activities.

Questions for Activities Design	Subject Module Design (Teacher)	Aspects to Evaluate (Teacher and Students)
What	What is the object of the learning process? What competences are to be developed in the students?	Learning goals. Design of Knowledge.
How	Design of learning tasks.	Test its effectiveness for the achievement of the proposed learning aims
Who	To whom is it directed? Gain knowledge of the characteristics of the students.	In the students - Prior knowledge of the learning material. - Metacognitive skills that the teacher employs.
When and Where	Chronogram of timing of the tasks and the moments and spaces in which they will take place. Behavior of (individual and group) learners on the platform.	Teacher Gradual sequencing of the difficulty of the learning tasks. ✓ Planning of process-oriented feedback in each of the learning experiences. ✓ Evaluation of student behavior in the various activities that have been designed and in (individual and group) teacher feedback through the platform.

Nevertheless, computational techniques are required to conduct a conclusive analysis of student behavior in LMS. As previously mentioned, at present a broad percentage of learning is done in virtual environments, in what is called blended learning teaching. A lot of data can be recorded by LMS and accessed through logs. However, educational data mining (EDM) [12,13] is needed to study them precisely. Machine learning techniques can be applied to EDM. Subsequently, possible applications of those techniques will be presented in the analysis of learning data in LMS environments.

1.2. Application of Artificial Intelligence Techniques to Analyze the Teaching and Learning Process

Development of the internet and information and communications technology (ICT) has expanded learner access to information, and they have changed the way that information is taught and the way it is learned [14]. A learning management system (LMS) is an interactive learning environment that facilitates both teaching and learning. In addition, these software environments record all the actions performed by the teacher and by the students, under individual and group headings. However, those logs store a lot of data and learning analytics have to be used in order to study them in a flexible and accurate manner. These techniques can be simple, such as the ones usually found in LMS (descriptive statistics). However, more complex analytical techniques can be used, such as machine learning techniques (a subset of artificial intelligence). The latter are analogous to the computational thought of the human brain and operate with what is known as artificial intelligence. Machine learning techniques of classification and clustering [15] are among the most widely applied techniques for data analysis in educational environments. The use of these techniques for the analysis of both student and teacher behaviors will provide the teacher and those responsible for educational institutions with ideas to introduce improvements into the learning environment [11].

In brief, machine learning techniques are used, as these techniques are currently considered to provide the researcher with more data in the field of cognitive psychology and learning than traditional statistical techniques [16,17]. In particular, machine learning techniques permit personalized learning and provide individualized information on the development of student learning. Prediction techniques facilitate early detection of at-risk students and, therefore, personalized [18] help from the teacher [19,20]. Machine learning techniques also provide information on the effects of predicting the independent variable over each of the dependent variables in percent effects [21].

1.3. Design of the Blended-Learning Space in Nursing Instruction

Blended teaching, increasingly present in educational scenarios, is done through a blend of face-to-face (F2F) and virtual learning on LMS, known as blended learning. However, there is no generalized agreement on the taxonomy of blended learning [22]. Nevertheless, its differences with blended learning are accepted; in the blended learning environment, the student completes 80% with LMS and 20% is F2F, hereafter referred to as Blended Learning type 1. In contrast, blended learning (80% interaction in the LMS) is a space where feedback is done 80% of the time through F2F and 20% through LMS [18,23], hereafter referred to as Blended Learning type 2. Recent investigations have found that the replacement blended environment accompanied by the use of active methodologies (e.g., PBL, use of hypermedia resources, flipped learning experiences, and quizzes, or all at once) improved the learning results of students [3,24]. These achievements are especially significant in university environments [25,26] because future graduates will have to develop collaborative work skills, problem-solving independence, and the use of new technologies. These skills are essential for good development of entrepreneurship.

Along these lines, recent studies have shown that [27] an educational intervention that applies blended learning methodology can easily be added into nursing curricula. This type of learning enhances learning in this field. Recent systematic research indicated that blended learning together with PBL is a methodology that ensures effective learning among nursing students [28]. This type of paradigm is more effective than traditional teaching such as face to face. The reasons are that students need to develop the knowledge and skills necessary in clinical practice. Several studies recommend nursing teachers to use multifaceted techniques (blended learning, learning based in projects, etc.) to promote effective learning beyond face-to-face teaching [29]. While these studies highlight the need to train teachers in these techniques [28], the main reason is that, traditionally, teaching has been done face to face, and an organized transfer towards the use of these methodological resources is needed. A recent systematic review showed that, since 2018, there has been a growing interest in the implementation of these experiences in nursing studies. However, an increase in these experiences and more research in this discipline of knowledge are needed [30].

Moreover, blended learning environments permit an evaluation of the whole teaching–learning process in a systematic and simple way. Thus, the suggestion is that there are different variables that influence successful learning in this line of investigation into e-evaluation models, especially the learning strategies employed by the students themselves [31,32], the environment in which the learning takes place [33], the teaching design that the teacher brings to the class [30], and the behavioral learning of the students in the LMS [23]. The prediction interval of these variables is situated around 56%-61% [34].

1.4. Extraction and Analysis of Information on the Teaching–Learning Process Recorded in LMS

As we have mentioned earlier, development of the teaching through LMS will facilitate the student in learning recording and follow-up behaviours [35]. Many of these learning managers use supervised machine learning techniques, techniques such as multiple regression analysis (MRA), neural network, and SVM. Those techniques help with the detection and subsequent prediction of successful and risk behaviours. Behaviours of the students in LMS that have been related to successful learning are, among others [23]:

- the time that is used in carrying out the tasks;
- student time expended on studying theoretical content;
- the results in the self-evaluation test (quiz efforts);
- the quality of forum discussions (type and length of message);
- time employed in analysing the feedback given by the teacher;
- the number and type of messages sent;
- the frequency of access to LMS;

- contribution to content creation;
- files opened; and
- delivery time of the activities.

Therefore, the frequency and systematicness of student interactions and their interactions with LMS are directly related to effective learning [36]. Along these lines, recent investigations [23] have revealed differences in predicting learning results in relation to the variable "teaching methodology" (understood in terms of the pedagogic structure of the teaching, the evaluation procedures, and feedback). The type of activities and the evaluation tests (quizzes, tests, projects, presentations …) are understood to determine the effectiveness of behavioural learning logged on the LMS.

As previously mentioned, application of machine learning techniques to study the logs will allow the teachers to analyze the behavioural learning of their students and to detect at-risk students. In these cases, early intervention will presumably improve student learning responses. Recent studies have confirmed [17,35] that following up with student behavioural learning in the LMS facilitates the identification of at-risk students with an explained variance of 67.2%.

In summary, the use of machine learning techniques will permit the study of behavioral learning of both students and teachers on the platform, which will facilitate the application of prediction techniques to the learning results [37]. Reviewing the investigations presented earlier, we consider it important to study the behavior of PBL in the LMS. As has been indicated, there are few studies in that field, and more information is needed that will help to improve teaching practices in these environments [38]. Project work and personalization of learning in LMS have been proven to have significant effects on the quality of learning. Particular relevance has been in Health Science degrees, such as nursing or medicine, etc., since it facilitates work on clinical cases in a collaborative way and optimizes the results applied to real learning contexts [39].

This research study was performed to analyze data of students' online and face-to-face (F2F) activity in a blended nursing learning course. We applied two types of blended learning: Blended Learning type 1 [in which the interaction between the teacher and students is 80% in the LMS and 20% Face to Face (F2F)] and Blended Learning type 2 [in which the interaction between the teacher and students is 20% in the LMS and 80% Face to Face (F2F)].

In light of the above, the hypotheses in this study were the following:

H 1: The types of blended learning (Blended Learning type 1 vs. Blended Learning type 2) used will predict student learning outcomes;

H 2: The types of blended learning (Blended Learning type 1 vs. Blended Learning type 2) used will predict the learning behaviours logged on the LMS; and

H 3: The type of clusters will be different for each type of blended learning used (Blended Learning type 1 vs. Blended Learning type 2)

2. Materials and Methods

2.1. Design

A quasi-experimental post-treatment design with an equal control group (in terms of metacognitive skill) was used. Likewise, learning outcomes (learning outcomes in the development of project-based learning; learning outcomes in exhibition of project-based learning; learning outcomes in the test; and learning outcomes total) and behavioral learning in the LMS were the dependent variables (access to complementary information; Access to guidance to prepare PBL; Access to theoretical information; Access to teacher feedback; and mean visits per day).

2.2. Participants

A sample of 120 university students was assembled following the third year of their nursery degree in Spain (the degree has four years) during one semester (9 weeks): 63 followed the Blended Learning type 1 methodology and 57 followed the Blended Learning type 2 methodology (see Table 2).

The students were assigned to each blended learning group (Blended Learning type 1 vs. Blended Learning type 2) by means of convenience sampling. The work was developed in the subject of "Quality management methodology of nursing services."

Table 2. Group assignment and descriptive statistics for age, [a]n = 60. [b]n = 62.

Groups	Men			Women		
	n	M_{age}	SD_{age}	n	M_{age}	SD_{age}
Experimental Group, Blended Learning type 1 ([a]n)	7	23.29	2.56	56	22.30	2.13
Control Group, Blended Learning type 2 ([b]n)	9	24.67	4.12	48	23.83	5.13

Note. M_{age} = Mean Age; SD_{age} = Standard Deviation.

2.3. Instruments

a. *LMS UBUVirtual version 3.1.* A Moodle-based learning management system (LMS) was used that began with a constructivist approach and was developed through a modular system. It is a personalized Moodle-based LMS. An LMS is a modular learning environment that permits interaction and feedback between teacher and students, in many cases in real time, and in addition it facilitates the process of automated feedback.

b. The (ACRAr) *Scales of Learning Strategies* by Román & Poggioli [40]. This widely tested instrument identifies 32 strategies at different points in the information processing cycle. The reliability indicators on the scale were between α = 0.75 to α = 0.90 and the indicators of content validity were between r = 0.85 and r = 0.88. The subscale of metacognitive skills was applied in this study; this scale incorporated 17 strategies about the use of metacognitive skills into the problem solving tasks. A reliability index of α = 0.80 was obtained in this study; the reliability indicator on this subscale was α = 0.90 and the indicator of validity was r = 0.88.

c. *Student learning results: the results were recorded in the different evaluation procedures.* (1) Multiple-choice tests on the theoretical contents of the subject (test) were assigned a weight of 30% of the final grade. The test had 10 multiple-choice questions (four possible answers) with only one correct response. As well, five questionnaire-type quizzes were administered, one for each thematic unit. Cronbach´s Alpha reliability of the test was α = 81. (2) Development of PBL, with a weight of 25%, was measured with a rubric, which can be seen in Supplemental Material Table S1. (3) Likewise, the exhibition of the PBL, with a weight of 20%, was also measured with a rubric and can be seen in Supplemental Material Table S2. In the final mark, Cronbach´s Alpha reliability of PBL was α = 62. This result is lower because there was less dispersion among the scores in this type of evaluation test. Since the performance of the groups was quite uniform, this aspect can be checked in the results section and it is in accordance with the philosophy of PBL. Finally, the learning outcomes total covered the weighted scores of all the results (over 10 points). 4) The students solved five practices, and this part was 25% of the final grade. However, in this part all students had the highest qualification since the teacher reviewed the practices continuously, and if they were not correct the teacher ordered them to be repeated. Therefore, because it is not discriminate it has not been included in the analysis. Examples of the PBLs developed can be found at this link https://riubu.ubu.es/handle/10259/3753/discover.

2.4. Procedure

Convenience sampling was followed for the choice of the sample. This was due to the possibility of working with this methodology by a specialist teacher who attended to both groups, and in this way the "type of teacher" effect was avoided. Before the instructional intervention, the two groups (Blended Learning type 1 vs. Blended Learning type 2) were scored on the metacognitive skills Scale of ACRAr [40], with the aim of establishing the similarities between both groups in terms of metacognitive skills.

As stated in the introduction, Blended Learning type 1 was applied to the experimental group, a learning environment in which the interactions between teacher and student were 20% F2F and 80%

LMS. Likewise, Blended Learning type 2 was applied to the control group, a learning environment in which the interactions between teacher and students were 20% LMS and 80% F2F. In the experimental Group, hypermedia resources were used such as videos, and feedback was through the LMS. In contrast, classroom interactions between teacher and students and feedback in the control group were all F2F. In both groups, PBL methodology was followed. The difference, as has been pointed out, consisted of the type of blended learning in use (Blended Learning type 1 vs. Blended Learning type 2). Project development was done in both (the control and the experimental) groups in a collaborative way. The project work was completed in small groups of students of between 2 and 5 members.

2.5. Data Analysis

The following statistical analyses were applied: (1) Analysis of asymmetry and kurtosis; (2) analysis of the variance of a fixed-effect factor (ANOVA); (3) multiple regression analysis (MRA) [appropriate Tolerance (T) values were considered close to one and, with respect to the variance inflation factor, the values were between 1–10]; (4) cluster analysis. Package for the Social Sciences (SPSS) v.24 was used to perform the different analyses [41]. Likewise, the Goodness-of-fit indices were measured by structural equation modeling (SEM) and was used to study the settings of the machine learning technique to predict the learning results. The calculations were performed with the Statistical Package for the Social Sciences (SPSS) AMOS v.24 [42]. (5) Finally, to visualize the results in a cluster analysis, RapidMiner Studio software [43] was used.

2.6. Ethical Considerations

The research project was approved by the Ethics Committee of the University of Burgos. Previously, at the start of the project, the students were informed of the objectives, and their participation was at all times on a voluntary basis. Likewise, informed consent of each participant was recorded in writing.

3. Results

3.1. Previous Statistical Normalcy Analysis in the Sample

Before starting the research, the indicators of normality were studied. The results obtained from earlier statistical analyses with regard to the normality of the sample are presented below (values higher than |2.00| indicate extreme asymmetry, the lowest values indicate normality, and the values of between |8.00| and |20.00| suggest extreme kurtosis [44]). The results of metacognitive skills on the ACRAr subscale in both groups were acceptable for both indicators (see Table 3). Therefore, parametric statistics were used. Descriptive statistics are also shown in Tables A1 and A2 (see Appendix A).

Table 3. Indicators of asymmetry and kurtosis in the experimental group and control group.

Blended Learning Type 1 (Experimental Group)						Blended Learning Type 2 (Control Group)					
M	*SD*	*A*	*ASE*	*K*	*SEK*	*M*	*SD*	*A*	*AES*	*K*	*SEK*
80	23.85	−0.464	0.441	−0.973	0.858	75	28.75	−0.333	0.306	−0.957	0.604

Note. *M* = Mean Age; *SD* = Standard Deviation; *A* = Asymmetry; *K* = Kurtosis; *ASE* = Asymmetry Standard Error; *SEK* = Kurtosis Standard Error.

3.2. Previous Statistical Analysis of Homogeneity between the Groups before the Intervention

Significant differences between both groups (experimental and control) in their use of metacognitive strategies were anlayzed before application of the different types of blended learning (Type 1 vs. Type 2). To do so, a single-factor ANOVA with fixed-effects was performed (blended learning type) on the results. No significant differences were found between both, so they can be considered similar groups ($F_{1,119} = 0.276$; $p = 0.601$; $\eta^2 = 0.002$) in the ACRAr subscale of metacognitive skills.

Similarly, in order to study which type of supervised learning technique would be the most appropriate, the Goodness-of-fit indices were measured in the structural equation modeling (SEM) that was used to study the settings of the machine learning technique to predict the learning results. The calculations were performed with the Statistical Package for the Social Sciences (SPSS) AMOS v.24, as may be seen in Table 4, and no dependent relations between the observed values and the different prediction methods (LR, DT, RBFN, and kNN) were found for any of the four prediction models. Among these possibilities, the following were applied in the MRA.

Table 4. Goodness-of-fit indices.

Goodness of Fit Index	LR	RBFN	kNN	Accepted Value
df	5	5	5	
χ^2	174.121 ($p = 0.000$)	98.279 ($p = 00.00$)	106.532($p = 0.00$)	$p > 0.05$ $\alpha = 0.05$
RAMSEA	0.769	0.616	0.683	>0.05–0.08
RAMSEA interval	0.722–0.817	0.568–0.664	0.636–0.732	
SRMR	0.1602	0.1086	0.1152	>0.05–0.08
TLI	0.000	0.000	0.000	0.85–0.90<
CFI	0.000	0.000	0.000	0.95–0.97<
AIC	730.199	474.186	580.261	The lowest value
ECVI	6.085	3.956	4.836	The lowest value
ECVI interval (90%)	5.382–6.849	3.960–4.574	4.214–5.518	The lowest value

Note. df = degrees of liberty; χ^2 = Chi squared; LR = Linear Regression; DT = Decision Trees; RBFN = Radial basis function network; kNN = k-Nearest Neighbor classification; NFI = normed-fit-index; RMSEA = Root-Mean-Square Error of Approximation; SRMR = Standardized Root-Mean-Square Residual; TLI = Tucker–Lewis index; CFI = comparative fit index; AIC = Akaike Information criterion; ECVI = parsimony index.

3.3. Hypothesis 1.

MRA was performed to study the predictive value of the variable blended learning type applied to the student learning outcomes. An $R^2 = 0.404$ was found, which indicates that this variable explained 40.04% of the variance in the learning results. The Tolerance (*T*) values were within an interval of 0.106 and 0.336 and the Variance Inflation Factor (*VIF*) between 3.491 and 9.45, so none of the variables had to be removed. Likewise, the highest partial correlation was found in the Learning Outcomes Total ($r = 0.586$; $p = 0.000$), see Table A3.

3.4. Hypothesis 2.

MRA yielded a figure of $R^2 = 0.719$ in the study of the predictive value of blended learning applied to student behaviors on the platform. This figure indicated that the blended learning type in use explained 71.19% of the variance in the learning behaviors of students on the platform. The Tolerance (T) values were situated within an interval between 0.136 and 0.539 and the Variance Inflation Factor (VIF) between 1.472 and 7.346, so that no variable had to be removed. The highest partial correlation was found in Access to Teacher Feedback ($r = 0.448$), see Table A4.

3.5. Hypothesis 3.

A k-means clustering technique was applied in each type of blended learning in use (Blended Learning type 1 vs. Blended Learning type 2), as seen in Table 5. Three clusters are shown in Table 5 that were found in the two types of blended learning (Cluster 1, Sufficient; Cluster 2, Intermediary; and Cluster 3, Excellent. The classification of Cluster type was according to the maximum possible value in each learning outcome and number of accesses obtained). Higher values for performance were found in the Blended Learning type 1 rather than the Blended Learning type 2 in all three clusters, specifically in Learning Outcomes Total. Likewise, with regard to the learning behaviors developed by students in the type of blended learning in use (Blended Learning type 1 vs. Blended Learning type 2), as may be seen in Table 5, a higher number of log-ons to the platform in the Blended Learning type 1 rather than the Blended Learning type 2 environment were found, except for student queries on theoretical information provided by the teacher (see Table 6).

Table 5. Centers of final clusters for the learning results variable in Blended Learning type 1 and type 2, Blended Learning type 1: [a]$n = 1$; [b]$n = 45$; [c]$n = 17$; Blended Learning type 2: A lost value is observed. [a]$n = 9$; [b]$n = 30$; [c]$n = 18$

	Maximum	Cluster 1 Sufficient	Cluster 2 Intermediary	Cluster 3 Excellent
Blended Learning type 1				
Learning outcomes in PBLD	2.50	1.75	2.00	2.34
Learning outcomes in PBLE	2.00	1.00	1.62	1.80
Learning outcomes in test	3.00	2.30	2.24	2.50
Learning outcomes Total	10	7.00	8.62	9.26
Blended Learning type 2				
Learning outcomes in PBLD	2.50	1.88	2.09	2.32
Learning outcomes in PBLE	2.00	1.50	1.59	1.87
Learning outcomes in test	3.00	1.70	1.82	2.39
Learning outcomes Total	10	6.08	8.00	9.08

Note. PBLD = Project-Based Learning Development; PBLE = Project-Based Learning Exhibition.

Table 6. Centers of final clusters and the variable behavioral learning on the LMS in Blended Learning type 1 and type 2. Blended Learning type 1: a lost value is observed. [a]$n = 31$; [b]$n = 27$; [c]$n = 5$; Blended Learning type 2: Two lost values were observed. [a]$n = 36$; [b]$n = 16$; [c]$n = 6$.

	Interval	Cluster 1 Sufficient	Cluster 2 Intermediate	Cluster 3 Excellent
Blended Learning type 1				
Access to Complementary Information	0–14	9	14	14
Access to guidance to prepare PBL	0–6	10	9	6
Access to Theoretical Information	0–14	12	18	14
Access to Teacher Feedback	0–158	69	103	158
Mean Visits per day	0–7	2.48	3.40	4.51
Blended Learning type 2				
Access to Complementary Information	0–7	4	6	7
Access to guidance to prepare PBL	0–5	3	5	5
Access to Theoretical Information	0–14	12	18	14
Access to Teacher Feedback	0–66	5	30	66
Mean Visits per day	0–2	0.84	1.30	1.93

Note; PBL = Project-Based Learning Development.

Figure 1 shows the scores in the two groups: experimental group (red color) and control group (blue color). As can be seen, there was a greater homogeneity of higher scores in the experimental group for different types of Learning outcomes. Similarly, Figure 2 points to the distributions of LMS behavioral learning scores in different resources.

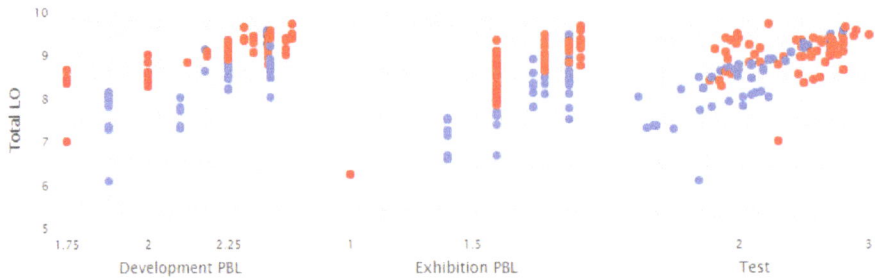

Figure 1. Distribution of scores in the different types of Learning outcomes. Note. Development PBL = Development Project-Based Learning outcomes; Exhibition PBL = Exhibition Project-Based Learning outcomes; Test = Test Learning outcomes; Total LO = Learning outcomes Total.

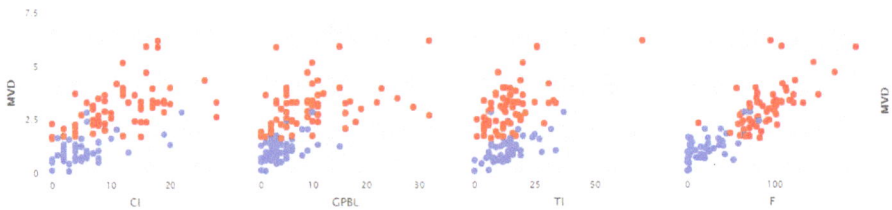

Figure 2. Distribution of scores in the different types of behavioral learning in the LMS. Note. CI = Access to Complementary Information scores; CPBL = Access to guidance to prepare PBL scores; TI = Access to Theoretical Information scores; F = Access to Teacher Feedback; MVD = Mean Visits per day.

4. Discussion

In the blended learning environments, the type of teaching design appears to be a predictive factor in both the learning results and the learning behaviors that the students develop in the LMS. blended learning with 80% of interactions in LMS appeared to be more effective, both with respect to the learning results of the students and the effectiveness of the learning behaviors that they develop. This type of pedagogic design includes the use of hypermedia resources that strengthen teacher feedback in real time, which furthers the development of SRL strategies [24,35]. This aspect is of special relevance for teachers in nursing higher education, and the implicit message is that they would be well advised to design their materials for use in a blended learning environment [27–30], as those environments appear to have increased the effectiveness of active methodologies, especially PBL with hypermedia resources in LMS [38]. In addition, Blended Learning type 1 (80% the interaction in the LMS) strengthens students' use of learning-based projects that have been considered more effective in the LMS [2,23]. These behaviors range from access to feedback given by the teacher to tasks carried out by the student or the collaborative groups and the average number of visits per day [23]. All of this indicates that the Blended Learning type 1 design increases the interaction of the student in the LMS and that interaction also facilitates student access to feedback from the teacher, as the LMS can be consulted as many times as necessary when learning, an aspect that is less feasible with F2F instruction [9,10,18]. In this way, the teachers can structure their help and prepare specific materials for each group.

In addition, machine learning techniques have been used in this study, in view of their effective use with what is known as data mining [13,18,36]. In particular, supervised and unsupervised machine learning techniques have been used (linear regression and clustering K-means methods, respectively). Prediction and clustering studies, among others, can be conducted with these techniques, which help the teacher to gain knowledge of the learning characteristics of students and to predict at-risk students [23,34,38]. Even so, it is true that these techniques should be used throughout the whole teaching process to be able to develop personalized actions for student learning [35,36]. In subsequent studies, therefore, development of the learning process among students at the start, in the middle, and at the end of the study module will be analyzed with machine learning techniques [12,13].

5. Limitations

This study has limitations, but the results of this study should, nevertheless, be given prudent consideration. Limitations include the following: methodological intervention was in one university, the students were from a specific country, convenience sampling was applied, the knowledge area of the students was specific, and the type of design (quasi-experimental) was also specific. Although, it must be taken into consideration that there are few specific studies to test the effectiveness of this type of methodology in nursing students. Studies that have been carried out have similar characteristics that are justified from the specificity of this research [28–30].

Therefore, future studies will be directed at increasing the size of the sample and the diversity of the nursing degree course level. Therefore, this profession is subject to continuous theoretical and technological advances that require systematic research on how to teach better in order to learn more effectively.

6. Conclusions

This research study has identified the characteristics to design an effective LMS in the nursing degree. The use of prediction and clustering techniques is very important to facilitate personalized learning and to analyze how resources are better utilized in the blended learning space. This type of analysis can be automatically generated in LMS environments, such as Moodle, and could be integrated in modules and plugins. These tools would facilitate rapid and straightforward generation of those analyses, which would be of great utility for the teacher and would assist with the early detection of at-risk students, as well as behavioral analyses of both the individual student and the collaborative groups of students, which would foreseeably increase the teaching quality and learning outcomes. This need has been underlined in such studies as those by Peña-Ayala [12] and Romero et al. [17], and they have to be approved by university management, but they will virtually be a necessity in 21st century teaching as we move closer to personalized on-line teaching, both in F2F teaching and in virtual learning environments. In summary, this teaching design is especially significant in the nursing degree since project work is a practice that has proved very effective in the training of future professionals.

Good results have been obtained in all assessment tests in the two types of blended learning. However, the type of blended learning that applied automated feedback and hypermedia resources obtained even better results (more percentage of work in the LMS) [28–30]. One explanation may be that the student can access information in the LMS at any time, which is not possible for F2F interaction, and this facilitates personalization of learning and motivates the student [7,8,39]. Therefore, incorporating these forms of work in teaching in the field of health is a very effective option.

The results obtained are in line with those found in the research of Oh & Lee [28]. The use of PBL methodology in blended learning environments empowers nursing students to acquire practical skills that are of great help for nursing work in real intervention environments [28]. This form of teaching is flexible [30] because it facilitates development and tests hypotheses in the resolution of tasks similar to those they will encounter in a working environment, and in addition, group work facilitates the acquisition of collaborative work skills, which they will also encounter in such working environments. All this increases the self-efficacy and critical thinking skills of these professionals. Recent studies recommend the application of this methodology within the nursing degree curricula [27].

In sum, it can be concluded that this way of teaching seems to be effective for nursing students. Although, more studies are needed in this field aimed at studying the effectiveness of blended learning in teaching in the nursing degree.

Int. J. Environ. Res. Public Health **2020**, *17*, 1589

Supplementary Materials: The following are available online at http://www.mdpi.com/1660-4601/17/5/1589/s1, Table S1: Rubric to evaluate development of Project-Based Learning, Table S2: Rubric to evaluate Exhibition of Project-Based Learning.

Author Contributions: Conceptualization, M.C.S.M., and M.d.C.E.L.; methodology, M.C.S.M.; software, Á.A.G.; validation, M.C.S.M., and Á.A.G.; formal analysis, M.C.S.M.; investigation, M.C.S.M., and M.D.C.E.L.; resources, M.C.S.M.; data curation, M.C.S.M.; writing—original draft preparation, M.C.S.M. and M.D.C.E.L. and Á.A.G.; writing—review and editing, M.C.S.M., and M.D.C.E.L. and Á.A.G.; visualization, Á.A.G.; supervision, M.C.S.M., and M.D.C.E.L.; project administration, M.C.S.M.; funding acquisition, M.C.S.M. and M.D.C.E.L. All authors have read and agreed to the published version of the manuscript.

Funding: This research was funded by the of Consejería de Educación de la Junta de Castilla y León (Spain) (Department of Education of the Junta de Castilla y León), Grant number BU032G19, and grants from the University of Burgos for the dissemination and the improvement of teaching innovation experiences of the Vice-Rectorate of Teaching and Research Staff, the Vice-Rectorate for Research and Knowledge Transfer, 2020, at the University of Burgos (Spain).

Acknowledgments: Thanks to all the students who participated in this study and the Committee of Bioethics of University of Burgos (Spain).

Conflicts of Interest: The authors declare no conflicts of interest.

Appendix A

Table A1. Descriptive statistics for the Learning outcomes.

Learning Outcomes	Blended Learning Type 1 (Experimental Group)					Blended Learning Type 2 (Control Group)				
	Minimum	*Maximum*	*M*	*SD*	*α*	*Minimum*	*Maximum*	*M*	*SD*	*α*
Learning outcomes in the preparation of PBL	1.75	2.45	2.23	0.21	0.79	1.88	2.38	2.25	0.17	0.81
Learning outcomes in presentation of PBL	1.00	1.95	1.74	0.17	0.76	0	1.90	1.75	0.19	0.75
Learning outcomes in test	1.78	3.00	2.43	0.35	0.80	1.23	2.80	2.17	0.42	0.78
Learning Outcomes Total	7.00	0.72	9.03	0.44	0.73	6.08	9.57	8.64	0.66	0.70

Note: M = Mean; SD = Standard Deviation; PBL = Project-Based Learning; $α$ = Reliability index of Cronbach's Alpha.

Table A2. Descriptive statistics for Behavioral learning in the LMS.

Behavioral Learning in the LMS	Blended Learning Type 1 (Experimental Group)				Blended Learning Type 2 (Control Group)			
	Minimum	*Maximum*	*M*	*SD*	*Minimum*	*Maximum*	*M*	*SD*
Access to Complementary Information	0	28	5.07	11.60	0	22	5.07	4.60
Access to Guidance for the Preparation of PBL	0	32	9.46	7.59	0	15	3.60	3.01
Access to Theoretical Information	1	70	14.84	10.23	0	37	13.81	7.49
Access to Teacher Feedback	0	194	90.90	29.21	0	82	18.43	21.14
Mean Visits per day	0.41	6.15	3.04	1.02	0.06	2.81	1.08	0.58

Note: M = Mean; SD = Standard Deviation

Table A3. Coefficients in the prediction of learning outcomes with variable types of Blended Learning.

	Unstandardized Coefficients		Standardized Coefficients	t	p	Correlations			Collinearity Statistics	
	B	Standard Error	Beta			Zero Order	Partial	Part	Tolerance	VIF
(Constant)	-2.52	0.64		-3.93	0.00					
Learning outcomes Elaboration PBL	-1.22	0.32	-0.48	-3.87	0.00	0.01	-0.34	-0.28	0.34	3.00
Learning outcomes PBL Exhibition	-2.29	0.37	-0.82	-6.18	0.00	-0.06	-0.50	-0.44	0.29	3.49
Learning outcomes in test	-0.69	0.17	-0.56	-4.00	0.00	0.32	-0.35	-0.28	0.26	3.91
Learning outcomes Total	1.39	0.19	1.64	7.49	0.00	0.33	0.57	0.53	0.11	9.45

Note: Dependent variable: Blended Learning type; PBL = Project-Based Learning; VIF = Variance Inflation Factor.

Table A4. Coefficients in the prediction of Behavioral learning with variable types of Blended Learning.

	Unstandardized Coefficients		Standardized Coefficients	t	p	Correlations			Collinearity Statistics	
	B	Standard Error	Beta			Zero Order	Partial	Part	Tolerance	VIF
(Constant)	1.02	0.05		19.53	0.00					
Access to Complementary Information	0.002	0.01	0.03	0.38	0.71	0.51	0.035	0.02	0.54	1.85
Access to guidance for the Preparation of PBL	0.02	0.01	0.20	3.14	0.002	0.45	0.28	0.15	0.60	1.66
Access to Theoretical Information	-0.01	0.003	-0.21	-3.49	0.001	0.06	-0.31	-0.17	0.68	1.47
Access to Teacher Feedback	0.01	0.001	0.60	5.37	0.00	0.82	0.45	0.26	0.19	5.25
Mean Visits per day	0.08	0.05	0.20	1.55	0.13	0.76	0.14	0.08	0.14	7.35

Note: Dependent variable: Blended Learning type; VIF = Variance Inflation Factor.

References

1. Siddiq, F.; Scherer, R. Revealing the processes of students' interaction with a novel collaborative problem solving task: An in-depth analysis of think-aloud protocols. *Comput. Human Behav.* **2017**, *76*, 509–525. [CrossRef]
2. Sáiz, M.C.; Escolar, M.C.; Marticorena, R.; García-Osorio, C.I.; Queiruga, M.A. Aprendizaje Basado en Proyectos utilizando LMS: una experiencia en Ciencias de la Salud [Project Based Learning using LMS: an experience in Health Sciences]. In *Temas actuales de investigación en áreas de la Salud y de la Educación [Current research topics in the areas of Health and Education]*; SCINFOPER: Almería, Spain, 2017; pp. 739–746.
3. Lau, C.; Sinclair, J.; Taub, M.; Azevedo, R.; Jang, E.E. Transitioning Self-regulated Learning Profiles in Hypermedia-learning Environments. In Proceedings of the Seventh International Learning Analytics & Knowledge Conference, 17 March 2017, Vancouver, BC, Canada; Association for Computing Machinery: New York, NY, USA, 2017; pp. 198–202. [CrossRef]
4. Krathwohl, D.R. A Revision of Bloom's Taxonomy: An Overview. *Theory Pract.* **2002**, *41*, 212–218. [CrossRef]
5. le Roux, I.; Nagel, L. Seeking the best blend for deep learning in a flipped classroom—viewing student perceptions through the Community of Inquiry lens. *Int. J. Educ. Technol. High* **2018**, *15*, 1–28. [CrossRef]
6. Scoular, C.; Care, E.; Hesse, F.W. Designs for operationalizing collaborative problem solving for automated assessment. *J. Educ. Meas.* **2017**, *54*, 12–35. [CrossRef]
7. Sung, T.-W.S.; Wu, T.-T. Learning With E-books and Project-based Strategy in a Community Health Nursing Course. *Comput. Inform. Nurs.* **2018**, *36*, 140–146. [CrossRef]
8. Feather, R.; Carr, D.; Reising, D.; Garletts, D. Team-Based Learning for Nursing and Medical Students: Focus Group Results From an Interprofessional Education Project. *Nurse Educ.* **2016**, *41*, E1–E5. [CrossRef]
9. Sáiz, M.C.; Montero, E. *Metodologías activas en docencia universitaria: Diseño de una asignatura de Ciencias de la Salud en la plataforma virtual*; [Actives Methodologies at the university: Design of a subject of Health Sciences in the virtual platform]; Servicio de Publicaciones de la Universidad de Burgos: Burgos, Spain, 2016.
10. Von Davier, A.A. Computational psychometrics in support of collaborative educational assessments. *J. Educ. Meas.* **2017**, *54*, 3–11. [CrossRef]
11. Oh, Y.; Oh, Y.K. A computational model of design critiquing. *Artif. Intell. Rev.* **2017**, *48*, 529–555. [CrossRef]
12. Peña-Ayala, A. Educational data mining: A survey and a data mining-based analysis of recent works. *Expert. Syst. Appl.* **2014**, *41*, 1432–1462. [CrossRef]
13. Romero, C.; Ventura, S. Educational data mining: A survey from 1995 to 2005. *Expert. Syst. Appl.* **2007**, *33*, 135–146. [CrossRef]
14. Bernard, P.; Broś, P.; Migdał-Mikuli, A. Influence of blended learning on outcomes of students attending a general chemistry course: summary of a five-year-long study. *Chem. Educ. Res. Pract.* **2017**, *18*, 682–690. [CrossRef]
15. Asif, R.; Merceron, A.; Ali, S.B.; Haider, N.G. Analyzing undergraduate students' performance using educational data mining. *Comput. Educ.* **2017**, *113*, 177–194. [CrossRef]
16. Condell, J.; Wade, J.; Galway, L.; McBride, M.; Gormley, P.; Brennan, J. Problem solving techniques in cognitive science. *Artif. Intell. Rev.* **2010**, *34*, 221–234. [CrossRef]
17. Romero, C.; Espejo, P.G.; Zafra, A.; Romero, J.R.; Ventura, S. Web Usage Mining for Predicting Final Marks of Students That Use Moodle Courses. *Comput. Appl. Eng. Educ.* **2013**, *21*, 135–146. [CrossRef]
18. Sáiz, M.C.; Marticorena, R.; García-Osorio, C.I.; Díez-Pastor, J.F. How Do B-Learning and Learning Patterns Influence Learning Outcomes? *Front. Psychol.* **2017**, *8*, 1–13.
19. Mozer, M.C.; Lindsey, R.V. Predicting and improving memory retention: Psychological theory matters in the big data era. In *Big Data in Cognitive Science*; Jones, M., Ed.; Oxford University Press: Oxford, UK, 2017; pp. 34–64.
20. Dramiński, M. ADX Algorithm for Supervised Classification. In *Challenges in Computational Statistics and Data Mining*; Matwin, S., Mielniczuk, J., Eds.; Springer: Basel, Switzerland, 2016; pp. 39–52.
21. Hu, H.; Wen, Y.; Chua, T.S.; Li, X. Toward scalable systems for big data analysis: A technology tutorial. *IEEE Access* **2014**, *2*, 652–687.
22. Margulieux, L.E.; McCracken, W.M.; Catrambone, R. A taxonomy to define courses that mix face-to-face and online learning. *Educ. Res. Rev.* **2016**, *19*, 104–118. [CrossRef]

23. Cerezo, R.; Sánchez-Santillan, M.; Paule-Ruiz, M.P.; Núñez, J.C. Students´ LMS interaction patterns and their relationship with achievement: A case study in higher education. *Comput. Educ.* **2016**, *96*, 42–54. [CrossRef]

24. Moos, D.C.; Bonde, C. Flipping the Classroom: Embedding Self-Regulated Learning Prompts in Videos. *Technol. Knowl. Learn.* **2016**, *21*, 225–242. [CrossRef]

25. Järvelä, S.; Malmberg, J.; Koivuniemi, M. Recognizing socially shared regulation by using the temporal sequences of online chat and logs in CSCL. *Learn. Instr.* **2016**, *42*, 1–11. [CrossRef]

26. Sáiz, M.C.; Marticorena, R. Metacognition, self-regulation and feedback for Object-Oriented Programming problem-solving. In *Metacognition: Theory Performance and Current Research*; Benson, J., Ed.; Nova Science Publishers: New York, NY, USA, 2016; pp. 43–94.

27. Álvarez-García, C.; Álvarez-Nieto, C.; Kelsey, J.; Carter, R.; Sanz-Martos, S.; López-Medina, I.M. Effectiveness of the e-NurSus Children Intervention in the Training of Nursing Students. *Int. J. Environ. Res. Public Health* **2019**, *16*, 4288. [CrossRef] [PubMed]

28. Oh, E.G.; Yang, Y.L. Evidence-based nursing education for undergraduate students: A preliminary experimental study. *Nurse Educ. Pract.* **2019**, *38*, 45–51. [CrossRef] [PubMed]

29. Häggman-Laitila, A.; Mattila, L.R.; Melender, H.-L. Educational interventions on evidence-based nursing in clinical practice: A systematic review with qualitative analysis. *Nurse Educ. Today* **2016**, *43*, 50–59. [CrossRef] [PubMed]

30. Leidl, D.M.; Ritchie, L.; Moslemi, N. Blended learning in undergraduate nursing education – A scoping review. *Nurse Educ. Today* **2020**, *86*, 1–9. [CrossRef]

31. Pitigala-liyanage, M.P.; Lasith-Gunawardena, K.S.; Hirakawa, M. Detecting Learning Styles in Learning Management Systems Using Data Mining. *J. Inf. Process.* **2016**, *24*, 740–749.

32. Sáiz, M.C.; Montero, E.; Bol, A.; Carbonero, M.Á. An analysis of Learning to Learning competencies at the University. *Electron. J. Res. Educ. Psychol.* **2012**, *10*, 253–270.

33. Harrati, N.; Bouchrika, I.; Tari, A.; Ladjailia, A. Exploring user satisfaction for e-learning systems via usage-based metrics and system usability scale analysis. *Comput. Human Behav.* **2016**, *61*, 463–471. [CrossRef]

34. Sáiz, M.C.; Marticorena, R.; García-Osorio, C.I.; Díez-Pastor, J.F. Does the Use of Learning Management Systems With Hypermedia Mean Improved Student Learning Outcomes? *Front. Psychol.* **2019**, *10*, 1–14.

35. Strang, K.D. Beyond engagement analytics: which online mixed-data factors predict student learning outcomes? *Educ. Inf. Technol.* **2016**, *22*, 917–937. [CrossRef]

36. Yücel, Ü.A.; Usluel, Y.K. Knowledge building and the quantity, content and quality of the interaction and participation of students in an online collaborative learning environment. *Comput. Educ.* **2016**, *97*, 31–48. [CrossRef]

37. Jones, M.N. *Big Data in Cognitive Science*; Routledge: New York, NY, USA, 2017. [CrossRef]

38. Saqr, M.; Fors, U.; Tedre, M. How learning analytics can early predict under-achieving students in a blended medical education course. *Med. Teach.* **2017**, *39*, 757–767. [CrossRef] [PubMed]

39. Hodges, H.F.; Massey, A.T. Interprofessional Problem-Based Learning Project Outcomes Between Prelicensure Baccalaureate of Science in Nursing and Doctor of Pharmacy Programs. *J. Nurs. Educ.* **2015**, *54*, 201–206. [CrossRef] [PubMed]

40. Román, J.M.; Poggioli, L. *ACRA (r): Escalas de Estrategias de Aprendizaje*; [Learning Strategies Scales]; Publicaciones UCAB (Postgraduate Doctorate in Education): Caracas, Venezuela, 2013.

41. IBM Corp. *SPSS Statistical Package for the Social Sciences (SPSS), Version 24*; IBM: Madrid, Spain, 2016.

42. IBM Corp. *AMOS Statistical Package for the Structural Equation Modeling (AMOS), Version 24*; IBM: Madrid, Spain, 2016.

43. RapidMiner Studio. Available online: https://rapidminer.com/why-rapidminer/ (accessed on 6 September 2019).

44. Bandalos, D.L.; Finney, S.J. Item parceling issues in structural equation modeling. In *New Development and Techniques in Structural Equation Modeling*; Marcoulides, G.A., Schumacker, R.E., Eds.; Lawrence Erlbaum Associates: Mahwah, NJ, USA, 2001; pp. 269–296.

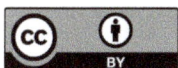

International Journal of
Environmental Research and Public Health

MDPI

Article

Kinesiophobia and Pain Intensity Are Increased by a Greater Hallux Valgus Deformity Degree- Kinesiophobia and Pain Intensity in Hallux Valgus

Patricia Palomo-López [1], Ricardo Becerro-de-Bengoa-Vallejo [2], Marta Elena Losa-Iglesias [3], Daniel López-López [4], David Rodríguez-Sanz [2], Carlos Romero-Morales [5], César Calvo-Lobo [2,*] and Victoria Mazoteras-Pardo [2]

[1] University Center of Plasencia, Universidad de Extremadura, 10600 Badajoz, Spain; patibiom@unex.es
[2] Facultad de Enfermería, Fisioterapia y Podología, Universidad Complutense de Madrid, 28040 Madrid, Spain; ribebeva@ucm.es (R.B.-d.-B.-V.); davidrodriguezsanz@ucm.es (D.R.-S.); vmazoter@ucm.es (V.M.-P.)
[3] Faculty of Health Sciences, Universidad Rey Juan Carlos, 28922 Alcorcon, Spain; marta.losa@urjc.es
[4] Research, Health and Podiatry Group, Department of Health Sciences, Faculty of Nursing and Podiatry, Universidade da Coruña, 15403 Ferrol, Spain; daniellopez@udc.es
[5] Faculty of Sport Sciences, Universidad Europea de Madrid, Villaviciosa de Odón, 28670 Madrid, Spain; carlos.romero@universidadeuropea.es
* Correspondence: cescalvo@ucm.es

Received: 1 December 2019; Accepted: 16 January 2020; Published: 18 January 2020

check for updates

Abstract: Background: Hallux valgus (HV) has been previously associated with psychological disorders. Thus, the purposes of this study were to associate kinesiophobia and pain intensity with HV deformity degrees, as well as predict kinesiophobia and pain intensity based on HV deformity and demographic features. Methods: A cross-sectional study was carried out recruiting 100 subjects, who were divided into HV deformity degrees, such as I-no HV (n = 25), II-mild (n = 25), III-moderate (n = 25), and IV-severe (n = 25) HV. Kinesiophobia total and domains (activity avoidance and harm) scores and levels were self-reported by the Tampa Scale of Kinesiophobia (TSK-11). Pain intensity was self-reported by the numeric rating scale (NRS). Results: Statistically significant differences ($p < 0.01$; $\eta^2 = 0.132$–0.850) were shown for between-groups comparison of kinesiophobia total and domain scores (activity avoidance and harm) and levels, as well as pain intensity among HV deformity degrees. Post hoc comparisons showed statistically significant differences with a large effect size ($p < 0.05$; $d = 0.85$–4.41), showing higher kinesiophobia symptoms and levels and pain intensity associated with greater HV deformity degrees, especially for III-moderate and/or IV-severe HV deformity degrees versus I-no HV and/or II-mild deformity degrees. Both statistically significant prediction models ($p < 0.05$) for kinesiophobia ($R^2 = 0.300$) and pain intensity ($R^2 = 0.815$) were predicted by greater HV deformity degree and age. Conclusions: Greater kinesiophobia symptoms and levels and pain were associated with higher HV deformity degrees, especially severe and/or moderate HV with respect to no and/or mild HV. The kinesiophobia and pain intensity were predicted by greater HV deformity degree and age.

Keywords: chronic pain; hallux valgus; musculoskeletal diseases; psychology

1. Introduction

The affectation of the toe body region may comprise up to 14% of the non-traumatic primary care consultations of the foot and ankle, being hallux valgus (HV) considered as one of the 10 most commonly documented non-traumatic conditions [1]. This condition may reach a prevalence of up to 23% in adults, showing an increase in female sex or higher age distribution [2]. HV may be defined as a complex deformity of the 1st metatarsophalangeal joint composed of great toe lateral drift and linked to joint subluxation [3]. Indeed, HV may impair quality of life related to foot health, increase depression, and alter muscle or connective tissue morphology of the plantar region, which seems to be linked to its degree of deformity [4–7].

Several psychological disorders, such as depression or sociability and vigor linked to general health-related quality of life alterations, have been associated with musculoskeletal conditions, which may increase with greater age ranges [8–13]. In addition, musculoskeletal disorders of the lower limbs may alter body stability, showing a greater instability in older adults [14–16]. Combining both factors, kinesiophobia and pain intensity seem to play a key role in musculoskeletal disorders prognosis [17–19]. Among these conditions, patellofemoral pain has been linked to greater higher kinesiophobia levels [20]. Currently, there is a lack of research studies detailing kinesiophobia and pain intensity in subjects suffering from HV deformity. Pain and kinesiophobia, defined as fear of movement under a painful condition [21,22], could be linked to a greater HV deformity degree as the higher HV deformity has been related to a worse foot health-related quality of life, greater depression, and presence of foot posture, pressure patterns, and function alterations [4–7,23,24].

Greater HV deformity degree has shown higher radiographic first metatarsophalangeal joint osteoarthritis severity in conjunction with physical and psychological conditions [4–7,23–25]. Thus, the purpose of this study was to find the association between kinesiophobia and pain intensity with HV deformity degrees. In addition, the secondary aim was to predict kinesiophobia and pain intensity based on HV deformity and demographic features. We hypothesized that higher kinesiophobia and pain intensity could be shown and predicted by a greater HV deformity degree.

2. Materials and Methods

2.1. Design

A cross-sectional study was performed according to the STrengthening the Reporting of OBservational studies in Epidemiology (STROBE) criteria [26]. Thus, kinesiophobia and pain intensity were compared under different HV deformity degrees. Furthermore, the ethics committee of Extremadura University (code: 175/2019) approved this research, and all subjects signed the informed consent form before the beginning of the study. Finally, the Helsinki declaration and all human experimentation rules were respected [27].

2.2. Sample Size Calculation

Kinesiophobia score was used as the main outcome measurement to carry out the sample size calculation because prior lower limb musculoskeletal conditions were linked to higher kinesiophobia symptoms [20]. Kinesiophobia total score assessed with the Spanish validated version of the Tampa Scale of Kinesiophobia–11 items (TSK-11) [21,22] of a pilot study (n = 40 subjects) with 4 groups of HV deformity degree (n; TSK-11 mean ± SD), divided into I–no HV (n = 10 participants; 21.70 ± 5.41 points), II–mild (n = 10; 20.70 ± 4.62 points), III–moderate (n = 10; 22.60 ± 3.83 points), and IV–severe (n = 10; 24.80 ± 4.18 points) HV deformity degree, was used for the sample size calculation by the one-way, omnibus, and fixed-effects analysis of variance (ANOVA) F test using G*Power 3.1.9.2 software version. Indeed, a partial Eta-squared (η^2) of 0.109, an effect size of 0.349, an α error probability of 0.05, a number of 4 groups, and a power (1-β error probability) of 0.80 were used for this sample size calculation procedure. Thus, a total sample size of 96 subjects, 24 for each group, was calculated with an actual power of 0.813. Finally, a total sample size of 100 subjects, 25 for each group, was included in the present study.

2.3. Sample

A total sample of 100 subjects with different HV deformity degrees was recruited by a consecutive convenience sampling method in an outpatient clinic from March to November 2019 [4–7]. Inclusion criteria comprised subjects older than 18 years old, being healthy subjects for the control group classified as I degree–no HV presence (n = 25), as well as patients with HV deformity for cases groups, such as II degree–mild HV (n = 25), III degree–moderate HV (n = 25), and IV degree–severe HV (n = 25) [28,29].

Systemic diseases, neurological conditions, arthritis, neoplasm, autoimmune pathology, vascular alterations, neuropathic disorders or radiculopathies, sprains, fractures, tendinopathies, surgeries, presence of dysmetria with length difference greater than 1 cm between both lower extremities, mental disorders, or cognitive conditions were considered as exclusion criteria according to the medical record [7,30].

2.4. HV Deformity Degrees

A specialized podiatrist carried out the HV deformity degree diagnosis by the Manchester Scale [28]. This tool might be considered as a non-invasive technique in order to measure the HV deformity degree using a standardized photograph set, divided into I degree (no HV), II degree (mild HV), III degree (moderate HV), and IV degree (severe HV). This scale showed an excellent inter-examiner repeatability (κ = 0.86) [29]. Also, excellent inter-examiner reliability and validity were shown for the HV angle between photographic measures and radiographs. Intraclass correlation coefficients (ICCs > 0.96) and the Pearson's correlation coefficient (r = 0.96) were categorized as excellent. Despite this method was recommended in order to avoid the cost and radiation exposure secondary to radiographs, foot radiographs might be considered as the current standard in clinical practice, and thus HV angle clinical measurements have been recommended if it is not possible or necessary to perform radiographs [29].

2.5. Demographic Data

Demographic data comprised age (years), sex (female or male), body mass index (kg/cm^2) [31], height (cm), weight (kg), and pain chronicity, measured as duration in months with painful HV [7,30].

2.6. Outcome Measurements

Kinesiophobia total score was considered as the main outcome measurement and evaluated with the Spanish validated version of the Tampa Scale of Kinesiophobia–11 items (TSK-11) [21,22]. Secondary outcome measures were activity avoidance and harm domains scores of kinesiophobia, as well as fear of movement or kinesiophobia levels categorized by the TSK-11 score [21,22], and the pain intensity score measured by the numeric rating scale (NRS) [32,33]. According to these scales, both tools were self-reported by the study's subjects.

2.6.1. TSK-11

The Spanish validated version of the TSK-11 was self-reported by all study's subjects in order to detail kinesiophobia symptoms total scores, activity avoidance and harm domains scores of kinesiophobia, and levels fear of movement or kinesiophobia [21,22]. Kinesiophobia was considered as an adaptive response to the threat, which might consequently generate maladaptive or avoidance behaviors with an increase of fear and/or pain as well as activities limitation and/or fear of movement [34–36]. Future disability of a musculoskeletal condition might be predicted by fear or movement or kinesiophobia [34]. This scale was composed of total kinesiophobia symptoms score and two domains, including activity avoidance and harm under kinesiophobia. This scale was scored using 4 points Likert-type scale, indicating higher scores as an increase of fear of pain, movement, or damage. In addition, TSK-11 total scores were categorized into kinesiophobia levels of fear of movement, including no fear of movement (0–17 points), slight fear of movement (18–24 points), moderate fear of movement (25–31 points), severe fear of movement (32–38 points), and maximum fear of movement (39–44 points) [21,22]. Adequate psychometric properties were reported for this scale, showing an internal consistency with Cronbach's α of 0.78, test-retest with ICC of 0.82, standard error of measurement with SEM of 3.16, responsiveness of −1.19, minimum clinical important difference with MCID of 4.80, and minimum detectable change with MDC of 5.60 [21,22,37–39].

2.6.2. NRS

Pain intensity was measured by the NRS. This tool showed 11 points ranged from 0 (no pain) to 10 (highest pain intensity) points. Subjects were asked to mark the subjective pain intensity of the painful HV (Hallux valgus) by a finger on the scale composed of a graphic representation with 11 spaces. This scale was stated as a valid and reliable scale to evaluate subjective pain intensity in adults and older adults [32,33]. High convergent validity (0.79–0.95) was shown with respect to the VAS (Visual Analogue Scale) [40]. The MDC and MCID were set at 2 points for lower limb musculoskeletal conditions [41–43].

2.7. Statistical Analysis

The software version 24th of the Statistical Package for Social Sciences (from IBM Corp; Armonk, NY, USA) was utilized to carry out all data analyses by an α error of 0.05, a p-value < 0.05 as statistically significant, and a 95% confidence interval (CI).

First, quantitative data analyses were performed by the Shapiro–Wilk test to determine normality distributions. Second, all data were described by the mean ± standard deviation (SD). Third, one-way analysis of variance completed with Bonferroni's correction post hoc analyses was used to assess between-group differences for parametric data. Fourth, Kruskal–Wallis test completed with Bonferroni's correction post hoc analyses were used to assess between-groups differences for non-parametric data. For outcome measurements, effect size was calculated by Eta-squared (η^2) coefficients for comparisons among all groups, as well as Cohen's d coefficients for comparisons between paired groups and categorized into very small effect size ($d < 0.20$), small effect size ($d = 0.20$–0.49), medium effect size ($d = 0.50$–0.79), and large effect size ($d > 0.8$) [44,45]. Finally, categorical data were described as frequency (n) and percentage (%). In addition, Chi-square tests were applied to assess differences among all groups.

Furthermore, multivariate predictive analyses were performed by means of two linear regression models. Both models were carried out by the stepwise selection method; as well as R^2 coefficients were determined to show the quality of adjustment [46]. The 1st linear regression model included demographic data, pain intensity (NRS), chronicity, and HV deformity degree as independent variables, as well as kinesiophobia total score (TSK-11) as the dependent variable. The 2nd linear regression model included demographic data, kinesiophobia total score, levels of fear of movement of kinesiophobia, activity avoidance, and harm domains of kinesiophobia (TSK-11), and HV deformity degree as independent variables, as well as pain intensity (NRS) as the dependent variable. F probability pre-established parameters ranged from $p_{in} = 0.05$ to $p_{out} = 0.10$, and p-values < 0.05 for statistical significance with a 95% CI were considered for these analyses.

3. Results

3.1. Demographic Data

Statistically significant differences ($p < 0.05$) were shown for demographic data, except for weight ($p = 0.608$), showing that a higher HV deformity degree was associated with greater age, height, body mass index (BMI), and chronicity, as well as female sex (Table 1).

Table 1. Demographic data among different HV deformity degrees.

Sociodemographic Characteristics		No HV Degree-I (n = 25)	Mild HV Degree-II (n = 25)	Moderate HV Degree-III (n = 25)	Severe HV Degree-IV (n = 25)	*p*-Value
Age (years)		37.52 ± 15.19	37.16 ± 19.53	59.24 ± 18.35	68.40 ± 14.60	<0.001 †
Weight (kg)		75.80 ± 16.12	70.80 ± 15.03	72.92 ± 10.57	73.08 ± 13.03	0.608 †
Height (m)		1.70 ± 0.07	1.69 ± 0.08	1.64 ± 0.05	1.61 ± 0.08	<0.001 *
BMI (kg/cm^2)		26.01 ± 4.52	24.34 ± 3.32	26.87 ± 3.49	27.92 ± 3.65	0.003 †
Chronicity (months)		0	15.37 ± 37.13	88.32 ± 55.62	190.08 ± 160.20	<0.001 †
Sex	male	12 (48%)	13 (52%)	7 (28%)	4 (16%)	0.025 ‡
	female	13 (52%)	12 (48%)	18 (72%)	21 (84%)	

Abbreviations: BMI: body mass index; CI: confidence interval; HV: hallux valgus; SD: standard deviation. * Mean ± SD and one-way analysis of variance (ANOVA) were used. † Mean ± SD and the Kruskal–Wallis test were used. ‡ Frequency, percentage (%), and the Chi-squared test (χ^2) were utilized. In all analyses, *p* < 0.05 (with a 95% CI) was considered statistically significant.

3.2. Kinesiophobia Total Score

Statistically significant differences (*p* < 0.001; η^2 = 0.203) were shown for between-groups comparison of kinesiophobia total scores among HV deformity degrees by the one-way ANOVA test. Post hoc comparisons showed statistically significant differences with a large effect size (*p* < 0.05; *d* = 0.85–1.44), showing higher kinesiophobia symptoms for III-moderate and IV-severe HV deformity degrees with respect to I-no HV deformity degree, as well as for IV-severe HV deformity degree versus II-mild HV deformity degree. The rest of the post hoc comparisons did not show statistically significant differences (*p* < 0.05) (Table 2).

Table 2. Comparisons of outcome measurement scores among different HV deformity degrees.

Outcome Measurements	No HV Degree-I (n = 25)	Mild HV Degree-II (n = 25)	Moderate HV Degree-III (n = 25)	Severe HV Degree-IV (n = 25)	p-Value (η^2)	Bonferroni p-Value (d) (1) I vs. II (2) I vs. III (3) I vs. IV (4) II vs. III (5) II vs. IV (6) III vs. IV
Kinesiophobia total score (TSK-11)	19.64 ± 4.81	21.60 ± 6.07	23.64 ± 4.56	26.36 ± 4.49	<0.001* (η^2 = 0.203)	(1) (d = 0.35) (2) (d = 0.85) (3) <0.001 (d = 1.44) (4) 0.928 (d = 0.38) (5) (d = 0.89) (6) 0.353 (d = 0.60)
Activity avoidance score (TSK-11)	12.84 ± 3.11	13.76 ± 4.56	15.44 ± 3.96	17.24 ± 3.41	<0.001 † (η^2 = 0.168)	(1) (d = 0.23) (2) 0.127 (d = 0.87) (3) (d = 1.34) (4) 0.392 (d = 0.39) (5) (d = 0.86) (6) 0.851 (d = 0.48)
Harm score (TSK-11)	6.80 ± 2.29	7.84 ± 2.19	8.20 ± 2.16	9.12 ± 2.02	0.002 † (η^2 = 0.132)	(1) 0.599 (d = 0.46) (2) 0.205 (d = 0.62) (3) (d = 1.07) (4) (d = 0.16) (5) 0.177 (d = 0.60) (6) 0.530 (d = 0.43)
Pain intensity (NRS)	0	1.12 ± 1.26	6.40 ± 1.87	7.36 ± 1.55	<0.001 † (η^2 = 0.850)	(1) 0.420 (d = N/A) (2) <0.001 (d = N/A) (3) <0.001 (d = N/A) (4) <0.001(d = 3.31) (5) <0.001 (d = 4.41) (6) 1.000 (d = 0.55)

Abbreviations: CI, confidence interval; d, Cohen d coefficient; HV, hallux valgus; η^2, Eta-squared coefficient; N/A, not applicable; NRS, numeric rating scale; SD, standard deviation; TSK-11, Tampa Scale of Kinesiophobia–11 items. * Mean ± SD and one-way analysis of variance (ANOVA) completed with Bonferroni's correction were used. † Mean ± SD and Kruskal—allis test completed with Bonferroni's correction were used. In all analyses, $p < 0.05$ (with a 95% CI) was considered statistically significant.

3.3. Activity Avoidance Score (TSK-11)

Statistically significant differences ($p < 0.001$; $\eta^2 = 0.168$) were shown for between-groups comparison for the activity avoidance domain of kinesiophobia among HV deformity degrees by the Kruskal–Wallis test. Post hoc comparisons showed statistically significant differences with a large effect size ($p < 0.01$; $d = 0.86$–1.34), showing higher activity avoidance kinesiophobia symptoms for IV-severe HV deformity degree with respect to I-no HV and II-mild HV deformity degrees. The rest of the post hoc comparisons did not show statistically significant differences ($p < 0.05$) (Table 2).

3.4. Harm Score (TSK-11)

Statistically significant differences ($p = 0.002$; $\eta^2 = 0.132$) were shown for between-groups comparison for the harm domain of kinesiophobia among HV deformity degrees by the Kruskal–Wallis test. Post hoc comparisons showed statistically significant differences with a large effect size ($p = 0.001$; $d = 1.07$), showing higher harm kinesiophobia symptoms for IV-severe HV deformity degree with respect to I-no HV deformity degree. The rest of the post hoc comparisons did not show statistically significant differences ($p < 0.05$) (Table 2).

3.5. Pain Intensity (NRS)

Statistically significant differences ($p < 0.001$; $\eta^2 = 0.850$) were shown for between-groups comparison for the pain intensity among HV deformity degrees by the Kruskal–Wallis test. Post hoc comparisons showed statistically significant differences with a large effect size ($p < 0.001$; $d = 3.31$–4.41), showing higher pain intensity for III-moderate and IV-severe HV deformity degree with respect to I-no HV and II-mild HV deformity degree. The rest of the post hoc comparisons did not show statistically significant differences ($p < 0.05$) (Table 2).

3.6. Kinesiophobia Levels of Fear of Movement (TSK-11)

Statistically significant differences ($p = 0.007$; $\chi^2 = 22.556$) were shown for between-groups comparison for the kinesiophobia levels of fear of movement among HV deformity degrees by the Chi-squared test, showing higher kinesiophobia levels with greater HV deformity degree, especially for moderate kinesiophobia level (Figure 1).

3.7. Prediction Models

Kinesiophobia total score (TSK-11) showed one statistically significant prediction model ($R^2 = 0.300$) based on age (R2 = 0.271; $\beta = +0.101$; F[1,98] = 35.978; P < 0.001) and HV deformity degrees (R2 = 0.029; $\beta = +1.050$; F[1,97] = 4.033; P = 0.047), predicting higher kinesiophobia total scores based on greater age and HV deformity degree. Therefore, this prediction model excluded the rest of independent variables (P > 0.05) as the kinesiophobia total score (dependent variable) was not predicted by sex, height, weight, BMI, chronicity, and pain intensity (independent variables) according to the pre-established parameters for F probability (Table 3).

Table 3. Linear regression model for the kinesiophobia total score multivariate among HV deformity degrees.

Parameter	Model	R^2 Change	Model R^2
Kinesiophobia total score (TSK-11)	15.136		
	+0.101 * Age (years)	0.271 ‡	
	+0.050 * HV deformity degrees	0.029 †	0.300

Abbreviations: HV, hallux valgus; TSK-11, Tampa Scale of Kinesiophobia–11 items. * Multiplay: HV deformity degrees (I degree (no HV) = 1; II degree (mild HV) = 2; III degree (moderate HV) = 3; IV degree (severe HV) = 4). † *p*-value < 0.05 for a 95% confidence interval was shown, ‡ *p*-value < 0.001 for a 95% confidence interval was shown.

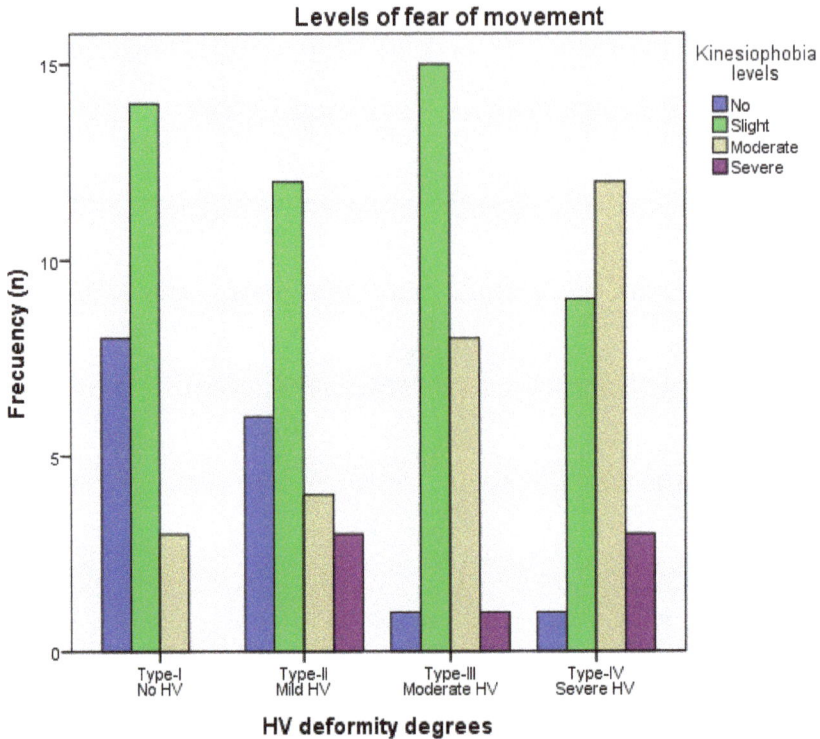

Figure 1. Bar graph showing the kinesiophobia levels of fear of movement (TSK-11), such as no fear (0–17 points), slight (18–24 points), moderate (25–31 points), severe (32–8 points), and maximum (39–4 points) kinesiophobia levels among different HV deformity degrees. Abbreviations: HV, hallux valgus; TSK-11, Tampa Scale of Kinesiophobia–11 items.

Pain intensity (NRS) showed one statistically significant prediction model ($R^2 = 0.815$) based on HV deformity degrees ($R^2 = 0.776$; $\beta = +0.276$; F[1,98] = 339.076; P < 0.001) and age (R2 = 0.040; $\beta = +1.050$; F[1,97] = 20.782; P < 0.001), predicting higher pain intensity based on greater HV deformity degree and age. Therefore, this prediction model excluded the rest of independent variables (P > 0.05) as the pain intensity (dependent variable) was not predicted by sex, height, weight, BMI, kinesiophobia total scores, kinesiophobia activity avoidance and harm domain scores, and kinesiophobia levels of fear of movement (TSK-11) according to the pre-established parameters for F probability (Table 4).

Table 4. Linear regression model for the pain intensity multivariate among HV deformity degrees.

Parameter	Model	R^2 Change	Model R^2
Pain intensity (NRS)	−3.993 +2.276 * HV deformity degrees +0.040 * Age (years)	0.776 ‡ 0.040 ‡	0.815

Abbreviations: HV: hallux valgus; NRS: numeric rating scale. * Multiplay: HV deformity degrees (I degree (no HV) = 1; II degree (mild HV) = 2; III degree (moderate HV) = 3; IV degree (severe HV) = 4). ‡ *p*-value < 0.001 for a 95% confidence interval was shown.

4. Discussion

Despite higher HV deformity degree has been previously associated with psychological disorders [4,5,47], this study might be considered as the first cross-sectional study detailing greater kinesiophobia symptoms, total scores as activity avoidance and harm domains scores, as well as pain intensity associated with higher HV degree deformity, especially for severe and/or moderate HV deformity degrees with respect to non-presence of HV and/or mild HV deformity degrees. Indeed, moderate kinesiophobia level deformity showed a clear increase according to greater HV deformity degrees. Thus, pain and fear of movement under HV condition might be linked to III and IV deformity degrees compared to I and II deformity degrees according to prior studies associating greater HV deformity with worse quality of life related to foot health, higher depression, as well as foot posture, pressure patterns, and function alterations [4–7,23,24]. Our findings were in line with prior research studies detailing kinesiophobia and pain in different musculoskeletal conditions, such as patellofemoral pain [20], temporomandibular conditions [48], chronic fatigue syndrome and/or fibromyalgia [49], whiplash-associated conditions and/or low back pain [50], chronic mechanical neck pain [51], or migraine [52].

In addition, our study showed that age and the HV deformity degree were shown as predictors for kinesiophobia symptoms and pain intensity. These findings were in accordance with prior studies reporting that psychological disorders were linked to musculoskeletal conditions, increasing this association with greater age distribution [8–13]. In addition, greater instability was shown in older adults under musculoskeletal disorders [14–16]. Finally, higher HV deformity was associated with worse physical and psychological factors [4–7,23,24].

4.1. Future Studies

Future studies should propose interventions in order to reduce kinesiophobia and pain intensity in patients with HV, such as myofascial pain interventions [53,54], neural mobilization techniques [55], or surgical procedures [47]. In addition, other outcome measurements should be evaluated in order to determine the influence of HV mechanical soft tissue properties on pain and kinesiophobia, such as myofascial trigger points evaluation [56], sonoelastography [57], pressure pain threshold [58], or thermography [59]. Finally and most importantly, an x-ray should be included in future studies as the gold stand, as well as ultrasound imaging could be used in advance to decline other possible pathologies [29].

4.2. Limitations

The following limitations could be acknowledged in this study. Firstly, socio-economic, civil, or working status should be considered for future studies. In spite of the pain intensity of HV was measured by the NRS [32,33], pain location, distribution, or type (neurological or musculoskeletal) were not collected. Second, despite the presented prediction models determined the influence of demographic data on our findings, future studies should detail the influence of age ranges on kinesiophobia and pain intensity according to our multivariate regression analyses. Thirdly, pregnant women could influence the psychological status and should be considered in future research studies [60]. Finally, despite exclusion criteria were considered according to the medical record, imaging examination was not performed (i.e., ultrasound and/or x-ray) to rollout other underlying pathologies (i.e., Morton neuroma, stress fracture, metatarsal bursitis, and others), which should be included in future studies. In addition, foot x-ray might provide additional information about the other metatarsal angles, sesamoid displacement, or underlying pathologies [29].

5. Conclusions

Greater kinesiophobia symptoms and levels and pain were associated with higher HV deformity degrees, especially severe and/or moderate HV with respect to no and/or mild HV. The kinesiophobia and pain intensity were predicted by greater HV deformity degree and age.

Author Contributions: Conceptualization, R.B.-d.-B.-V., M.E.L.-I., D.L.-L., C.C.-L., and V.M.-P.; Data curation, P.P.-L. and C.C.-L.; Formal analysis, R.B.-d.-B.-V., M.E.L.-I., D.R.-S., and C.C.-L.; Investigation, P.P.-L. and V.M.-P.; Methodology, P.P.-L., R.B.-d.-B.-V., M.E.L.-I., D.L.-L., D.R.-S., C.R.-M., C.C.-L., and V.M.-P.; Supervision, D.L.-L. and

C.R.-M.; Writing—original draft, D.L.-L. and C.C.-L.; Writing—review and editing, P.P.-L., R.B.-d.-B.-V., M.E.L.-I., D.R.-S., C.R.-M., C.C.-L., and V.M.-P. All authors have read and agreed to the published version of the manuscript.

Funding: This research received no external funding.

Conflicts of Interest: The authors declare no conflict of interest.

References

1. Menz, H.B.; Jordan, K.P.; Roddy, E.; Croft, P.R. Characteristics of primary care consultations for musculoskeletal foot and ankle problems in the UK. *Rheumatology* **2010**, *49*, 1391–1398. [CrossRef]

2. Nix, S.; Smith, M.; Vicenzino, B. Prevalence of hallux valgus in the general population: A systematic review and meta-analysis. *J. Foot Ankle Res.* **2010**, *3*, 21. [CrossRef] [PubMed]

3. Hecht, P.J.; Lin, T.J. Hallux valgus. *Med. Clin. N. Am.* **2014**, *98*, 227–232. [CrossRef] [PubMed]

4. López, D.L.; González, L.C.; Iglesias, M.E.L.; Canosa, J.L.S.; Sanz, D.R.; Lobo, C.C.; de Bengoa Vallejo, R.B. Quality of Life Impact Related to Foot Health in a Sample of Older People with Hallux Valgus. *Aging Dis.* **2016**, *7*, 45. [CrossRef]

5. López, D.L.; Fernández, J.M.V.; Iglesias, M.E.L.; Castro, C.Á.; Lobo, C.C.; Galván, J.R.; de Bengoa Vallejo, R.B. Influence of depression in a sample of people with hallux valgus. *Int. J. Ment. Health Nurs.* **2016**, *25*, 574–578. [CrossRef] [PubMed]

6. Palomo-López, P.; Becerro-de-Bengoa-Vallejo, R.; Losa-Iglesias, M.E.; Rodríguez-Sanz, D.; Calvo-Lobo, C.; López-López, D. Impact of Hallux Valgus related of quality of life in Women. *Int. Wound J.* **2017**, *14*. [CrossRef] [PubMed]

7. Lobo, C.C.; Marin, A.G.; Sanz, D.R.; Lopez, D.L.; Lopez, P.P.; Morales, C.R.; Corbalan, I.S. Ultrasound evaluation of intrinsic plantar muscles and fascia in hallux valgus: A case-control study. *Medicine* **2016**, *95*, e5243. [CrossRef]

8. Calvo-Lobo, C.; Fernández, J.M.V.; Becerro-de-Bengoa-Vallejo, R.; Losa-Iglesias, M.E.; Rodríguez-Sanz, D.; López, P.P.; López, D.L. Relationship of depression in participants with nonspecific acute or subacute low back pain and no-pain by age distribution. *J. Pain Res.* **2017**, *10*, 129–135. [CrossRef]

9. Lobo, C.C.; Morales, C.R.; Sanz, D.R.; Corbalán, I.S.; Romero, E.A.S.; Carnero, J.F.; López, D.L. Comparison of hand grip strength and upper limb pressure pain threshold between older adults with or without non-specific shoulder pain. *PeerJ* **2017**, *5*, e2995. [CrossRef]

10. Palomo-López, P.; Becerro-de-Bengoa-Vallejo, R.; Losa-Iglesias, M.E.; Rodríguez-Sanz, D.; Calvo-Lobo, C.; López-López, D. Footwear used by older people and a history of hyperkeratotic lesions on the foot. *Medicine* **2017**, *96*, e6623. [CrossRef]

11. López-López, D.; Vilar-Fernández, J.M.; Calvo-Lobo, C.; Losa-Iglesias, M.E.; Rodriguez-Sanz, D.; Becerro-De-Bengoa-Vallejo, R. Evaluation of depression in subacute low back pain: A case control study. *Pain Physician* **2017**, *20*, E499–E505. [CrossRef] [PubMed]

12. Rodríguez-Sanz, D.; Tovaruela-Carrión, N.; López-López, D.; Palomo-López, P.; Romero-Morales, C.; Navarro-Flores, E.; Calvo-Lobo, C. Foot disorders in the elderly: A mini-review. *Dis. Mon.* **2017**, *64*, 64–91. [CrossRef] [PubMed]

13. Palomo López, P.; Rodríguez-Sanz, D.; Becerro de Bengoa Vallejo, R.; Losa-Iglesias, M.E.; Guerrero Martín, J.; Calvo Lobo, C.; Lopez Lopez, D. Clinical aspects of foot health and their influence on quality of life among breast cancer survivors: A case–control study. *Cancer Manag. Res.* **2017**, *9*, 545–551. [CrossRef] [PubMed]

14. Kazemi, K.; Arab, A.M.; Abdollahi, I.; López-López, D.; Calvo-Lobo, C. Electromyography comparison of distal and proximal lower limb muscle activity patterns during external perturbation in subjects with and without functional ankle instability. *Hum. Mov. Sci.* **2017**, *55*, 211–220. [CrossRef]

15. Romero Morales, C.; Calvo Lobo, C.; Rodríguez Sanz, D.; Sanz Corbalán, I.; Ruiz Ruiz, B.; López López, D. The concurrent validity and reliability of the Leg Motion system for measuring ankle dorsiflexion range of motion in older adults. *PeerJ* **2017**, *5*, e2820. [CrossRef]

16. Velázquez-Saornil, J.; Ruíz-Ruíz, B.; Rodríguez-Sanz, D.; Romero-Morales, C.; López-López, D.; Calvo-Lobo, C. Efficacy of quadriceps vastus medialis dry needling in a rehabilitation protocol after surgical reconstruction of complete anterior cruciate ligament rupture. *Medicine* **2017**, *96*, e6726. [CrossRef]

17. Oosterhoff, J.H.F.; Bexkens, R.; Vranceanu, A.-M.; Oh, L.S. Do Injured Adolescent Athletes and Their Parents Agree on the Athletes' Level of Psychologic and Physical Functioning? *Clin. Orthop. Relat. Res.* **2018**, *476*, 767–775. [CrossRef]

18. Goubert, L.; Crombez, G.; Van Damme, S. The role of neuroticism, pain catastrophizing and pain-related fear in vigilance to pain: A structural equations approach. *Pain* **2004**, *107*, 234–241. [CrossRef]

19. Hoch, J.M.; Houston, M.N.; Baez, S.E.; Hoch, M.C. Fear-Avoidance Beliefs and Health-Related Quality of Life in Post-ACL Reconstruction and Healthy Athletes: A Case-Control Study. *J. Sport Rehabil.* **2019**, 1–5. [CrossRef]

20. Priore, L.B.; Azevedo, F.M.; Pazzinatto, M.F.; Ferreira, A.S.; Hart, H.F.; Barton, C.; de Oliveira Silva, D. Influence of kinesiophobia and pain catastrophism on objective function in women with patellofemoral pain. *Phys. Ther. Sport* **2019**, *35*, 116–121. [CrossRef]

21. Gómez-Pérez, L.; López-Martínez, A.E.; Ruiz-Párraga, G.T. Psychometric Properties of the Spanish Version of the Tampa Scale for Kinesiophobia (TSK). *J. Pain* **2011**, *12*, 425–435. [CrossRef] [PubMed]

22. Woby, S.R.; Roach, N.K.; Urmston, M.; Watson, P.J. Psychometric properties of the TSK-11: A shortened version of the Tampa Scale for Kinesiophobia. *Pain* **2005**, *117*, 137–144. [CrossRef] [PubMed]

23. Hagedorn, T.J.; Dufour, A.B.; Riskowski, J.L.; Hillstrom, H.J.; Menz, H.B.; Casey, V.A.; Hannan, M.T. Foot disorders, foot posture, and foot function: The Framingham foot study. *PLoS ONE* **2013**, *8*, e74364. [CrossRef] [PubMed]

24. Galica, A.M.; Hagedorn, T.J.; Dufour, A.B.; Riskowski, J.L.; Hillstrom, H.J.; Casey, V.A.; Hannan, M.T. Hallux valgus and plantar pressure loading: The Framingham foot study. *J. Foot Ankle Res.* **2013**, *6*, 42. [CrossRef] [PubMed]

25. Menz, H.B.; Roddy, E.; Marshall, M.; Thomas, M.J.; Rathod, T.; Myers, H.; Thomas, E.; Peat, G.M. Demographic and clinical factors associated with radiographic severity of first metatarsophalangeal joint osteoarthritis: Cross-sectional findings from the Clinical Assessment Study of the Foot. *Osteoarthr. Cartil.* **2015**, *23*, 77–82. [CrossRef]

26. Vandenbroucke, J.P.; von Elm, E.; Altman, D.G.; Gøtzsche, P.C.; Mulrow, C.D.; Pocock, S.J.; Poole, C.; Schlesselman, J.J.; Egger, M.; STROBE Initiative. Strengthening the Reporting of Observational Studies in Epidemiology (STROBE): Explanation and elaboration. *Int. J. Surg.* **2014**, *12*, 1500–1524. [CrossRef]

27. World Medical Association. World Medical Association Declaration of Helsinki. Ethical principles for medical research involving human subjects. *J. Am. Coll. Dent.* **2014**, *81*, 14–18.

28. Menz, H.B.; Fotoohabadi, M.R.; Wee, E.; Spink, M.J. Validity of self-assessment of hallux valgus using the Manchester scale. *BMC Musculoskelet. Disord.* **2010**, *11*, 215. [CrossRef]

29. Nix, S.; Russell, T.; Vicenzino, B.; Smith, M. Validity and reliability of hallux valgus angle measured on digital photographs. *J. Orthop. Sports Phys. Ther.* **2012**, *42*, 642–648. [CrossRef]

30. Lobo, C.C.; Morales, C.R.; Sanz, D.R.; Corbalán, I.S.; Marín, A.G.; López, D.L. Ultrasonography Comparison of Peroneus Muscle Cross-sectional Area in Subjects With or Without Lateral Ankle Sprains. *J. Manip. Physiol. Ther.* **2016**, *39*, 635–644. [CrossRef]

31. Garrow, J.S. Quetelet index as indicator of obesity. *Lancet* **1986**, *1*, 1219. [CrossRef]

32. Williamson, A.; Hoggart, B. Pain: A review of three commonly used pain rating scales. *J. Clin. Nurs.* **2005**, *14*, 798–804. [CrossRef] [PubMed]

33. Taylor, L.J.; Harris, J.; Epps, C.D.; Herr, K. Psychometric evaluation of selected pain intensity scales for use with cognitively impaired and cognitively intact older adults. *Rehabil. Nurs.* **2005**, *30*, 55–61. [CrossRef] [PubMed]

34. Swinkels-Meewisse, I.E.J.; Roelofs, J.; Schouten, E.G.W.; Verbeek, A.L.M.; Oostendorp, R.A.B.; Vlaeyen, J.W.S. Fear of movement/(re)injury predicting chronic disabling low back pain: A prospective inception cohort study. *Spine* **2006**, *31*, 658–664. [CrossRef]

35. Ferrer-Peña, R.; Moreno-López, M.; Calvo-Lobo, C.; López-de-Uralde-Villanueva, I.; Fernández-Carnero, J. Relationship of Dynamic Balance Impairment with Pain-Related and Psychosocial Measures in Primary Care Patients with Chronic Greater Trochanteric Pain Syndrome. *Pain Med.* **2019**, *20*, 810–817. [CrossRef]

36. Costa, L.d.C.M.; Maher, C.G.; McAuley, J.H.; Hancock, M.J.; Smeets, R.J.E.M. Self-efficacy is more important than fear of movement in mediating the relationship between pain and disability in chronic low back pain. *Eur. J. Pain* **2011**, *15*, 213–219. [CrossRef]

37. Chmielewski, T.L.; Zeppieri, G.; Lentz, T.A.; Tillman, S.M.; Moser, M.W.; Indelicato, P.A.; George, S.Z. Longitudinal changes in psychosocial factors and their association with knee pain and function after anterior cruciate ligament reconstruction. *Phys. Ther.* **2011**, *91*, 1355–1366. [CrossRef]

38. George, S.Z.; Valencia, C.; Beneciuk, J.M. A psychometric investigation of fear-avoidance model measures in patients with chronic low back pain. *J. Orthop. Sports Phys. Ther.* **2010**, *40*, 197–205. [CrossRef]

39. Hapidou, E.G.; O'Brien, M.A.; Pierrynowski, M.R.; de Las Heras, E.; Patel, M.; Patla, T. Fear and Avoidance of Movement in People with Chronic Pain: Psychometric Properties of the 11-Item Tampa Scale for Kinesiophobia (TSK-11). *Physiother. Can.* **2012**, *64*, 235–241. [CrossRef]

40. Kahl, C.; Cleland, J.A. Visual analogue scale, numeric pain rating scale and the McGill pain Questionnaire: An overview of psychometric properties. *Phys. Ther. Rev.* **2005**, *10*, 123–128. [CrossRef]

41. Katz, N.P.; Paillard, F.C.; Ekman, E. Determining the clinical importance of treatment benefits for interventions for painful orthopedic conditions. *J. Orthop. Surg. Res.* **2015**, *10*. [CrossRef] [PubMed]

42. Salaffi, F.; Stancati, A.; Silvestri, C.A.; Ciapetti, A.; Grassi, W. Minimal clinically important changes in chronic musculoskeletal pain intensity measured on a numerical rating scale. *Eur. J. Pain* **2004**, *8*, 283–291. [CrossRef] [PubMed]

43. Devji, T.; Guyatt, G.H.; Lytvyn, L.; Brignardello-Petersen, R.; Foroutan, F.; Sadeghirad, B.; Buchbinder, R.; Poolman, R.W.; Harris, I.A.; Carrasco-Labra, A.; et al. Application of minimal important differences in degenerative knee disease outcomes: A systematic review and case study to inform BMJ Rapid Recommendations. *BMJ Open* **2017**, *7*, e015587. [CrossRef] [PubMed]

44. Kelley, K.; Preacher, K.J. On Effect Size. *Psychol. Methods* **2012**, *17*, 137–152. [CrossRef]

45. Lakens, D. Calculating and reporting effect sizes to facilitate cumulative science: A practical primer for *t*-tests and ANOVAs. *Front. Psychol.* **2013**, *4*. [CrossRef]

46. Austin, P.C.; Steyerberg, E.W. The number of subjects per variable required in linear regression analyses. *J. Clin. Epidemiol.* **2015**, *68*, 627–636. [CrossRef]

47. Shakked, R.; McDonald, E.; Sutton, R.; Lynch, M.K.; Nicholson, K.; Raikin, S.M. Influence of Depressive Symptoms on Hallux Valgus Surgical Outcomes. *Foot Ankle Int.* **2018**, *39*, 795–800. [CrossRef]

48. Gil-Martínez, A.; Grande-Alonso, M.; López-de-Uralde-Villanueva, I.; López-López, A.; Fernández-Carnero, J.; La Touche, R. Chronic Temporomandibular Disorders: Disability, pain intensity and fear of movement. *J. Headache Pain* **2016**, *17*, 103. [CrossRef]

49. Malfliet, A.; Van Oosterwijck, J.; Meeus, M.; Cagnie, B.; Danneels, L.; Dolphens, M.; Buyl, R.; Nijs, J. Kinesiophobia and maladaptive coping strategies prevent improvements in pain catastrophizing following pain neuroscience education in fibromyalgia/chronic fatigue syndrome: An explorative study. *Physiother. Theory Pract.* **2017**, *33*, 653–660. [CrossRef]

50. Reis, F.; Guimarães, F.; Nogueira, L.C.; Meziat-Filho, N.; Sanchez, T.A.; Wideman, T. Association between pain drawing and psychological factors in musculoskeletal chronic pain: A systematic review. *Physiother. Theory Pract.* **2019**, *35*, 533–542. [CrossRef]

51. Saavedra-Hernández, M.; Castro-Sánchez, A.M.; Cuesta-Vargas, A.I.; Cleland, J.A.; Fernández-de-las-Peñas, C.; Arroyo-Morales, M. The contribution of previous episodes of pain, pain intensity, physical impairment, and pain-related fear to disability in patients with chronic mechanical neck pain. *Am. J. Phys. Med. Rehabil.* **2012**, *91*, 1070–1076. [CrossRef]

52. Benatto, M.T.; Bevilaqua-Grossi, D.; Carvalho, G.F.; Bragatto, M.M.; Pinheiro, C.F.; Lodovichi, S.S.; Dach, F.; Fernandez-de-Las-Penas, C.; Florencio, L.L. Kinesiophobia is associated with migraine. *Pain Med.* **2019**, *20*, 846–851. [CrossRef] [PubMed]

53. Calvo-Lobo, C.; Pacheco-da-Costa, S.; Hita-Herranz, E. Efficacy of Deep Dry Needling on Latent Myofascial Trigger Points in Older Adults With Nonspecific Shoulder Pain: A Randomized, Controlled Clinical Trial Pilot Study. *J. Geriatr. Phys. Ther.* **2017**, *40*, 63–73. [CrossRef] [PubMed]

54. Segura-Pérez, M.; Hernández-Criado, M.T.; Calvo-Lobo, C.; Vega-Piris, L.; Fernández-Martín, R.; Rodríguez-Sanz, D. A Multimodal Approach for Myofascial Pain Syndrome: A Prospective Study. *J. Manip. Physiol. Ther.* **2017**, *40*, 397–403. [CrossRef] [PubMed]

55. Rodríguez-Sanz, D.; Calvo-Lobo, C.; Unda-Solano, F.; Sanz-Corbalán, I.; Romero-Morales, C.; López-López, D. Cervical Lateral Glide Neural Mobilization Is Effective in Treating Cervicobrachial Pain: A Randomized Waiting List Controlled Clinical Trial. *Pain Med.* **2017**, *18*, 2492–2503. [CrossRef]

56. Sanz, D.R.; Lobo, C.C.; López, D.L.; Morales, C.R.; Marín, C.S.; Corbalán, I.S. Interrater Reliability in the Clinical Evaluation of Myofascial Trigger Points in Three Ankle Muscles. *J. Manip. Physiol. Ther.* **2016**, *39*, 623–634. [CrossRef]

57. Calvo-Lobo, C.; Diez-Vega, I.; Martínez-Pascual, B.; Fernández-Martínez, S.; de la Cueva-Reguera, M.; Garrosa-Martín, G.; Rodríguez-Sanz, D. Tensiomyography, sonoelastography, and mechanosensitivity differences between active, latent, and control low back myofascial trigger points: A cross-sectional study. *Medicine* **2017**, *96*, e6287. [CrossRef]

58. Romero-Morales, C.; Jaén-Crespo, G.; Rodríguez-Sanz, D.; Sanz-Corbalán, I.; López-López, D.; Calvo-Lobo, C. Comparison of Pressure Pain Thresholds in Upper Trapezius and Temporalis Muscles Trigger Points Between Tension Type Headache and Healthy Participants: A Case–Control Study. *J. Manip. Physiol. Ther.* **2017**, *40*, 609–614. [CrossRef]

59. Rodríguez-Sanz, D.; Losa-Iglesias, M.E.; López-López, D.; Calvo-Lobo, C.; Palomo-López, P.; Becerro-de-Bengoa-Vallejo, R. Infrared thermography applied to lower limb muscles in elite soccer players with functional ankle equinus and non-equinus condition. *PeerJ* **2017**, *5*, e3388. [CrossRef]

60. López-López, D.; Rodríguez-Vila, I.; Losa-Iglesias, M.E.; Rodríguez-Sanz, D.; Calvo-Lobo, C.; Romero-Morales, C.; Becerro-De-Bengoa-Vallejo, R. Impact of the quality of life related to foot health in a sample of pregnant women: A case control study. *Medicine* **2017**, *96*, e6433. [CrossRef]

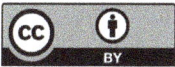

MDPI

St. Alban-Anlage 66

4052 Basel

Switzerland

Tel. +41 61 683 77 34

Fax +41 61 302 89 18

www.mdpi.com

International Journal of Environmental Research and Public Health Editorial Office

E-mail: ijerph@mdpi.com

www.mdpi.com/journal/ijerph

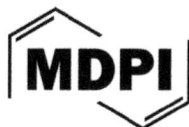

MDPI

www.ingramcontent.com/pod-product-compliance
Lightning Source LLC
Chambersburg PA
CBHW051925190326

41458CB00026B/6410